D1499146

Progress in Pain Research and Management
Volume 4

Temporomandibular Disorders and Related Pain Conditions

Mission Statement of IASP Press

The International Association for the Study of Pain (IASP) is a nonprofit, interdisciplinary organization devoted to understanding the mechanisms of pain and improving the care of patients with pain through research, education, and communication. The organization includes scientists and health care professionals dedicated to these goals. The IASP sponsors scientific meetings and publishes newsletters, technical bulletins, the journal *Pain*, and books.

The goal of IASP Press is to provide the IASP membership with timely, high-quality, attractive, low-cost publications relevant to the problem of pain. These publications are also intended to appeal to a wider audience of scientists and clinicians interested in the problem of pain.

We will achieve high-quality publications through careful selection of subjects and authors, well-focused editorial work at several levels of production, and a smooth flow of materials. In addition, we believe that we can restrain costs and prices by employing the administrative resources of the IASP central office and by obtaining grant support for selected publications.

Because we will keep the price of our books low and their value high, they will reach a wider audience than do similar books published by for-profit companies. Furthermore, our access to leaders in the field of pain research and treatment guarantees an outstanding selection of material and excellent editorial oversight.

Previous volumes in the series
Progress in Pain Research and Management

Pharmacological Approaches to the Treatment of Chronic Pain: New Concepts and Critical Issues, edited by Howard L. Fields and John C. Liebeskind

Proceedings of the 7th World Congress on Pain, edited by Gerald F. Gebhart, Donna L. Hammond, and Troels S. Jensen

Touch, Temperature, and Pain in Health and Disease: Mechanisms and Assessments, edited by Jörgen Boivie, Per Hansson, and Ulf Lindblom

Progress in Pain Research and Management
Volume 4

Temporomandibular Disorders and Related Pain Conditions

Editors

Barry J. Sessle, MDS, PhD

Faculty of Dentistry
University of Toronto
Toronto, Ontario, Canada

Patricia S. Bryant, PhD

National Institute of Dental Research
National Institutes of Health
Bethesda, Maryland, USA

Raymond A. Dionne, DDS, PhD

National Institute of Dental Research
National Institutes of Health
Bethesda, Maryland, USA

IASP PRESS • SEATTLE

Library of Congress Cataloging-in-Publication Data

Temporomandibular disorders and related pain conditions / editors, Barry J. Sessle,
    Patricia S. Bryant, Raymond A. Dionne.
        p.   cm. — (Progress in pain research and management ; v. 4)
    Includes bibliographical references and index.
    ISBN 0-931092-09-4
    1. Temporomandibular joint—Diseases—Congresses. 2. Orofacial pain—
Congresses. I. Sessle, Barry J., 1941–   . II. Bryant, Patricia. III. Dionne,
Raymond. IV. Series.
    [DNLM: 1. Temporomandibular Joint Diseases—congresses.
W1 PR677BL v.4 1995 / WU 140.5 T288 1995]
RK470.T437 1995
617.5'22—dc20
DNLM/DLC
for Library of Congress   95-3084

Published by:

IASP Press
International Association for the Study of Pain
909 NE 43rd St., Suite 306
Seattle, WA 98105 USA
Fax: 206-547-1703

Printed in the United States of America

Contents

Contributing Authors

Alexia Antczak-Bouckoms, D.M.D., Sc.D., M.P.H. *Harvard School of Public Health, Boston, Massachusetts, USA*

Walter Bowles, D.D.S., M.S. *Division of Endodontics, University of Minnesota Schools of Dentistry and Medicine, Minneapolis, Minnesota, USA*

Laurence A. Bradley, Ph.D. *Division of Clinical Immunology and Rheumatology, The University of Alabama at Birmingham, Birmingham, Alabama, USA*

Phyllis A. Browne, Ph.D., P.T. *Division of Physical Therapy, Chapman University, Orange, California, USA*

Patricia S. Bryant, Ph.D. *National Institute of Dental Research, National Institutes of Health, Bethesda, Maryland, USA*

Gunnar E. Carlsson, L.S., Odont. Dr. *Department of Prosthetic Dentistry, Faculty of Odontology, Göteborg University, Göteborg, Sweden*

Jae-Kap Choi, D.D.S., Ph.D. *University of California Los Angeles Dental Research Institute, Los Angeles, California, USA*

Glenn T. Clark, D.D.S., M.S. *University of California Los Angeles Dental Research Institute, Los Angeles, California, USA*

Pierre Clavelou, M.D., Ph.Cert.Neurol. *Faculté de médecine dentaire and Centre de recherche en sciences neurologiques, Université de Montréal, Québec, Canada*

Lambert G.M. de Bont, D.D.S., Ph.D. *Department of Oral and Maxillofacial Surgery, University Hospital Groningen, Groningen, The Netherlands*

Timothy A. DeRouen, Ph.D. *Departments of Biostatistics and Dental Public Health Sciences, University of Washington, Seattle, Washington, USA*

Raymond A. Dionne, D.D.S., Ph.D. *Neurobiology and Anesthesiology Branch, National Institute of Dental Research, National Institutes of Health, Bethesda, Maryland, USA*

M. Franklin Dolwick, D.M.D., Ph.D. *Department of Oral and Maxillofacial Surgery, University of Florida, Gainesville, Florida, USA*

Samuel F. Dworkin, D.D.S., Ph.D. *Department of Oral Medicine, School of Dentistry, University of Washington, Seattle, Washington, USA*

Mark G. Fontenot, D.D.S., M.Eng. *Department of Biomedical Engineering, Tulane University, New Orleans, Louisiana, USA*

James R. Fricton, D.D.S., M.S. *Department of Diagnostic and Surgical Sciences, University of Minnesota School of Dentistry, Minneapolis, Minnesota, USA*

Robert J. Gatchel, Ph.D. *Deptartment of Psychiatry, Division of Psychology, University of Texas Southwestern Medical Center at Dallas, Texas, USA*

Alan G. Glaros, Ph.D. *School of Dentistry, University of Missouri–Kansas City, Kansas City, Missouri, USA*

Ernest G. Glass, D.D.S., M.S., M.S.D. *School of Dentistry, University of Missouri–Kansas City, Kansas City, Missouri, USA*

Alan G. Hannam, B.D.S., Ph.D., FDSRCS *Department of Oral Biology, University of British Columbia, Vancouver, British Columbia, Canada*

Kenneth M. Hargreaves, D.D.S., Ph.D. *Division of Endodontics and Department of Pharmacology, University of Minnesota Schools of Dentistry and Medicine, Minneapolis, Minnesota, USA*

Charles H. Henry, D.D.S. *Private practice, Keene, New Hampshire, USA*

Susan W. Herring, Ph.D. *Department of Orthodontics, University of Washington, Seattle, Washington, USA*

Howard A. Israel, D.D.S. *Division of Oral and Maxillofacial Surgery, Columbia University, New York, New York, USA*

Douglass L. Jackson, D.M.D., M.S. *Division of Endodontics, University of Minnesota Schools of Dentistry and Medicine, Minneapolis, Minnesota, USA*

Rigmor Jensen, M.D. *Department of Neurology, Rigshospitalet,Copenhagen University Hospital, Copenhagen, Denmark*

David A. Keith, B.D.S., D.M.D. *Department of Oral and Maxillofacial Surgery, Massachusetts General Hospital, and Harvard Center for Orofacial Pain and Temporomandibular Disorders, Harvard School of Dental Medicine, Boston, Massachusetts, USA*

Sigvard Kopp, D.D.S., Ph.D. *Department of Clinical Oral Science, Section of Clinical Oral Physiology, School of Dentistry, Karolinska Institutet, Huddinge, Sweden*

Daniel M. Laskin, D.D.S., M.S. *Department of Oral and Maxillofacial Surgery, Medical College of Virginia, Richmond, Virginia, USA*

Jack E. Lemons, Ph.D. *Departments of Surgery and Biomaterials, Division of Orthopaedic Surgery, Schools of Medicine and Dentistry, University of Alabama at Birmingham, Birmingham, Alabama, USA*

Linda LeResche, Sc.D. *Department of Oral Medicine, University of Washington, Seattle, Washington, USA*

Jon D. Levine, M.D., Ph.D. *Department of Medicine, University of California, San Francisco, California, USA*

James P. Lund, B.D.S., Ph.D. *Faculté de médecine dentaire and Centre de recherche en sciences neurologiques, Université de Montréal, Québec, Canada*

Joseph J. Marbach, D.D.S. *Department of Psychiatry and School of Public Health, Columbia University New York, New York, USA*

James A. McNamara, Jr., D.D.S., Ph.D. *Department of Orthodontics and Pediatric Dentistry and Center for Human Growth and Development, The University of Michigan, Ann Arbor, Michigan, USA*

Siegfried Mense, Prof. Dr. med. *Institut für Anatomie und Zellbiologie, Universität Heidelberg, Heidelberg, Germany*

Louis G. Mercuri, D.D.S., M.S. *Division of Oral and Maxillofacial Surgery and Dental Medicine, Stritch School of Medicine, Loyola University Medical Center, Maywood, Illinois, USA*

Stephen B. Milam, D.D.S., Ph.D. *University of Texas Health Science Center, San Antonio, Texas, USA*

Norman D. Mohl, D.D.S., Ph.D. *Department of Oral and Diagnostic Sciences, State University of New York, Buffalo, New York, USA*

Thomas C. Namey, M.D. *Departments of Medicine, Pediatrics, Nutrition, and Exercise Science, University of Tennessee Graduate School of Medicine, and Department of Medicine, University of Tennessee, Knoxville, Tennessee, USA*

Joseph T. Newman, Ph.D. *Department of Immunology, Baylor University Medical Center, Dallas, Texas, USA*

Afzal Nikaein, Ph.D. *Transplantation Immunology Laboratory, Baylor University Medical Center, Dallas, Texas, USA*

Jeffrey P. Okeson, D.M.D. *Orofacial Pain Center, University of Kentucky College of Dentistry, Lexington, Kentucky, USA*

Jes Olesen, M.D., Ph.D. *Department of Neurology, Glostrup Hospital, University of Copenhagen, Copenhagen, Denmark*

Anthony Ratcliffe, Ph.D. *Department of Orthopaedic Surgery, Columbia University, New York, New York, USA*

Jennelle Durnett Richardson, B.A. *Department of Pharmacology, University of Minnesota Schools of Dentistry and Medicine, Minneapolis, Minnesota, USA*

Mark T. Roszkowski, D.D.S. *Division of Endodontics, University of Minnesota Schools of Dentistry and Medicine, Minneapolis, Minnesota, USA*

Thomas E. Rudy, Ph.D. *Department of Anesthesiology/CCM and Pain Evaluation and Treatment Institute, University of Pittsburgh Medical Center, Pittsburgh, Pennsylvania, USA*

Gordon Schwartz, M.Sc., D.D.S. *Faculté de médecine dentaire and Centre de recherche en sciences neurologiques, Université de Montréal, Québec, Canada*

Donald A. Seligman, D.D.S. *Section of Orofacial Pain and Occlusion, School of Dentistry, University of California Los Angeles, Los Angeles, California, USA*

Barry J. Sessle, M.D.S, Ph.D. *Faculty of Dentistry, University of Toronto, Toronto, Ontario, Canada*

Christian S. Stohler, D.M.D., Dr.Med.Dent. *University of Michigan School of Dentistry and Center for Human Growth and Development, Ann Arbor, Michigan, USA*

Arthur Storey, D.D.S., Ph.D. *Department of Orthodontics, School of Dentistry, University of Texas Health Science Center, San Antonio, Texas, USA*

James Q. Swift, D.D.S. *Division of Oral and Maxillofacial Surgery, University of Minnesota Schools of Dentistry and Medicine, Minneapolis, Minnesota, USA*

Dennis C. Turk, Ph.D. *Department of Psychiatry and Pain Evaluation and Treatment Institute, University of Pittsburgh Medical Center, Pittsburgh, Pennsylvania, USA*

Michael Von Korff, Sc.D. *Center for Health Studies, Group Health Cooperative of Puget Sound, Seattle, Washington, USA*

Karl-Gunnar Westberg, D.D.S., Ph.D. *Faculté de médecine dentaire and Centre de recherche en sciences neurologiques, Université de Montréal, Québec, Canada*

Charles G. Widmer, D.D.S., M.S. *Department of Oral and Maxillofacial Surgery, University of Florida, Gainesville, Florida, USA*

Frederick Wolfe, M.D. *Department of Internal Medicine and Family and Community Medicine, University of Kansas School of Medicine, and Wichita Arthritis Research and Clinical Centers, Wichita, Kansas, USA*

Larry M. Wolford, D.D.S. *Department of Oral and Maxillofacial Surgery, Baylor College of Dentistry, Dallas, Texas, USA*

Preface

The craniofacial region is not only one of the most densely innervated areas of the body but also the focus of some of the most common pains (e.g., toothache, headache) and some of the most bizarre and puzzling pains (e.g., trigeminal neuralgia) that afflict humans. One of the pain conditions that reflects all these features is that group of conditions now collectively termed temporomandibular disorders (TMDs). The etiology and pathogenesis of TMDs are still unclear, and clinicians frequently experience difficulty in differentiating TMDs from other craniofacial pain conditions or neuromuscular disturbances as well as in managing the many patients who present with these conditions. Perhaps not surprisingly then, there has evolved a plethora of diagnostic aids and therapeutic approaches directed at dental clinicians and specialists and advocated with their traditional training in mind, namely that they should be able to "treat what they see." Practitioners called upon to deal with TMDs often may also "see what they treat" and use clinical approaches with which they are comfortable but which have little if any foundation in scientific fact. As a consequence, the field of "TMJ" is currently characterized by a variety of concepts and approaches, many of which have little scientific basis, regarding how best to diagnose TMDs and how best to treat them. These are almost matched in number, and certainly are matched in the zeal of those who advocate them, by the numerous theories advocated on the etiology and pathogenesis of TMDs. Despite their limited scientific basis, many of these clinical approaches are in widespread use, at considerable financial, and in some cases functional, cost to the patient population.

The need to review the clinical approaches currently in use for TMDs and the current state of scientific knowledge bearing on the TMDs was the impetus for this book and the meeting upon which it is based. Dr. Harold Löe, who served as Director of the National Institute for Dental Research from January 1983 through June 1994, provided the vision and leadership that made this meeting and book possible. Recognizing parallels between the current state of TMD research and the state of periodontal research before the first World Workshop on Periodontal Diseases, and discerning the role that an international meeting could play in accelerating progress, he provided both fiscal resources and invaluable encouragement and insights that helped to make these efforts successful.

The organizers of the meeting saw the need to point out what is known and proven about TMDs and, equally important, to emphasize what is not proven and what remains to be investigated. The meeting, entitled International Workshop on the Temporomandibular Disorders and Related Pain Conditions, was held in April 1994 at Hunt Valley, Maryland, USA. It assembled many of the world's leading experts in scientific and clinical areas relevant to understanding conditions associated with persistent pain or dysfunction in the temporomandibular joint (TMJ), masticatory muscles, or associated tissues.

This workshop was planned and co-sponsored by the National Institute of Dental Research of the National Institutes of Health, the National Institute of Arthritis and Musculoskeletal and Skin Diseases, the Office of Research on Women's Health, and the Food and Drug Administration, all of the United States. Its two primary objectives were to synthesize available information from both the United States and abroad on TMDs and associated conditions, and to identify major research needs in this field. A supplementary workshop held later in 1994 generated additional research recommendations specific to the serious health problems resulting from the use of TMJ alloplastic implants.

Although the term *temporomandibular disorders* is included in the title of the original workshop and the title of this volume, the editors candidly admit to a certain discomfort with this terminology. This convenient though somewhat vague term almost invites misinterpretation. In this book the authors and editors clearly intend its use to denote an array of conditions, likely to be distinctive in etiology and clinical presentation. Thus, specific chapters address discrete topics, for example, masticatory muscle disorders, degenerative and inflammatory TMJ disorders, and cross-cutting basic science issues. We would be neither surprised nor disappointed if within the decade specific terms referring to different disorders with distinct etiologies begin to supplant the current TMD nomenclature.

Sincere thanks are due to all the authors, whose excellent papers, provocative insights, and commitment to ensuring sound research on these perplexing and challenging issues, as well as their diligence, have made editing this book a genuine pleasure. We join them in hoping that the knowledge summarized here, and new knowledge resulting from the research recommendations generated, will ultimately benefit those patients suffering with TMDs, the clinicians attempting to help them, and the research scientists trying to provide new insights into these conditions. We also gratefully acknowledge the expert guidance and efforts of Dr. Howard L. Fields, Editor-in-Chief, and the editorial staff of IASP Press.

Part I

Muscle Pain and Pathophysiology

Temporomandibular Disorders and Related Pain Conditions, Progress in Pain Research and Management, Vol. 4, edited by B.J. Sessle, P.S. Bryant, and R.A. Dionne, IASP Press, Seattle, © 1995.

1

Clinical Perspectives on Masticatory and Related Muscle Disorders

Christian S. Stohler

University of Michigan School of Dentistry and Center for Human Growth and Development, Ann Arbor, Michigan, USA

It is not uncommon that patients with facial pain are told that cramps, spasms, hyperactivity, or increased tone of the muscles of mastication are the reasons for their discomfort. Electromyographic instrumentation is still promoted to document the purported altered state of contraction of the musculature and the diagnosis of pain. In fact, the view that such phenomena cause pain is so widely shared that the need to revisit the issue may come as a surprise to many clinicians. However, given the rather frequent and potentially disabling presentation of muscle pains in combination with the insufficient level of support of many claims used to explain the underlying causes, a renewed look at the problem is warranted.

The literature is quite substantial because the boundaries between local, regional, and widespread myalgia are indistinct. This chapter focuses specifically on clinical matters of masticatory and related muscle pain, so references are limited to work on humans. Basic aspects of muscle pains are purposely omitted because they are addressed elsewhere in this volume.

PHYSICAL DIAGNOSIS

CLINICAL PRESENTATION

While muscle disorders can be painful or nonpainful, this chapter discusses only painful conditions that form the most prevalent clinical entity afflicting the masticatory apparatus. In a sample of 525 consecutive patients seen in a facial pain referral center, 52.9% were classified as having myofascial pain (Marbach and Lipton 1982).

Various forms of muscle pain range from a response to simple injury to complaints of localized, regional, or even generalized muscle soreness and pain. Except for some aspects of ischemic muscle pain, drug-induced muscle pain, and postexercise muscle soreness, much is unknown about the etiology and natural history of the more chronic forms. Pain of muscular origin is typically described as a diffuse ache, and the coexisting muscle tenderness represents the most obvious finding of the physical examination. Compared with pain arising from ectodermal tissue, pain originating from muscle cannot be localized with the same level of precision. A carefully chosen vocabulary, involving words such as aching, tender, and throbbing, appears to be used by a significant portion of subjects to describe the sensation of persistent jaw muscle pain (Stohler and Lund 1994).

A few reports note that a painful masticatory muscle condition is not necessarily limited to the muscles of mastication. In an epidemiologic data set, tenderness to palpation of masticatory muscles corresponds well with clinically tender neck and shoulder muscles (Krogstad et al. 1992). Retrospective data of sequential patients seen in a temporomandibular joint (TMJ) clinic also suggest that the condition is not necessarily localized to the head region (Blasberg and Chalmers 1989). Because nonmasticatory muscles are tender as often as masticatory muscles, it was suggested that masticatory myofascial pain is part of a larger group of muscle conditions, involving the pericranial, jaw, middle ear, and cervical musculature (Heiberg et al. 1978; Curtis 1980). There is additional evidence that masticatory myofascial pain also can occur with widespread muscle involvement. In a sample of eight patients with fibromyalgia, six demonstrated moderate to severe dysfunction of the stomatognathic system according to the Helkimo anamnestic dysfunction index (Eriksson et al. 1988).

In this author's tertiary care pain patient population, patients who are diagnosed with myofascial pain may well experience muscle pains in body parts other than the face. However, their chief complaint may not necessarily reflect the involvement of other body parts. Fig. 1 illustrates this fact in pain drawings of four consecutive subjects who fulfilled the criteria for myofascial pain with limitation of mouth opening according to research diagnostic criteria for temporomandibular disorders (TMDs) (Dworkin and LeResche 1992). While in a dental environment, a patient may report only symptoms to the face, the condition cannot be reduced to a simple "jaw problem." Such a reporting bias may exist because the patient does not expect services beyond the scope of dentistry from a general dental practitioner.

Boundaries between the diagnostic labels of myofascial pain and fibromyalgia have traditionally been vague. Criteria such as localized, regional, and generalized pain and tenderness represent a continuum with arbi-

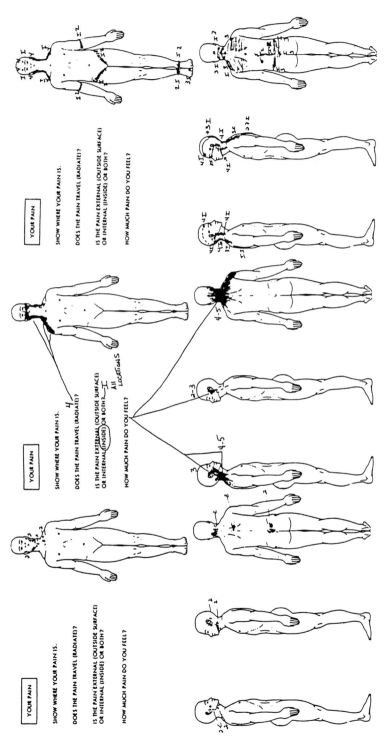

Fig. 1. Pain drawings of three consecutive subjects with the chief complaint of facial pain. Subjects were classified as having myofascial pain with limited mouth opening according to the research diagnostic criteria for TMD. Subject 3 (far right) also fulfilled the 1990 American College of Rheumatology criteria for fibromyalgia. Note the patients' reporting bias when seen in a facial pain clinic.

trary cutoff points between categories. Given these vague distinctive criteria, a high reliability of the diagnostic labeling cannot be expected. A second level of uncertainty is introduced when different diagnostic criteria are applied to the same clinical presentation, such as the requirement of either taut bands or trigger points. In the absence of validated markers that permit distinction, identification of diagnostic subsets remains a problem of pattern recognition. For better delineation, the American College of Rheumatology (ACR) proposed that criteria such as widespread pain with tenderness at 11 or more of 18 specific examination sites is required for the positive classification of fibromyalgia (Wolfe et al. 1990). While the recent introduction of the research diagnostic criteria for fibromyalgia is already improving case definition in the literature, the diagnostic label is still based on a simple count of tender points, scattered over the body surface at specified sites, rather than on unique features of pathogenic significance.

EXAMINATION

History and clinical examination are essential to establishing the diagnosis. Reliance on diagnostic tools is not an option given the insufficient specificity of available tests (Widmer 1989; Widmer et al. 1990). Palpatory tenderness of muscle remains the essential element of diagnostic significance, whether we are dealing with persistent localized, regional, or general muscle pain. It is routinely identified as discrete palpatory hypersensitivity within muscle and its fascia. Tender points are present in normal subjects but are less frequent and less tender than in patients. Clinic cases with TMDs exhibit more pain during muscle palpation of their jaw muscles than do community controls (Dworkin et al. 1990). Sometimes these areas of increased sensitivity to palpation exhibit palpable abnormality in consistency. On other occasions, pain is elicited in a part of the body other than the site of pressure application. Such sites, commonly referred to as trigger points, produce a referral pain pattern that is believed to be specific to each muscle. Documentation of the phenomenon is primarily based upon case reports (Jaeger 1989; Reeh and elDeeb 1991). Our findings using experimental muscle pain support in part the widely publicized referral patterns of Travell and Simons (1983) for the masseter muscle. However, neither pain radiation nor pain referral to a particular tissue different from the site of stimulation represents a phenomenon that occurs in every case (Stohler and Lund 1994).

If tenderness to palpation is a key component in diagnostic reasoning, the need for reproducible and reliable clinical measurement should be of concern. Acceptable agreement has been reported for the muscles of mastication among untrained examiners, and following training, the interexaminer agreement for the palpation of extraoral muscle sites is even better (Dworkin et al. 1990). Based on the careful study of an area by pressure algometry, sensitive areas appear as discrete locations of focal tenderness within the muscle under investigation (Reeves et al. 1986). While equally reliable, digital examination results in higher tender point counts than does dolorimetry (Cott et al. 1992). This finding is important because the number of tender points is critical in the diagnostic process in both the research diagnostic criteria for TMDs and the 1990 ACR criteria for fibromyalgia (see below). It is quite likely that different diagnoses are assigned to a particular case depending on the technique used.

Greater concerns regarding the reliability of findings arise when assessing aspects of tissue compliance in the clinical context. The measurement of trigger points or tissue compliance can reveal alteration in soft tissue resistance; however, the discrimination of scar tissue, fibrositic nodules, or spasticity from presumed "taut bands" has not been convincingly resolved. Indeed, problems with the reliability of assessment have been documented for taut bands. While blinded as to the diagnosis, eight clinicians performed trigger and tender point examinations on patients with fibromyalgia or myofascial pain, and on healthy subjects. Taut bands were about equally distributed, occurring in about 50% of cases in the three groups (Wolfe et al. 1992). Given the multipennate structure of the human masseter muscle with muscle fiber lengths of about 15 mm, it can be questioned whether the diagnosis of "taut band" would be possible at all, even if it existed. Should it be discarded because it is so unreliable? The low inter-rater reliability of the judgment (kappa coefficients, ranging from .29 to .38) of whether trigger points in the region of the lumbar spine exist in patients with low back pain suggests problems with the operational definition even in an anatomically more favorable location than the masticatory system (Nice et al. 1992).

Are there specific predilection sites for muscle pain? The low pressure-pain thresholds observed at tender sites of fibromyalgia patients are paralleled by a more general lowering of thresholds at nontender points as well (Quimby et al. 1988; Tunks et al. 1988). In fact, the increased frequency of tender sites reflects increased pain sensitivity and does not appear to represent a distinct pathology with a specific regional distribution. Similarly, children who meet the ACR diagnostic criteria for fibromyalgia have lower thresholds for tenderness both at control and tender points compared with subjects without fibromyalgia (Buskila et al. 1993).

When pressure is applied transcutaneously to muscle, the question arises regarding the contribution of the skin to the outcome of the clinical assessment of whether a particular site is painful to palpation. Skinfold tenderness was present in 95% of fibromyalgia patients and 33% of controls. Similarly, palpation sites overlying bone demonstrate lower pressure-pain thresholds in fibromyalgia patients than in healthy controls (Mikkelsson et al. 1992). This tenderness exists in both painful and nonpainful sites (Granges and Littlejohn 1993). However, the cutaneous sensory thresholds from skin overlying the masseter muscles and right ventral forearm were not significantly different in a group of 12 myofascial pain patients when compared with matched controls (Davidson and Gale 1983). The answer to this question is crucial to future research. If the sensitivity is not limited to muscle, it is possible that this condition represents a form of connective tissue disease rather than a condition specifically involving muscle. Of course, central nervous system phenomena also could explain a generally increased pain sensitivity.

CLASSIFICATION AND DIAGNOSIS

Authors of diagnostic systems for TMDs have recognized for some time the need for a delineation of muscle conditions from other musculoskeletal afflictions. However, most earlier diagnostic systems were limited due to lack of clinically suitable criteria that would permit reliable distinction of their proposed subsets. Concordance between classification schemes does not exist for masticatory muscle disorders (Ohrbach and Stohler 1992). Notable is Block's classification scheme of craniofacial-cervical pain, the first to call attention to the significant similarities between the painful muscle conditions of the jaw and those of other body parts (Block 1980). In response to the weakness of earlier diagnostic systems, the research diagnostic criteria for TMD were constructed to favor a more reliable assignment of cases to diagnostic subsets by avoidance of ambiguous terms and testing of the proposed criteria for their logic and internal consistency (Dworkin and LeResche 1992). Construct validation of the proposed diagnostic system must be regarded as the next step of this endeavor.

Using the most common diagnostic label to describe chronic pain conditions involving muscle, the research diagnostic criteria for TMDs propose two subsets of masticatory muscle disorders: (1) myofascial pain without limited mouth opening, and (2) myofascial pain with limited mouth opening. The criteria for inclusion into one or the other category are defined in an unambiguous way; the relatively rare conditions such as muscle spasm, myositis, and contracture are ruled out. Limited criteria for exclusion of these rare conditions are provided, and it remains to be seen whether they are effective in screening for these disorders (Dworkin and LeResche 1992). In contrast to the widely held view that trigger points are an essential feature of myofascial pain, trigger points are not discriminant criteria in the decision tree of the research diagnostic criteria for TMDs. Given the size and multipennate complexity of the muscles of mastication, including the limited palpatory access, trigger points may be difficult to detect, even if present. The same holds true for taut bands.

The question arises whether a research diagnostic system should discriminate between a painful muscle condition limited to the masticatory apparatus from an affliction involving, for example, the jaw, neck, and even the shoulders. Should we separately process cases that demonstrate "tension headache" in combination with masticatory muscle pain? How are these cases reliably recognized? What boundaries should be applied between conditions? Does widespread involvement suggest the presence of different risk factors, natural history, treatment response, or prognosis? Due to lack of information, the current version of the research diagnostic criteria for TMDs does not address these issues (Dworkin and LeResche 1992). While this is clearly an important matter, the answer to these questions can only come from research.

Based on case studies, the 1990 American College of Rheumatology proposed that criteria such as (1) pain for at least three months and (2) tenderness at 11 or more of 18 specific examination sites be required for the positive classification of fibromyalgia (Wolfe et al. 1990). The Guidelines of the American Academy of Orofacial Pain state that fibromyalgia should *not* be considered a specific masticatory muscle disorder even though there may be concurrent masticatory muscle pain (McNeill 1993). No information is given with respect to the establishment of this diagnosis in a dental environment, raising legal concerns in a number of states. In contrast, because some nonmasticatory muscles were found to be tender as frequently as masticatory muscles, it was proposed that the myofascial pain dysfunction syndrome is not necessarily limited to the muscles of mastication (Curtis 1980). Should the diagnosis of myofascial pain (as listed in the research diagnostic criteria for TMD) be assigned to cases that fulfill the 1990 ACR criteria for fibromyalgia? If not, what protocol is to be followed to exclude such patients from receiving the diagnosis of myofascial pain with or without mouth opening?

Very recent evidence suggests that the extent of involvement of other body systems in a pain problem of muscular origin deserves attention. Psychologically distressed persons were more likely to report pain at multiple anatomical sites (Von Korff et al. 1991). The number of reported pain conditions is significantly associated with elevated levels of somatization as measured by the Symptom Checklist 90-Revised (SCL-90-R) (Dworkin et al. 1990c). Comparisons between groups of patients with fibromyalgia, widespread myalgia, or regional myalgia showed that unspecific symptoms such as sleep disturbance, subjective swelling, intolerance to cold and exercise, and low self-reported physical conditioning surfaced more frequently in the fibromyalgia group than in the others (Jacobsen et al. 1993b). Patients with more widespread muscle pains used outpatient medical services more often than did controls, and national averages are consistent with other rheumatic disorders such as osteoarthritis and lower back pain (Cathey et al. 1986). These findings suggest that prognostic differences between such patient populations may indeed exist.

In summary, the formulation of unambiguous case definitions, such as the research diagnostic criteria for TMDs and the ACR criteria for fibromyalgia, have significantly affected the literature and current research trends in a positive fashion. Case definition is no longer as vague as it used to be. While we now need to learn more about the reliability of diagnostic assignment, construct validation must follow. Besides the more general issues, studies should address the question of whether it is warranted to distinguish among local, regional, and widespread muscle pains.

LABORATORY FINDINGS

Diagnosis remains a clinical judgment call in the absence of confirmatory laboratory tests. The search for distinctive laboratory findings has followed several approaches

Algometry. Tenderness to palpation constitutes the most distinctive feature of patients with myofascial pain and fibromyalgia, so it is not surprising that algometry is capable of showing consistent differences between groups with and without muscle pain. A study by Simms and colleagues (1988) showed that the mean pressure required to elicit tenderness at 19 sites, which were mostly different from the ones included in the operational ACR definition of fibromyalgia (Wolfe et al. 1990), was significantly lower than in controls. Notably, this sensitivity is not limited to areas overlying muscle. Pressure pain thresholds and tolerances on nontrigger point muscle and bone are lower in fibromyalgia patients than in healthy controls (Mikkelsson et al. 1992), which can be explained by a generalized increase in pain sensitivity. Issues related to reliability of algometry measurement and its comparison with digital palpation have been discussed above.

Biopsy studies. Although numerous hypotheses have been proposed to explain pain originating from muscle, studies have demonstrated no reproducible tissue abnormality with the exception of the condition of postexercise muscle soreness (Armstrong et al. 1983; Friden et al. 1983; Newham et al. 1983).

No evidence of muscle disease in muscle biopsies can be detected using light microscopy, or histochemical and immunoenzymatic methods (Drewes et al. 1993). Muscle biopsies of subjects with work-related trapezius myalgia and healthy volunteers showed a similar fiber type composition for both groups (Elert et al. 1992). No significant differences could be found in the blinded, ultrastructural examination of trapezius muscle biopsies of fibromyalgia patients and healthy controls (Yunus et al. 1989). No evidence of inflammation could be found in biopsies of the upper medial trapezius muscle from 12 fibromyalgia patients (Kalyan-Raman et al. 1984). In addition, serum creatine kinase, a marker of muscle damage, is not elevated in a group of facial pain patients when compared with controls (Cox and Rothwell 1984).

One report indicated light-microscopic tissue variations in at least some subjects. Routine histopathologic and histochemical methods revealed that more than half of muscle biopsies from patients with fibromyalgia appeared normal, while the remaining samples showed discrete pathological changes involving degeneration, regeneration, inflammatory infiltrates, ragged red fibers, or "moth-eaten" fibers (Bengtsson et al. 1986). Limited ultrastructural observation demonstrated pathologic findings that included empty sleeves of basal membrane, many lipofuscin bodies, or other degenerative changes (Drewes et al. 1993). Finally, in preliminary work, attachment of IgG to collagen bundles in the extracellular matrix has been observed in skin biopsies of patients with widespread muscle pain. Control skin biopsies were negative but showed intense reactivity for IgG following collagenase treatment (Enestrom et al. 1990). Such differences in IgG deposition between patients and controls were reported in a second study (Caro et al. 1986). In summary, no specific tissue abnormality can be linked reproducibly to myofascial pain and fibromyalgia at this time. The findings of differences in IgG deposition between patients and controls requires further work to determine whether it is of any causative significance.

Imaging studies. Skeletal uptake of technetium 99 pyrophosphate permits localization of leg muscle damage associated with postexercise muscle soreness (Matin et al. 1983; Newham et al. 1986); however, no study is available with respect to the masticatory muscles. Another study reports on a reduced radiologic density of the erector spinae muscles in 45 to 55-year-old men with chronic lower back pain when compared with subjects with no or intermittent back pain (Hultman et al. 1993). Again, no such reports are available for the jaw musculature, and it is conceivable that this finding could be responsive rather than linked to causation.

Resting and postural muscle activity. Electromyography has been used widely to evaluate the chronicity of pain of muscular origin based on the hypothesis that pain and abnormal muscle function are reciprocally linked. Muscle hyperactivity during rest is supposed to cause pain, which in turn reinforces abnormal muscle function, setting up a vicious cycle that perpetuates pain (Travell et al. 1942). A logical extension of this line of thought was the idea to use electromyography to obtain information on the level of resting activity in a given muscle in pain. However, the literature is rather contradictory on this subject, causing significant confusion among clinicians. Even a recently published conclusion such as "lengthy disclusion time leading to excessive muscle activity that introduce spasm and fatigue of the masseter and temporal muscle" (Kerstein and Wright 1991) is neither supported by the presented results, nor does the study design allow such a conclusion.

What can be said about the electromyographic (EMG) findings of painful muscles at rest? No change in EMG activity of sore muscles was observed in the situation of delayed muscle soreness (Abraham 1977). Surface electromyograms obtained before, during, and after perceptual-motor tasks failed to discriminate between women with fibromyalgia and matched healthy controls (Svebak et al. 1993). EMG examination of the paraspinal biceps brachii, trapezius, and anterior tibial muscles did not show evidence of any pain-related muscle activity in muscles that were reported as painful (Zidar et al. 1990). No differences in EMG measures were found between painful and nonpainful sides in 11 subjects with unilateral muscle pain in the anterior temporal region (Majewski and Gale 1984). These findings also are supported by experimental work using tonic muscle pain (Lund et al. 1991; Zhang et al. 1993).

It is, however, not surprising to find small differences when surface electrodes are used in the face, particularly when the electrodes are adapted over the mimic musculature. Rather than attributing such differences to the jaw musculature, Lund and colleagues (1993) suggest that pain could evoke distinct facial expressions. Indeed, facial expressions in pain are correlated with pain report but appear to be unrelated to depression or anxiety (LeResche and Dworkin 1988). Therefore, it is not surprising to find reports of myofascial pain patients showing higher resting EMG levels at four of six facial muscle sites than shown by matched controls (Kapel et al. 1989). In this context, observed increases in surface EMG resting muscle activity of 1–2 μV over the sternocleidomastoid muscle following the introduction of experimental pain can be explained by platysma effects (Ashton-Miller et al. 1990).

Conflicting results are available with respect to spontaneous activity or motor unit activity in tender points or trigger points. However, a recent study in 25 subjects presents convincing evidence for the lack of focal motor unit activity in tender points, trigger points, or associated muscle bands (Durette et al. 1991). In summary, despite lack of strong supporting evidence, muscle hyperactivity continues to be quoted as the single most likely cause of muscle pain.

Muscle strength, muscular endurance, and fatigue. Based on an analysis of the clinical literature, Lund and collaborators conclude that there is a decrease in activity of agonist muscles during pain (Lund et al. 1991, 1993; Lund and Stohler 1994). This conclusion is supported by reports of reduced amplitudes of agonist EMG muscle bursts from subjects with chronic musculoskeletal pain, such as TMDs (Molin 1972), chronic lower back pain (Thorstensson and Arvidson 1982; Suzuki and Endo 1983), and fibromyalgia (Bengtsson et al. 1986a; Jacobsen and Danneskiold-Samsoe 1987, 1989) when compared with controls. When compared with normative data of healthy women, grip strength is reduced by 40% in fibromyalgia patients (Nordenskiold and Grimby 1993). Muscle strength, measured with an isokinetic dynamometer, decreases with the increase in the number of tender points (Jacobsen and Danneskiold-Samsoe 1989). It is also consistent with the observation of contraction-induced pain, limiting the sustained jaw-closing effort (Jow and Clark 1989), and the high correlation between the reduction of bite strength following wisdom tooth extraction and pain measures recorded by the McGill pain questionnaire (High et al. 1988). The pain-adaptation model unifies these findings and proposes a neural network underlying the pain-induced reduction of muscle strength. It incorporates the idea that chronic pain from a variety of tissues exhibits the same consequences, which include a diminished capacity to perform work against loads and a reduction in the amplitude and speed of movement. Recent reviews of this subject matter (Lund et al. 1991, 1993; Lund and Stohler 1994) provide more details.

Not infrequently, muscle fatigue due to muscle hyperactivity is believed to be the cause of muscle pain. However, due to the lack of evidence in support of resting muscle hyperactivity, and good evidence for reduced muscle activity during agonistic function, the assumption of an "overworked," fatigued musculature is difficult to accept. Another line of thought considers that fatigability is, at least in part, due to pain (Bengtsson et al. 1989). This hypothesis is consistent with the idea of nociceptive reflex pathways that facilitate inhibitory interneurons, which in turn inhibit agonist motoneurons. Muscle fatigue has been defined in operational terms as an inability to sustain further exercise, or a loss of the capacity to generate force. When compared with healthy controls, myofascial pain patients have shorter endurance time when clenching at their 30% maximum contraction level (Clark et al. 1984). A significantly lower dynamic muscular endurance was observed in the fibromyalgia cases when compared with controls who were matched for age, gender, height, weight, peak torque, and contractional work (Jacobsen and Danneskiold-Samsoe 1992). Ten subjects with unilateral myofascial shoulder pain showed a reduced endurance on the painful side (Hagberg and Kvarnstrom 1984).

The literature is inconclusive when EMG parameters are used as a measure of fatigue. Parameters that have been selected to reflect the fatigued state of muscle have either not proven valid, or are likely confounded by the pain-related reduction in bite force and/or endurance (see above). Paraspinal muscle fatigue, measured with a standardized isometric endurance test in 14 fibromyalgia patients and 14 age- and sex-matched controls, did not demonstrate differences in the integrated surface electromyogram between groups (Stokes et al. 1993). Rather than concluding that no difference in endurance exists, we need to recognize that the integrated surface electromyogram has not proven to be a sufficiently valid parameter of fatigue. Spectral analysis of EMG activity during fatiguing muscle contraction in jaw and other muscles, however, has consistently shown an increase in the low-frequency content that occurs in synchrony with the perception of muscle fatigue or the loss of the capacity of the muscle to generate force of a certain level (Palla and Ash 1981b; Sadoyama and Miyano 1981; Kroon et al. 1986; Bouissou et al. 1989; Yaar and Niles 1992). This shift in the power spectrum to lower frequencies with fatigue might reflect physiological processes such as increased motor unit synchronization (Buchthal and Madsen 1950), slowing of the propagation velocity of the muscle action potential (Mortimer et al. 1970; Arendt-Nielsen and Mills, 1985; Eberstein and Beattie 1985; Christensen 1986), metabolic changes within the muscle (Mills et al. 1982), or changes in motor control (DeLuca and Creigh 1985). Given that muscle pain patients demonstrate reduced muscle strength and endurance, likely as a consequence of pain, findings of mean frequency shifts should not come as a surprise. Indeed, the power spectrum is influenced by bite force (Palla and Ash 1981a). However, given the absence of a good understanding of the neuromuscular phenomena involved in this frequency shift under experimental conditions, any difference in group mean frequency of the power spectrum in subjects with masticatory muscle pain (Kroon and Naeije 1992) cannot be explained in terms of defined pathophysiological processes.

Activity of antagonistic muscles. Subjects with orofacial pain frequently report a reduced mouth opening capacity. After oral surgery, a sudden and substantial increase in EMG activity of jaw closing muscles occurs when subjects are asked to open their mouth in their painful range (Greenfield and Moore 1969). When compared with unmatched controls, increased activity levels of antagonists are reported for subjects with painful temporomandibular disorders during empty mouth opening and the jaw opening phase of chewing (Moller et al. 1984; Stohler et al. 1985, 1988). In studies using both matched and unmatched control subjects, the phenomenon of significantly increased antagonistic co-contraction has been observed in other musculoskeletal conditions, such as lower back pain patients (Floyd and Silver 1955; Suzuki and Endo 1983; Triano and Schultz 1987; Ahern et al. 1988) and patients with fibromyalgia (Jacobsen and Danneskiold-Samsoe 1987; Backman et al. 1988). Lund and colleagues have proposed that reflex pathways facilitate the action of excitatory interneurons to antagonist motoneurons, resulting in reduced speed and amplitude of movement (Lund et al. 1991, 1993; Lund and Stohler

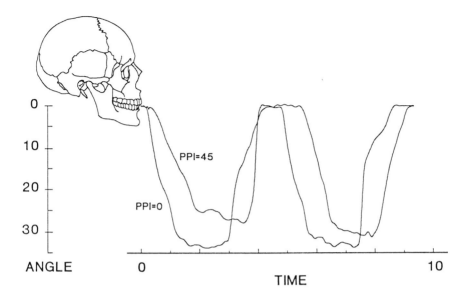

Fig. 2. Metronome-timed, maximum open-close movements in the absence and presence of experimental masseter muscle pain, induced by intramuscular infusion of hypertonic saline. PPI refers to present pain intensity and is expressed by the score on the visual analog scale. Maximum mouth opening is given in angular gape measurements. The movement of the incisal point is plotted against time using the Jaw-3D tracking system for data acquisition. Note the reduced range of motion associated with a pain intensity of 45.

1994). A reduced range of motion would be the consequence for the jaw. An example of the phenomenon obtained under experimental conditions is given in Fig. 2.

Studies of metabolic aspects. The literature on possible metabolic markers also is not conclusive. Jaw and other muscle pain conditions have been postulated to involve either a peripheral or central cause, so it is not surprising that both aspects have been explored.

Fatigue has empirically been associated with hypoxic conditions and the formation of free oxygen radicals in muscle. Reduced high-energy phosphate levels (adenosine triphosphate, adenosine diphosphate, and phosphoryl creatine) have been observed in biopsy samples of painful trapezius muscles. This finding has been associated with increased levels of adenosine monophosphate and creatine (Bengtsson et al. 1986c). However, ^{31}P magnetic resonance spectroscopy (MRS) reveals no evidence of changes in the high-energy phosphate metabolism at the site of tender points in the trapezius muscle of patients with fibromyalgia (de Blecourt et al. 1991). Another MRS study convincingly concludes that differences in painful calf muscles of 12 fibromyalgia patients and seven healthy volunteers appear to be related to the reduced muscle power produced by patients rather than specific biochemical changes to work and recovery (Jacobsen et al. 1992). It also has been hypothesized that impaired glycogenolysis is responsible for the development and maintenance of pain. However, impaired glycogenolysis does not appear to be the reason for myalgia because the ischemic forearm test in a group of fibromyalgia patients did not provide evidence for this assumption (Bengtsson et al. 1986a). Related to this finding is the report that assays of phosphorylase, glycolytic enzymes, and isocitrate dehydrogenase were in the normal range in 11 patients with chronic fatigue and myalgia (Byrne and Trounce 1987).

A strong association between joint hypermobility and myalgia has been observed in school children (Gedalia et al. 1993). However, markers of connective tissue disease have not been extensively investigated in the context of masticatory or other forms of persistent myalgia. Changes in bone metabolism could be hypothesized because physical activity is prevalent among patients with fibromyalgia. Due to an increased 24-hour pyrophosphate retention, an accelerated bone metabolism has been suggested in patients with widespread muscle pain (Appelboom and Schoutens 1990), and the urinary excretion of hydroxyproline and calcium relative to urinary creatinine is significantly higher in patients than in controls. However, when considering the lower urinary creatinine excretion in patients (likely due to lower physical activity), the bone turnover does not appear to be affected by the condition (Jacobsen et al. 1993a).

The clinical impression that antidepressants are beneficial in the management of chronic masticatory and other muscle pain has led to the hypothesis that persistent muscle pain results from a deficiency in the brain serotonin metabolism. Serotonin is a member of the indolamine class of neurotransmitters, which are synthesized from the amino acid tryptophan. Serotonergic neurons possess the enzymes for conversion of the molecule to 5-hydroxytryptophan and serotonin. Indeed, a few reports suggest differences in serotonin metabolism between subjects with and without persistent myalgia. A significantly lower serum concentration of serotonin (5-HT) was found in 31 patients with fibromyalgia when compared with 20 healthy volunteers (Stratz et al. 1993). Low levels of free tryptophan also occur in patients with severe fibromyalgia (Yunus et al. 1992), and metabolites of serotonin, identified by liquid chromatography from samples of the cerebrospinal fluid, are lower in patients with fibromyalgia than in controls (Russell et al. 1992). However, studies using ^{3}H-imipramine binding as a biochemical indicator of serotonin uptake revealed that women with fibromyalgia are not significantly different from control women (Kravitz et al. 1992).

The view that persistent muscle pain could possibly represent a disorder of pain modulation has triggered a few comparative studies into endogenous opioids. The endogenous opioid peptides are believed to suppress pain and to play a role in the modulation of mood and the regulation of pituitary hormone release. All endogenous opioids are the products of three large precursors, each encoded by a separate gene. The possibility of explaining the existing hyperalgesia via a mechanism of reduced endorphin secretion does not appear to be strong, given the limited data in the literature. In patients with fibromyalgia, the cerebrospinal fluid level of the pain modulatory neuropeptide beta-endorphin is not significantly different from the level of controls (Vaeroy et al. 1988). Similarly, the blinded analysis of assays of serum beta-endorphin did not show differences between these groups (Yunus et al. 1986). Levels of dynorphin A and met-enkephalin-arg6-phe7 are elevated in the cerebrospinal fluid of fibromyalgia patients when compared with levels available for comparison groups (Vaeroy et al. 1991).

Notable is the absence of any systematic study of the estrogen metabolism in patients with persistent muscle pain despite the up to 10:1 ratio of female sufferers in the childbearing years. A recent preliminary, controlled report suggests that the use of postmenopausal estrogen increases significantly the risk of seeking treatment for TMDs (LeResche et al. 1994). A few other studies suggest a possible connection between hormones and persistent pain of muscular origin. Myalgic symptoms resolved in 75% of patients with chemical evidence of hypothyroidism following initiation of treatment with low-dose thyroid replacement (Wilke et al. 1981). However, the prevalence of fibromyalgia in 100 patients with subclinical or biochemical hypothyroidism is low (Carette and Lefrancois 1988) and not strikingly different from expected values (see above). Laboratory tests revealed normal levels of 25-hydroxyvitamin D, cobalamin, folate, myoglobin, and most notably, estrogen and testosterone in a sample of patients with fibromyalgia (Bengtsson et al. 1986a). Preliminary reports suggest low levels of somatomedin C (Bennett et al. 1992), altered interleukin-2 secretion (Hader et al. 1991), and an increased adrenocorticotropic hormone release (Griep et al. 1993) in patients with persistent and widespread muscle pain.

Studies of autonomic nervous system function. Another hypothesis states that increased muscle sympathetic nerve discharge is contributory to or causative of chronic muscle pain. It needs to be emphasized that the role of the autonomic nervous system in these or other pain conditions is far from understood. At present, these data cannot be viewed as having causal significance nor can they be regarded with any degree of certainty as a consequence of persistent pain. Compared with controls, patients with fibromyalgia exhibit a significantly larger overall increase in the skin electrical conductance and reduced vasoconstriction during cold pressor tests (Vaeroy et al. 1989; Qiao et al. 1991). Mechanically induced vasodilatation of the skin, which is believed to be a neurogenically mediated axon reflex, is significantly greater in patients with fibromyalgia than in controls (Littlejohn et al. 1987). Autonomic function, such as pupil size, heart rate, and skin conductance, appears to be altered in chronic pain patients with inflammatory arthritis or myofascial pain (Perry et al. 1989). At the therapeutic level, sympathetic activity may in some patients contribute to the experience of focal tenderness because complete stellate ganglion blockade reduces the number of tender points and decreases pain at rest (Bengtsson and Bengtsson 1988). However, rarely are such reports of the beneficial effect of stellate ganglion blockade adequately placebo-controlled.

Immunologic studies. While no infection has been linked to masticatory myalgia, a few reports have listed either similarities in symptom presentation or laboratory tests between established infections and fibromyalgia. However, given the limited number of cases, the possibility of a pure coincidence cannot be rejected. Three patients developed fibromyalgia after documented episodes of acute parvovirus B19 infections (Leventhal et al. 1991). In areas endemic for Lyme disease, a high incidence of false-positive serologic results in patients with nonspecific myalgia has been observed (Lightfoot et al. 1993). However, fibromyalgia associated with Lyme disease is not favorably influenced by antibiotics (Dinerman and Steere 1992). Finally, the absence of abnormal Epstein-Barr virus serology in patients with widespread myalgia is noteworthy (Buchwald et al. 1987; Fye et al. 1988).

PSYCHOLOGICAL STATUS AND PAIN-RELATED DISABILITY

PSYCHOLOGICAL STATUS

Is there a particular psychopathology that predisposes a subject to experience masticatory muscle pain? If these muscle pain conditions represent a variant of a psychiatric disease, evidence of a particular psychopathology should be established by now. The hypothesis that distinct psychopathology is linked to these painful muscle conditions, however, can safely be rejected on the basis of the current and rather impressive body of literature. Fibromyalgia or myofascial pain patients do not distinguish themselves on any psychological dimensions, nor is there any evidence of an overt psychological response that increases the likelihood of these pains. Similar to the physical presentation, where a number of motor-dysfunctional aspects appear to be a consequence of pain, convincing data suggest that many of the emotional sequelae can be considered as a response to chronic pain rather than its cause.

Chronic pain patients and cancer patients report higher visual analog scale (VAS) affective ratings when compared with VAS sensory ratings for their pain. This is not the case for labor pain, indicating that the experience of pain is influenced by contextual factors (Price et al. 1987). While mostly sensory cues are given by subjects exposed to acute muscle pain stimuli of short duration, words of the affective dimension can surface in the situation of tonic pain (Stohler and Lund 1994). No differences on the Zung Self-Rating Depression scale were found when comparing the group responses of 45 fibromyalgia with 29 rheumatoid arthritis patients, thereby not supporting the hypothesis that the presentation of chronic pain in the absence of known organic pathology is a variant of a depressive illness (Ahles et al. 1987). The Psychiatric Diagnostic Interview also fails to discriminate between patients with primary fibromyalgia and rheumatoid arthritis (Ahles et al. 1991). The psychological make-up of chronic pain patients and fibromyalgia patients as measured with psychological questionnaires (Illness Behavior Questionnaire [IBQ], Symptom Checklist-90 revised [SCL-90R]) proved to be similar; both these groups were easily distinguished from a group of nonchronic pain patients (Birnie et al. 1991). Patients with fibromyalgia are not significantly more likely than arthritis patients to report depressive symptoms or to receive a lifetime diagnosis of major depression. The fibromyalgia patients reported more somatic symptoms, however, which has been interpreted as a process of somatization rather than a discrete psychiatric disorder (Kirmayer et al. 1988). Because trait measures are less predictive of pain ratings than are measures of the current pain state, chronic pain appears to influence mood more likely than the reverse (Gaskin et al. 1992).

The psychological response to chronic pain is also not mandatory. The extent or severity of pathological/pathophysiological findings does not translate into a corresponding amount of psychological response (Turk and Rudy 1987). In fact, a large portion of patients who present with persistent pain without obvious pathology do not demonstrate psychopathology as evidenced by their MMPI findings (Ahles et al. 1986). In addition, psychopathology as measured by the Beck Depression Inventory, the Spielberger State and Trait Anxiety Inventory, and the SCL-90R does not appear to be an essential feature of fibromyalgia (Clark et al. 1985). One study comparing fibromyalgia patients with rheumatoid arthritis patients and healthy controls reported no differences for the Assertiveness-Aggressiveness Inventory but significantly higher scores on the Life Events Inventory (Ahles et al. 1984).

NONSPECIFIC PHYSICAL SYMPTOMS

Nonmusculoskeletal symptoms such as exhaustion, poor sleep, irritable bowel symptoms, chronic headaches, and irritability are common among chronic pain patients (Smythe 1986; Yunus et al. 1988; Veale et al. 1991; Hudson et al. 1992). High lifetime rates of migraines, irritable bowel syndrome, chronic fatigue syndrome, major depression, and panic disorders have been loosely associated with fibromyalgia (Campbell et al. 1983; Yunus et al. 1989; Hudson et al. 1992). Contrary to these findings, sleep disturbances, irritable bowel syndrome, or morning stiffness were not reported in any great frequency in a national health survey in Sweden among subjects who fulfilled the research diagnostic criteria of fibromyalgia (Prescott et al. 1993).

DISABILITY

Excellent recent reviews provide the underlying construct of chronic pain-related illness behavior and dysfunction (Dworkin 1991, 1994). Some information is available on global disability measures in patients with fibromyalgia. However, specific data on orofacial disability associated with chronic masticatory muscle disorders are not yet available. It is conceivable that orofacial disability affects activities such as chewing, drinking, exercising, eating various foods, smiling/laughing, sexual activities, cleaning teeth or face, yawning, swallowing, talking, and having the usual facial appearance (Von Korff et al. 1992).

Disability in chronic muscle pain conditions, reflected in family/home responsibilities, recreation, social activity, occupation, and sexual behavior is significant and similar to other chronic musculoskeletal conditions. Assessment of the disability of 1,522 patients with rheumatic disease, involving seven distinct disorders, showed that disability in activities of daily living was as high in fibromyalgia as in rheumatoid arthritis cases (Hawley and Wolfe 1991). Comparison of 20 fibromyalgia patients with 23 rheumatoid arthritis patients on measures of somatic symptomatology, pain, and disability demonstrated greater somatic symptomatology and smaller physical disability for the fibromyalgia group, but with equivalent pain levels between groups (Robbins et al. 1990).Conversely, another study reports greater limitations with regard to activities of daily living in the fibromyalgia than rheumatoid arthritis patients (Gaston-Johansson et al. 1990).

Chronic pain of muscular origin appears to be particularly persistent. Patients with herniated discs are more likely to experience periodic pain relief than are patients with myofascial pain (Cassisi et al. 1993). However, when compared with myofascial pain patients, low back pain patients are less active, are more likely to use opioids or sedatives, and exhibit more pain-related motor behaviors, such as guarding, rubbing, and bracing (Keefe and Dolan 1986).

DIAGNOSIS

Preliminary data suggest that an improved treatment outcome prediction for TMDs can be achieved when both biological and psychological factors are considered (Gerke et al. 1989). Besides the reliable measurement of physical findings, the dimension of psychological status and pain-related disability is quantified in the research diagnostic criteria for TMDs. This diagnostic system employs a second axis (Axis II) to assess the global severity of the pain condition in terms of: (1) pain intensity, (2) pain-related orofacial disability, (3) depression, and (4) nonspecific physical symptoms (see Von Korff et al. 1992 for more details regarding construct and assessment methods). Axis II is comprised of a seven-item questionnaire for grading chronic pain severity, an orofacial disability checklist, and a subscale of the SCL-90-R. It permits more reliable and comprehensive characterization of subjects with myofascial pain with and without limited mouth opening.

CONCLUSIONS

The use of terms such as myofascial pain suggests that we are dealing with a defined disease entity of the masticatory system. However, this has not been proven. Diagnostic criteria are descriptive and include a history of pain of muscular origin and the clinical documentation of palpatory tenderness as main features. Basic understanding has not yet reached a level that would permit a diagnostic assignment based upon knowledge of the involved pathophysiological processes. For this very reason, a high priority should be assigned to investigations that enhance our understanding of the peripheral and central processes involved in these conditions.

Based on this review, research topics focusing on matters of central modulatory effects of pain and the role of estrogens appear to provide the most promising leads for discovering the causes of these clinical muscle pains seen most commonly in women of child-bearing age. Experimental models of muscle pain are expected to allow better description and understanding of mechanisms underlying painful function. For example, when and under what conditions does pain change the use of agonist and antagonist muscles, how long does it take after pain subsides for the usual muscle recruitment patterns to return to the control state, and what are the effects of various analgesics?

Review of the literature does not identify any marker for myofascial pain or fibromyalgia of acceptable diagnostic validity. Most notably, electronic instrumentation used for establishing the resting EMG activity does not appear to have any scientific support for diagnosing pain of muscular origin.

Attention should be given to the indistinct boundaries between local and regional myofascial pain and fibromyalgia. Do these conditions distinguish themselves by their natural history, psychological response to pain, disability, response to intervention, or prognostic features? How should a case be treated that receives the assignment "myofascial pain" using the research diagnostic criteria for TMDs (Dworkin and LeResche 1992) and that fulfills the requirements of the ACR (Wolfe et al. 1990) at the same time?

The significant continuing controversy about the etiology of these painful jaw muscle conditions is particularly apparent in the clinical literature. Factors such as occlusal relationships, muscle-occlusion imbalance, inadequate posture among the neuromuscular system, temporomandibular joints and dental occlusion, faulty vertical dimension, or lack of radiographic condyle-fossa concentricity, among others, have been proposed as being of causal significance. However, neither systematic studies nor epidemiological data support hypotheses that any of these conditions increase the likelihood of persistent muscle pain by a factor of 1000, 50, or even 10 times. All these presumed causes occur with similar frequencies in subjects without pain. There is also lack of agreement between studies as to which specific factors exhibit a statistically significant relationship with the occurrence of persistent pain. Such agreement must be expected if pathogenic significance is assumed. Although none of these prevailing theories are convincing based on our current knowledge, they continue to influence decisions related to issues of care. The existing controversy and professional insecurity represent an educational challenge that must be dealt with in a fashion comparable to many medical situations where safe clinical decision-making has to be taught despite the absence of a comprehensive understanding of the underlying disease mechanisms. The abandonment of unproven and disproved explanations has to be accepted as scientific progress for the better of the profession and the public.

ACKNOWLEDGMENT

This work was supported by National Institute of Health/National Institute of Dental Research grant 5RO1-DE8606-06.

REFERENCES

Abraham, W.M., Factors in delayed muscle soreness, Med. Sci. Sports, 9 (1977) 11–20.

Ahern, D.K., Follick, M.J., Council, J.R., Laser-Wolston, N. and Litchman, H., Comparison of lumbar paravertebral EMG patterns in chronic low back pain patients and non-patient controls, Pain, 34 (1988) 153–160.

Ahles, T.A., Yunus, M.B., Riley, S.D., Bradley, J.M. and Masi, A.T., Psychological factors associated with primary fibromyalgia syndrome, Arthritis Rheum., 27, (1984) 1101–1106.

Ahles, T.A., Yunus, M.B., Gaulier, B., Riley, S.D. and Masi, A.T., The use of contemporary MMPI norms in the study of chronic pain patients, Pain, 24 (1986) 159–163.

Ahles, T.A., Yunus, M.B. and Masi, A.T., Is chronic pain a variant of depressive disease? The case of primary fibromyalgia syndrome, Pain, 29 (1987) 105–111.

Ahles, T.A., Khan, S.A., Yunus, M.B., Spiegel, D.A. and Masi, A.T., Psychiatric status of patients with primary fibromyalgia, patients with rheumatoid arthritis, and subjects without pain: a blind comparison of DSM-III diagnoses, Am. J. Psychiatry, 148 (1991) 1721–1726.

Appelboom, T. and Schoutens, A., High bone turnover in fibromyalgia, Calcif. Tissue Int., 46 (1990) 314–317.

Arendt-Nielsen, L. and Mills, K.R., The relationship between mean power frequency of the EMG spectrum and muscle fibre conduction velocity, Electroencephalogr. Clin. Neurophysiol., 60 (1985) 130–134.

Armstrong, R.B., Ogilvie, R.W. and Schwane, J.A., Eccentric exercise-induced injury to rat skeletal muscle, J. Appl. Physiol., 54 (1983) 80–93.

Ashton-Miller, J.A., McGlashen, K.M., Herzenberg, J.E. and Stohler, C.S., Cervical muscle myoelectric response to acute experimental sternocleidomastoid pain, Spine, 15 (1990) 1006–1012.

Backman, E., Bengtsson, A., Bengtsson, M., Lennmarken, C. and Henriksson, K.G., Skeletal muscle function in primary fibromyalgia. Effect of regional sympathetic blockade with guanethidine, Acta Neurol. Scand., 77 (1988) 187–191.

Bengtsson, A. and Bengtsson, M., Regional sympathetic blockade in primary fibromyalgia, Pain, 33 (1988) 161–167.

Bengtsson, A., Henriksson, K.G., Jorfeldt, L., Kagedal, B., Lennmarken, C. and Lindstrom, F., Primary fibromyalgia: a clinical and laboratory study of 55 patients, Scand. J. Rheumatol., 15 (1986a) 340–347.

Bengtsson, A., Henriksson, K.G. and Larsson, J., Muscle biopsy in primary fibromyalgia: lightmicroscopical and histochemical findings, Scand. J. Rheumatol., 15 (1986b) 1–6.

Bengtsson, A., Henriksson, K.G. and Larsson, J., Reduced high-energy phosphate levels in the painful muscles of patients with primary fibromyalgia, Arthritis Rheum., 29 (1986c) 817–821.

Bengtsson, M., Bengtsson, A. and Jorfeldt, L., Diagnostic epidural opioid blockade in primary fibromyalgia at rest and during exercise, Pain, 39 (1989) 171–180.

Bennett, R.M., Clark, S.R., Campbell, S.M. and Burckhardt, C.S., Low levels of somatomedin C in patients with the fibromyalgia syndrome: a possible link between sleep and muscle pain, Arthritis Rheum., 35 (1992) 1113–1116.

Birnie, D.J., Knipping, A.A., van Rijswijk, M.H., de Blecourt, A.C. and de Voogd, N., Psychological aspects of fibromyalgia compared with chronic and nonchronic pain, J. Rheumatol., 18 (1991) 1845–1848.

Blasberg, B. and Chalmers, A., Temporomandibular pain and dysfunction syndrome associated with generalized musculoskeletal pain, a retrospective study, J. Rheumatol. Suppl., 19 (1989) 87–90.

Block, S.L., Differential diagnosis of craniofacial-cervical pain. In B.G. Sarnat and D.M. Laskin (Eds.), The Temporomandibular Joint, C.C. Thomas, Springfield, Ill., 1980, pp. 348–421.

Bouissou, P., Estrade, P.Y., Goubel, F., Guezennec, C.Y. and Serrurier, B., Surface EMG power spectrum and intramuscular pH in human vastus lateralis muscle during dynamic exercise, J. Appl. Physiol., 67 (1989) 1245–1249.

Buchthal, F. and Madsen, A., Synchronous activity in normal and atrophic muscle, Electroencephalogr. Clin. Neurophysiol., 2 (1950) 425–444.

Buchwald, D., Goldenberg, D.L., Sullivan, J.L. and Komaroff, A.L., The "chronic, active EpsteinBarr virus infection" syndrome and primary fibromyalgia, Arthritis Rheum., 30 (1987) 1132–1136.

Buskila, D., Press, J., Gedalia, A., Klein, M., Neumann, L., Boehm, R. and Sukenik, S., Assessment of nonarticular tenderness and prevalence of fibromyalgia in children, J. Rheumatol., 20 (1993) 368–370.

Byrne, E. and Trounce, I., Chronic fatigue and myalgia syndrome: mitochondrial and glycolytic studies in skeletal muscle, J. Neurol. Neurosurg. Psychiatry, 50 (1987) 743–746.

Campbell, S.M., Clark, S., Tindall, E.A., Forehand, M.E. and Bennett, R.M., Clinical characteristics of fibrositis. I. A "blinded," controlled study of symptoms and tender points, Arthritis Rheum., 26 (1983) 817–824.

Carette, S. and Lefrancois, L., Fibrositis and primary hypothyroidism, J. Rheumatol, 15 (1988) 1418–1421.

Caro, X.J., Wolfe, F., Johnston, W.H. and Smith, A.L., A controlled and blinded study of immunoreactant deposition at the dermal-epidermal junction of patients with primary fibrositis syndrome, J. Rheumatol., 13 (1986) 1086–1092.

Cassisi, J.E., Sypert, G.W., Lagana, L., Friedman, E.M. and Robinson, M.E., Pain, disability, and psychological functioning in chronic low back pain subgroups: myofascial versus herniated disc syndrome, Neurosurgery, 33 (1993) 379–385.

Cathey, M.A., Wolfe, F., Kleinheksel, S.M. and Hawley, D.J., Socioeconomic impact of fibrositis: a study of 81 patients with primary fibrositis, Am. J. Med., 81 (1986) 78–84.

Christensen, H., Muscle activity and fatigue in the shoulder muscles of assembly-plant employees, Scand. J. Work. Environ. Health, 12 (1986) 582–587.

Clark, G.T., Beemsterboer, P.L. and Jacobson, R., The effect of sustained submaximal clenching on maximum bite force in myofascial pain dysfunction patients, J. Oral Rehabil., 11 (1984) 387–391.

Clark, S., Campbell, S.M., Forehand, M.E., Tindall, E.A. and Bennett, R.M., Clinical characteristics of fibrositis. II. A "blinded," controlled study using standard psychological tests, Arthritis Rheum., 28 (1985) 132–137.

Cott, A., Parkinson, W., Bell, M.J., Adachi, J., Bedard, M., Cividino, A. and Bensen, W., Interrater reliability of the tender point criterion for fibromyalgia, J. Rheumatol., 19 (1992) 1955–1959.

Cox, P.J. and Rothwell, P.S., Serum creatine kinase studies in mandibular pain dysfunction, J. Oral Rehabil., 11 (1984) 45–52.

Curtis, A.W., Myofascial pain-dysfunction syndrome: the role of nonmasticatory muscles in 91 patients, Otolaryngol. Head Neck Surg., 88 (1980) 361–367.

Davidson, R.M. and Gale, E.N., Cutaneous sensory thresholds from skin overlying masseter and forearm in MPD patients and controls, J. Dent. Res., 62 (1983) 555–558.

de Blecourt, A.C., Wolf, R.F., van Rijswijk, M.H., Kamman, R.L., Knipping, A.A. and Mooyaart, E.L., In vivo 31P magnetic resonance spectroscopy (MRS) of tender points in patients with primary fibromyalgia syndrome, Rheumatol. Int., 11 (1991) 51–54.

DeLuca, C.J. and Creigh, J.L., Do the firing statistics of motor units modify the frequency content of the EMG signal during sustained contractions? In: D.A.Winter (Ed.), Biomechanics IXA, Human Kinetics Publishers, Champaign, Ill., 1985, pp.358–362.

Drewes, A.M., Andreasen, A., Schroder, H.H., Hogasa, B. and Jebbum, P., Pathology of skeletal muscle in fibromyalgia: a histo-immuno-chemical and ultrastructural study, Br. J. Rheumatol., 32 (1993) 479–483.

Durette, M.R., Rodriquez, A.A., Agre, J.C. and Silverman, J.L., Needle electromyographic evaluation of patients with myofascial or fibromyalgic pain, Am. J. Phys. Med. Rehabil., 70 (1991) 154–156.

Dworkin, S.F., Illness behavior and dysfunction: review of concepts and application to chronic pain, Can. J. Physiol. Pharmacol., 69 (1991) 662–671.

Dworkin, S.F., Behavioral, emotional, and social aspects of orofacial pain. In: C.S. Stohler and D.S. Carlson (Eds.), Biological and Psychological Aspects of Orofacial Pain, Craniofacial Growth Series, Vol. 29, Center for Human Growth and Development, The University of Michigan, Ann Arbor, Mich., 1994, pp. 93–112.

Dworkin, S.F. and LeResche, L., Research diagnostic criteria for temporomandibular disorders: review, criteria, examinations and specifications, critique, J. Craniomandib. Disord., 6 (1992) 301–355.

Dworkin, S.F., Huggins, K.H., LeResche, L., Von Korff, M., Howard, J., Truelove, E. and Sommers, E., Epidemiology of signs and symptoms in temporomandibular disorders: clinical signs in cases and controls, J. Am. Dent. Assoc., 120 (1990a) 273–281.

Dworkin, S.F., LeResche, L., DeRouen, T. and Von Korff, M., Assessing clinical signs of temporomandibular disorders: reliability of clinical examiners, J. Prosthet. Dent., 63 (1990b) 574–579.

Dworkin, S.F., Von Korff, M. and LeResche, L., Multiple pains and psychiatric disturbance: an epidemiologic investigation, Arch. Gen. Psychiatry, 47 (1990c) 239–244.

Eberstein, A. and Beattie, B., Simultaneous measurement of muscle conduction velocity and EMG power spectrum changes during fatigue, Muscle Nerve, 8 (1985) 768–773.

Elert, J.E., Rantapaa-Dahlqvist, S.B., Henriksson-Larsen, K., Lorentzon, R. and Gerdle, B.U., Muscle performance, electromyography and fibre type composition in fibromyalgia and work-related myalgia, Scand. J. Rheumatol., 21 (1992) 28–34.

Enestrom, S., Bengtson, A., Lindstrom, F. and Johan, K., Attachment of IgG to dermal extracellular matrix in patients with fibromyalgia, Clin. Exp. Rheumatol., 8 (1990) 127–135.

Eriksson, P.O., Lindman, R., Stal, P. and Bengtsson, A., Symptoms and signs of mandibular dysfunction in primary fibromyalgia syndrome (PFS) patients, Swed. Dent. J., 12 (1988) 141–149.

Floyd, W.F. and Silver, P.H.S., The function of the erectores spinae muscles in certain movements and postures in man, J. Physiol. (Lond.), 129 (1955) 184–203.

Friden, J., Sjostrom, M. and Ekblom, B., Myofibrillar damage following intense eccentric exercise in man, Int. J. Sports Med., 4 (1983) 170–176.

Fye, K.H., Whiting-O'Keefe, Q.E., Lennette, E.T. and Jessop, C., Absence of abnormal Epstein-Barr virus serologic findings in patients with fibrositis (letter), Arthritis Rheum., 31 (1988) 1455–1456.

Gaskin, M.E., Greene, A.F., Robinson, M.E. and Geisser, M.E., Negative affect and the experience of chronic pain, J. Psychosom. Res., 36 (1992) 707–713.

Gaston-Johansson, F., Gustafsson, M., Felldin, R. and Sanne, H., A comparative study of feelings, attitudes and behaviors of patients with fibromyalgia and rheumatoid arthritis, Soc. Sci. Med., 31 (1990) 941–947.

Gedalia, A., Press, J., Klein, M. and Buskila, D., Joint hypermobility and fibromyalgia in schoolchildren, Ann. Rheum. Dis., 52 (1993) 494–496.

Gerke, D.C., Richards, L.C. and Goss, A.N., Discriminant function analysis of clinical and psychological variables in temporomandibular joint pain dysfunction, Aust. Dent. J., 34 (1989) 44–48.

Granges, G. and Littlejohn, G.O., A comparative study of clinical signs in fibromyalgia/fibrositis syndrome, healthy and exercising subjects, J. Rheumatol., 20 (1993) 344–351.

Greenfield, B.E. and Moore, J.R., Electromyographic study of postoperative trismus, J. Oral Surg., 27 (1969) 92–98.

Griep, E.N., Boersma, J.W. and de Kloet, E.R., Altered reactivity of the hypothalamic-pituitary-adrenal axis in the primary fibromyalgia syndrome [see comments], J. Rheumatol., 20 (1993) 469–474.

Hader, N., Rimon, D., Kinarty, A. and Lahat, N., Altered interleukin-2 secretion in patients with primary fibromyalgia syndrome, Arthritis Rheum., 34 (1991) 866–872.

Hagberg, M. and Kvarnstrom, S., Muscular endurance and electromyographic fatigue in myofascial shoulder pain, Arch. Phys. Med. Rehabil., 65 (1984) 522–525.

Hawley, D.J. and Wolfe, F., Pain, disability, and pain/disability relationships in seven rheumatic disorders: a study of 1,522 patients, J. Rheumatol., 18 (1991) 1552–1557.

Heiberg, A.N., Heloe, B. and Krogstad, B.S., The myofascial pain dysfunction: dental symptoms and psychological and muscular function. An overview. A preliminary study by team approach, Psychother. Psychosom., 30 (1978) 81–97.

High, A.S., MacGregor, A.J., Tomlinson, G.E. and Salkouskis, P.M., A gnathodynanometer as an objective means of pain assessment following wisdom tooth removal, Br. J. Oral Maxillofac. Surg., 26 (1988) 284–291.

Hudson, J.I., Goldenberg, D.L., Pope, H.G., Jr., Keck, P.E., Jr. and Schlesinger, L., Comorbidity of fibromyalgia with medical and psychiatric disorders, Am. J. Med., 92 (1992) 363–367.

Hultman, G., Nordin, M., Saraste, H. and Ohlsen, H., Body composition, endurance, strength, cross-sectional area, and density of MM erector spinae in men with and without low back pain, J. Spinal Disord., 6 (1993) 114–123.

Jacobsen, S. and Danneskiold-Samsoe, B., Isometric and isokinetic muscle strength in patients with fibrositis syndrome: new characteristics for a difficult definable category of patients, Scand. J. Rheumatol., 16 (1987) 61–65.

Jacobsen, S. and Danneskiold-Samsoe, B., Inter-relations between clinical parameters and muscle function in patients with primary fibromyalgia, Clin. Exp. Rheumatol., 7 (1989) 493–498.

Jacobsen, S. and Danneskiold-Samsoe, B., Dynamic muscular endurance in primary fibromyalgia compared with chronic myofascial pain syndrome, Arch. Phys. Med. Rehabil., 73 (1992) 170–173.

Jacobsen, S., Jensen, K.E., Thomsen, C., Danneskiold-Samsoe, B. and Henriksen, O., 31P magnetic resonance spectroscopy of skeletal muscle in patients with fibromyalgia, J. Rheumatol., 19 (1992) 1600–1603.

Jacobsen, S., Gam, A., Egsmose, C., Olsen, M., Danneskiold-Samsoe, B. and Jensen, G.F., Bone mass and turnover in fibromyalgia, J. Rheumatol., 20 (1993a) 856–859.

Jacobsen, S., Petersen, I.S. and Danneskiold-Samsoe, B., Clinical features in patients with chronic muscle pain—with special reference to fibromyalgia, Scand. J. Rheumatol., 22 (1993b) 69–76.

Jaeger, B., Are "cervicogenic" headaches due to myofascial pain and cervical spine dysfunction? Cephalalgia, 9 (1989) 157–164.

Jow, R.W. and Clark, G.T., Endurance and recovery from a sustained isometric contraction in human jaw-elevating muscles, Arch. Oral Biol., 34 (1989) 857–862.

Kalyan-Raman, U.P., Kalyan-Raman, K., Yunus, M.B. and Masi, A.T., Muscle pathology in primary fibromyalgia syndrome: a light microscopic, histochemical and ultrastructural study, J. Rheumatol., 11 (1984) 808–813.

Kapel, L., Glaros, A.G. and McGlynn, F.D., Psychophysiological responses to stress in patients with myofascial pain-dysfunction syndrome, J. Behav. Med., 12 (1989) 397–406.

Keefe, F.J. and Dolan, E., Pain behavior and pain coping strategies in low back pain and myofascial pain dysfunction syndrome patients, Pain, 24 (1986) 49–56.

Kerstein, R.B. and Wright, N.R., Electromyographic and computer analyses of patients suffering from chronic myofascial pain-dysfunction syndrome: before and after treatment with immediate complete anterior guidance development, J. Prosthet. Dent., 66 (1991) 677–686.

Kirmayer, L.J., Robbins, J.M. and Kapusta, M.A., Somatization and depression in fibromyalgia syndrome, Am. J. Psychiatry, 145 (1988) 950–954.

Kravitz, H.M., Katz, R., Kot, E., Helmke, N. and Fawcett, J., Biochemical clues to a fibromyalgia-depression link: imipramine binding in patients with fibromyalgia or depression and in healthy controls, J. Rheumatol., 19 (1992) 1428–1432.

Krogstad, B.S., Dahl, B.L., Eckersberg, T. and Ogaard, B., Sex differences in signs and symptoms from masticatory and other muscles in 19-year-old individuals, J. Oral Rehabil., 19 (1992) 435–440.

Kroon, G.W. and Naeije, M., Electromyographic evidence of local muscle fatigue in a subgroup of patients with myogenous craniomandibular disorders, Arch. Oral Biol., 37 (1992) 215–218.

Kroon, G.W., Naeije, M. and Hansson, T.L., Electromyographic power-spectrum changes during repeated fatiguing contractions of the human masseter muscle, Arch. Oral Biol., 31 (1986) 603–608.

LeResche, L. and Dworkin, S.F., Facial expressions of pain and emotions in chronic TMD patients, Pain, 35 (1988) 71–78.

LeResche, L., Dworkin, S.F., Saunders, K., Von Korff, M. and Barlow, W., Is postmenopausal hormone use a risk factor for TMD? J. Dent. Res., 73 (spec. iss.) (1994) 186.

Leventhal, L.J., Naides, S.J. and Freundlich, B., Fibromyalgia and parvovirus infection, Arthritis Rheum., 34 (1991) 1319–1324.

Lightfoot, R.W., Jr., Luft, B.J., Rahn, D.W., Steere, A.C., Sigal, L.H., Zoschke, D.C., Gardner, P., Britton, M.C. and Kaufman, R.L., Empiric parenteral antibiotic treatment of patients with fibromyalgia and fatigue and a positive serologic result for Lyme disease: a cost-effectiveness analysis [see comments], Ann. Intern. Med., 119 (1993) 503–509.

Littlejohn, G.O., Weinstein, C. and Helme, R.D., Increased neurogenic inflammation in fibrositis syndrome, J. Rheumatol., 14 (1987) 1022–1025.

Lund, J.P. and Stohler, C.S., Effect of pain on muscular activity in temporomandibular disorders and related conditions. In: C.S. Stohler and D.S. Carlson (Eds.), Biological and Psychological Aspects of Orofacial Pain, Craniofacial Growth Series, Vol. 29, Center for Human Growth and Development, The University of Michigan, Ann Arbor, Mich., 1994, pp. 75–91.

Lund, J.P., Donga, R., Widmer, C.G. and Stohler, C.S., The pain-adaptation model: a discussion of the relationship between chronic musculoskeletal pain and motor activity, Can. J. Physiol. Pharmacol., 69 (1991) 683–694.

Lund, J.P., Stohler, C.S. and Widmer, C.G., The relationship between pain and muscle activity in fibromyalgia and similar conditions. In: H. Vaeroy and H. Merskey (Eds.), Progress in Fibromyalgia and Myofascial Pain, Elsevier, Amsterdam, 1993.

Majewski, R.F. and Gale, E.N., Electromyographic activity of anterior temporal area pain patients and non-pain subjects, J. Dent. Res., 63 (1984) 1228–1231.

Marbach, J.J. and Lipton, J.A., Treatment of patients with temporomandibular joint and other facial pain by otolaryngologists, Arch. Otolaryngol., 108 (1982) 102–107.

Matin, P., Lang, G., Carretta, R. and Simon, G., Scintigraphic evaluation of muscle damage following extreme exercise: concise communication, J. Nucl. Med., 24 (1983) 308–311.

McNeill, C., Temporomandibular Disorders: Guidelines for Classification, Assessment, and Management, Quintessence, Chicago, 1993.

Mikkelsson, M., Latikka, P., Kautiainen, H., Isomeri, R. and Isomaki, H., Muscle and bone pressure pain threshold and pain tolerance in fibromyalgia patients and controls, Arch. Phys. Med Rehabil., 73 (1992) 814–818.

Mills, K.R., Newham, D.J. and Edwards, R.H., Force, contraction frequency and energy metabolism as determinants of ischaemic muscle pain, Pain, 14 (1982) 149–154.

Molin, C., Vertical isometric muscle forces of the mandible: a comparative study of subjects with and without manifest mandibular pain dysfunction syndrome, Acta Odontol. Scand., 30 (1972) 485–499.

Moller, E., Sheikholeslam, A. and Lous, I., Response of elevator activity during mastication to treatment of functional disorders, Scand. J. Dent. Res., 92 (1984) 64–83.

Mortimer, J.T., Magnusson, R. and Petersen, I., Conduction velocity in ischemic muscle: effect on EMG frequency spectrum, Am. J. Physiol., 219 (1970) 1324–1329.

Newham, D.J., McPhail, G., Mills, K.R. and Edwards, R.H., Ultrastructural changes after concentric and eccentric contractions of human muscle, J. Neurol. Sci., 61 (1983) 109–122.

Newham, D.J., Jones, D.A., Tolfree, S.E. and Edwards, R.H., Skeletal muscle damage: a study of isotope uptake, enzyme efflux and pain after stepping, Eur. J. Appl. Physiol., 55 (1986) 106–112.

Nice, D.A., Riddle, D.L., Lamb, R.L., Mayhew, T.P. and Rucker, K., Intertester reliability of judgments of the presence of trigger points in patients with low back pain [see comments], Arch. Phys. Med. Rehabil., 73 (1992) 893–898.

Nordenskiold, U.M. and Grimby, G., Grip force in patients with rheumatoid arthritis and fibromyalgia and in healthy subjects: a study with the Grippit instrument, Scand. J. Rheumatol., 22 (1993) 14–19.

Ohrbach, R. and Stohler, C.S., Current diagnostic systems. In: S.F. Dworkin and L. LeResche (Eds.), Research diagnostic criteria for temporomandibular disorders, review, criteria, examinations and specifications, critique, J. Craniomandib. Disord. Facial Oral Pain, 6 (1992) 307–317.

Palla, S. and Ash, M.M., Jr., Effect of bite force on the power spectrum of the surface electromyogram of human jaw muscles, Arch. Oral Biol., 26 (1981a) 287–295.

Palla, S. and Ash, M.M., Jr., Power spectral analysis of the surface electromyogram of human jaw muscles during fatigue, Arch. Oral Biol., 26 (1981b) 547–553.

Perry, F., Heller, P.H., Kamiya, J. and Levine, J.D., Altered autonomic function in patients with arthritis or with chronic myofascial pain, Pain, 39 (1989) 77–84.

Prescott, E., Jacobsen, S., Kjoller, M., Bulow, P.M., Danneskiold-Samsoe, B. and Kamper-

Jorgensen, F., Fibromyalgia in the adult Danish population: II. A study of clinical features, Scand. J. Rheumatol., 22 (1993) 238–242.

Price, D.D., Harkins, S.W. and Baker, C., Sensory-affective relationships among different types of clinical and experimental pain, Pain, 28 (1987) 297–307.

Qiao, Z.G., Vaeroy, H. and Morkrid, L., Electrodermal and microcirculatory activity in patients with fibromyalgia during baseline, acoustic stimulation and cold pressor tests, J. Rheumatol., 18 (1991) 1383–1389.

Quimby, L.G., Block, S.R. and Gratwick, G.M., Fibromyalgia: generalized pain intolerance and manifold symptom reporting, J. Rheumatol., 15 (1988) 1264–1270.

Reeh, E.S. and elDeeb, M.E., Referred pain of muscular origin resembling endodontic involvement: case report, Oral Surg. Oral Med. Oral Pathol., 71 (1991) 223–227.

Reeves, J.L., Jaeger, B. and Graff-Radford, S.B., Reliability of the pressure algometer as a measure of myofascial trigger point sensitivity, Pain, 24 (1986) 313–321.

Robbins, J.M., Kirmayer, L.J. and Kapusta, M.A., Illness worry and disability in fibromyalgia syndrome, Int. J. Psychiatry Med 20 (1990) 49–63.

Russell, I.J., Vaeroy, H., Javors, M. and Nyberg, F., Cerebrospinal fluid biogenic amine metabolites in fibromyalgia/fibrositis syndrome and rheumatoid arthritis [see comments], Arthritis Rheum., 35 (1992) 550–556.

Sadoyama, T. and Miyano, H., Frequency analysis of surface EMG to evaluation of muscle fatigue, Eur. J. Appl. Physiol., 47 (1981) 239–246.

Simms, R.W., Goldenberg, D.L., Felson, D.T. and Mason, J.H., Tenderness in 75 anatomic sites: distinguishing fibromyalgia patients from controls, Arthritis Rheum., 31 (1988) 182–187.

Smythe, H., Referred pain and tender points, Am. J. Med., 81 (1986) 90–92.

Stohler, C.S. and Lund, J.P., Effects of noxious stimulation of the jaw muscles on the sensory experience of volunteer human subjects. In: C.S. Stohler and D.S. Carlson (Eds.), Biological and Psychological Aspects of Orofacial Pain, Craniofacial Growth Series, Vol. 29, Center for Human Growth and Development, The University of Michigan, Ann Arbor, Mich., 1994, pp. 55–74.

Stohler, C., Yamada, Y. and Ash, M.M., Jr., Antagonistic muscle stiffness and associated reflex behaviour in the pain-dysfunctional state, Schweiz. Monatsschr. Zahnmed., 95 (1985) 719–726.

Stohler, C.S., Ashton-Miller, J.A. and Carlson, D.S., The effects of pain from the mandibular joint and muscles on masticatory motor behaviour in man, Arch. Oral Biol., 33 (1988) 175–182.

Stokes, M.J., Colter, C., Klestov, A. and Cooper, R.G., Normal paraspinal muscle electromyographic fatigue characteristics in patients with primary fibromyalgia, Br. J. Rheumatol., 32 (1993) 711–716.

Stratz, T., Samborski, W., Hrycaj, P., Pap, T., Mackiewicz, S., Mennet, P. and Muller, W., [Serotonin concentration in serum of patients with generalized tendomyopathy (fibromyalgia) and chronic polyarthritis](in German), Med. Klin., 88 (1993) 458–462.

Suzuki, N. and Endo, S., A quantitative study of trunk muscle strength and fatigability in the low-back-pain syndrome, Spine, 8 (1983) 69–74.

Svebak, S., Anjia, R. and Karstad, S.I., Task-induced electromyographic activation in fibromyalgia subjects and controls, Scand. J. Rheumatol., 22 (1993) 124–130.

Thorstensson, A. and Arvidson, A., Trunk muscle strength and low back pain, Scand. J. Rehabil. Med., 14 (1982) 69–75.

Travell, J.G. and Simons, D.G., Myofascial Pain and Dysfunction, The Trigger Point Manual, The Upper Extremities, Vol. 1, Williams and Wilkins, Baltimore, 1983.

Travell, J.G., Rinzler, S. and Herman, M., Pain and disability of the shoulder and arm. Treatment by intramuscular infiltration with procaine hydrochloride, JAMA, 120 (1942) 417–422.

Triano, J.J. and Schultz, A.B., Correlation of objective measure of trunk motion and muscle function with low-back disability ratings, Spine, 12 (1987) 561–565.

Tunks, E., Crook, J., Norman, G. and Kalaher, S., Tender points in fibromyalgia, Pain, 34 (1988) 11–19.

Turk, D.C. and Rudy, T.E., Toward a comprehensive assessment of chronic pain patients: a multiaxial approach, Behav. Res. Ther., 25 (1987) 237–249.

Vaeroy, H., Helle, R., Forre, O., Kass, E. and Terenius, L., Cerebrospinal fluid levels of beta-endorphin in patients with fibromyalgia (fibrositis syndrome), J. Rheumatol., 15 (1988) 1804–1806.

Vaeroy, H., Qiao, Z.G., Morkrid, L. and Forre, O., Altered sympathetic nervous system response in patients with fibromyalgia (fibrositis syndrome), J. Rheumatol., 16 (1989) 1460–1465.

Vaeroy, H., Nyberg, F. and Terenius, L., No evidence for endorphin deficiency in fibromyalgia following investigation of cerebrospinal fluid (CSF) dynorphin A and Met-enkephalin-Arg6-Phe7, Pain, 46 (1991) 139–143.

Veale, D., Kavanagh, G., Fielding, J.F. and Fitzgerald, O., Primary fibromyalgia and the irritable bowel syndrome: different expressions of a common pathogenetic process, Br. J. Rheumatol., 30 (1991) 220–222.

Von Korff, M., Wagner, E.H., Dworkin, S.F. and Saunders, K.W., Chronic pain and use of ambulatory health care, Psychosom. Med., 53 (1991) 61–79.

Von Korff, M.R., Dworkin, S.F., Fricton, J.R. and Ohrbach, R., Research diagnostic criteria. B. Axis II: Pain-related disability and psychological status, J. Craniomandib. Disord. Facial Oral Pain, 6 (1992) 330–334.

Widmer, C.G., Temporomandibular joint sounds: a critique of techniques for recording and analysis, J. Craniomandib. Disord., 3 (1989) 213–217.

Widmer, C.G., Lund, J.P. and Feine, J.S., Evaluation of diagnostic tests for TMD, J. Calif. Dent. Assoc., 18 (1990) 53–60.

Wilke, W.S., Sheeler, L.R. and Makarowski, W.S., Hypothyroidism with presenting symptoms of fibrositis, J. Rheumatol., 8 (1981) 626–631.

Wolfe, F., Smythe, H.A., Yunus, M.B., Bennett, R.M., Bombardier, C., Goldenberg, D.L., Tugwell, P., Campbell, S.M., Abeles, M., Clark, P., et al., The American College of Rheumatology 1990 Criteria for the Classification of Fibromyalgia. Report of the Multicenter Criteria Committee [see comments], Arthritis Rheum., 33 (1990) 160–172.

Wolfe, F., Simons, D.G., Fricton, J., Bennett, R.M., Goldenberg, D.L., Gerwin, R., Hathaway, D., McCain, G.A., Russell, I.J., Sanders, H.O., et al., The fibromyalgia and myofascial pain syndromes: a preliminary study of tender points and trigger points in persons with fibromyalgia, myofascial pain syndrome and no disease, J. Rheumatol., 19 (1992) 944–951.

Yaar, I. and Niles, L., Muscle fiber conduction velocity and mean power spectrum frequency in neuromuscular disorders and in fatigue, Muscle Nerve, 15 (1992) 780–787.

Yunus, M.B., Denko, C.W. and Masi, A.T., Serum beta-endorphin in primary fibromyalgia syndrome: a controlled study, J. Rheumatol., 13 (1986) 183–186.

Yunus, M.B., Kalyan-Raman, U.P. and Kalyan-Raman, K., Primary fibromyalgia syndrome and myofascial pain syndrome: clinical features and muscle pathology, Arch. Phys. Med. Rehabil., 69 (1988) 451–454.

Yunus, M.B., Kalyan-Raman, U.P., Masi, A.T. and Aldag, J.C., Electron microscopic studies of muscle biopsy in primary fibromyalgia syndrome: a controlled and blinded study, J. Rheumatol., 16 (1989a) 97–101.

Yunus, M.B., Masi, A.T. and Aldag, J.C., A controlled study of primary fibromyalgia syndrome: clinical features and association with other functional syndromes, J. Rheumatol. Suppl., 19 (1989b) 62–71.

Yunus, M.B., Dailey, J.W., Aldag, J.C., Masi, A.T. and Jobe, P.C., Plasma tryptophan and other amino acids in primary fibromyalgia: a controlled study, J. Rheumatol., 19 (1992) 90–94.

Zhang, X., Ashton-Miller, J.A. and Stohler, C.S., A closed-loop system for maintaining constant experimental muscle pain in man, IEEE Trans. Biomed. Eng., 40 (1993) 344–352.

Zidar, J., Backman, E., Bengtsson, A. and Henriksson, K.G., Quantitative EMG and muscle tension in painful muscles in fibromyalgia, Pain, 40 (1990) 249–254.

Correspondence to: Christian S. Stohler, DMD, Dr. Med. Dent., The University of Michigan School of Dentistry, Ann Arbor, MI 48109, USA. Tel: 313-747-4242; Fax: 313-747-2110.

Temporomandibular Disorders and Related Pain Conditions, Progress in Pain Research and Management, Vol. 4, edited by B.J. Sessle, P.S. Bryant, and R.A. Dionne, IASP Press, Seattle, © 1995.

2

Fibromyalgia

Frederick Wolfe

Department of Internal Medicine and Family and Community Medicine, University of Kansas School of Medicine, and Wichita Arthritis Research and Clinical Centers, Wichita, Kansas, USA

Usually, when I go to see a doctor I tell them about the pain that's worst. If I tell them about everything they think I'm nuts.
— Fibromyalgia patient

FIBROMYALGIA AND TEMPOROMANDIBULAR DISORDERS

The fibromyalgia syndrome is a disorder characterized primarily by widespread pain, decreased pain threshold, sleep disturbance, fatigue and, often, psychological distress. Anecdotally, a disproportionate number of persons with fibromyalgia report having had "TMJ syndrome," although few reports have described or attempted to investigate this relationship (McCain and Scudds 1988; Eriksson et al. 1988; Blasberg and Chalmers 1989; Block 1993). McCain and Scudds hypothesized, using Venn diagrams, that fibromyalgia and temporomandibular disorders (TMDs) overlapped, with a minority of TMD patients also having fibromyalgia (McCain and Scudds 1988). A review of the fibromyalgia concept also noted similarities between the two syndromes (Block 1993), but there have been few studies. A retrospective review of TMD patients noted that more than expected had features associated with generalized distress (Blasberg and Chalmers 1989), but specific examinations for fibromyalgia were not performed. In a dental clinic eight patients with fibromyalgia were examined, and six had "severe mandibular dysfunction" (Eriksson et al. 1988). Jaw pain was reported in 35.5% of fibromyalgia patients in a Swiss investigation (Müller 1991), and was found in 18% by U.S. investigators (Leavitt et al. 1986). Lautenschläger and co-workers (1991) studied pain threshold in the masseter in fibromyalgia and normal controls. They noted decreased pain threshold among patients, but, in comparison to other tender points, somewhat decreased in controls as well. Thus, only limited data exist on the relationship between fibromyalgia and TMDs. In rheumatology clinics, almost all of the patients with TMDs have fibromyalgia, excluding those with rheumatoid arthritis. But it is likely that such a finding is the result of referral and selection bias: rheumatologists tend to see individuals with generalized pain and musculoskeletal complaints.

Recent studies from TMD centers have indicated that many TMD patients have more diffuse muscle tenderness than ordinarily would be expected within the hypothesis of a "local" TMD disorder (Dworkin et al. 1990), suggesting the possibility that some patients might fulfill fibromyalgia criteria (Wolfe et al. 1990). Symptoms of fibromyalgia appear to be common in chronic TMDs (Fricton et al. 1985; Wolfe et al. 1992), but just as there have been no studies of TMDs in fibromyalgia, there have been no systematic studies of fibromyalgia in TMDs. Such studies are needed and will enhance understanding of both conditions. Finally, continuously complicating understanding are publications that use terminology incorrectly. One recent paper, entitled "Head and neck fibromyalgia and temporomandibular arthralgia," used a definition totally at variance with current concepts and diagnostic criteria (Truta and Santucci 1989).

THE NATURE OF FIBROMYALGIA

As indicated above, fibromyalgia is a disorder characterized primarily by widespread pain, decreased pain threshold, sleep disturbance, fatigue and, often, psychological distress, and is diagnosed when widespread pain, decreased pain threshold to palpation, and characteristic symptoms are all present together. Fibromyalgia has been called a disorder of "pain modulation" (Smythe 1979; Moldofsky 1982; Simons and Travell 1983; Yunus 1992), "pain amplification" (Smythe 1979, 1985), and the "irritable everything syndrome" (Smythe 1985). Conceptually, it can be thought of as a syndrome in which not only pain but all stimuli appear to be amplified. Fig. 1 presents a model of fibromyalgia.

One consequence of the amplification process is that nociceptive stimuli that are normally below the pain threshold may be perceived as pain, and that mild pain is perceived as being more than mild, and often severe. Associated with the change in pain threshold is an unexpected increase in the distribution of pain, which becomes wider and more generalized. Fig. 2 displays pain drawings from four patients with fibromyalgia and emphasizes the characteristic distribution of fibromyalgia pain: widespread, axial, radiating, and joint associated. The extent of the pain is often surprising, and may, in and of itself, suggest the diagnosis. Note that one patient in Fig. 2 clearly has facial (TMJ)

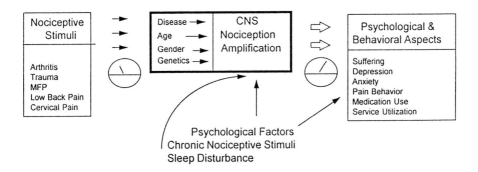

Fig. 1. A model of fibromyalgia pathogenesis and clinical expression. (Wolfe and Hawley 1993)

pain. When patients with such widespread pain complaints consult clinicians who are not aware of fibromyalgia, the diagnosis may depend on the specific complaint or the specific clinician chosen. As noted above, one patient reported, "Usually, when I go to see a doctor I tell them about the pain that's worst. If I tell them about everything they think I'm nuts." Perhaps patients in whom facial pain is worst are diagnosed with TMDs, while those with neck or back pain are referred to neurosurgeons or orthopedic surgeons, respectively.

While the distribution of pain can suggest fibromyalgia, the key clinical and diagnostic feature is decreased pain threshold as manifested by tenderness (tender points) at specific anatomic locations. Fig. 3 presents the 18 tender point sites used by the American College of Rheumatology 1990 Criteria for the Classification of Fibromyalgia (Wolfe et al. 1990). Tender point sites represent specific areas of muscle, tendon, and fat pads that are considerably more tender to palpation than surrounding sites. In patients with fibromyalgia, a positive tender point is identified by palpating the tender point site with approximately 4 kg of force. Usually the second and/or third fingers or the thumb are used for palpation, and a rolling motion may be helpful in eliciting tenderness. A positive examination is one in which the patient states that the examination caused pain (not just "tenderness"). The American College of Rheumatology (ACR) criteria for the classification of fibromyalgia (Table I) require that 11 of 18 specified sites be painful on palpation (61%). The presence of 11 tender points together with widespread pain constitutes the ACR definition and criteria for fibromyalgia (Wolfe et al. 1990). These criteria have superseded older criteria, and for reasons of performance and uniformity, should be used.

In addition to widespread pain and generalized tenderness, a series of symptoms commonly are found in fibromyalgia and tend to further define the syndrome. Table II describes the symptoms and their prevalence. The core

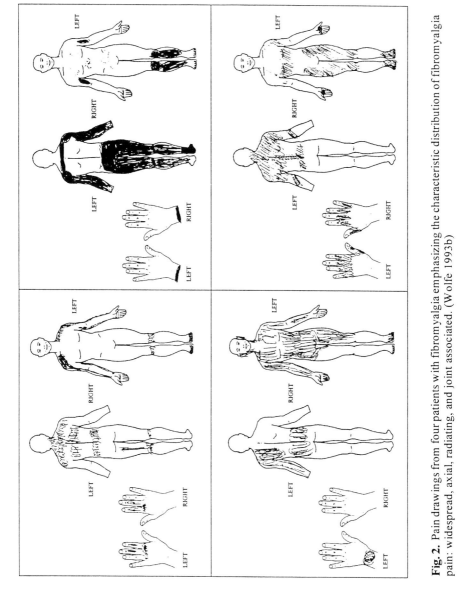

Fig. 2. Pain drawings from four patients with fibromyalgia emphasizing the characteristic distribution of fibromyalgia pain: widespread, axial, radiating, and joint associated. (Wolfe 1993b)

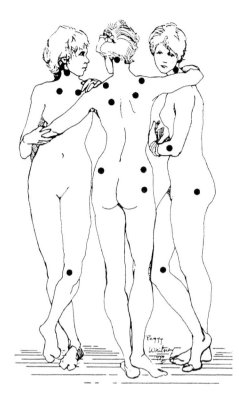

Fig. 3. The 18 tender point sites of the American College of Rheumatology 1990 criteria for the classification of fibromyalgia. Eleven of 18 tender points satisfies the tenderness criterion. (Wolfe et al. 1990)

symptoms are usually considered to be fatigue, sleep disturbance, and stiffness.

Fatigue. Defined as (usually or often) being "too tired during the day to do what I want to do," fatigue is among the most common of symptoms and was found in 77% of patients in the ACR study (Wolfe et al. 1990).

Sleep disturbance. Moldofsky originally described the sleep disturbance of fibromyalgia in terms of "alpha delta intrusion" observable in EEGs during sleep studies (Moldofsky et al. 1975). In the clinic the concept of "awaking unrefreshed" has been adopted as the most effective way of ascertaining the clinical complaint (Campbell et al. 1983; Wolfe et al. 1985). In the ACR study 74.6% reported this symptom (Wolfe et al. 1990).

Morning stiffness. This symptom has been reported in 75% (Wolfe and Cathey 1983; Goldenberg 1987; Wolfe et al. 1990; Ledingham et al. 1993) to 100% (Campbell et al. 1983) of cases.

Headache. Chronic headache, as either migraine (Yunus et al. 1981, 1989;) or other headache, has been reported in 44–58% of patients with fibromyalgia (Yunus et al. 1981, 1989; Campbell et al. 1983; Wolfe and Cathey 1983; Bengtsson et al. 1986; Goldenberg 1987; Wolfe et al. 1990).

Paresthesia. Paresthesias were among the most common findings (62%)

Table I
The 1990 American College of Rheumatology criteria
for the classification of fibromyalgia

1. History of Widespread Pain

Definition: Pain is considered widespread when all of the following are present: pain in the left side of the body, pain in the right side of the body, pain above the waist, and pain below the waist. In addition, axial skeletal pain (cervical spine or anterior chest or thoracic spine or low back) must be present. In this definition shoulder and buttock pain is considered as pain for each involved side. "Low back" pain is considered lower segment pain.

2. Pain in 11 of 18 Tender Point Sites on Digital Palpation

Definition: Pain, on digital palpation, must be present in at least 11 of the following 18 tender point sites:

Occiput: bilateral, at the suboccipital muscle insertions.

Low cervical: bilateral, at the anterior aspects of the inter-transverse spaces at C5–C7.

Trapezius: bilateral, at the midpoint of the upper border.

Supraspinatus: bilateral, at origins, above the scapula spine near the medial border.

Second rib: bilateral, at the second costochondral junctions, just lateral to the junctions on upper surfaces.

Lateral epicondyle: bilateral, 2 cm distal to the epicondyles.

Gluteal: bilateral, in upper outer quadrants of buttocks in anterior fold of muscle.

Greater trochanter: bilateral, posterior to the trochanteric prominence.

Knees: bilateral, at the medial fat pad proximal to the joint line.

Digital palpation should be performed with an approximate force of 4 kg.

For a tender point to be considered "positive" the subject must state that the palpation was painful. "Tender" is not to be considered painful.

Source: Wolfe et al. 1990.
Note: For classification purposes, patients will be said to have fibromyalgia if both criteria are satisfied. Widespread pain must have been present for at least three months. The presence of a second clinical disorder does not exclude the diagnosis of fibromyalgia.

in the ACR study (Wolfe et al. 1990) and have been noted by others at rates varying from 26% (Yunus et al. 1981) to 71% (Bengtsson et al. 1986).

   Irritable bowel syndrome (IBS). The prevalence of IBS is dependent upon referral pattern of the clinic, the definition of IBS, and the interest of the examiner. It has been reported in 34–53% of studies (Yunus et al. 1981; Campbell et al. 1983; Wolfe and Cathey 1983; Goldenberg 1987; Yunus et al. 1989), including 35.7% in the ACR criteria study (Wolfe et al. 1990). But GI symptoms may be even more pervasive when a less strict definition is

Table II
Prevalence of pain and symptoms in the 1990 American College of
Rheumatology study of criteria for the classification of fibromyalgia

Criterion	Positive (%)	Classification Accuracy (%)
Pain symptoms		
Pain posterior thorax	72.3	73.9
15+ painful sites	55.6	70.6
Neck pain	85.3	67.5
Low back pain	78.8	66.6
Widespread pain	97.6	65.9
Symptoms		
Sleep disturbance	74.6	73.8
"Pain all over"	67.0	73.6
Fatigue	81.4	71.7
Morning stiffness > 15 minutes	77.0	67.2
Paresthesias	62.8	63.6
Anxiety	47.8	62.9
Headache	52.8	62.3
Prior depression	31.5	58.0
Irritable bowel syndrome	29.6	57.1
Sicca symptoms	35.8	55.4
Urinary urgency	26.3	54.2
Dysmenorrhea history	40.6	53.4
Raynaud's phenomenon	16.7	51.6
Modulating factors		
Noise	24.0	68.5
Cold	79.3	66.6
Poor sleep	76.0	65.2
Anxiety	69.0	63.7
Humidity	59.6	63.6
Stress	63.0	60.4
Fatigue	76.7	60.3
Weather change	66.1	60.3
Warmth	78.0	50.8

Source: Modified from Wolfe et al. 1990 with permission.

used. Using a validated self-administered questionnaire, Triadafilopoulos and co-workers (1991) reported "altered bowel function" in 73% and "abdominal pain" in 64% of subjects.

Irritable bladder syndrome. This aspect of fibromyalgia has not been widely studied (Wallace 1990). It may manifest as reports of frequent urinary tract infections or as urinary urgency. Urinary urgency was found in 26.3% of fibromyalgia patients as compared with 15.5% of controls in the ACR criteria study (Wolfe et al. 1990).

PSYCHOLOGICAL ABNORMALITY

No factor in fibromyalgia has been more intensively studied than psychological status. This interest has been fueled by the almost universal clinical observation of increased psychological abnormality in those with fibromyalgia compared with other patients, an observation supported by a multitude of studies (Ahles et al. 1984; Wolfe et al. 1984; Hudson et al. 1985; Leavitt et al. 1986; Scudds et al. 1987; Egle et al. 1989; Leavitt and Katz 1989; Piergiacomi et al. 1989; Uveges et al. 1990; Anch et al. 1991; Birnie et al. 1991; Samborski et al. 1991; Hudson et al. 1992; Hawley and Wolfe 1993). In the face of such observations it is often easy to forget the other truth, that many, perhaps most, patients with fibromyalgia are psychologically normal. Hawley and Wolfe (1993) have studied the extent to which fibromyalgia patients differ from those with other rheumatic diseases. They noted that 48.6% of unselected clinic fibromyalgia patients (N = 543) had Arthritis Impact Measurement Scales (AIMS) (Hawley and Wolfe 1993) depression scores indicating possible (score ≥ 3.0) clinical depression and 29.3% had scores indicating probable (score ≥ 4.0) clinical depression compared with 34.5% and 19.1%, respectively, of all other clinic patients (N = 5610).

Thus depression, variously defined, is 10–15% more common in those with fibromyalgia. Another insight into fibromyalgia patients' adjustment comes from a study of marital status in rheumatic disease. Divorce rate was higher among fibromyalgia patients (10.1%) compared with all other rheumatic conditions (6.6%) (Hawley et al. 1991).

Only a few studies have not found evidence of psychological abnormality compared to other rheumatic disease and general medical patients (Clark et al. 1985; Ahles et al. 1991; Birnie et al. 1991), or have suggested a history of past major depression and increased family depression but not current psychiatric diagnosis (Hudson et al. 1985; Goldenberg 1986).

Many studies have found increased prevalence of psychological abnormalities among fibromyalgia patients for anxiety (Wolfe et al. 1984; Hudson et al. 1984; Hudson et al. 1985; Anch et al. 1991), depression (Wolfe et al. 1984; Alfici et al. 1989; Piergiacomi et al. 1989; Robbins et al. 1990; Anch et al. 1991; Hawley and Wolfe 1993), somatization or emphasis on bodily concerns including hypochondriasis (Scudds et al. 1987; Kirmayer et al. 1988;

Leavitt and Katz 1989; Robbins et al. 1990; Birnie et al. 1991), coping (Uveges et al. 1990), daily hassles (Dailey et al. 1990; Uveges et al. 1990), and history of major depression (Hudson et al. 1984, 1985; Goldenberg 1986; Alfici et al. 1989). Evidence of psychopathology has been hypothesized using the Minnesota Multiphasic Personality Inventory (MMPI) (Payne et al. 1982; Wolfe et al. 1984; Ahles et al. 1986; Arnett et al. 1988), the Symptom Check List-90-R (SCL-90-R) scales (Kirmayer et al. 1988; Anch et al. 1991), and the Basic Personality Inventory (BPI) (Scudds et al. 1987).

PHYSICAL FINDINGS

Swelling. Patients frequently complaint about swelling, often in characteristic locations—around the elbows, in the hands, and in the medial aspect of the knees. This complaint originally was called "subjective swelling" (Yunus et al. 1981) because it is often not observed by physicians. But patients can point out tightness of their wristwatch band and the loss of the skin lines over the metacarpophalangeal (MCP) joints (observable by physicians). Swelling is nonarticular and often improves during the course of the day. It is possible that such swelling is related causally to complaints of carpal tunnel symptoms among fibromyalgia patients.

Neurogenic inflammation. Reactive hyperemia (Smythe and Moldofsky 1977; Astrand 1987), the presence of erythema in the skin following mechanical (palpation) or chemical (capsaicin) stimulation, was demonstrated by Littlejohn, who showed increased erythema in those with fibromyalgia compared with controls (Littlejohn et al. 1987) and normals (Granges and Littlejohn 1993). This finding as determined during routine clinical examination, however, does not have sufficient specificity to be used for diagnosis because it is seen (in lesser proportion) in others with rheumatic diseases (Wolfe et al. 1990). When carefully quantitated it accurately classifies 74.5% of patients compared with normal controls (Granges and Littlejohn 1993).

Tissue compliance. Tissue compliance is significantly lower in patients with fibromyalgia and has good diagnostic specificity (Granges and Littlejohn 1993).

Skin fold tenderness. Originally suggested by Smythe and Moldofsky (Smythe and Moldofsky 1977), the assessment of tenderness at the upper border of the trapezius had a diagnostic accuracy of 71.2% in the ACR criteria study (Wolfe et al. 1990). When applied to the thoracic region, however, sensitivity was 96.6% and diagnostic accuracy 92.5% against normal controls (Granges and Littlejohn 1993).

Laboratory studies. In general, routine laboratory studies are normal in fibromyalgia unless the patient has an additional disorder that is associated with laboratory abnormalities.

EPIDEMIOLOGY OF FIBROMYALGIA

Socio-demographic factors. Fibromyalgia is largely a disorder of women (85–90% of cases, or greater), both in the clinic and in the community. Although the syndrome is often found in younger persons (20–40 years of age), when concomitant illnesses are excluded, data from our recent population survey in Wichita indicate that fibromyalgia prevalence increases with age, with an approximate mean age of 54 years for persons with the syndrome. Fibromyalgia has been linked to several socio-demographic factors. In the clinic (Hawley et al. 1991) and in the general population fibromyalgia is associated with increased divorce rates (Wolfe et al. 1995). Failure to graduate from high school is more common among those with fibromyalgia in the general population compared to those without fibromyalgia, and persons with fibromyalgia have lower family incomes (Wolfe et al. 1995). Unpublished data from our clinic indicate that the body mass index of 770 consecutive patients with fibromyalgia is 28.1, a value that is abnormally high. Thus, obesity also may be linked to fibromyalgia. Persons with fibromyalgia are frequent users of medical and surgical services, well in excess of the expected proportion.

Prevalence and characteristics. In rheumatology clinics fibromyalgia is present in 12% (Wolfe and Cathey 1983) to 20% (Yunus et al. 1981) of new patients. The prevalence is lower in general medical clinics (5.7%) (Campbell et al. 1983) and family practice settings (2.1%) (Hartz and Kirchdoerfer 1987). Our group has recently performed the first prevalence study of fibromyalgia in the general population in North America, interviewing 3,066 persons (Wolfe et al. 1995). We noted chronic regional pain in 20.1% (18.7–21.5) and chronic widespread pain in 10.6% (9.5–11.7) and found an estimated fibromyalgia prevalence in Wichita of 2.0% (1.4–2.7), for women 3.4% (2.3–4.6) and for men 0.5% (0.0–1.0). These data are generally consistent with reports from non–North American sources (Wolfe 1993a). The population study data, showing an increasing association with age, suggest that fibromyalgia is more common in those with other medical and musculoskeletal disorders. The community data also found significant increases in depression and other psychological abnormalities in the fibromyalgia group, as well as inverse associations with health satisfaction and global health perception (Wolfe 1993a). These observations suggest that, for some in the community, fibromyalgia can be conceived of as a general distress disorder.

COURSE AND OUTCOME

Persistence of symptoms. At our present state of knowledge from clinical data, most observations suggest that fibromyalgia is a chronic, rather
unchanging disorder that rarely ends in remission (Bengtsson et al. 1986;
Cathey et al. 1986; Felson and Goldenberg 1986; Hawley et al. 1988;
Henriksson et al. 1992; Ledingham et al. 1993). In the most detailed report
(Ledingham et al. 1993), four years after initial examination, 97% still had
symptoms and 85% fulfilled diagnostic criteria. Half had significant levels of
functional disability measured by the Health Assessment Question (HAQ), as
indicated by a median HAQ score of 1. Many patients had abnormal scores
for depression and anxiety. Even so, such reports may be wrong because for
the most part they have focused on patients with disease of long duration who
have been referred to specialty clinics. In addition, it is clear that improvement generally occurs in a wide spectrum of chronic pain patients (Crook et
al. 1989; Whitney and Von Korff 1992). Fibromyalgia related to trauma also
appears to be chronic as well as severe (Greenfield et al. 1992).

Functional disability. Functional problems, as measured by self-report,
are a common finding. Using the HAQ, one center (Hawley and Wolfe 1991)
in the United States and another study in the United Kingdom (Ledingham et
al. 1993) found significantly abnormal scores averaging approximately 1.00
(0–3 scale). The HAQ scores and ability to perform work tasks were correlated at $r = -0.61$ in one U.S. study (Cathey et al. 1988).

Work disability. Work disability and compensation is related to country
and social system. After an average of seven years, 55% of Swedish patients
were unable to do necessary household tasks and 24% were receiving disability pensions (Bengtsson et al. 1986). In separate reports from one center in
the United States, 6.3% (Cathey et al. 1986) and 9.3% of patients reported
being disabled (Cathey et al. 1988), while 5.7% were receiving disability
payments, 30.4% reported having to change jobs because of their illness, and
17% retired because of fibromyalgia (Cathey et al. 1988). In another center
22% reported being disabled and 33% changed jobs because of the illness
(Mason et al. 1989). A 1990 multicenter study of 620 patients indicated that
14.9% had received disability payments; 8.8% of these patients received Social Security disability payments (Cathey et al.1990).

POSSIBLE RELATIONSHIPS BETWEEN FIBROMYALGIA
AND TMDs

The association between TMDs and fibromyalgia is probably not fortu-
itous. Some of the possible links are suggested below.

Model 1—Decreased pain threshold of fibromyalgia results in facial and TMJ pain and symptoms. This model suggests that the general lowering of the pain threshold causes below-threshold nociception to become a clinical problem. In addition, mild pain is amplified and becomes very disturbing. In the statement "When I go to see a doctor I tell them about the pain that's worst," we would see TMD as only one of the possible medical disorders that the patient might have. Direction of causation: fibromyalgia to TMD; fibromyalgia is the predominant problem, TMD is the diagnosis.

Model 2—Fibromyalgia and TMDs are linked by psychological distress. This model suggests that in some patients psychological distress is linked causally to the development of two common and related syndromes. Direction of causation: no causal relationship; psychological distress is the problem, fibromyalgia and TMDs are the diagnoses.

Model 3—The psychological distress noted in some fibromyalgia patients leads to increased somatic concern, medical visits, and diagnostic prevalence. This model suggests that some patients diagnosed with TMDs will have less evidence of disease than would be expected. Direction of causation: fibromyalgia to TMDs; fibromyalgia is the problem, TMDs are not a necessary diagnosis.

Model 4—All pain disorders are associated in an increased prevalence of fibromyalgia. Various clinic and community survey data suggest that fibromyalgia prevalence is at least twice expected values in those with other pain disorders such as rheumatoid arthritis and osteoarthritis. Mechanisms are unknown but might be related to an increase in nociceptive stimuli in patients with pain disorders (Wolfe 1993a), with psychological distress secondary to chronic pain, or to both. Direction of causation: TMDs to fibromyalgia; TMDs are the primary problem, TMD and fibromyalgia are the diagnoses.

FUTURE DIRECTIONS

Clarification of these hypotheses, and better understanding of both conditions, require clinic studies of patients with fibromyalgia and patients with TMDs that consider both diagnoses. No such studies have been done, but without these investigations knowledge will remain only anecdotal. Longitudinal studies also are required to observe the development and course of the syndromes. Clinic studies, however, are limited by the selection and filtration process of the clinic, and major increases in understanding can come from studies of both conditions in the community.

REFERENCES

Ahles, T.A., Yunus, M.B., Riley, S.D., Bradley, J.M. and Masi, A.T., Psychological factors associated with primary fibromyalgia syndrome, Arthritis Rheum., 27 (1984) 1101–1106.

Ahles, T.A., Yunus, M.B., Gaulier, B., Riley, S.D. and Masi, A.T., The use of contemporary MMPI norms in the study of chronic pain patients, Pain., 24 (1986) 159–163.

Ahles, T.A., Khan, S.A., Yunus, M.B., Spiegel, D.A. and Masi, A.T., Psychiatric status of patients with primary fibromyalgia, patients with rheumatoid arthritis, and subjects without pain: a blind comparison of DSM-III diagnoses, Am. J. Psychiatry, 148 (1991) 1721–1726.

Alfici, S., Sigal, M. and Landau, M., Primary fibromyalgia syndrome: a variant of depressive disorder?, Psychother. Psychosom., 51 (1989) 1056–161.

Anch, A.M., Lue, F.A., MacLean, A.W. and Moldofsky, H., Sleep physiology and psychological aspects of the fibrositis (fibromyalgia) syndrome, Can. J. Psychol., 45 (1991) 179–184.

Arnett, F.C., Edworthy, S.M., Bloch, D.A., McShane, D.J., Fries, J.F., Cooper, N.S., Healy, L.A., Caplan, S.R., Liang, M.H., Luthra, H.S., Medsger, T.A., Jr., Mitchell, D.M., Neustadt, D.H., Pinals, R.S., Schaller, J.G., Sharp, J.T., Wilder, R.L. and Hunder, G.G., The American Rheumatism Association 1987 revised criteria for the classification of rheumatoid arthritis, Arthritis Rheum., 31 (1988) 315–324.

Astrand, P.O., Exercise physiology and its role in disease prevention and in rehabilitation, Arch. Phys. Med. Rehabil., 68 (1987) 305–309.

Bengtsson, A., Henriksson, K.G., Jorfeldt, L., Kagedal, B., Lennmarken, C. and Lindstrom, F., Primary fibromyalgia: a clinical and laboratory study of 55 patients, Scand. J. Rheumatol., 15 (1986) 340–347.

Birnie, D.J., Knipping, A.A., van Rijswijk, M.H., de Blëcourt, A.C. and de Voogd, N., Psychological aspects of fibromyalgia compared with chronic and nonchronic pain, J. Rheumatol., 18 (1991) 1845–1848.

Blasberg, B. and Chalmers, A., Temporomandibular pain and dysfunction syndrome associated with generalized musculoskeletal pain: a retrospective study, J. Rheumatol., 16, Suppl. 19 (1989) 87–90.

Block, S.R., Fibromyalgia and the rheumatisms: common sense and sensibility, Rheum. Dis. Clin. North Am., 19 (1993) 61–78.

Campbell, S.M., Clark, S., Tindall, E.A., Forehand, M.E. and Bennett, R.M., Clinical characteristics of fibrositis. I. A "blinded," controlled study of symptoms and tender points, Arthritis Rheum., 26 (1983) 817–824.

Cathey, M.A., Wolfe, F., Kleinheksel, S.M. and Hawley, D.J., Socioeconomic impact of fibrositis: a study of 81 patients with primary fibrositis, Am. J. Med., 81 (1986) 78–84.

Cathey, M.A., Wolfe, F., Kleinheksel, S.M., Miller, S. and Pitetti, K.H., Functional ability and work status in patients with fibromyalgia, Arthritis Care Res., 1 (1988) 85–98.

Cathey, M.A., Wolfe, F., Roberts, F.K., Bennett, R.M., Caro, X., Goldenberg, D.L., Russell, I.J. and Yunus, M.B., Demographic, work disability, service utilization and treatment characteristics of 620 fibromyalgia patients in rheumatologic practice (abstract), Arthritis Rheum., 33 (1990) S10.

Clark, S., Campbell, S.M., Forehand, M.E., Tindall, E.A. and Bennett, R.M., Clinical characteristics of fibrositis. II. A "blinded," controlled study using standard psychological tests, Arthritis Rheum, 28 (1985) 132–137.

Crook, J., Weir, R. and Tunks, E., An epidemiological follow-up survey of persistent pain sufferers in a group family practice and specialty pain clinic, Pain, 36 (1989) 49–61.

Dailey, P.A., Bishop, G.D., Russell, I.J. and Fletcher, E.M., Psychological stress and the fibrositis/fibromyalgia syndrome, J Rheumatol, 17 (1990) 1380–1385.

Dworkin, S.F., Huggins, K.H., LeResche, L., Von Korff, M., Howard, J., Truelove, E. and Sommers, E., Epidemiology of signs and symptoms in temporomandibular disorders: clinical signs in cases and controls, J. Am. Dent. Assoc., 10 (1990) 11–23.

44   *F. WOLFE*

Egle, U.T., Rudolf, M.L., Hoffmann, S.O., Konig, K., Schofer, M., Schwab, R. and von Wilmowsky, H., Personality markers, defense behavior and illness concept in patients with primary fibromyalgia, Z. Rheumatol., 48 (1989) 73–78.

Eriksson, P.O., Lindman, R., Stal, P. and Bengtsson, A., Symptoms and signs of mandibular dysfunction in primary fibromyalgia syndrome (PSF) patients, Swed. Dent. J., 12 (1988) 141–149.

Felson, D.T. and Goldenberg, D.L., The natural history of fibromyalgia, Arthritis. Rheum., 29 (1986) 1522–1526.

Fricton, J.R., Kroening, R., Haley, D. and Siegert, R., Myofascial pain syndrome of the head and neck: a review of clinical characteristics of 164 patients, Oral. Surg., 60 (1985) 615–623.

Goldenberg, D.L., Psychologic studies in fibrositis, Am. J. Med., 81 (1986) 67–70.

Goldenberg, D.L., Fibromyalgia syndrome: an emerging but controversial condition, JAMA, 257 (1987) 2782–2787.

Granges, G. and Littlejohn, G.O., A comparative study of clinical signs in fibromyalgia/fibrositis syndrome, healthy and exercising subjects, J. Rheumatol., 20 (1993) 344–351.

Greenfield, S., Fitzcharles, M.A. and Esdaile, J.M., Reactive fibromyalgia syndrome, Arthritis Rheum., 35 (1992) 678–681.

Hartz, A. and Kirchdoerfer, E., Undetected fibrositis in primary care practice, J. Fam. Pract., 25 (1987) 365–369.

Hawley, D.J. and Wolfe, F., Pain, disability, and pain/disability relationships in seven rheumatic disorders: a study of 1522 patients, J. Rheumatol., 18 (1991) 1552–1557.

Hawley, D.J. and Wolfe, F., Depression is not more common in rheumatoid arthritis: a 10 year longitudinal study of 6,608 rheumatic disease patients, J. Rheumatol., 20 (1993) 2025–2031.

Hawley, D.J., Wolfe, F. and Cathey, M.A., Pain, functional disability, and psychological status: a 12-month study of severity in fibromyalgia, J. Rheumatol., 15 (1988) 1551–1556.

Hawley, D.J., Wolfe, F., Cathey, M.A. and Roberts, F.K., Marital status in rheumatoid arthritis and other rheumatic disorders: a study of 7,293 patients, J. Rheumatol., 18 (1991) 654–660.

Henriksson, C., Gundmark, I., Bengtsson, A. and Ek, A.C., Living with fibromyalgia: consequences for everyday life, Clin. J. Pain, 8 (1992) 138–144.

Hudson, J.I., Pliner, L.F., Hudson, M.S., Goldenberg, D.L. and Melby, J.C., The dexamethasone suppression test in fibrositis, Biol. Psychiatry, 19 (1984) 1489–1493.

Hudson, J.I., Hudson, M.S., Pliner, L.F., Goldenberg, D.L. and Pope, H.G.J., Fibromyalgia and major affective disorder: a controlled phenomenology and family history study, Am. J. Psychiatry., 142 (1985) 441–446.

Hudson, J.I., Goldenberg, D.L., Pope, H.G., Keck, P.E. and Schlesinger, L., Comorbidity of fibromyalgia with medical and psychiatric disorders, Am. J. Med., 92 (1992) 363–367.

Kirmayer, L.J., Robbins, J.M. and Kapusta, M.A., Somatization and depression in fibromyalgia syndrome, Am. J. Psychiatry, 145 (1988) 950–954.

Lautenschläger, J., Brückle, W. and Müller, W., Untersuchen über druckschmerzhafte Puncte bei Patienten mit generalisierte Tendomyopathie. In: W. Müller (Ed.), Generalisierte Tendomyopathie (Fibromyalgie), Steinkopff Verlag Darmstadt, Darmstadt, 1991, pp. 105–114.

Leavitt, F. and Katz, R.S., Is the MMPI invalid for assessing psychological disturbance in pain related organic conditions? J. Rheumatol., 16 (1989) 521–526.

Leavitt, F., Katz, R.S., Golden, H.E., Glickman, P.B. and Layfer, L.F., Comparison of pain properties in fibromyalgia patients and rheumatoid arthritis patients, Arthritis Rheum., 29 (1986) 775–781.

Ledingham, J., Doherty, S. and Doherty, M., Primary fibromyalgia syndrome: an outcome study, Br. J. Rheumatol., 32 (1993) 139–142.

Littlejohn, G.O., Weinstein, C. and Helme, R.D., Increased neurogenic inflammation in fibrositis syndrome, J. Rheumatol., 14 (1987) 1022–1025.

Mason, J.H., Simms, R.W., Goldenberg, D.L. and Meenan, R.F., The impact of fibromyalgia on work: a comparison with RA, Arthritis Rheum., 32 (1989) S197 (Abstract)

McCain, G.A. and Scudds, R.A., The concept of primary fibromyalgia (fibrositis): clinical value, relation and significance to other chronic musculoskeletal pain syndromes, Pain, 33 (1988) 273–287.

Moldofsky, H., Rheumatic pain modulation syndrome: the interrelationships between sleep, central nervous system serotonin, and pain, Adv. Neurol., 33 (1982) 51–57.

Moldofsky, H., Scarisbrick, P., England, R. and Smythe, H.A., Musculosketal symptoms and non-REM sleep disturbance in patients with "fibrositis syndrome" and healthy subjects, Psychosom. Med., 37 (1975) 341–351.

Müller, W., Der Verlauf der primarin generalisierten Tendomyopathie (GTM). In: W. Muller (Ed.), Generalisierte Tendomyopathie (Fibromyalgie), Stenkopff Verlag, Darmstadt, 1991, pp. 29–43.

Payne, T.C., Leavitt, D.C., Garron, D.C., Katz, R.S., Golden, H.E., Glickman, P.B. and Vanderplate, C., Fibrositis and psychologic disturbance, Arthritis Rheum., 25 (1982) 213–217.

Piergiacomi, G., Blasetti, P., Berti, C., Ercolani, M. and Cervini, C., Personality pattern in rheumatoid arthritis and fibromyalgic syndrome: psychological investigation, Z. Rheumatol., 48 (1989) 288–293.

Robbins, J.M., Kirmayer, L.J. and Kapusta, M.A., Illness worry and disability in fibromyalgia syndrome, Int. J. Psychiatry Med., 20 (1990) 49–63.

Samborski, W., Stratz, T., Kretzmann, W.M., Mennet, P. and Müller, W., Comparative studies of the incidence of vegetative and functional disorders in backache and generalized tendomyopathies, Z. Rheumatol., 50 (1991) 378–381.

Scudds, R.A., Rollman, G.B., Harth, M. and McCain, G.A., Pain perception and personality measures as discriminators in the classification of fibrositis, J. Rheumatol., 14 (1987) 563–569.

Simons, D.G. and Travell, J.G., Myofascial origins of low back pain, Postgrad. Med., 73 (1983) 66–108.

Smythe, H.A., Fibrositis as a disorder of pain modulation, Clin. Rheum. Dis., 5 (1979) 823–832.

Smythe, H.A., "Fibrositis" and other diffuse musculoskeletal syndromes. In: W.N. Kelley, E.D. Harris Jr., S. Ruddy and C.B. Sledge (Eds.), Textbook of Rheumatology, Vol. 2, W.B. Saunders, Philadelphia, 1985, pp. 481–489.

Smythe, H.A. and Moldofsky, H., Two contributions to understanding of the "fibrositis" syndrome, Bull. Rheum. Dis., 28 (1977) 928–931.

Triadafilopoulos, G., Simms, R.W. and Goldenberg, D.L., Bowel dysfunction in fibromyalgia syndrome, Dig. Dis. Sci., 36 (1991) 59–64.

Truta, M.P. and Santucci, E.T., Head and neck fibromyalgia and temporomandibular arthralgia, Otolaryngol. Clin. North Am., 22 (1989) 1159–1171.

Uveges, J.M., Parker, J.C., Smarr, K.L., McGowan, J.F., Lyon, M.G., Irvin, W.S., Meyer, A.A., Buckelew, S.P., Morgan, R.K., Delmonico, R.L., et al., Psychological symptoms in primary fibromyalgia syndrome: relationship to pain, life stress, and sleep disturbance, Arthritis Rheum., 33 (1990) 1279–1283.

Wallace, D.J., Genitourinary manifestations of fibrositis: an increased association with the female urethral syndrome, J. Rheumatol., 17 (1990) 238–239.

Whitney, C.W. and Von Korff, M., Regression to the mean in treated versus untreated chronic pain, Pain, 50 (1992) 281–285.

Wolfe, F., The epidemiology of fibromyalgia, Journal of Musculoskeletal Medicine, 1 (1993a) 137–148.

Wolfe, F., Fibromyalgia and problems in classification of musculoskeletal disorders. In: H. Vaeroy and H. Merskey (Eds.), Progress in Fibromyalgia and Myofascial Pain, Elsevier, Amsterdam, 1993b, pp. 217–235.

Wolfe, F. and Cathey, M.A., Prevalence of primary and secondary fibrositis, J. Rheumatol., 10 (1983) 965–968.

Wolfe, F. and Hawley, D.J., Fibromyalgia. In: W.N. Kelley, E.D. Harrk, Jr., S. Ruddy and C.B. Sledge (Eds.), Textbook of Rheumatology (Suppl.), W.B. Saunders, Philadelphia, 1993.

Wolfe, F., Cathey, M.A., Kleinheksel, S.M., Amos, S.P., Hoffman, R.G., Young, D.Y. and Hawley, D.J., Psychological status in primary fibrositis and fibrositis associated with rheumatoid arthritis, J. Rheumatol., 11 (1984) 500–506.

Wolfe, F., Hawley, D.J., Cathey, M.A., Caro, X. and Russell, I.J., Fibrositis: symptom frequency and criteria for diagnosis. An evaluation of 291 rheumatic disease patients and 58 normal individuals, J. Rheumatol., 12 (1985) 1159–1163.

Wolfe, F., Smythe, H.A., Yunus, M.B., Bennett, R.M., Bombardier, C., Goldenberg, D.L., Tugwell, P., Abeles, M., Campbell, S.M., Clark, P., Fam, A.G., Farber, S.J., Fiechtner, J.J., Franklin, C.M., Gatter, R.A., Hamaty, D., Lessard, J., Lichtbroun, A.S., Masi, A.T., McCain, G.A., Reynolds, W.J., Romano, T.J., Russell, I.J. and Sheon, R.P., The American College of Rheumatology 1990 Criteria for the Classification of Fibromyalgia: report of the Multicenter Criteria Committee, Arthritis. Rheum., 33 (1990) 160–172.

Wolfe, F., Simons, D.G., Fricton, J.R., Bennett, R.M., Goldenberg, D.L., Gerwin, R., Hathaway, D., McCain, G.A., Russell, I.J., Sanders, H.O. and Skootsky, S.A., The fibromyalgia and myofascial pain syndromes: a preliminary study of tender points and trigger points in persons with fibromyalgia, myofascial pain syndrome and no disease, J. Rheumatol., 19 (1992) 944–951.

Wolfe, F., Ross, K., Anderson, J., Russell, I.J. and Hebert, L., The prevalence and characteristics of fibromyalgia in the general population, Arthritis. Rheum., 38 (1995) 19–28.

Yunus, M.B., Towards a model of pathophysiology of fibromyalgia: aberrant central pain mechanisms with peripheral modulation, J. Rheumatol., 19 (1992) 846–850.

Yunus, M.B., Masi, A.T., Calabro, J.J., Miller, K.A. and Feigenbaum, S.L., Primary fibromyalgia (fibrositis): clinical study of 50 patients with matched normal controls, Semin. Arthritis. Rheum., 11 (1981) 151–171.

Yunus, M.B., Masi, A.T. and Aldag, J.C., A controlled study of primary fibromyalgia syndrome: clinical features and association with other functional syndromes, J. Rheumatol., 19 (suppl.) (1989) 62–71.

Correspondence to: Frederick Wolfe, MD, Arthritis Research and Clinical Centers, 1035 N. Emporia, Suite 230, Wichita, KS 67214, USA. Tel: 316-263-2125; Fax: 316-256-0761.

Temporomandibular Disorders and Related Pain Conditions, Progress in Pain Research and Management, Vol. 4, edited by B.J. Sessle, P.S. Bryant, and R.A. Dionne, IASP Press, Seattle, © 1995.

3

Masticatory Muscle Disorders: Basic Science Perspectives

Barry J. Sessle

Faculty of Dentistry, University of Toronto, Ontario, Canada

Pain commonly arises from deep structures, such as muscular and articular tissues, yet research into the neural mechanisms underlying pain has focused on the processing of nociceptive information from spinally innervated superficial tissues such as skin. However, some recent studies have provided some initial insights into the peripheral and central processes underlying musculoskeletal pain, and this chapter will review recent advances in our knowledge of the neural processes involved in musculoskeletal pain of the craniofacial region and identify where major gaps in knowledge still occur.

PRIMARY AFFERENTS

This section will be brief in view of the detailed review by Hargreaves et al. in this volume. Peripheral tissues contain several types of sense organs or receptors, and several types of small-diameter, slowly conducting primary afferents are associated with free nerve endings, many of which respond to noxious stimuli (Dubner 1985; Willis 1985). More complex endings are generally associated with larger-diameter, faster-conducting primary afferents. These corpuscular or encapsulated endings, as well as some free nerve endings, function as mechanoreceptors. Articular and myofascial tissues are also innervated by small-diameter, slow-conducting nociceptive afferents (see below) as well as by large-diameter, fast-conducting primary afferents. In articular tissues, the latter are associated with low-threshold receptors that respond to non-noxious mechanical stimuli or movements; in most muscles, some of these large, fast-conducting afferents are also associated with other specialized receptors, e.g., muscle spindles and Golgi tendon organs. These various low-threshold receptors are considered to play a role in perceptual and reflex responses related to muscular and articular stimuli. Their specific contribution to the senses of joint position and movement is, however, a subject of some controversy.

The temporomandibular joint (TMJ) contains numerous free nerve endings but lacks an abundance of the more specialized endings; indeed, such specialized receptors may be nonexistent in some species. Most of the afferents supplying these specialized and nonspecialized receptors are less than 10 microns in diameter (i.e., Groups II, III, and IV), especially in those species lacking specialized receptors (Dubner et al. 1978; Rossignol et al. 1988; Dreesen et al. 1990; Widenfalk and Wiberg 1990; Kido et al. 1993). Many of these small-diameter afferents contain substance P and other neuropeptides involved in nociception and neurogenic inflammation, and some of the innervating fibers are not afferents but efferents of the sympathetic nervous system. The masticatory muscles also are supplied by sensory nerve fibers and sympathetic efferents, as well as by motor axons, but a major gap in knowledge exists in the functional properties of the smaller-diameter afferents, many of which appear to be nociceptive, that supply these muscles and the TMJ (for review, see Dubner et al. 1978; Rossignol et al. 1988; Hannam and Sessle 1994).

The more extensive literature on spinal afferents provides insights into the likely properties of TMJ and jaw muscle nociceptive afferents (Mense 1986, 1993; Schaible and Grubb 1993). In the limbs, for example, while the precise morphological features of the different nociceptive endings have yet to be resolved, the endings of many of the small-diameter Group III and IV afferents that innervate joint and muscle respond to stimuli that cause pain in humans, e.g., heavy pressure, algesic chemicals, and inflammatory agents. Ischemia also is an effective stimulus if it is prolonged and associated with muscle contractions. Some afferents are associated with "silent nociceptors" that respond only to frank noxious stimuli of inflamed tissues; they have not been found in muscles. The nociceptive afferents can be excited by a wide range of stimuli, but their sensitivity may increase following mild injury. This feature, so-called peripheral sensitization, is thought to be a major factor in producing hyperalgesia, and together with central sensitization (see below), can explain why the tissues become tender and hurt after injury or disease. The chapter by Hargreaves et al. (this volume) reviews the neurochemical processes involved in the responsiveness and sensitivity of peripheral nociceptive afferents and the role that the autonomic nervous system may play in modulating these properties.

BRAIN STEM SENSORY PROCESSING OF NOCICEPTIVE INFORMATION

The central projection sites within the trigeminal (cranial nerve V) brain stem complex of TMJ and craniofacial muscle nociceptive afferents have received little attention, although the technique of intracellular labeling of functionally identified afferents is now available. In spinal afferents, with such techniques, the projection of Group III deep afferents to laminae I, IV and V have been documented, although the laminar projection of Group IV deep nociceptive afferents is not yet resolved (Mense 1993; Schaible and Grubb 1993). Nonetheless, bulk labeling studies have shown that deep afferents project to one or more subdivisions of the V brain stem complex (Fig. 1), and the termination sites of TMJ afferents, jaw, or tongue muscle afferents (Shigenaga et al. 1988; Nazruddin et al. 1989; Capra and Dessem 1992) include the superficial laminae of V subnucleus caudalis as well as its deeper laminae, i.e., sites where V nociceptive neurons responsive to deep afferent stimulation are located (see below).

Electrophysiological data acquired in the last two decades generally support the view that subnucleus caudalis of the V spinal tract nucleus is an

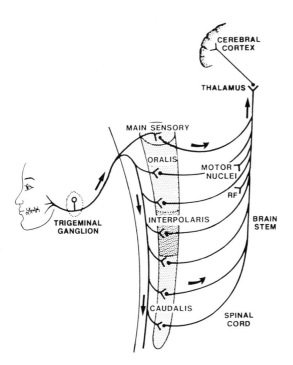

Fig. 1. The major pathways transmitting sensory information from the mouth, TMJ, jaw muscles, and face. Primary afferents project through the gasserian (trigeminal) ganglion to second-order neurons (in the trigeminal brain stem complex), which may project to neurons in higher levels of the central nervous system (e.g., in thalamus) or in brain stem regions such as the cranial nerve motor nuclei or reticular formation (RF). (Sessle 1986)

essential V brain stem relay for orofacial pain. These findings are consistent with observations that V tractotomy near the obex in humans or analogous lesions in experimental animals produce a profound orofacial analgesia (and thermanesthesia), with much less complete loss of tactile sensibility (although see below). Like the rest of the V brain stem complex, subnucleus caudalis does contain low-threshold mechanoreceptive (LTM) neurons, especially in its laminae III/IV, but nociceptive neurons also have been documented in anesthetized, decerebrate, or unanesthetized animals, concentrated in the superficial (laminae I/II) and deep (laminae V/VI) laminae of caudalis (for review, see Dubner 1985; Yokota 1985; Sessle 1987; Hannam and Sessle 1994). The morphological and physiological similarities of subnucleus caudalis with the spinal dorsal horn, which is the integral component of spinal nociceptive mechanisms, have led to its designation as the medullary dorsal horn.

As in the spinal dorsal horn, the two types of neurons that are responsive to noxious *cutaneous* stimuli are wide dynamic range (WDR) neurons, which respond to both noxious and innocuous stimulation of skin in a graded fashion as intensities increase into the noxious range, and nociceptive-specific (NS) neurons, which only respond to noxious stimuli. The properties of both neuron types are consistent with their receipt of cutaneous nociceptive small-diameter (groups III and/or IV) afferent inputs, and specifically in the case of WDR neurons, of inputs also from larger-diameter afferents conveying low-threshold mechanosensitive information from the skin. These two types of *cutaneous* nociceptive neurons can code the spatial localization and intensity of noxious cutaneous stimuli, and many have been shown, on the basis of antidromic activation, to project directly to the thalamus (see Dubner 1985; Yokota 1985; Sessle 1987; Hannam and Sessle 1994). Other output sites include the pontine parabrachial area, periaqueductal gray, and more rostral components of the V brain stem complex. However, caudalis and especially the rostral V subnuclei and adjacent regions (e.g., supratrigeminal nucleus, intertrigeminal nucleus) also have been implicated as sites of interneurons serving in craniofacial muscle reflex pathways, autonomic reflexes, and more complex integrative motor functions (see below).

It is noteworthy that while these WDR neurons are sometimes termed convergent neurons, many NS as well as WDR neurons also can be excited by stimulation of afferents other than cutaneous afferents (see Sessle 1987; Hannam and Sessle 1994). These include tooth pulp and cerebrovascular afferents, and also high-threshold, small-diameter afferent inputs from articular or muscular tissues (Fig. 2). Neurons responsive to noxious mechanical stimuli or to algesic chemicals applied to articular and/or muscular tissues predominate in the superficial and deep laminae of subnucleus caudalis, where anatomical studies indicate that projections of deep afferent inputs terminate. Neurons responsive

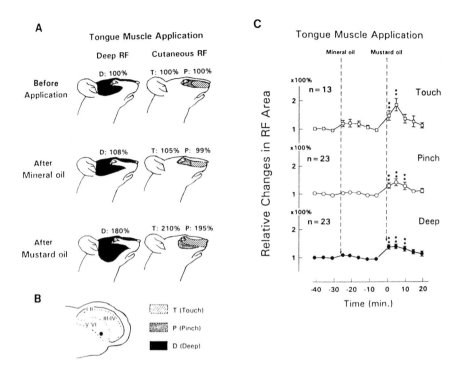

Fig. 2. Mechanoreceptive field (RF) expansion of nociceptive neurons after application of mustard oil to masticatory musculature. In **A**, the deep (D) RF (blackened area) of a wide dynamic range neuron is shown separately on the *left;* the cutaneous RF is shown on the *right.* The neuron could be activated by pinch as well as tactile stimulation of the touch (T) component of the cutaneous RF, and by pinch only from the pinch (P) component. The two drawings in the top row show the RF of the neuron before application of mineral oil; changes in the areas of the D and P RF components of the neuron after mineral oil or mustard oil application are expressed relative to the control (pre-application) values. **B** shows the location within the V subnucleus caudalis of the neuron. **C** shows time course of RF changes in caudalis nociceptive neurons as a result of the application of mineral oil and mustard oil to muscle. Values indicate changes in mean (± SE) area of each RF component relative to mean control (preapplication) areas (100%), i.e., areas before the vehicle (mineral oil) was applied (n = number of neurons tested). Differences in RF area that were statistically significant at $P < 0.01$ are shown as **. (Yu et al. 1993)

to low-threshold inputs from TMJ or associated muscles have received little attention, but some do appear to occur, at least in the rostral V brain stem regions (Capra and Dessem 1992; Hannam and Sessle 1994).

The TMJ differs from most other joints in the body in that its condyle not only rotates but also translates, and so it is conceivable that nociceptive as well as non-nociceptive afferent inputs from the TMJ and associated masticatory muscles into the central nervous system (CNS) might be associated with central integrative processes that are somewhat different from those in other joints. However, at least at the levels of the early relay stations, data so far indicate that analogous nociceptive processes apparently occur in the spinal dorsal horn and subnucleus caudalis, and in both structures few neurons appear to relay exclusively deep nociceptive information (Mense 1986, 1993; Sessle and Hu 1991; Schaible and Grubb 1993; Hannam and Sessle 1994); the relevance of this finding to deep pain mechanisms is considered later in this chapter.

Despite the importance of subnucleus caudalis in nociceptive processing, electrophysiological and behavioral (e.g., lesion) studies also have implicated more rostral components of the V brain stem complex as well as the subnucleus caudalis in orofacial pain mechanisms (Sessle 1987; Hannam and Sessle 1994). Evidence is emerging that the role of subnucleus caudalis in pain is primarily related to processing of nociceptive information from facial skin and deep tissues, whereas the more rostral components such as subnucleus oralis may be more involved in intraoral and perioral pain mechanisms. However, little attention has been directed to possible deep nociceptive inputs to the rostral components of the V brain stem complex, and indeed, the relative importance of the rostral and caudal components in craniofacial pain is still a crucial issue to address. Space limitations preclude discussion of other important issues related to brain stem nociceptive processing, such as the relative contribution to craniofacial pain of WDR compared to NS neurons, the relative importance of the different projection pathways, and the various neurochemicals involved in the excitatory transmission process; these issues apply to processing of deep as well as cutaneous nociceptive information.

THALAMOCORTICAL PROCESSING OF NOCICEPTIVE INFORMATION

The somatosensory thalamus is a major projection site for neurons at all levels of the V brain stem sensory nuclear complex and analogous regions of the spinal somatosensory system. This input to the thalamus is partly direct, especially from the V main sensory nucleus and subnucleus caudalis, but a portion of the projection involves multisynaptic pathways relaying in the reticular formation and adjacent brain stem areas. As noted above, the relative importance of these direct and indirect pathways for deep craniofacial pain is unclear.

The ventrobasal complex (VB) or ventroposterior nucleus, the posterior group of nuclei (PO), and parts of the medial thalamus are especially involved in receiving and relaying somatosensory information (Willis 1985). Those VB neurons receiving and relaying tactile information from the face and mouth (i.e., LTM neurons) are concentrated in the medial half of the VB (the nucleus ventralis posteromedialis), have localized mechanoreceptive fields, and are somatotopically organized. The neurons in the PO and medial thalamus appear to be much less specific in the information they relay.

WDR and NS neurons also occur in these various parts of the thalamus, although their spatial distribution within VB is a matter of controversy (Willis 1985; Yokota 1985). Those nociceptive neurons associated with the VB have properties (e.g., localized receptive field, somatotopic organization) more indicative of a role in pain localization and discrimination, whereas those in the PO and medial thalamus have properties more suggestive of a role in the affective-motivational dimensions of pain; recent studies have, however, raised some doubt about this generalization (Bushnell and Duncan 1989).

Some WDR and NS thalamic neurons as well as LTM neurons also project directly to the overlying cortex. WDR and NS neurons have been reported in somatosensory cortex (especially areas 1 and 3b) with properties indicative of a role in pain localization and discrimination of noxious stimulation, including that of the facial skin and tooth pulp (Willis 1985; Sessle 1987; Iwata et al. 1992; Kenshalo et al. 1992).

Low-threshold muscle afferent inputs activate neurons in the VB thalamus, somatosensory cortex, and primary motor cortex, and are primarily operational in mandibular kinesthesia and as peripheral feedback mechanisms involved in sensorimotor control of orofacial movements (Hannam and Sessle 1994; Lund and Enomoto 1988). Only limited information is available, however, on the thalamocortical processing of deep nociceptive information. Neurons can be activated in the medial and VB thalamus and primary somatosensory (SI) and secondary somatosensory (SII) cortex by noxious mechanical or algesic chemical stimulation and by electrical stimulation of Group II or III afferents supplying deep tissues of the forelimb and hindlimb (Guilbaud 1991; Mense 1993). However, the projection sites and neuronal properties related to the thalamocortical processing of nociceptive information from craniofacial musculoskeletal tissues is virtually unexplored, except for a brief description of high-threshold XII afferent inputs to the cat's SII cortex (Hanson 1985).

REFLEX RESPONSES TO NOCICEPTIVE INPUTS

Orofacial somatosensory inputs into the CNS may access brain stem motor and autonomic systems as well as ascending sensory systems (Fig. 1). Reflex activity in the craniofacial muscles and autonomic reflex changes (e.g., in blood pressure, respiration, salivation) have been studied extensively by stimulating afferent inputs from cutaneous, mucosal, dental pulp, and periodontal sources (Dubner et al. 1978; Rossignol et al. 1988; Lund 1991; Hannam and Sessle 1994). However, reflex responses specifically evoked by stimulating articular and muscle receptors have not been investigated to any great extent, although a jaw-opening reflex (transient jaw-closing muscle inhibition and jaw-opening muscle activation) as well as a tongue protrusive reflex can be elicited (Dubner et al. 1978; Lowe 1990). Hannam and Sessle (1994) have pointed out that although jaw opening may be an appropriate avoidance behavior following noxious intraoral stimulation, it is hard to rationalize this in the case of TMJ and jaw muscle stimulation. Moreover, any potential reflex effects may be modulated by the brain stem masticatory pattern generator and higher brain centers. Modulation of jaw-opening reflexes during mastication is well established and is considered essential to suppress unwanted reflexes and to favor those that enhance motor performance (Dubner et al. 1978; Lund 1991; Hannam and Sessle 1994; Lund and Sessle 1994).

Sustained stimulation of high-threshold articular and muscle receptors can produce jaw reflex effects that are longer-lasting, and perhaps more clinically relevant, than the transient responses referred to above. For example, algesic chemicals applied to the TMJ of cats reflexly produce sustained EMG activity, especially in the jaw-opening (and tongue) muscles (Broton and Sessle 1988). Again, it is difficult to rationalize how jaw opening in this situation can be protective, even though it can be considered analogous to flexion withdrawal in the limbs, which has been viewed as a nociceptive reflex response serving to protect the limb from further noxious stimulation and counteracting excessive movement that could further damage articular or muscular tissues (Mense 1986, 1993; Schaible and Grubb 1993). However, as Hannam and Sessle (1994) have pointed out, given the relative cross-sectional sizes of the jaw muscles, strong jaw-opening EMG activity coupled with weakly increased jaw-closing EMG activity might provide sufficient coactivation of normally antagonistic muscles to immobilize and attempt to protect the joint, an example of so-called muscle splinting. Such coactivation indeed occurs, at least in the rat, because significant and reversible increases in EMG activity in jaw-closing as well as jaw-opening muscles occurred when mustard oil, an inflammatory irritant, was injected into the TM region (Yu et al. 1994). However, Stohler et al. (1992) reported no increase in jaw-closing muscle activity in humans following painful hypertonic saline infusions into the masseter muscle, although an increase does occur during jaw-opening movements (also see below). In limb muscles, the predominant effect of Group III/IV nociceptive afferent input from muscle appears to be suppression of agonist extensor muscles accompanied by excitation of flexor muscles; gamma motoneurons also are predominantly inhibited, although an increase in alpha or gamma motoneuron excitability may occur as a result of injury to articular tissues (Mense 1993). The involvement of sympathetic reflexes in such effects is still unclear (Mense 1993; Schaible and Grubb 1993) and has received little study in relation to mechanisms of craniofacial musculoskeletal pain.

These reflex changes have been studied mainly in the "resting" state; the extent to which these effects also manifest during functional movements (e.g., chewing) needs more intensive investigation to clarify the relation of these reflex effects to any neuromuscular changes that may occur in functional disturbances such as those seen in temporomandibular disorders (TMDs). Indeed, recent studies have revealed that in the presence of noxious craniofacial stimulation, alterations in the normal alternating activity of the jaw-opening and jaw-closing muscles can occur during mastication; this includes an enhancement of jaw-closing EMG activity during jaw-opening, and vice versa (Lund 1991; Lund et al. 1991; Stohler et al. 1992). However, the long-term effects of such stimulation, especially of musculoskeletal tissues, still require investigation given the chronicity of the TMDs and other conditions manifesting pain and neuromuscular changes. Lund et al. (1991) have viewed these and other findings as being inconsistent with many current and long-held concepts related to the etiologies underlying the TMDs, and specifically the association of muscle hyperactivity and pain (e.g., the so-called vicious cycle). While heavy exercise appears to lead to microtrauma in muscles and connective tissue (Mense 1993), usually followed by pain that peaks in about 24 hours (i.e., postexercise muscle soreness), it is unclear that such processes characterize TMDs (Lund et al. 1991; Lund and Sessle 1994). Lund and colleagues have pointed out that most elements of the vicious cycle have not been experimentally tested or proven; moreover, the mechanisms involved in trigger points and their influences are equally unclear (see Mense 1993). They have instead proposed a concept of pain adaptation and suggested that pain results in agonist muscles becoming less active during a movement (e.g., mastication) and antagonist muscles more active, which reduces movement and thus may aid healing. Their critique clearly underscores the need to test and determine further the relationships between muscle activity and pain, especially long-term pain, and the role of factors such as ischemia, the autonomic nervous system, and peripheral and central sensitization (see below) in these relationships and in the etiology and pathogenesis of TMDs.

CENTRAL CONTROL MECHANISMS

SENSORIMOTOR CONTROL

The musculoskeletal and other orofacial afferent inputs that access the brain stem, thalamus, and cerebral cortex are involved not only in perceptual and reflex responses but also may be involved at each of these levels in sensorimotor integration and pain control. The areas involved include the sensorimotor cortex and adjacent cortical masticatory, swallow, and speech areas, as well as the amygdala and other parts of the limbic system, lateral hypothalamus, basal ganglia, red nucleus, cerebellum, and brain stem reticular formation. There is little information available related specifically to nociceptive inputs from craniofacial musculoskeletal tissues, but the central processes responsible for sensorimotor control of the craniofacial muscles have been studied extensively and reviewed in detail (Dubner et al. 1978; Lund and Enomoto 1988; Rossignol et al. 1988; Lund 1991; Hannam and Sessle 1994); page limitations allow for only a few examples. The somatosensory and motor areas of the cerebral cortex may use orofacial afferent inputs to guide, correct, and control movement by using sensory cues prior to movement and sensory information generated during movement. The processes involved include intracortical processing, cortical gating and transfer of somatosensory information and the subcortical modulation and selection of ascending somatosensory information, for example, through the V brain stem complex. Another example is the masticatory central pattern generator in the brainstem. The pattern generator not only generates rhythmical bursts in selected masticatory motoneurons, but also, as a consequence of its afferent inputs and extensive connections with other brain stem neurons, modulates other systems such as reflex pathways so that undesirable reflexes can be suppressed and desirable ones enhanced.

MODULATION OF NOCICEPTIVE TRANSMISSION

The excitatory responses of nociceptive neurons and the autonomic and muscle reflex responses to deep as well as cutaneous (or mucosal) afferent inputs also are subject to modulation from higher brain centers as well as other sensory inputs. Low- or high-intensity electrical stimulation of sensory nerves or noxious stimulation of sites remote from the orofacial area (e.g., limb) can suppress nociceptive responses of V brain stem neurons and related reflexes; such inhibitory effects have been implicated in the analgesic effects attributed to certain therapeutic procedures such as acupuncture, transcutaneous electrical nerve stimulation (TENS), and counter-irritation (Sessle 1987; Hu 1990; Bushnell et al. 1991).

Electrical stimulation of central sites including the sensorimotor cortex, hypothalamus, periaqueductal gray, nucleus raphe magnus, anterior pretectal nucleus, and parabrachial area of the pons also can inhibit both V brain stem neuronal and related reflex responses to noxious (and non-noxious) stimuli, including TMJ and muscle stimuli (Sessle et al. 1992; Chiang et al. 1994);

analogous mechanisms appear to exist in the spinal system (Mense 1993; Schaible and Grubb 1993). A variety of recently instituted techniques have been used (e.g., immunocytochemistry, in situ hybridization, in vitro nerve/ neuronal preparations or spinal cord/brainstem slices, microiontophoresis) to identify several endogenous neurochemicals involved in the excitatory process of nociceptive transmission or in these intrinsic modulatory effects that operate through presynaptic as well as postsynaptic inhibitory processes. These neurochemicals include substance P, enkephalin, serotonin, and gamma-aminobutyric acid (GABA) (Wilcox 1991; Woolf 1991; Dubner 1992). This is a fertile area for further study to delineate the underlying neurochemical processes and to define the sites within or adjacent to the V brain stem complex where these influences are exerted. There has been little definition, however, of intrinsic brain stem modulatory mechanisms specifically related to deep craniofacial pain, or of comparable processes at higher somatosensory levels of the CNS accessed by deep nociceptive craniofacial inputs.

THE NEUROPLASTICITY OF NOCICEPTIVE NEURONS

As noted above, some neurons in the V brain stem complex are responsive to non-noxious stimulation of TMJ and muscle, but many others can be activated by noxious deep stimuli. Such observations have led to the suggestion that these neurons, so far documented for subnucleus caudalis, are critical neural elements in deep pain in the craniofacial region (Sessle and Hu 1991; Hannam and Sessle 1994). Yet, a particular characteristic of nearly all these neurons transmitting deep nociceptive information is that they receive additional inputs from afferents supplying other tissues, including skin. Such features are thought to underlie the poor localization, spread, and referral of pain that are characteristic of pain conditions involving the TMJ and associated musculature (Sessle and Hu 1991; Sessle et al. 1993). Similar suggestions for deep pain and its spread and referral also have been made for the convergent afferent inputs documented in spinal dorsal horn neurons transmitting deep nociception (Cervero 1993; Mense 1993; Schaible and Grubb 1993).

Convergent inputs also appear to be involved in so-called central sensitization of nociceptive neurons, a process thought to contribute (along with peripheral sensitization) to hyperalgesia. The injection of algesic chemicals into deep tissues, or the presence of acute localized inflammation or chronic arthritis, can result in neuroplastic changes in the cutaneous as well as the deep receptive field properties of neurons of the spinal dorsal horn, thalamus, and somatosensory cortex; these changes include prolonged responsiveness to afferent inputs, increased receptive field size, and spontaneous bursts of activity (Woolf and Wall 1986; Guilbaud 1991; Dubner 1992; Mense 1993;

Schaible et al. 1993). C-fibers appear to be especially important for inducing these effects, which can occur even when peripheral sensitization is experimentally bypassed.

Similar neuroplastic effects appear to occur in cutaneous nociceptive neurons in the V brain stem complex (Sessle and Hu 1991; Hu et al 1992; Sessle et al. 1993). For example, a brief train of high-intensity electrical stimulation of XII muscle afferents can enhance neuronal responses of WDR and NS neurons in the subnucleus caudalis of the rat, particularly those evoked by C-fiber cutaneous afferents; this effect may last for 15 to 30 minutes. A more natural activation of small-fiber afferents from deep tissues by injecting mustard oil into the masseter muscle, TMJ, or tongue has similar effects, and can induce a reversible expansion of the neuronal cutaneous mechanoreceptive field and a lowering of the mechanical threshold (Fig. 2).

As in the spinal dorsal horn, these neuroplastic changes are not restricted to alterations in cutaneous receptive field properties, and it is significant that the neuroplastic changes in the deep receptive field properties may be even greater (Sessle et al. 1993). Furthermore, deep afferent inputs appear to be more effective than cutaneous inputs in inducing these changes in caudalis neurons. These findings may underlie the apparently greater sensory disturbances in pain conditions involving deep tissues than in those involving cutaneous tissues, but this possibility warrants detailed clinical experimentation in pain patients. These changes also have a time course of minutes or hours, and represent the acute alterations that can ensue from a short-acting inflammatory agent such as mustard oil. Profound and prolonged alterations might result when an inflamed TMJ or muscle generates days of continuous nociceptive afferent input, but this hypothesis is speculative and needs to be tested in animal models of chronic craniofacial pain conditions. Unfortunately, few of the new chronic pain models developed in the spinal somatosensory system have been specifically developed for the craniofacial region, and investigation is needed of the effects and underlying mechanisms of longer-term alterations in afferent inputs (e.g., inflammation, nerve injury, deafferentation) that mimic more closely chronic craniofacial pain conditions in humans. Such studies would provide important insights not only into the pathogenesis of the pain, but also into improved therapeutic approaches.

Some preliminary insights into the neurochemical mechanisms involved in these neuroplastic changes induced by deep nociceptive inputs have been gained. It appears that central N-methyl-D-aspartate (NMDA) receptors may be involved in the increased jaw activity and V neuronal receptive field changes evoked by deep noxious stimuli (e.g., the TM injection of mustard oil) and that a central opioid depressive effect may be triggered by such stimuli and serve to limit the neuroplastic changes (Sessle et al. 1993; Yu et al. 1994).

These findings are in keeping with recent spinal dorsal horn studies of injury or inflammation-induced changes in neuronal properties and the involvement of NMDA and opioid receptor mechanisms (Dubner 1992; Mense 1993; Schaible and Grubb 1993). In addition, recent in vitro studies further implicate substance P in such neuroplastic changes (Woolf 1991; Mense 1993). Alterations in the efficacy of the various intrinsic modulatory influences and neurochemical processes briefly described in the previous section also must be considered as possible factors contributing to the changes in receptive field and response properties of central nociceptive neurons and related motor changes that can result from damage or inflammation of deep tissues. Such findings point to the need for further studies of the underlying neurochemical mechanisms to clarify the basis of the central neuronal and neuromuscular changes that may occur in craniofacial pain and inflammatory conditions.

Finally, these recent findings of the remarkable neuroplasticity of V and spinal nociceptive neurons that follows damage and the stimulation of small-diameter afferent fibers from muscle, joints, and other deep tissues indicate that peripheral and central sensitization and associated neuromuscular adjustments can explain the hyperalgesia, spread and referral of pain, and the limitation of mandibular movement that characterize conditions such as TMDs (Lund and Sessle 1994). What remains unclear is the site(s) and mechanism(s) of action by which peripheral damage of deep craniofacial tissues results in TMDs.

REFERENCES

Broton, J.G. and Sessle, B.J., Reflex excitation of masticatory muscles induced by algesic chemicals applied to the temporomandibular joint of the cat, Arch. Oral Biol., 33 (1988) 741–747.

Bushnell, M.C. and Duncan, G.H., Sensory and affective aspects of pain perception: is medial thalamus restricted to emotional issues? Exp. Brain Res., 78 (1989) 415–418.

Bushnell, M.C., Marchand, S., Tremblay, N. and Duncan, G.H., Electrical stimulation of peripheral and central pathways for the relief of musculoskeletal pain, Can. J. Physiol. Pharmacol., 69 (1991) 697–703.

Capra, N.F. and Dessem, D., Central connections of trigeminal primary afferent neurons: topographical and functional considerations, Crit. Rev. Oral Biol. Med., 4 (1992) 1–52.

Cervero, F., Pathophysiology of referred pain and hyperalgesia from viscera. In: L. Vecchiet, D. Albe-Fessard and U. Lindblom (Eds.), New Trends in Referred Pain and Hyperalgesia, Pain Research and Clinical Management, Vol. 7, Elsevier, Amsterdam, 1993, pp. 35–46.

Chiang, C.Y., Hu, J.W. and Sessle, B.J., Parabrachial area and nucleus raphe magnus-induced modulation of nociceptive and nonnociceptive trigeminal subnucleus caudalis neurons activated by cutaneous or deep inputs, J. Neurophysiol., 71 (1994) 2430–2445.

Dreesen, D., Halata, Z. and Strasmann, T., Sensory innervation of the temporomandibular joint in the mouse, Acta Anat., 139 (1990) 154–160.

Dubner, R., Recent advances in our understanding of pain. In: I. Klineberg and B. Sessle (Eds.), Oro-facial Pain and Neuromuscular Dysfunction: Mechanisms and Clinical Correlates, Pergamon, Oxford, 1985, pp. 3–19.

Dubner, R., Neuronal plasticity in the spinal dorsal horn following tissue inflammation. In: R.

Inoki, Y. Shigenaga and M. Tohyama (Eds.), Processing and Inhibition of Nociceptive Information, Excerpta Medica, Tokyo, 1992, pp. 35–41.

Dubner, R., Sessle, B.J. and Storey, A.T., The Neural Basis of Oral and Facial Function, Plenum, New York, 1978, 483 pp.

Guilbaud, G., Central neurophysiological processing of joint pain on the basis of studies performed in normal animals and in models of experimental arthritis, Can. J. Physiol. Pharmacol., 69 (1991) 637–646.

Hannam, A.G. and Sessle, B.J., Temporomandibular neurosensory and neuromuscular physiology. In: G.A. Zarb, G.E. Carlsson, B.J. Sessle and N. Mohl (Eds.), Temporomandibular Joint and Masticatory Muscle Disorders, Munksgaard, Copenhagen, 1994, pp. 67–100.

Hanson, J., Hypoglossal high threshold afferents projecting to the secondary somatosensory area in the cat, Arch. Ital. Biol., 123 (1985) 63–68.

Hu, J.W., Response properties of nociceptive and non-nociceptive neurons in the rat's trigeminal subnucleus caudalis (medullary dorsal horn) related to cutaneous and deep craniofacial afferent stimulation and modulation by diffuse noxious inhibitory controls, Pain, 41 (1990) 331–345.

Hu, J.W., Sessle, B.J., Raboisson, P., Dallel, R. and Woda, A., Stimulation of craniofacial muscle afferents induces prolonged facilitatory effects in trigeminal nociceptive brain-stem neurones, Pain, 48 (1992) 53–60.

Iwata, K., Tsuboi, Y., Kamogawa, H., Kawasaki, K. and Sumino, R., Morphology of tooth pulp-driven neurons identified electrophysiologically in the SI cortex. In: R. Inoki, Y. Shigenaga and M. Tohyama (Eds.), Processing and Inhibition of Nociceptive Information, Excerpta Medica, Amsterdam, 1992, pp. 203–206.

Kenshalo, D.R., Jr., Iwata, K. and Thomas, D.A., Differences in the distribution of nociceptive neurons in SI cortex of the monkey. In: R. Inoki, Y. Shigenaga and M. Tohyama (Eds.), Processing and Inhibition of Nociceptive Information, Excerpta Medica, Tokyo, 1992, pp. 141–146.

Kido, M.A., Kiyoshima, T., Kondo, T., Ayasaka, N., Moroi, R., Terada, Y. and Tanaka, T., Distribution of substance P and calcitonin gene-related peptide-like immunoreactive nerve fibers in the rat temporomandibular joint, J. Dent. Res., 72 (1993) 592–598.

Lowe, A.A., Neural control of tongue posture. In: A. Taylor (Ed.), Neurophysiology of the Jaws and Teeth, Macmillan, London, 1990, pp. 322–368.

Lund, J.P., Mastication and its control by the brainstem, Crit. Rev. Oral Biol. Med., 2 (1991) 33–64.

Lund, J.P. and Enomoto, S., The generation of mastication by the mammalian nervous system. In: A. Cohen, S. Rossignol and S. Grillner (Eds.), Neural Control of Rhythmic Movements in Vertebrates, John Wiley and Sons, New York, 1988, pp. 41–72.

Lund, J.P. and Sessle, B.J., Neurophysiological mechanisms. In: G.A. Zarb, G.E. Carlsson, B.J. Sessle and N. Mohl (Eds.), Temporomandibular Joint and Masticatory Muscle Disorders, Munksgaard, Copenhagen, 1994, pp. 188–207.

Lund, J.P., Donga, R., Widmer, C.G. and Stohler, C.S., The pain-adaptation model: a discussion of the relationship between chronic musculoskeletal pain and motor activity, Can. J. Physiol. Pharmacol., 69 (1991) 683–694.

Mense, S., Slowly conducting afferent fibers from deep tissues: neurobiological properties and central nervous actions, Prog. Sens. Physiol., 6 (1986) 140–219.

Mense, S., Nociception from skeletal muscle in relation to clinical muscle pain, Pain, 54 (1993) 241–289.

Nazruddin, Suemune, S., Shirana, Y., Yamauchi, K. and Shigenaga, Y., The cells of origin of the hypoglossal afferent nerves and central projections in the cat, Brain Res., 490 (1989) 219–235.

Rossignol, S., Lund, J.P. and Drew, T., The role of sensory inputs in regulating patterns of rhythmical movements in higher vertebrates: a comparison between locomotion, respiration and mastication. In: A. Cohen, S. Rossignol and S. Grillner (Eds.), Neural Control of Rhythmic Movements in Vertebrates, John Wiley and Sons, New York, 1988.

Schaible, H.-G. and Grubb, B.D., Afferent and spinal mechanisms of joint pain, Pain, 55 (1993) 5–54.

Sessle, B.J., Recent developments in pain research: central mechanisms of orofacial pain and its control, J. Endodontics, 12 (1986) 435–444.

Sessle, B.J., The neurobiology of facial and dental pain: present knowledge, future directions, J. Dent. Res., 66 (1987) 962–981.

Sessle, B.J. and Hu, J.W., Mechanisms of pain arising from articular tissues, Can. J. Physiol. Pharmacol., 69 (1991) 617–626.

Sessle, B.J., Chiang, C.Y., and Dostrovsky, J.O., Interrelationships between sensorimotor cortex, anterior pretectal nucleus and periaqueductal gray in modulation of trigeminal sensorimotor function in the rat. In: R. Inoki, Y. Shigenaga and M. Tohyama (Eds.), Processing and Inhibition of Nociceptive Information, Excerpta Medica, Tokyo, 1992, pp. 77–82.

Sessle, B.J., Hu, J.W. and Yu, X.-M., Brainstem mechanisms of referred pain and hyperalgesia in the orofacial and temporomandibular region. In: L. Vecchiet, D. Albe-Fessard and U. Lindblom (Eds.), New Trends in Referred Pain and Hyperalgesia, Pain Research and Clinical Management, Vol. 7, Elsevier, Amsterdam, 1993, pp. 59–71.

Shigenaga, Y., Sera, M., Nishimori, T., Suemune, S., Nishimura, M., Yoshida, A. and Tsuru, K., The central projection of masticatory afferent fibers to the trigeminal sensory nuclear complex and upper cervical spinal cord, J. Comp. Neurol., 268 (1988) 489–507.

Stohler, C.S., Zhang, X., and Ashton-Miller, J.A., An experimental model of jaw muscle pain in man. In: Z. Davidovitch (Ed.), The Biological Mechanisms of Tooth Movement and Craniofacial Adaptation, Ohio State University, Columbus, Ohio, 1992, pp. 503–511.

Widenfalk, B. and Wiberg, M., Origin of sympathetic and sensory innervation of the temporomandibular joint: a retrograde axonal tracing study in the rat, Neurosci. Lett., 109 (1990) 30–35.

Wilcox, G.L., Excitatory neurotransmitters and pain. In: M.R. Bond, J.E. Charlton and C.J. Woolf (Eds.), Proceedings of the VIth World Congress on Pain, Pain Research and Clinical Management, Vol. 4, Elsevier, Amsterdam, 1991, pp. 97–117.

Willis, W.D., The Pain System, Karger, Basel, 1985.

Woolf, C.J., Central mechanisms of acute pain. In: M.R. Bond, J.E. Charlton and C.J. Woolf (Eds.), Proceedings of the VIth World Congress on Pain, Pain Research and Clinical Management, Vol. 4, Elsevier, Amsterdam, 1991, pp. 25–34.

Woolf, C.J. and Wall, P.D., Relative effectiveness of C primary afferent fibers of different origins in evoking a prolonged facilitation of the flexor reflex in the rat, J. Neurosci., 6 (1986) 1433–1442.

Yokota, T., Neural mechanisms of trigeminal pain. In: H.L. Fields, R. Dubner and F. Cervero (Eds.), Proceedings of the Fourth World Congress on Pain, Advances in Pain Research and Therapy, Vol. 9, Raven Press, New York, 1985, pp. 221–232.

Yu, X.-M., Sessle, B.J. and Hu, J.W., Differential effects of cutaneous and deep application of inflammatory irritant on mechanoreceptive field properties of trigeminal brain stem nociceptive neurons, J. Neurophysiol., 70 (1993) 1704–1707.

Yu, X.-M., Hu, J.W., Vernon, H. and Sessle, B.J., Effects of inflammatory irritant application to the rat temporomandibular joint on jaw and neck muscle activity, Pain (1994) in press.

Correspondence to: Barry J. Sessle, MDS, PhD, Faculty of Dentistry, University of Toronto, 124 Edward St., Toronto, ON, Canada M5G 1G6. Tel: 416-979-4921; Fax: 416-979-4937.

Temporomandibular Disorders and Related Pain Conditions, Progress in Pain Research and Management, Vol. 4, edited by B.J. Sessle, P.S. Bryant, and R.A. Dionne, IASP Press, Seattle, © 1995.

4

Mechanisms of Pain in Hindlimb Muscles: Experimental Findings and Open Questions

Siegfried Mense

Institut für Anatomie und Zellbiologie, Universität Heidelberg, Heidelberg, Germany

The following contribution discusses the neurobiological background of some clinical symptoms associated with temporomandibular disorders and adds data obtained in animal studies on hindlimb muscles and neurons of the lumbar spinal cord. Despite differences in organization between the spinal cord and brain stem, many of the basic mechanisms that control neuronal events at both levels appear to be similar. Therefore, data obtained at the spinal level can contribute to the understanding of brain stem mechanisms.

PRIMARY AFFERENT LEVEL

Sensitization of nociceptive endings by endogenous substances such as bradykinin (BK) and prostaglandins is a well-established neurophysiological mechanism that occurs in muscle, joint, and other tissues. Sensitization of a receptive ending leads to lowering of its mechanical threshold into the innocuous range and thus represents a peripheral mechanism explaining the tenderness of inflamed or otherwise pathologically altered tissue. In the skin and joints, so-called silent receptors have been reported; they cannot be activated by mechanical stimuli under normal conditions but acquire a mechanical sensitivity if the surrounding tissue is inflamed (Grigg et al. 1986; Häbler et al. 1988; Meyer and Campbell, 1988; Handwerker et al. 1991). Whether these receptors are also present in skeletal muscle has not been studied yet. The recruitment of formerly silent receptors during inflammation may contribute to the hyperalgesia of arthritic joints, thereby increasing nociceptive input into the central nervous system.

Systemic administration of nonsteroidal anti-inflammatory drugs such as acetylsalicylic acid (ASA) in animals with experimental myositis abolishes the raised activity in some—but not all—free nerve endings (Diehl et al. 1993). The finding that ASA does not act equally well on all sensitized nociceptors suggests that sensitizing substances other than prostaglandins also are present in inflamed tissues. One is substance P (SP), which increases the background activity of mechanically high-threshold (presumably nociceptive) nerve endings in vitro (Reinert et al. 1992) without sensitizing them to mechanical stimuli. Apparently, nociceptive neurons can change their background activity without altering their mechanical excitability, and vice versa (see below).

In patients, an increase in background activity of nociceptive neurons is probably associated with spontaneous pain, whereas a change in mechanical excitability is likely to lead to an altered threshold and intensity of pain (e.g., allodynia or hyperalgesia).The failure of ASA to abolish all inflammation-induced changes in nociceptive muscle afferents may explain why administration of this drug in patients with arthritis or myositis often does not result in complete pain relief.

Recent data indicate that in chronically inflamed muscle the innervation density of afferent nerve endings—probably including nociceptive ones—is higher than in intact tissue. This means that in inflamed muscle a given noxious stimulus will activate more receptive endings. Therefore, the higher innervation density is probably associated with an increase in the afferent activity from inflamed tissue and thus could contribute to the hyperalgesia. Moreover, the increase in the number of receptive endings is a true neuroplastic change of the peripheral nervous system, which could be an important peripheral factor in the transition from acute to chronic pain.

SPINAL CORD MECHANISMS

FEATURES OF SPINAL CORD NEURONS WITH DEEP INPUT

Dorsal horn neurons processing nociceptive input from deep somatic tissues are mainly located in lamina I and laminae IV–VI of the cat and rat (Hoheisel and Mense 1990; Yu and Mense 1990a). A typical—but surprising—feature of these cells is that they receive little excitatory input via C-fibers from muscle, although these fibers substantially outnumber the myelinated ones in the gastrocnemius-soleus (GS) muscle nerve (Mitchell and Schmidt 1983). This observation raises the question about the normal spinal action of an input from muscle C-fibers. A speculative answer is that it induces neuroplastic changes rather than eliciting fast synaptic potentials.

CONVERGENCE

Dorsal horn neurons with input from nociceptors in deep tissues typically have convergent input from other sources as well, e.g., from the skin and viscera (Schaible et al. 1987; Hoheisel and Mense 1990). No major spinal pathway seems to be specific for joint or muscle pain. The input from joint and muscle nociceptors is fed into a neuron population that simultaneously processes information from receptors in other tissues. This makes it difficult to understand how higher central nervous centers extract the information about noxious stimulation of deep tissue and elicit the sensations typical of muscle or joint pain. The extensive convergence at the spinal level may be the neurobiological basis of the diffuse nature of muscle pain, because it reduces the spatial resolution of the dorsal horn as an information processing system.

The convergence from muscle and skin receptors is probably not related to the referral of muscle pain, because this type of pain is usually referred to other deep tissues and not to the skin. On the other hand, input convergence from muscle and other deep tissues on the same dorsal horn cell—which could explain the pattern of referral of muscle pain—is rare.

Recent studies have shown that the degree of input convergence to dorsal horn neurons is not fixed but changes within minutes following noxious stimulation of hindlimb muscles with injections of BK (Hoheisel et al. 1993). A general problem for animal experimentation is that the surgical preparation of the animal is likely to change the pattern of convergence at the spinal or brain stem level.

Under the influence of nociceptive input from muscle, many cells acquire new receptive fields (RFs) in deep tissues far away from the site of stimulation. Thus, following a muscle lesion the neurons can be stimulated from body regions that are somatotopically inappropriate for that neuron. For instance, a neuron in the medial dorsal horn that is responsible for sensations from deep tissues in the distal hindlimb (Yu and Mense 1990b) may now be excited by noxious stimulation of the proximal limb. Transferred to the clinical situation, this observation could mean that a lesion in the proximal leg leads to pain sensations in the distal leg, i.e., the pain is referred distally. Because the newly formed RFs are also deep, the input convergence has the pattern required for pain referral from muscle to other deep tissues.

This mechanism differs from the original convergence-projection theory of pain referral (Ruch 1949) in that the convergent input is not present from the beginning but is unmasked acutely as a result of the noxious stimulus.

SPINAL REFLEXES

In many textbooks on pain, a vicious cycle is hypothesized that includes a pain-spasm-pain mechanism. At the lumbar level, the hypothesis that muscle pain leads to reflex spasm of the affected muscle, which causes pain and thus perpetuates the cycle, has never been proven. In fact, the bulk of available experimental data suggests that following a muscle lesion reflex muscle inhibition is more likely to occur than reflex spasm. Prominent examples of reflex inhibition of muscles following noxious stimulation of deep tissues is the weakness and atrophy of the quadriceps muscle as a sequel to traumatic or surgical knee joint lesion, and the Chassaignac (1856) syndrome in infants. The neurophysiological basis of these inhibitions may be a reflex reduction in the activity of gamma-motoneurons supplying the affected muscle (Mense and Skeppar 1991).

A basic difference between spinal and masticatory motor reflexes is that the ipsilateral flexor reflex is associated with a contralateral extensor reflex at the spinal level, whereas at the brainstem level such an antagonistic organization of the masticatory reflexes is not present. For instance, during the jaw-opening reflex the muscles of both sides must be inhibited (or activated) together.

NEUROPLASTIC CHANGES

The term neuroplasticity is mainly used for neuronal changes that outlast a triggering stimulus, but changes accompanying a subchronic or chronic peripheral disturbance (probably associated with ongoing pathological afferent activity) are often included. The acute changes in RF configuration following intramuscular BK injections (see above) often last for more than 30 minutes, whereas the afferent input elicited by the BK injection is known to be over within a few minutes (Mense and Meyer 1988). Apparently, the nociceptive input changes the responsiveness of the dorsal horn neurons for a prolonged period of time, possibly by releasing modulator substances from the spinal terminals of the muscle afferents.

During a longer-lasting nociceptive input such as follows the induction of an acute experimental arthritis or myositis, several effects with different time courses are triggered. Fig. 1 shows data obtained from experiments in which the influence of an acute myositis of the gastrocnemius-soleus (GS) muscle on the excitability of lumbar dorsal horn neurons was studied. In the figure, the effects observed 2–8 hours after the induction of a myositis are compared with those present 20–25 hours after the lesion (in the latter case the myositis was induced one day before the electrophysiological measurements started). The proportion of neurons activated by A-fiber stimulation of the GS nerves and

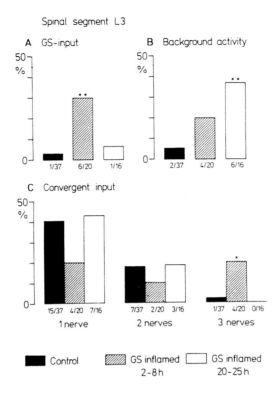

Fig. 1. Time course of myositis-induced effects in dorsal horn neurons in the spinal segment L3. **A**, proportion of neurons having A-fiber input from the GS nerves. **B**, proportion of cells exhibiting background activity. **C**, proportion of cells having input from one nerve only (left), two nerves (middle), and three nerves (right). The figures underneath the columns are the numbers of neurons from which the columns were constructed. The asterisks mark significant differences between control and myositis animals (* $P < 0.05$; ** $P < 0.01$; chi^2 test, two-tailed). In **A** and **B** the myositis-induced effects were gone 20–25 hours after induction of the inflammation; the only persisting change was the increase in the proportion of cells having background activity.

the degree of convergence from three hindlimb nerves were increased during the acute inflammation (2–8 hours), but both effects had returned to about normal values 20–25 hours after the induction of the inflammation. Only the proportion of neurons exhibiting background activity (defined as discharges in the absence of acute stimulation) still rose one day after onset of the inflammation. The data suggest that the development of background activity is controlled by mechanisms different from those leading to excitability changes.

Two more lines of evidence obtained in recent experiments support the hypothesis that changes in excitability and background activity are caused by different mechanisms: (1) Superfusion of the spinal cord with antagonists of neurokinin-1 and neurokinin-2 receptors (GR 82 334; spantide; spantide II) as well as with antagonists of ionotropic NMDA receptors (MK-801, AP-5) prevents the myositis-induced increase in electrical excitability of dorsal horn neurons, but not the myositis-induced change in background activity. (2) Blocking the electrical activity from the inflamed GS muscle by local anesthesia of the dorsal roots L4 and L5 prevents the increase in electrical excitability but not the change in background activity.

If similar events also occur in patients, it is conceivable that the mechanisms underlying spontaneous pain (probably elicited by background activity in nociceptive neurons) and those underlying hyperalgesia (probably caused by excitability changes in the spinal cord) are different and, therefore, sensitive to different forms of treatment.

DESCENDING CONTROLS

Previous work of this laboratory has shown that the dorsal horn neurons processing input from deep nociceptors are subjected to a powerful descending inhibition that is tonically active and operates with opioidergic synapses at the supraspinal level (Yu et al. 1991). Of possible clinical interest is the finding that descending inhibition in neurons with convergent input from cutaneous and deep nociceptors abolishes background activity and acts more strongly on deep input than on input from the skin. Thus, a reduced activity of the descending system could lead to widespread spontaneous pain and hyperalgesia in deep tissues because of a disinhibition of neurons mediating deep pain. The above combination of symptoms resembles fibromyalgia in some aspects. The available evidence is not sufficient to suggest that the pain and tenderness of fibromyalgia are due to a disturbance of the antinociceptive descending system; however, other findings such as increase in SP (Vaeroy et al. 1988) and change in serotonin turnover (Russell et al. 1992) in the cerebrospinal fluid of fibromyalgia patients likewise indicate that the central nervous processing of nociceptive information is changed.

REFERENCES

Chassaignac, C.M.E., De la paralysie douloureuse des jeunes enfants, Arch. Gén. Méd., 5, Ser. I (1856) 653–669.

Diehl, B., Hoheisel, U. and Mense, S., The influence of mechanical stimuli and of acetylsalicylic acid on the discharges of slowly conducting afferent units from normal and inflamed muscle in the rat, Exp. Brain Res., 92 (1993) 431–440.

Grigg, P., Schaible, H.-G. and Schmidt, R.F., Mechanical sensitivity of group III and IV afferents from posterior articular nerve in normal and inflamed cat knee, J. Neurophysiol., 55 (1986) 635–643.

Häbler, H.J., Jänig, W. and Koltzenburg, M., A novel type of unmyelinated chemosensitive nociceptor in the acutely inflamed urinary bladder, Agents Actions, 25 (1988) 219–221.

Handwerker, H.O., Kilo, S. and Reeh, P.W., Unresponsive afferent nerve fibres in the sural nerve of the rat, J. Physiol., 435 (1991) 229–242.

Hoheisel, U. and Mense, S., Response behaviour of cat dorsal horn neurones receiving input from skeletal muscle and other deep somatic tissues, J. Physiol., 426 (1990) 265–280.

Hoheisel, U., Mense, S., Simons, D.G. and Yu, X.-M., Appearance of new receptive fields in rat dorsal horn neurons following noxious stimulation of skeletal muscle: a model for referral of muscle pain? Neurosci. Lett., 153 (1993) 9–12.

Mense, S. and Meyer, H., Bradykinin-induced modulation of the response behaviour of different types of feline group III and IV muscle receptors, J. Physiol., 398 (1988) 49–63.

Mense, S. and Skeppar, P., Discharge behaviour of feline gamma-motoneurones following induction of an artificial myositis, Pain, 46 (1991) 201–210.

Meyer, R.A. and Campbell, J.N., A novel electrophysiological technique for locating cutaneous nociceptive and chemospecific receptors, Brain Res., 441 (1988) 81–86.

Mitchell, J.H. and Schmidt, R.F., Cardiovascular reflex control by fibers from skeletal muscle. In: J.T. Shepherd and F.M. Abboud (Eds.), Handbook of Physiology, Section 2: The Cardiovascular System, Volume III: Peripheral Circulation and Organ Blood Flow, Part 2. American Physiological Society, Bethesda, 1983, pp. 623–658.

Reinert, A., Vitek, M. and Mense, S., Effects of substance P on the activity of high- and low-threshold mechanosensitive receptors of the rat diaphragm in vitro, Pflügers Arch., 420, Suppl. 1 (1992) R 47.

Ruch, T.C. Visceral sensation and referred pain. In: J.F. Fulton (Ed.), Howell's Textbook of Physiology, 16th ed., Saunders, Philadelphia, 1949, pp. 385–401.

Russell, I.J., Vaeroy, H., Javors, M. and Nyborg, F., Cerebrospinal fluid biogenic amine metabolites in fibromyalgia/fibrositis syndrome and rheumatoid arthritis, Arthritis Rheum., 35 (1992) 550–556.

Schaible, H.-G., Schmidt, R.F. and Willis, W.D., Convergent inputs from articular, cutaneous and muscle receptors onto ascending tract cells in the cat spinal cord, Exp. Brain Res., 66 (1987) 479–488.

Vaeroy, H., Helle, R., Forre, 0., Kass, E. and Terenius, L., Elevated CSF levels of substance P and high incidence of Raynaud's phenomenon in patients with fibromyalgia: new features for diagnosis, Pain, 33 (1988) 21–26.

Yu, X.-M. and Mense, S., Response properties and descending control of rat dorsal horn neurons with deep receptive fields, Neuroscience, 39 (1990a) 823–831.

Yu, X.-M. and Mense, S., Somatotopical arrangement of rat spinal dorsal horn cells processing input from deep tissues, Neurosci. Lett., 108 (1990b) 43–47.

Yu, X.-M., Hua, M. and Mense, S., The effects of intracerebroventricular injection of naloxone, phentolamine and methysergide on the transmission of nociceptive signals in rat dorsal horn neurones with convergent cutaneous-deep input, Neuroscience, 44 (1991) 715–723.

Correspondence to: S. Mense, Prof. Dr.med., Institut für Anatomie und Zellbiologie, Im Neuenheimer Feld 307, D-69120, Heidelberg, Germany. Tel: 37-6221-564193; Fax: 37-6221-563071.

Temporomandibular Disorders and Related Pain Conditions, Progress in Pain Research and Management, Vol. 4, edited by B.J. Sessle, P.S. Bryant, and R.A. Dionne, IASP Press, Seattle, © 1995.

Reaction Paper to Chapters 1–4

James P. Lund, Pierre Clavelou, Karl-Gunnar Westberg, and Gordon Schwartz

Faculté de médecine dentaire and Centre de recherche en sciences neurologiques, Université de Montréal, Québec, Canada

CLINICAL AND EPIDEMIOLOGICAL FINDINGS

Both Stohler (this volume) and Wolfe (this volume) suggest that chronic muscle pain is much more prevalent in women than in men. This is definitely true, but in at least two conditions this observation does not seem to apply—painful bruxism and chronic lower back pain (CLBP). More men than women are given a diagnosis of CLBP (Praemer et al. 1991), while the prevalence of signs of bruxism in the general population (with and without pain) is about the same in the two sexes (Goulet et al. 1992). Although bruxism and other oral habits are thought by many to be an etiological factor in temporomandibular disorders (TMDs), a recent study found that only six of a group of 19 patients given a diagnosis of bruxism (on the basis of sleep lab recordings) reported pain. Three were women, three were men. Furthermore, their pain was worst during the morning, as opposed to myofascial pain, which peaks in the evening in most patients (Dao et al. 1994). This finding supports the suggestion that trigeminal myofascial pain and painful bruxism are separate disorders (Lund 1992).

Stohler and Wolfe stress the similarities in the symptoms reported by TMD, myofascial pain, and fibromyalgia patients, and both authors comment on the arbitrary nature of the distinctions made between these and other similar diseases. When a patient visits the dentist, there is a tendency for both participants in the diagnostic process to concentrate on the head and neck, while at the rheumatologist's office, the therapist may not look for tenderness in the muscles of mastication because none of the 18 specified sites for fibromyalgia are found there. A striking example of the tendency for specialists to concentrate on their "bread and butter" is seen in a recent American

Academy of Orthopaedic Surgeons survey of musculoskeletal conditions. According to this survey, chronic musculoskeletal pain above C1 does not exist in the United States, and CLBP is classified as a joint condition (Praemer et al. 1991).

One fact contradicts the hypothesis that temporomandibular (TM) myofascial pain is a variant of fibromyalgia; the prevalence of TMDs seems to decrease with age, while Wolfe quotes several studies that the prevalence of fibromyalgia increases with age. Wolfe and colleagues also have data that fibromyalgia patients tend to be heavier than normal. How does this observation compare to TM myofascial pain? A problem that must be faced is the lack of a diagnostic category for patients who appear to have a chronic myofascial pain condition but do not have enough tender sites for a positive diagnosis.

ETIOLOGY

Both fibromyalgia and TM myofascial pain are characterized by tenderness over muscle, joints, and bone. The pressure-pain threshold of these patients is lower than normal. Wolfe and others have proposed that there are abnormalities of modulation or amplification of pain and other stimuli in fibromyalgia. This suggestion is in line with the data on the central processing of pain presented by Sessle and by Mense (this volume).

However, it is also possible that connective tissue or the nerve endings and capillaries within the connective tissue are abnormally susceptible to damage. The finding of differences in immunoglobulin G (IgG) deposition on collagen bundles from skin biopsies in fibromyalgia patients and controls in the absence of evidence of an abnormal immunological response (Wolfe, this volume) suggests that the collagen of fibromyalgia patients is not normal. If this makes connective tissue more susceptible to damage, it could explain the work intolerance, decrease in pain threshold to palpation, skinfold tenderness, swelling, lower tissue compliance, and greater reactive hyperemia seen in fibromyalgia (Wolfe, this volume; Granges and Littlejohn 1993).

REPRESENTATION OF DEEP PAIN IN THE THALAMUS AND CORTEX

Sessle has reviewed the few findings on the projection of nociceptors from deep tissues to the thalamus and cortex. At the moment, we do not know which areas receive inputs from the muscles of mastication. However, many of the neurons in the thalamus and cortex that are activated by cutaneous nociceptors should respond to high-threshold muscle afferents because of convergence of these inputs on the nociceptive specific (NS) and wide dynamic range (WDR) neurons in the medullary dorsal horn that provide their somatosensory inputs.

Positron emission tomography has been used to identify cortical areas in which metabolic activity increases during cutaneous pain. As a result, several groups have become interested in the roles of the anterior cingulate gyrus and insula in pain perception (e.g., Talbot et al. 1991). As usual, data on deep pain is lacking.

We suggest that there is one little-known region of S1 cortex that may have an important role in trigeminal (V) muscle pain—the upper head area. Woolsey and his colleagues (1942) were the first to show that stimulation of the face evoked potentials in this region, which lies at the medial end of the arm area, and lateral to the representation of the trunk in monkeys and man. These inputs definitely come from the V nerve, because they remain after all the cervical nerves are cut (Bioulac and Lamarre 1979). It was recently shown that the central part of the face is not represented here. The neurons have receptive fields on the lower lip and jaw, posterior parts of the face, and on the forehead, including the eyebrows (Lund et al. 1994). To explain this finding, it was suggested that the upper face area receives its inputs only from the upper cervical dorsal horn, and not from the more rostral trigeminal nuclei. This hypothesis is based on the observations of Denny-Brown and Yanagisawa (1973) that the section of the descending V tract just caudal to the obex causes sensory deficits that are confined to the lower jaw, outer face, and forehead (their Fig. 4), exactly the same regions that are represented in the upper head area.

PROJECTION OF MUSCLE NOCICEPTORS TO THE BRAIN STEM

Although small-diameter muscle afferents terminate in the caudal part of the V subnucleus interpolaris (NVspo-alpha) and the adjacent interstitial nucleus of Cajal (Shigenaga et al. 1988), the more rostrally located subnucleus-gamma, as well as the intra- and supratrigeminal areas, receive few terminals from group III and IV jaw muscle afferents (Nishimori et al 1986). In addition, the responses of neurons in the rostral subnuclei to high-threshold inputs from muscle are significantly longer in latency than are those caused by high-threshold inputs from cutaneous nerves (Olsson et al 1986; Westberg and Olsson 1991). We have infused 5% saline into the masseter muscle in anesthetized or decerebrate and paralyzed rabbits and shown that neurons in these regions are insensitive to nociceptive inputs. Although the rate of delivery of the saline was much higher than that necessary to cause pain in humans

(Stohler and Lund 1994), neurons in the oral subnucleus and adjacent supra- and intertrigeminal areas did not change their resting firing rate. In contrast, the same rate of infusion activated WDR neurons recorded in medullary dorsal horn, consistent with the medullary and spinal dorsal horn findings reported in the chapters by Sessle and Mense.

EFFECTS OF PAIN ON MOTOR PATTERNS

The same infusions of hypertonic saline that cause tonic pain reduce the frequency, amplitude, and velocity of mastication in humans (Stohler, this volume) and decerebrate rabbits (Schwartz et al. 1993), and we have recently found that the same infusions slow the rhythm of "fictive" mastication recorded from the trigeminal motor nucleus. These findings offer evidence that pain acts on brain stem and spinal cord circuits to change movements. Although neurons in subnucleus-gamma, many of which project to trigeminal motoneurons, do not respond to saline infusions at rest (see above), some do change their burst pattern when the saline is infused during fictive mastication. The onset is rapid and the effect outlasts the stimulus by several minutes, as does the fall in masticatory frequency (Fig. 1).

These data suggest that much of the nociceptive input from muscle to the premotor neurons in subnucleus-gamma and nearby regions is transmitted through the caudal nuclei via ascending polysynaptic pathways (Hockfield and Gobel 1982). Alternatively, the input could come from the few nociceptive afferents to the rostral V nuclei. In either case, these inputs must be under tonic inhibitory control because they have little effect except during movement. The new evidence presented by Mense that the increase in excitability of dorsal horn neurons caused by myositis can be blocked by N-methyl-D-aspartate (NMDA) and neurokinin antagonists, while changes in background activity cannot, is interesting in this regard.

High-threshold muscle afferents activate both NS and WDR neurons in the medullary and spinal dorsal horns. It is probable that long-lasting changes in the behavior of these neurons underlie many chronic pain states (Sessle and Mense, this volume). However, as Sessle points out, the evidence that the more rostral V subnuclei and adjacent cell groups such as the supratrigeminal and intertrigeminal nuclei are implicated in deep pain perception is limited. We suggest that the neurons in these areas have different roles, one of which is to adapt motor output to the presence of pain so as to minimize damage to tissues.

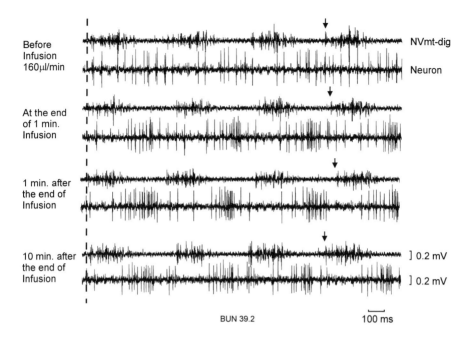

Fig. 1. Effects on the masticatory pattern of a decerebrated paralyzed rabbit following an injection of 5% saline into the anterior part of the masseter muscle. Fictive mastication was induced by repetitive stimulation of the corticobulbar tract (3 volts; 40 Hz; 0.1 msec.) and recorded in the digastric motoneuron pool (NVmt-dig). The interneuron (neuron) recorded at the same time was located in the rostral part of subnucleus oralis. The recordings are aligned to the start of a NVmt-dig burst. Note the increase of the duration of the masticatory cycle (the arrows indicate the end of three successive cycles) and the increased firing frequency of the neuron during the closing phase, when saline was injected (160 ml in 1 minute). There was a gradual decrease in firing of the neuron and in the masticatory cycle duration during the 10 minutes following the end of infusion.

REFERENCES

Bioulac, B. and Lamarre, Y., Activity of postcentral cortical neurons of the monkey during conditioned movements of a deafferented limb, Brain Res., 172 (1979) 427–437.

Dao, T.T.T., Lund, J.P. and Lavigne, G.J., Comparison of pain and quality of life in bruxers and patients with myofascial pain of the masticatory muscles, J. Orofacial Pain, 8 (1994) 350–356.

Denny-Brown, D. and Yanagisawa, N., The function of the descending root of the fifth nerve, Brain, 96 (1973) 783–814.

Goulet, J.P., Montplaisir, J., Lund, J.P. and Lavigne, G., Relations entre les habitudes parafonctionnelles, le stress et les symptômes temporomandibulaires. In: Méridien (Ed.), 9ᵉ Colloque de l'A.I.F.R.O., Université de Montréal, Faculté de Médecine Dentaire, Montréal, 1992, pp. 139–144.

Granges, G. and Littlejohn, G.O., A comparative study of clinical signs in fibromyalgia/fibrositis syndrome, healthy and exercising subjects, J. Rheumatol., 20 (1993) 344–351.

Hockfield, S. and Gobel, S., An anatomical demonstration of projections to the medullary dorsal

76 *J.P. LUND ET AL.*

horn (trigeminal nucleus caudalis) from rostral nuclei and the contralateral caudal medulla, Brain Res., 252 (1982) 203–211.

Lund, J.P., Review and commentary. In: S.F. Dworkin and L. LeResche, Research diagnostic criteria for temporomandibular disorders: review, criteria, examinations and specifications, critique, J. Craniomandib. Disord. Facial Oral Pain, 6 (1992) 301–355.

Lund, J.P., Donga, R., Widmer, C.G. and Stohler, C.S., The pain-adaptation model: a discussion of the relationship between chronic musculoskeketal pain and motor activity, Can. J. Physiol. Pharmacol., 69 (1991) 683–694.

Lund, J.P., Sun, G.-D. and Lamarre, Y., Cortical reorganization and deafferentation in adult macaques, Science, 265 (1994) 546–548.

Nishimori, T., Sera, M., Suemune, S., Yoshida, A., Tsuru, K., Tsuiki, Y., Akisaka, T., Okamoto, T., Daekota, Y. and Shigenaga, Y., The distribution of muscle primary afferents from the masseter nerve to the trigeminal sensory nuclei, Brain Res., 372 (1986) 375–381.

Olsson, K.Å., Landgren, S. and Westberg, K.G., Location of, and convergence on, the interneurone in the disynaptic path from the coronal gyrus of the cerebral cortex to the trigeminal motoneurones in the cat, Exp. Brain Res., 65 (1986) 83–97.

Praemer, A., Fumer, S. and Rice, P.R., Musculoskeletal Conditions in the United States, American Academy of Orthopedic Surgeons, Park Ridge, Ill. 1991.

Schwartz, G., Stohler, C.S. and Lund, J.P., An animal model to study the effects of pain on mandibular function, J. Orofacial Pain, 7 (1993) 107.

Shigenaga, Y., Sera, M., Nishimori, T., Suemune, S., Nishimura, M., Yoshida, A. and Tsuru, K., The cental projection of masticatory afferent fibers to the trigeminal sensory nuclear complex and upper cervical spinal cord, J. Comp. Neurol., 268 (1988) 489–507.

Stohler, C.S. and Lund, J.P., The effects of noxious stimulation of the jaw muscles on the sensory experience of human volunteers. In: D.S. Carlson and C.S. Stohler (Eds.), Biological and Psychological Aspects of Orofacial Pain, Vol. 29, Craniofacial Growth Series, Center for Human Growth and Development, University of Michigan, Ann Arbor, 1994, pp. 55–73.

Talbot, J.D., Marrett, S., Evens, A.C., Meyer, E., Bushnell, M.C. and Duncan, G.H., Multiple representations of pain in human cerebral cortex, Science, 251 (1991) 1355–1358.

Westberg, K.-G. and Olsson, K.Å., Integration in trigeminal premotor interneurones in the cat. 1. Functional characteristics of neurones located in the subnucleus-γ of the oral nucleus of the spinal trigeminal tract, Exp. Brain Res., 84 (1991) 102–114.

Woolsey, C.N., Marshall, W.H. and Bard, P., Representation of cutaneous tactile sensibility in the cerebral cortex of the monkey as indicated by evoked potentials, Bull. Johns Hopkins Hosp., 70 (1942) 399–441.

Correspondence to: James P. Lund, BDS, PhD, Faculté de médecine dentaire and Centre de recherche en sciences neurologiques, Université de Montréal, C.P. 6108, Succursale centreville, Montréal, Québec, Canada H3C 3J7. Tel: 514-343-2134; Fax: 514-343-2111.

Part II

Temporomandibular Joint
Disk Displacement

Temporomandibular Disorders and Related Pain Conditions, Progress in Pain Research and Management, Vol. 4, edited by B.J. Sessle, P.S. Bryant, and R.A. Dionne, IASP Press, Seattle, © 1995.

5

Temporomandibular Joint Disk Displacement: Clinical Perspectives

M. Franklin Dolwick

Department of Oral and Maxillofacial Surgery, University of Florida, Gainesville, Florida, USA

Internal derangement (disk displacement) of the temporomandibular joint (TMJ) was first identified by Annandale in 1887. Later, it was described as a causative factor in TMJ pain and dysfunction (Pringle 1918). Pringle stated that the disk "goes forward and inwards, so that its thick central ridge becomes displaced obliquely instead of lying in the coronal plane." Ireland described a progression of clinical symptoms ranging from nonpainful clicking, to painful clicking with intermittent locking, to locking of the TMJ (Ireland 1951). He related the clinical presentation to disk displacement and its progression. During the decades of the 1940s, 50s, and 60s, the literature periodically included papers on TMJ disk displacement (Bowman 1947; Burman and Sinberg 1946; Dingman and Moorman 1951; Kiehn 1952, 1962). They almost exclusively reported the surgical removal of the TMJ disk (diskectomy, meniscectomy) for the treatment of painful clicking and locking.

However, it was not until the 1970s that interest in TMJ disk derangement became widespread. The publications by Farrar (1971) relating TMJ signs and symptoms to disk displacement and the rediscovery of TMJ arthrography by Wilkes (1978a,b) stimulated this renewed interest in disk displacement. During the 1970s and 1980s numerous publications documenting disk displacement and its clinical presentation appeared in the literature. The supporting clinical evidence for disk displacement has come from diagnostic imaging and surgical observations correlated with clinical signs and symptoms.

While the term *internal derangement* literally refers to any abnormality within the joint, it is generally used to denote an abnormal relationship of the articular disk to the mandibular condyle and articular eminence. Generally, the disk is displaced in an anteromedial direction but also can be displaced posteriorly or sideways (medially or laterally). The terms disk displacement and internal derangement will be used interchangeably in this chapter.

CLINICAL PRESENTATIONS

The TMJ patient with internal derangement typically has pain localized to the joint. The pain becomes worse in association with movement or loading of the joint, e.g., during chewing. The patient also has either a clicking or locking joint and may seek treatment in any of several stages of the disorder (Ireland 1951; Dolwick and Riggs 1983; Farrar and McCarthy 1983).

In the first stage of TMJ internal derangement clicking begins suddenly and spontaneously or after an injury. The noise is quite often loud and may be audible to others. The patient may be aware of a feeling of obstruction within the joint during movement until the click occurs. The mandible frequently deviates toward the affected side until the click occurs and then returns to the midline after the click. Palpation or auscultation over the joint reveals that in addition to the click during opening, a faint click also occurs near the termination of closing. The opening and closing clicks were first reported by Ireland (Ireland 1951) and later termed reciprocal clicks by Farrar (Farrar and McCarthy 1983). Reciprocal clicking is considered to be pathognomonic for the first stage of disk displacement.

The second stage of disk derangement is reciprocal clicking with intermittent locking. The typical patient complains that the jaw becomes locked and that there is usually but not always severe pain over the affected joint. The patient may have the feeling of obstruction to opening within the joint. By making some maneuver of the jaw such as shifting it side to side or by applying pressure over the affected joint, the patient may be able to unlock the joint and restore normal movement. It is also possible for the joint to unlock spontaneously. In nearly all cases, there is a prior history of clicking of the affected joint.

The third stage of disk derangement is associated with limited opening and was called "closed lock" by Farrar (Farrar and McCarthy 1983). The patient typically has a limited opening of about 27 mm or less and severe pain over the affected joint. In most cases, the patient experienced clicking followed by intermittent locking, which became more frequent and increasingly difficult to unlock prior to the closed lock stage. The limited opening is associated with deviation of the mandible toward the affected side during opening and limited movement of the mandible toward the opposite side during lateral movements. The patient frequently has the awareness of fullness within the joint and/or the feeling of obstruction to movement.

Table I
Clinical stages of internal derangement

Stage 1	Disk displacement with reduction (reciprocal clicking)
Stage 2	Disk displacement with reduction associated with intermittent locking
Stage 3	Disk displacement without reduction (closed lock)
Stage 4	Disk displacement with perforation

The final stage of disk derangement is associated with an increase in opening and crepitus occurring within the joint during movement. The crepitant noise is believed to occur as a result of disk perforation. This stage is frequently less painful than the earlier stages of disk derangement.

Various terminology has been used to describe the clinical stages of internal derangement. The terminology was often confusing or misleading. At the sixth annual Temporomandibular Joint Research Seminar (Chicago, July 1979) disk displacement was subdivided into disk displacement with reduction (clicking joint) and disk displacement without reduction (closed lock) (Katzberg et al. 1980). This terminology has been generally accepted and is in widespread use today. Table I outlines the clinical stages of internal derangement.

TMJ DISK IMAGING

It was the rediscovery of TMJ arthrography by Wilkes (1978a,b) and its application to clinical diagnosis that stimulated widespread interest in TMJ disk derangement (Wilkes 1978). Zimmer (1941) first described arthrography of the TMJ, and Norgaard (1944) first described a standardized technique and demonstrated its potential value in diagnosing soft tissue abnormalities of the TMJ. However, TMJ arthrography had only limited clinical use until its application by Wilkes (1978a,b).

The reality of disk displacement was confirmed by numerous authors using a variety of arthrographic techniques (Farrar and McCarty 1979; Dolwick et al. 1979; Blaschke et al. 1980; Westesson 1983). The arthrographic findings were correlated with clinical signs and symptoms as well as surgical findings. The validity of arthrographic images was demonstrated by comparing the arthrographic images of postmortem TMJs with the anatomic findings of those joints (Westesson and Rohlin 1984a; Westesson et al. 1986). The accuracy of arthrography is approximately 85% for anteroposterior displacements (Westesson and Rohlin 1984). Its accuracy for sideways displacement is less.

Arthrography showed that during the clicking stage of internal derangement the disk is displaced anterior to its normal position. As opening occurs, the disk is pushed anteriorly by the condyle until a click occurs, at which time the disk returns to a normal relationship with the condyle. It also was observed that during closing the disk is again displaced anteriorly. Furthermore, the reduction and displacement of the disk correlated with the clinical finding of reciprocal clicking. Isberg et al. (1985) used high-speed cinematography on autopsy specimens to demonstrate the anatomic events associated with reciprocal clicking.

TMJ arthrography performed upon patients with closed-lock demonstrated that the disk was displaced anteriorly and remained displaced throughout the opening and closing cycle of movement. Varying degrees of disk deformity also were observed and appeared to be related to the severity of the derangement. Furthermore, it was confirmed that the joints associated with crepitus frequently had disk perforation.

Although most disk displacements occur in an anteromedial direction, other types of displacement have been demonstrated with coronal arthrography in combination with lateral images. Other forms of displacement include posterior as well as sideways displacement in either a medial or lateral direction.

Because TMJ arthrography is invasive and painful, requiring the injection of contrast material into the joint spaces followed by relatively large doses of radiation, clinicians have sought noninvasive, less painful diagnostic imaging procedures. Initially, computerized tomography of the TMJ was attempted, but proved less reliable than arthrography and never gained widespread application. Magnetic resonance imaging (MRI) became the technique of choice for imaging TMJ disk derangement following the development of surface coil technology (Harms et al. 1985; Katzberg et al. 1986).

The validity of MRI of the TMJ has been evaluated by imaging cadaver TMJs and comparing images obtained and anatomic findings. The MR images are 95% accurate in the assessment of disk position and form (Taski 1993). Despite these studies, some questions remain regarding imaging techniques and their interpretation. The observations of TMJ disk derangement seen with arthrography have been confirmed with MRI (Helms et al. 1984; Katzberg et al. 1985; Schellhas et al. 1988; Kaplan and Helms 1989). Again, disk displacements have been observed in all directions. Coronal imaging has improved the diagnosis of sideways displacement (Katzberg et al. 1989).

Magnetic resonance imaging is now the proven method of choice for the assessment of internal derangement. The major advantages of MRI in comparison with arthrography are: (1) MRI is noninvasive, (2) requires no radiation, (3) multiplanar imaging is readily obtained in an array of anatomic sections, and (4) new techniques permit evaluation of inflammation.

SURGICAL OBSERVATIONS

Since Annadale's 1987 report of disk displacement of the TMJ, numerous surgical papers have described disk derangements and correlated the findings with the clinical presentations of clicking and locking (McCarty and Farrar 1979; Dolwick et al. 1983). Correlations among clinical signs and symptoms, imaging observations, and surgical findings have been made (Dolwick and Sanders 1985). These clinical reports demonstrate a relationship between clicking and locking with disk displacement and deformity.

DISK DISPLACEMENT AND OSTEOARTHROSIS (DEGENERATIVE JOINT DISEASE)

Studies of human temporomandibular joints have provided evidence that disk displacement is associated with an increased incidence of osteoarthrosis (Westesson and Rohlin 1984b; Westesson 1985). Osteoarthrosis of the TMJ has been documented in more than 50% of patients with disk derangement. With imaging studies, osteoarthrosis is rarely observed in joints with normal disk position and is most often observed in joints with disk perforation and severe deformation (Katzberg et al. 1983). These results support the idea that disk displacement precedes osteoarthrosis and that disk displacement is a cause of osteoarthrosis. These observations suggest that the disk provides protection against excessive loading.

Alternatively, early osteoarthrotic changes such as articular cartilage softening and fibrillation have been observed arthroscopically in TMJs with normal disk position or minimally displaced disks. Additionally, de Bont (1986) observed histologic "osteoarthritic changes" affecting the articular surfaces of the TMJ in four of eight joints with normal disk-condyle relationships (de Bont et al. 1986). These results support the idea that osteoarthrotic changes precede disk displacement, which may be a sign of osteoarthrosis and not its cause.

RELATIONSHIP OF DISK DISPLACEMENT TO CLINICAL SYMPTOMS

Despite the clinical evidence supporting the existence of TMJ disk derangement, there remain many unanswered questions that raise doubt as to its significance. The most perplexing question concerns the relationship of disk displacement to pain. Because pain in patients with disk displacement is usually aggravated during jaw movements, it seems reasonable that the pain originates from pressure and traction on the disk attachments. In joints with anterior disk displacement, the loose tissue in the posterior attachment is displaced in between the condyle and fossa and could be compressed or stretched during function. However, there is still the perplexing question why many, perhaps most, patients with disk displacement have no pain while some have severe pain. Clicking occurs in 30–50% of the general population. Most persons with clicking joints probably have some form of disk displacement, yet most do not have pain. Arthrographic or MR imaging of normal TMJs free of signs and symptoms show that approximately 30% of the joints have evidence of disk displacement (Kircos et al. 1987; Westesson et al. 1989). Additionally, bilateral arthrograms performed on patients with unilateral symptoms demonstrate evidence of disk derangement in the nonpainful joint 88% of the time (Kozeniauskas and Ralph 1988). These findings make it obvious that disk displacement is not necessarily related to pain.

The relationship of disk displacement to reciprocal clicking, when the clicks occur at different positions during movement, is clear and the evidence supporting this relationship is strong. The relationship of disk displacement to limited opening (closed lock) is much less clear. The recent observations with arthroscopy (Sanders 1986; McCain 1988; Nitzan et al. 1990) and arthrocentesis (Nitzan et al. 1991) of the superior joint compartment in reestablishing normal mouth opening and reducing pain in patients with closed lock raises serious questions as to the relationship of disk displacement to closed lock and pain. Clearly, alternative explanations are plausible (Nitzan and Dolwick 1991).

It has been hypothesized that disk derangement is a progressive disorder, progressing from clicking to clicking with intermittent locking to closed lock and finally disk perforation (Ireland 1951; Boering 1966; Rasmussen 1983). While it is true that some symptomatic patients do progress through these stages of derangement, most do not. If TMJ internal derangement were progressive the symptom of pain should increase with age, but this is not observed. TMJ symptoms appear predominately during the second to fourth decades and occur less frequently in older age groups (Osterberg et al. 1992; Kordis et al. 1993). Therefore, it appears that disk derangement is not necessarily progressive, especially as it relates to pain (deLeeuw et al. 1994).

The relationship of disk displacement to osteoarthrosis is controversial. While it seems that they occur together, it is unclear as to whether disk displacement precedes or follows osteoarthrosis. While it also is possible that these conditions occur together but are unrelated, it seems unlikely. Hall and Nickerson (1994) recently stated that disk displacement is a significant cause of growth disturbance. Imaging studies demonstrated significant disk derangement in association with mandibular deficiency and asymmetry (Nickerson and Moystad 1982; Schellas and Keck 1989; Link and Nickerson 1992). These studies support earlier observations by Boering (1966) and Ricketts

(1966). Whether disk derangement is a cause of growth disturbance remains unclear, however, in that only symptomatic patients have been evaluated. This question is of obvious clinical importance and warrants further study.

The cause of internal derangement is uncertain. Although several possibilities, e.g., Class II deep bite malocclusion, posterior deflective contacts, hyperactivity of the superior belly of the lateral pterygoid, and bruxism and trauma have been proposed, none have been proven (Farrar and McCarty 1983). The mechanism(s) whereby the disk becomes displaced and/or deformed also has not been elucidated. It is apparent that no satisfactory understanding of internal derangement can be achieved until the causes and significance are understood.

In summary, the existence of disk displacement is a reality based on clinical evidence derived from patient evaluations, diagnostic imaging studies, and surgical findings. However, only symptomatic patients with pain have been studied which may have led to an overinterpretation of the importance of disk displacement. The relationship of disk displacement to pain, function, osteoarthrosis, and growth remain unclear. Further study of randomized populations of patients and nonpatients will be necessary to clarify these relationships.

REFERENCES

Annandale, T., Displacement of the inter-articular cartilage of the lower jaw, and its treatment by operation, Lancet, 1 (1887) 411.

Blaschke, D.D., Solberg, W.K. and Sanders, B., Arthrography of the temporomandibular joint: review of current status, J. Am. Dent. Assoc., 100 (1980) 388–395.

Boering, G., Temporomandibular joint arthrosis: an analysis of 400 cases, Thesis, University of Groningen, 1966.

Boman, K., Temporomandibular joint arthrosis and its treatment by extirpation of the disc, Acta Chir. Scand. (Suppl.), 118, 95 (1947) 1–225.

Burman, M. and Sinberg, S.E., Condylar movement in the study of internal derangement of the temporomandibular joint, J. Bone Joint Surg., 28 (1946) 351–373.

de Bont, L.G.M., Boering, G., Liem, R.S.B., Eulderink, F. and Westesson, P.L., Osteoarthritis and internal derangement of the temporomandibular joint: a light microscopic study, J. Oral Maxillofac. Surg., 44 (1986) 634–643.

de Leeuw, R., Boering, G, Stegenga, B. and de Bont, L.G.M., Clinical signs of TMJ osteoarthrosis and internal derangement 30 years after nonsurgical treatment, J. Orofac. Pain, 8 (1994) 18–24.

Dingman, R.O. and Moorman, W.C., Meniscectomy in the treatment of lesions of the temporomandibular joint, J. Oral Surg., 9 (1951) 214–224.

Dolwick, M.F. and Riggs, R.R., Diagnosis and treatment of internal derangements of the temporomandibular joint, Dent. Clin. North Am., 27 (1983) 561–572.

Dolwick, M.F. and Sanders, B., TMJ Internal Derangement and Arthrosis: Surgical Atlas. Mosby, St. Louis, 1985, pp 128–137.

Dolwick, M.F., Katzberg, R.W., Helms, C.A. and Bales, D.J., Arthro-tomographic evaluation of the temporomandibular joint, J. Oral Surg., 37 (1979) 793–799.

Dolwick, M.F., Katzberg, R.W. and Helms, C.A., Internal derangements of the temporomandibular joint: fact or fiction? J. Prosthet. Dent. 49 (1983) 415–418.

Farrar, W.B., Diagnosis and treatment of anterior dislocation of the articular disk, N.Y. J. Dent., 41 (1971) 348–351.

Farrar, W.B. and McCarty, W.L., Inferior joint space arthrography and characteristics of condylar path in internal derangements of the TMJ, J. Prosthet. Dent., 41 (1979) 548–555.

Farrar, W.B. and McCarty, W.L., A Clinical Outline of Temporomandibular Joint Diagnosis and Treatment, Normandie Publications, Montgomery, Ala., 1983, pp. 53–88.

Hall, H.D. and Nickerson, J.W., Is it time to pay more attention to disc position? J. Orofac. Pain, 8 (1994) 90–96.

Harms, S.E., Wilk, R.M., Wolford, L.M., Chiles, D.G. and Milam S.B, The temporomandibular joint: magnetic resonance imaging using surface coils, Radiology, 157 (1985) 133–136.

Helms, C.A., Richardson, M.L., Moon, K.L. and Ware, W.H., Nuclear magnetic resonance imaging of the temporomandibular joint: preliminary observations, J. Craniomandib. Pract., 2 (1984) 219–224.

Ireland, V.E., The problem of "the clicking jaw," Proc. R. Soc. Med. (Lond.), 44 (1951) 363–372.

Isberg, A., Widmainn, S.E. and Ivarsson, R., Clinical, radiographic, and electromyographic studies with internal derangement of the temporomandibular joint, Am. J. Orthod., 88 (1985) 453–460.

Kaplan, P.A. and Helms, C.A., Current status of temporomandibular joint imaging for diagnosis of internal derangements, AJR Am. J. Roentgenol., 152 (1989) 697–705.

Katzberg, R.W., Dolwick, M.F., Helms, C.A., Hopens, T., Bales, D.J. and Coggs, G.C., Arthrotomography of the temporomandibular joint, Am. J. Roentgenol., 134 (1980) 995–1003.

Katzberg, R.W., Keith, D.A., Guralnick, W.C., Manzione, J.V., Jr. and Ten Eick, W.R., Internal derangements and arthritis of the temporomandibular joint, Radiology, 146 (1983) 107–112.

Katzberg, R.W., Schneck, J., Roberts, B.A., Tallents, R.H., Menzione, J.V., Hart, H.R., Foster T.H., Wayne, W.S. and Bessette, R.M., Magnetic resonance imaging of the temporomandibular joint meniscus, Oral Surg. Oral Med. Oral Pathol., 59 (1985) 332–335.

Katzberg, R.W., Bessette, R.W., Tallents, R.H., Plewes, D.B., Manzione, J.V., Schenck, J.F., Foster, T.H. and Hart, H.R., Normal and abnormal temporomandibular joint: MR imaging with surface coil, Radiology, 158 (1986) 183–189.

Katzberg, R.W., Westesson, P.L., Tallents, R.H., Anderson, R., Kuritka, K. Manzione, J.F., Jr. and Totterman, S., Temporomandibular joint: MR assessment of rotational and sideways disk displacements, Radiology, 169 (1989) 741–748.

Kiehn, C.L., Meniscectomy for internal derangement of temporomandibular joint, Am. J. Surg., 83 (1952) 364–373.

Kiehn, C.L. and Des Prez, J.D., Meniscectomy for internal derangement of temporomandibular joint, Br. J. Plast. Surg., 15 (1962) 199–204.

Kircos, L.T., Ortendahl, D.A., Mark, A.S. and Arakawa, M., Magnetic resonance imaging of the TMJ disc in asymptomatic volunteers, J. Oral Maxillofac. Surg., 45 (1987) 852–854.

Kordis, P.T., Zarifi, A., Grigoriadou, E. and Garefis, P., Effect of age and sex on craniomandibular disorders, J. Prosthet. Dent. 69 (1993) 93–101.

Kozeniauskas, J.J. and Ralph, W.J., Bilateral arthrographic evaluation of unilateral temporomandibular joint pain and dysfunction, J. Prosth. Dent., 60 (1988) 98–105.

Link, J.J. and Nickerson, J.W., Temporomandibular joint internal derangements in an orthognathic surgery population, Int. J. Orthod. Orthognathic Surg., 7 (1992) 161–169.

McCain, J.P., Arthroscopy of the human temporomandibular joint, J. Oral Maxillofac. Surg., 46 (1988) 648–655.

McCarty, W.L. and Farrar, W.B., Surgery for internal derangements of the temporomandibular joint, J. Prosth. Dent., 42 (1979) 191–196.

Nickerson, J.W. and Moystad, A., Observations on individuals with radiographic bilateral condylar remodeling, J Craniomandib. Pract., 1 (1982) 21–36.

Nitzan, D.W. and Dolwick, M.F., An alternative explanation for the genesis of closed lock symptoms in the internal derangement process, J. Oral Maxillofac. Surg., 49 (1991) 810–815.

Nitzan, D.W., Dolwick, M.F. and Heft, M.W., Arthroscopic lavage and lysis of the temporomandibular joint: a change in perspective, J. Oral Maxillofac. Surg., 48 (1990) 798–801.

Nitzan, D.W., Dolwick, M.F. and Martinez, A., Temporomandibular joint arthrocentesis: a simplified treatment for severe, limited mouth opening, J. Oral Maxillofac. Surg., 49 (1991) 1163–1167.

Norgaard, F., Arthrography of the temporomandibular joint: preliminary report, Acta Radiol., 25 (1944) 679–685.

Osterberg, T., Carlsson, G.E., Wedel, A. and Johansson, U., A cross-sectional and longitudinal study of craniomandibular dysfunction in an elderly population, J. Craniomandib. Disord., 6 (1992) 237–245.

Pringle, J.H., Displacement of the mandibular meniscus and its treatment, Br. J. Surg., 6 (1918) 385–389.

Rasmussen, C.D., Temporomandibular arthropathy: clinical, radiologic, and therapeutic aspects with emphasis on diagnosis, Int. J. Oral Surg., 12 (1983) 365–397.

Ricketts, R.M., Clinical implications of the temporomandibular joint, Am. J. Orthod., 52 (1966) 416–439.

Sanders, B., Arthroscopic surgery of the temporomandibular joint: treatment of internal derangement with persistent closed lock, Oral Surg. Oral Med. Oral Pathol., 62 (1986) 361–372.

Schellhas, K.P. and Keck, R.J., Disorders of skeletal occlusion and temporomandibular joint disease, Northwest. Dent., 68 (1989) 35–42.

Schellhas, K.P., Fritts, H.M., Heitoff, K.B., Jahn, J.A., Wilkes, C.H. and Omlie, M.R., Temporomandibular joint: MR fast scanning, Cranio, 6 (1988) 209–216.

Taski, M.M. and Westesson, P.L., Temporomandibular joint: diagnostic accuracy with sagittal and coronal MR imaging, Radiology, 186 (1993) 723–729.

Westesson, P.L., Double-constant arthrotomography of the temporomandibular joint: introduction of an arthrographic technique for visualization of the disc and articular surfaces, J. Oral Maxillofac. Surg., 41 (1983) 163–172.

Westesson, P.L., Structural hard tissue changes in temporomandibular joints with internal derangment, Oral Surg. Oral Med. Oral Pathol., 59 (1985) 220–224.

Westesson, P.L. and Rohlin, M., Diagnostic accurracy of double-contrast arthrotomography of the temporomandibular joint: correlaton with postmortem morphology, AJNR Am. J. Neuroradiol., 5 (1984a) 463–468.

Westesson, P.L. and Rohlin, M., Internal derangement related to osteoarthrosis in temporomandibular joint autopsy specimens, Oral Surg. Oral Med. Oral Pathol., 57 (1984b) 17–22.

Westesson, P.L., Bronstein, S.L. and Liedberg, J., Temporomandibular joint: correlation between single contrast videoarthrography and postmortem morphology, Radiology, 160 (1986) 767–771.

Westesson, P.L., Ericksson, L. and Kurita, K., Reliability of a negative clinical temporomandibular joint examination: prevalence of disk displacement in asymptomatic temporomandibular joints, Oral Surg. Oral Med. Oral Pathol., 68 (1989) 551–554.

Wilkes, C.H., Structural and functional alterations of the temporomandibular joint, Northwest. Dent., 57 (1978a) 287–294.

Wilkes, C.H., Arthrography of the temporomandibular joint in patients with the TMJ pain-dysfunction syndrome, Minn. Med., 61 (1978b) 645–652.

Zimmer, E.A., Die Rontgenologie des Kiefergelenkes, Schweiz. Monatsschr. Zahnheild., 51 (1941) 12–24.

Correspondence to: M. Franklin Dolwick, DMD, PhD, Department of Oral and Maxillofacial Surgery, University of Florida, Box 100416 JHMHC, Gainesville, FL 32610-0416, USA. Tel: 904-392-4116; Fax: 904-392-7609.

Temporomandibular Disorders and Related Pain Conditions, Progress in Pain Research and Management, Vol. 4, edited by B.J. Sessle, P.S. Bryant, and R.A. Dionne, IASP Press, Seattle, © 1995.

6

Articular Disk Displacements and Degenerative Temporomandibular Joint Disease

Stephen B. Milam

University of Texas Health Science Center, San Antonio, Texas, USA

The articular disk of the temporomandibular joint (TMJ) is normally located between the articulating surfaces of the mandibular condyle and temporal bone. Displacement of the articular disk of the temporomandibular joint from its normal position was recognized as a potential clinical problem over 100 years ago (Annandale 1887). Subsequently, surgical repositioning of the disk (Annandale 1887) or its removal (Lanz 1909; Pringle 1918) were suggested as remedies for the condition. Since these early reports, several others have associated joint pain, limited mandibular movement, and joint sounds with articular disk displacement of the TMJ (Isberg et al. 1985; Rohlin et al. 1985; Gay et al. 1987; Isacsson et al. 1988; Stegenga et al. 1992; Sutton et al. 1992; Westesson and Brooks 1992; Widmalm et al. 1992).

The incidence of articular disk displacement in the general population is unknown, but is estimated at approximately 2–67% based on human cadaver studies (Westesson and Rohlin 1984; Castelli et al. 1985; Solberg et al. 1985; Westesson 1985; Liedberg et al. 1990; Nannmark et al. 1990). However, these studies do not provide information concerning the history of the subjects, so no conclusions can be made concerning the significance of articular disk displacements relative to temporomandibular dysfunction. Radiographic studies indicate that up to 70% of patients seeking treatment for a suspected TMJ disorder have articular disk displacements (Farrar and McCarty 1979). Yet, no causative relationship between articular disk displacement and patient symptoms can be determined from this study.

Articular disk displacements may alter the structure and biochemical composition of contacting surfaces of the TMJ. Disk deformation and/or perforation, atypical cellular architecture, osteophyte formation, subchondral bone resorption, disruption of the physical continuity of the articular surface of the mandibular condyle, and adhesion formation have all been observed in studies of human cadaver TMJs with articular disk displacements (Blackwood 1966; Castelli et al. 1985; Axelsson et al. 1987; Helmy et al. 1989; Kurita et al. 1989b; Nannmark et al. 1990). These anomalies have been described as degenerative changes. This implication of a disease process has influenced the clinical management of patients with signs of articular disk displacement. However, the significance of these structural changes must be interpreted in reference to our current knowledge of the molecular events that may underlie both adaptive and disease states affecting the TMJ.

ADAPTATION VERSUS DISEASE

Several studies have provided evidence of a remarkable adaptive capacity of the TMJ (Hinton 1987; Copray et al. 1988b; Hinton 1989; Block and Bouvier 1990; Hinton 1991; Scapino 1991; Kawamura et al. 1992). For example, Breitner (1940, 1941) altered occlusal patterns of adult rhesus monkeys and demonstrated marked adaptive changes in the TMJ. Similar adaptive changes of the articular surfaces of the TMJ have been documented in response to forced protrusion (Charlier et al. 1969; Petrovic 1972; Carlson et al. 1978; McNamara and Carlson 1979) or forced retrusion (Adams et al. 1972; Joho 1973) of the mandible. It has been suggested that articular tissues affected in this fashion may be better adapted to accommodate new mechanical stresses impacting the TMJ (Moffett et al. 1964; Meikle 1992).

Histological and arthroscopic studies of human TMJ have identified structural defects that are believed to represent a failure in the adaptive mechanism(s) of the joint (Westesson and Rohlin 1984; Castelli et al. 1985; Solberg et al. 1985; Westesson et al. 1985; Liedberg and Westesson 1988; Liedberg et al. 1990; Nannmark et al. 1990; Quinn 1992). However, the boundary between remodeling or adaptation and a disease state is, at present, ill-defined. Nevertheless, the adaptive capacity of the TMJ is not infinite. Several factors may directly or indirectly influence the adaptive capacity, including age, sex, psychological stress, systemic illness, and previous injury. Theoretically, these factors may reduce the adaptive capacity of the TMJ, leading to a disease state under conditions of "normal" joint function. In the pathological state, it is assumed that the delicate balance between catabolic and anabolic responses of affected articular tissue is perturbed and adaptation yields to disease (Moffett et al. 1964).

ARTICULAR DISK DISPLACEMENT AND DEGENERATIVE JOINT DISEASE

Structural changes of the mandibular condyle and temporal bone have been observed in animals following diskectomy, disk perforation, or disk displacement (Yaillen et al. 1979; Helmy et al. 1988; Block and Bouvier 1990; Axelsson et al. 1992; Hinton 1992; Macher et al. 1992; Axelsson 1993; Lang et al. 1993). Some of these changes have been dramatic (i.e., exposure of subchondral bone) and consistent with a degenerative process. In addition, studies of human TMJs have provided evidence that disk displacement is associated with an increased incidence of degenerative joint disease or osteoarthrosis (Westesson and Rohlin 1984; de Bont et al. 1986). These observations provide evidence that the articular disk affords some protection against excessive loading. These data also support the popular notion that articular disk displacements may contribute to degenerative joint disease by increasing functional demands on articular fibrocartilages of the TMJ.

Alternatively, degenerative joint disease may precede articular disk displacement. De Bont et al. (1986) conducted histological studies of 22 human TMJs. These investigators observed "osteoarthritic changes" affecting the articular surfaces of the TMJ in 50% (i.e., 4 of 8 joints) of joints with normal disk-condyle relationships. They also observed degenerative changes in 79%. (i.e., 11 of 14 joints) of the joints that had articular disk displacements. These investigators suggest that degenerative changes significantly affect the sliding properties of affected articulating surfaces of the joint. Subsequently, joint stiffness and friction may increase in osteoarthrotic joints, eventually leading to disk displacement. In this sense, articular disk displacement may be a sign of degenerative joint disease and not its cause.

The controversy concerning the significance of articular disk displacements in the TMJ is fueled by the lack of a suitable animal model to study the phenomenon. Nonprimate models are plagued by dissimilarities in joint structure and function. Also, in the majority of these animal studies, disk perforation or disk removal (i.e., diskectomy) is performed to initiate a response by articulating tissues. The biological response to these manipulations can be quite variable. Indeed, one may argue that the tissue response to a surgical wound may be quite different from that involved in degenerative joint disease. Furthermore, none of these studies have documented any functional limitations imposed on operated joints. Frequently, the majority of animals subjected to these procedures do not manifest any significant derangement in jaw function. Consequently, many of the structural changes observed in these models could represent remodeling or adaptive processes. Indeed, we should question the acceptance of even dramatic structural changes (i.e., fibrillation, fissuring, eburnation, and cystic alterations) as indicators of a disease process

(Moffett et al. 1964) in the absence of any detectable functional derangement in the joint. At present, no markers can reliably distinguish between an adaptive response and a disease process in the TMJ. Indeed, it is likely that many of the molecular events involved in normal remodeling are also involved in degenerative joint disease. A thorough understanding of these molecular processes will be required if were are to develop reliable indicators of disease.

While the relationship between articular disk displacement and degenerative joint disease is controversial, it appears that some persons do suffer from a degenerative process affecting the articular tissues of the TMJ. A model of the molecular processes involved would provide useful direction for future research. Much of our current thought regarding these molecular processes has been based on studies of other articular joints. However, there is evidence that the TMJ may be unique in some aspects. For example, the TMJ is unique with respect to its structure (i.e., gross structure and molecular composition) and function. The TMJ is a diarthroidial joint capable of both hinge and sliding motions. These functional differences may be important because biomechanical stimuli modulate various cellular activities in articular joints, including cell proliferation and matrix synthesis (Takano-Yamamoto et al. 1991). Furthermore, the fibrocartilages of the TMJ are described as secondary cartilages (Copray et al. 1988b). These specialized tissues differ from primary cartilages with respect to growth characteristics and response to specific growth factors. For example, parathyroid hormone (fragment 1-34) stimulates ^{3}H-thymidine incorporation by rat costal cartilage explants but not by mandibular condylar cartilage explants (Copray et al. 1988a). These differences undoubtedly contribute to the unpredictable growth patterns of primary cartilage grafts that have been used to reconstruct the TMJ. While, independent studies of the TMJ are warranted based on these observations, it is reasonable to assume that many of the molecular events that underlie degenerative processes in other joints are similar to those that may occur in the TMJ.

A MODEL OF DEGENERATIVE TMJ DISEASE

It is the consensus opinion that degenerative TMJ disease is the result of maladaptation to increased joint loading (Westesson and Rohlin 1984; Axelsson et al. 1987; Stegenga et al. 1990, 1991; Axelsson et al. 1992; Stegenga et al. 1992; Axelsson 1993; de Bont and Stegenga 1993). However, little is known about the actual forces that are transmitted to the articular surfaces of the human TMJ during function. There have been a few attempts to measure intracapsular pressures of the TMJ during function. Lower joint space forces up to 17.7 kg have been recorded in an adult monkey using an implanted piezoelectric foil (Boyd et al. 1990). During masticatory function, superior joint space pressures up to 20 mm Hg (i.e., 0.39 lb/in^2 or 0.31 gm/mm^2) were recorded in weanling pigs (Ward et al. 1990). More recently, intracapsular pressures ranging from slightly subatmospheric to 200 mm Hg (i.e., 3.9 lb/in^2 or 2.7 gm/mm^2) have been recorded in symptomatic human TMJs during function (Nitzan 1994).

Mathematical remodeling and limited animal data indicate that several factors may influence loading of the TMJ during function (Haskell et al. 1986; Faulkner et al. 1987; Throckmorton et al. 1990; Tuominen et al. 1993). These include the status of the dentition, the total bite force, ipsilateral and contralateral muscle force ratios, and the mechanical properties of food eaten (Hylander 1992). In addition, asymmetrical remodeling of the articular surfaces of both the mandibular condyle and temporal bone indicate that the articular structures of the human TMJ may be differentially loaded (Westesson and Rohlin 1984). However, these loads appear to be substantially smaller in magnitude than those observed in weight-bearing joints, though exact contact forces are unknown.

EFFECTS OF MECHANICAL LOADS ON ARTICULAR TISSUES

Excessive or protracted mechanical loads can affect articular tissues through several mechanisms. First, mechanical stress can alter synthetic functions in affected cell populations. Typically, chondrocytes subjected to compressive loads in a physiologic range increase their synthesis of cartilage matrix components (i.e., proteoglycans). For example, cells in the supporting tissues of the articular disk of the TMJ may synthesize glycosaminoglycans in response to compressive loading (Blaustein and Scapino 1986). Compressive loading of posterior supporting tissues could occur with anterior displacements of the articular disk. It has been suggested that newly synthesized glycosaminoglycans (proteoglycans) by cells in these tissues may afford increasing resiliency to compressive loads, thereby reflecting an adaptive process (Blaustein and Scapino 1986).

However, excessive or sustained mechanical loading may impair synthetic functions in affected tissues of the TMJ (Salo et al. 1993; Pirttiniemi et al. 1994). Haskin et al. (1993) provide evidence that chondroblast failure with excessive loading (i.e., 4 MPa for 20 minutes) may be associated with disruption of specific cytoskeletal elements, f-actin, and tubulin. The integrity of the cytoskeleton is required for various cell functions, including gene regulation and protein synthesis (Bissell et al. 1982). The induction of heat shock proteins has also been observed in MG-63 osteosarcoma cells subjected to a 20-minute continuous compressive force (Haskin et al. 1993). It is believed that heat shock proteins function primarily to preserve only vital cellular functions during stress in an attempt to conserve energy expenditure (Georgopoulos and Welch 1993). These changes could account for the decreased synthetic function observed in chondroblasts subjected to excessive loads in articular joints. Because adaptation or remodeling involves a delicate balance between catabolic and anabolic events, suppressed synthetic function in affected cell populations could contribute significantly to a maladaptive state.

Mechanical stresses can physically disrupt molecules in contact regions. Free radicals may be produced from molecular damage caused by excessive mechanical forces. For example, fingernail cutting generates a high yield of sulfur-centered free radicals by shearing keratin molecules (Chandra and Symons 1987). Free radicals are molecules or ions that contain an odd number (i.e., unpaired) of electrons. The presence of one or more unpaired electrons makes these molecules highly reactive. Free radicals can generate molecular chain reactions that can destroy molecules and inhibit and/or stimulate molecular activities.

The lubrication of articular surfaces by synovial fluid normally protects these surfaces from excessive frictional forces during joint movement. The articular disk of the TMJ further reduces mechanical stress by distributing contact forces over broad areas and by providing four lubricated surfaces. However, if these protective mechanisms are impaired (i.e., changes in the physical properties of synovial fluid and/or displacement or perforation of the articular disk), mechanical forces generated with joint movement could be sufficient to damage tissue, yielding free radicals in the process. Theoretically, these free radicals could cause additional damage to affected tissue.

Excessive joint loads could contribute to free radical generation in the TMJ via another mechanism. With unfavorable joint function, intra-articular pressures may exceed synovial capillary perfusion pressure and a period of hypoxia may result. Blake et al. observed a 33% reduction in synovial fluid pO_2 (i.e., from 61 mm Hg to 41 mm Hg) in arthritic human knee joints with isometric quadriceps contraction (Blake et al. 1989). An 87% reduction in synovial capillary perfusion was observed in these joints during this exercise (Blake et al. 1989). Likewise, intra-articular pressures have been recorded in the human TMJ during function that have exceeded capillary perfusion pressure (Nitzan 1994).

Transient hypoxia may result in significant alterations in the metabolism of affected cell populations as described by McCord (McCord and Fridovich 1968; McCord 1985; Fig. 1). When joint pressures decline (i.e., with muscular relaxation), tissue perfusion is reestablished. Metabolically transformed cells may then generate free radicals (i.e., superoxide anion and subsequently

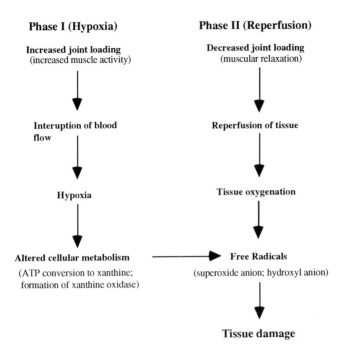

Phase I (Hypoxia)

Increased joint loading
(increased muscle activity)

Interuption of blood flow

Hypoxia

Altered cellular metabolism
(ATP conversion to xanthine; formation of xanthine oxidase)

Phase II (Reperfusion)

Decreased joint loading
(muscular relaxation)

Reperfusion of tissue

Tissue oxygenation

Free Radicals
(superoxide anion; hydroxyl anion)

Tissue damage

Fig. 1. Model of hypoxia-reperfusion injury, as proposed by McCord (1985) and Blake et al. (1989). Increased joint loading, which may occur with increased muscular activity and/ or unfavorable loading patterns (i.e., articular disk displacement), may produce regional pressures that exceed capillary perfusion pressure. As a result, blood flow to affected tissues decreases dramatically, resulting in hypoxia. Cells in these affected tissues respond to the change in oxygen tension by altering specific metabolic pathways including the conversion of ATP to xanthine and the formation of xanthine oxidase from xanthine dehydrogenase by action of a calcium-dependent enzyme (i.e., calpain). When joint loading subsides (i.e., muscular relaxation), blood flow returns and the affected tissues are reoxygenated. Metabolically altered cells generate free radicals from the replenished oxygen supply. These free radicals may damage local tissues or destroy important molecules (i.e., hyaluronic acid, collagens, proteoglycans), resulting in a weakened structure. Ultimately, these alterations could account for biomechanical changes in articular tissues that could predispose to articular disk displacements. (de Bont et al. 1986)

the hydroxyl radical) with replenished oxygen as a substrate. This type of injury, known as a hypoxia-reperfusion injury (McCord and Fridovich 1968; McCord 1985), could contribute to local tissue disruption during periods of excessive or sustained mechanical loads. For example, superoxide and hydroxyl radicals degrade hyaluronic acid from synovial fluid, thereby reducing its viscosity (McCord 1974). Free radicals also may damage cartilage matrix by both direct and indirect actions (Burkhardt et al. 1986). Also, oxygen-derived radicals may inhibit metabolic activities in articular chondrocytes (Vincent et al. 1994). These findings indicate that oxygen-derived free radicals may contribute to degenerative processes in affected joints by degrading important molecules and reducing the synthetic functions of chondrocytes. However, the relative contribution of these phenomena to degenerative TMJ disease has not been explored.

CHANGES IN THE MOLECULAR COMPOSITION OF ARTICULAR TISSUES IN DEGENERATIVE DISEASE

The articular fibrocartilages of the mandibular condyle and temporal bone are formed from a complex organization of extracellular matrix molecules and cells. A variety of extracellular matrix molecules have been identified in articular structures of the TMJ. These include collagens (Silbermann et al. 1987; Silbermann et al. 1990; Strauss et al. 1990; Ben et al. 1991; Milam et al. 1991b), cartilage proteoglycans (Ben et al. 1991; Milam et al. 1991b; Ben et al. 1992; Silbermann and Frommer 1973; Symons 1965), and glycoproteins (Silbermann et al. 1990; Strauss et al. 1990; Ben et al. 1991; Milam et al. 1991b; Tajima et al. 1991; Ben et al. 1993). Collagens and proteoglycans have received considerable attention because of their relative high abundance and their contribution to the biomechanical properties of articular cartilage. However, other matrical constituents also may contribute significantly to the continued health of these specialized tissues.

The most consistently observed changes in the extracellular matrix of articular cartilages obtained from degenerative joints are disruption of the collagenous matrix and a loss of glycosaminoglycans (Mankin and Lippiello 1971; Brandt and Radin 1987; Sandy et al. 1987; Helmy et al. 1988; Hinton 1992; Poole et al. 1993). However, these degradative events may not necessarily signal a disease process. As is the case for all connective tissues, these degradative events are a necessary component of normal tissue remodeling. It is likely that many of the molecular processes that have been observed in degenerative joint disease are also active in normal remodeling.

Articular disk perforation (or diskectomy) generally leads to an initial increase in the hydration of the articular cartilages of the TMJ (Hinton 1992; Lang et al. 1993). This phenomenon is commonly described in other joints with similar experimental manipulations (Hamerman 1989). The increased hydration may be attributed, in part, to a loss of the integrity of the collagen network of these tissues (Hamerman 1989). As the collagenous matrix becomes increasingly degraded, its restraining influence on large aggregating cartilage proteoglycans is lost. Large aggregating cartilage proteoglycans carry a significant negative charge by virtue of the large number of carboxyl and sulfate moieties found in these molecules. The net negative charge of these macromolecules attracts extracellular water molecules (Muir et al. 1969), accounting for 78% of the weight of the rabbit mandibular condylar fibrocartilage (Lang et al. 1993). The organization of extracellular matrix water around these molecules affords cartilage resiliency to compressive forces (Kempson et al. 1970). These negatively charged proteoglycan macromolecules expand like sponges, increasing water absorption when the restraining collagenous matrix is lost. As these molecules expand, they become increasingly vulnerable to enzymatic attack (Heinegard and Hascall 1974) and are eventually lost from affected tissues (Brandt and Radin 1987; Hamerman 1989; Poole et al. 1993). Thus, an early and key event in degenerative joint disease is the loss of the integrity of the collagenous matrix of articulating structures with subsequent loss of cartilage proteoglycans. With the loss of organized cartilage proteoglycans (i.e., intact large aggregating proteoglycans), affected articular tissues lose their resiliency to compressive loads. Mechanical forces transmitted to subchondral bone may increase under these conditions, leading to osteolysis.

The enzymatic events involved in this process are now being characterized. Several proteinases have been implicated in the degradation of cartilaginous matrices in degenerative joint disease. These include various members of the metalloproteinase family (Dean et al. 1989; McCachren 1991), serine proteases of the plasminogen/plasmin cascade (Campbell et al. 1988), and cysteine proteinases such as calpain and lysosomal cathepsins (Buttle and Saklatvala 1992; Suzuki et al. 1992). Products of these enzymatic processes have been recovered from synovial fluid (Heinegard and Saxne 1991; Xie et al. 1992; Lohmander et al. 1993; Saxne et al. 1993). These products might provide useful markers for evaluating cartilage matrix degradation in patients with suspected degenerative joint disease (Heinegard and Saxne 1991). However, these products may be generated from normal cartilage turnover (i.e., remodeling). Therefore, interpretation of these monitoring methods will require further studies to define abnormal matrix degradation rates for persons of different ages and gender.

ALTERATIONS IN THE SYNTHETIC CAPACITY OF CHONDROBLASTS

In degenerative joint disease, the degradative processes continue unchecked. It is likely that these degradative processes involve an increased synthesis of matrix-degrading enzymes, the generation of free radicals, and a reduction in the efficacy of fail-safe mechanisms that exist to limit proteolytic and nonproteolytic destruction of affected articular tissues. Failure of the structural integrity of affected articular surfaces may also be attributed, in part, to reduced synthetic function of local cell populations.

Chondroblasts are normally highly responsive to changes in their extracellular matrix. Embryonic chondroblasts can resynthesize a cartilage matrix depleted by enzymatic digestion in vitro in only a few days (Fritton Jackson 1970). The responsiveness of chondroblasts to changing functional demands significantly contributes to the adaptive capacity of articular tissues in the joint. However, the capacity of the chondroblast for repair may be limited. With continued and/or excessive loads, the chondroblast may fail as previously described.

Synthetic functions of chondroblasts (and other cell types) in the TMJ may also be adversely affected by other mechanisms. For example, mounting evidence indicates that changes in the molecular composition of the extracellular matrix may profoundly affect phenotypic expression of chondroblasts. Cells may receive "signals" from specific extracellular matrix molecules by way of transmembrane receptors, termed integrins (Milam et al. 1991a; Milam et al. 1991b; Ruoslahti 1991). Signaling through this mechanism may profoundly affect several important cell functions including proliferation and differentiation. One such cell-extracellular matrix interaction that could be important in growth regulation in the mandibular condyle is mediated by fibronectin and its principal cell surface receptor, the $\alpha 5\beta 1$ integrin (Milam 1990).

Fibronectins are glycoproteins that promote cell adhesion and facilitate cell migration in vitro (Milam et al. 1991a; Glukhova and Thiery 1993). In vitro studies have provided evidence that these molecules may inhibit chondrogenesis (Pennypacker et al. 1979; Pennypacker 1981) and may regulate proliferation of prechondroblasts in the TMJ (Milam 1990). Furthermore, specific binding events at the $\alpha 5\beta 1$ integrin may induce the synthesis and secretion of matrix-degrading enzymes including collagenase (MMP1) and stromelysin (MMP3) (Werb et al. 1989). These observations are particularly interesting given that a commonly observed change in the extracellular matrix of osteoarthrotic cartilages is an accumulation of fibronectins (i.e., up to a 10-fold increase) (Vilamitjana and Harmand 1990; Chevalier 1993). Several other important matrical molecules have been identified in articular tissues of the TMJ. Each undoubtedly contributes to the structural integrity and biomechanical properties of these specialized tissues. These recent observations indicate that the extracellular matrix may also profoundly affect specific cellular activities including gene expression. Therefore, disruption of the normal integrity or composition of the extracellular matrix can have a significant impact on *both* biomechanical properties *and* cellular activities of affected articular tissues.

CYTOKINES AND DEGENERATIVE JOINT DISEASE

Cytokines are polypeptide hormones that can evoke a variety of cellular responses. The cytokines implicated in degenerative joint disease are interleukin-1 (Chang et al. 1986; Goldring et al. 1988; Verschure and Van 1990; Chang et al. 1992; Davies et al. 1992), tumor necrosis factor (Campbell et al. 1990a,b; Pickvance et al. 1993), interleukin-6 (Bender et al. 1990), and interleukin-8 (DeMarco et al. 1991; Elford and Cooper 1991). Collectively, these cytokines increase fibrocartilage degradation by stimulating the synthesis of matrix-degrading enzymes by local cell populations. In addition, these cytokines may alter extracellular matrix synthesis and cell-extracellular matrix interactions that may be important to chondrogenesis. For example, interleukin-1 (IL-1) down-regulates the synthesis of cartilage-specific type II collagens (Goldring et al. 1988, 1990) and increases the synthesis of type I collagen (Goldring et al. 1988, 1990), fibronectin (Goldring et al. 1990), and several integrins including the $\alpha 5\beta 1$ integrin (Dedhar 1989; Milam et al. 1991b). IL-1 may also activate heat shock proteins in chondrocytes that could account, in part, for the inhibitory effect this cytokine has on glycosaminoglycan synthesis by chondrocytes (Cruz et al. 1991). These effects may be produced by incredibly low concentrations of IL-1. Primary cultures of chondrocytes obtained from primate mandibular condyles respond to femtomolar concentrations IL-1 in vitro (Milam 1990).

Cytokines may stimulate arachidonic acid metabolism and free radical production in articular tissues. IL-1 stimulates arachidonic acid metabolism by increasing phospholipase activity in chondrocytes (Chang et al. 1986; Milam 1990) and synoviocytes (Gilman et al. 1988). Nitric oxide may be produced by target cells in response to IL-1 (Corbett et al. 1992). IL-1 may also contribute to the production of oxygen-derived free radicals by stimulating arachidonic acid metabolism (Chang et al. 1986). Free radicals generated by the hypoxia/reperfusion mechanism stimulate IL-1 and IL-6 synthesis by cultured endothelial cells (Ala et al. 1992). Furthermore, the synthesis of these cytokines under experimental conditions is significantly inhibited in the presence of free radical scavengers (i.e., superoxide dismutase or glutathione peroxidase) (Ala et al. 1992). Therefore, it appears that both free radical production and inflammatory cytokine synthesis are involved in positive feedback mechanisms that perpetuate these signaling mechanisms.

Cytokines are likely to be involved in both remodeling and degenerative processes affecting the TMJ. Tumor necrosis factor has been detected in human TMJ synovial fluid (Rossomando et al. 1992). In a preliminary study, the levels of this cytokine in synovial fluid correlated with symptoms that were believed to be associated with articular disk displacements (Shafer et al. 1992). In addition, primary cultures of chondrocytes obtained from primate mandibular condyles respond to physiologic concentrations IL-1 in vitro (Milam 1990).

NEUROGENIC INFLAMMATION: NEUROPEPTIDES AND CYTOKINES

The articular disk of the TMJ is most commonly displaced in an anterior and medial direction. Displacement of the articular disk could result in traction and/or compression of nerve-rich regions of the TMJ. The capsular ligament and retrodiskal tissues of the TMJ are richly innervated by substance P- and CGRP-containing neurons (Johansson et al. 1986; Ichikawa et al. 1989; Kido et al. 1993). Stimulation of these nerve terminals by traction or compression could evoke a release of these neuropeptides into the surrounding tissue. Studies conducted by Holmlund and associates have provided evidence that is consistent with this hypothesis (Holmlund et al. 1991). These investigators have detected these neuropeptides in TMJ synovial fluid obtained from patients with articular disk displacements (Holmlund et al. 1991). In fact, compared with neuropeptide levels detected in the knee joint, significantly higher concentrations of substance P, CGRP, and neuropeptide Y were found in the TMJ (Holmlund et al. 1991). These neuropeptides evoke an intense inflammatory response when injected into articular joints (Kimball 1990).

Several studies have provided a substantial body of evidence that indicates that neuropeptides involved in neurogenic inflammation increase synthesis of both IL-1 (Kimball et al. 1988; Lotz et al. 1988; Laurenzi et al. 1990) and tumor necrosis factor (Lotz et al. 1988). Interestingly, IL-1 up-regulates the expression of substance P by affected neuronal populations, in what appears to be a positive response loop (Hart et al. 1991; Jonakait and Schotland 1990; Jonakait et al. 1990, 1991). The effect of interleukin-1 on substance P synthesis may be mediated by leukemia inhibitory factor (Shadiack et al. 1993). Leukemia inhibitory factor is produced by synoviocytes (Hamilton et al. 1993), chondrocytes (Campbell et al. 1993), and sympathetic neurons (Freidin and Kessler 1991; Shadiack et al. 1993) in response to interleukin-1 or tumor necrosis factor. In this regard, O'Byrne and colleagues have observed a dose-dependent increase in synovial fluid substance P levels following injection of IL-1 into the rabbit knee joint (O'Byrne et al. 1990). This signaling mechanism may be further amplified by the presence of prostaglandins and bradykinin. These substances may lower the response thresholds of nerve terminals in affected tissues, resulting in the release of these neuropeptides with lower intensity stimuli. Thus, cytokines and neuropeptides may self-perpetuate molecular events that could lead eventually to degenerative changes in tissues of affected joints.

FACTORS THAT MAY INFLUENCE THE ADAPTIVE CAPACITY OF THE TMJ

SEX HORMONES

Several epidemiological studies have provided evidence of a female predilection to temporomandibular dysfunction. In general, women tend to report more pain, and exhibit a higher incidence of joint noise and mandibular deflection with movement than do men. Histological studies of human cadaver TMJs also indicate that women have a incidence of articular disk displacements (Solberg et al. 1985).

Functional estrogen receptors have been identified in the female TMJ (Aufdemorte et al. 1986; Abubaker et al. 1993) but not in the male TMJ (Milam et al. 1987). High-affinity (Kd = 5×10^{-10} M) estrogen receptors have been identified in macrophage-like synoviocytes (Cutolo et al. 1993). In a model of osteoarthritis involving the rabbit knee joint (i.e., partial medial meniscectomy), systemically administered estradiol significantly reduced ^{35}S incorporation into affected cartilages compared to operated controls (Rosner et al. 1979). Furthermore, the authors noted that articular cartilages from estradiol-treated animals were more friable than cartilages obtained from control animals. In these studies, however, Safranin-O staining of affected articular tissue was not appreciably different between experimental groups. Safranin-O is a cationic dye that binds to anionic molecules such as glycosaminoglycans. These data indicate the estrogen may inhibit glycosaminoglycan degradation and synthesis. Estrogen may also promote degenerative changes in the TMJ by increasing the synthesis of specific cytokines. Estradiol enhances the synthesis of IL-1 and IL-6 by peripheral blood mononuclear cells (Li et al. 1993). On the other hand, testosterone may inhibit the release of these cytokines from stimulated monocytes (Li et al. 1993). In addition, prolactin, released from the pituitary in response to estrogen, exacerbates collagen-induced arthritis in mice (Whyte and Williams 1988). Prolactin also stimulates cytokine production by lymphocytes and macrophages. Bromocriptine, a dopaminergic agonist that inhibits prolactin release from the pituitary, markedly (50%) suppresses the severity of collagen-induced arthritis in postpartum (i.e., hyperprolactinemic) mice (Whyte and Williams 1988). Sex hormone regulation of cytokine production is complex and depends on other coexisting factors. It is likely that sex hormones profoundly influence several cell activities that may be associated with remodeling or degenerative processes in the TMJ.

AGE

With aging, it appears that the regenerative capacity of the articular tissues of the TMJ declines. Cell density in the prechondroblastic region decreases steadily with aging (Livne et al. 1985). Prechondroblasts are the sole source of daughter cells in the fibrocartilages of the mandibular condyle and temporal bone (Livne et al. 1989). With aging there is also a progressive loss of cartilaginous matrix from these fibrocartilages. The cartilaginous matrix is gradually replaced with fibrous tissue that is sparsely populated with cells. Degenerative changes that occur in increasing frequency with age probably reflect the reduced synthetic capacity of these aged tissues.

OTHER FACTORS

Levine et al. have suggested that sympathetic innervation may influence neurogenically mediated inflammatory responses (Levine et al. 1987). These investigators have provided evidence that conditions that reduce sympathetic tone can significantly decrease the severity of experimentally induced arthritis. It is conceivable from this model that heightened sympathetic tone (i.e., related to pain, psychological stress, etc.) could contribute to advancing degenerative joint disease. These factors may obviously aggravate a deteriorating condition by increasing mechanical loading of the joint (i.e., increased muscle activity). Other factors that may influence the adaptive capacity of the TMJ include diet, cigarette smoking (Miao et al. 1992), previous joint trauma (including surgical), and systemic illness (i.e., collagen vascular diseases, diabetes, etc.).

CONCLUSIONS AND FUTURE DIRECTIONS

In summary, the molecular events that may underlie TMJ remodeling and degenerative disease are complex and poorly understood. Structural changes that have been associated with articular disk displacement in the TMJ may be the result of a series of cascading molecular events that include neuropeptide synthesis and release, generation of free radicals, cytokine synthesis, increased arachidonic acid metabolism, activation of matrix-degrading enzymes, inhibition and/or reduced synthesis of protease inhibitors, and altered cell-extracellular matrix interactions (Fig. 2). These molecular events ultimately affect the structural and molecular composition of the affected tissue(s). Furthermore, these processes are probably modulated by other factors including sex hormones and psychological stress. For these reasons, some persons may experience a severe degenerative response to a physical stress imposed on the TMJ

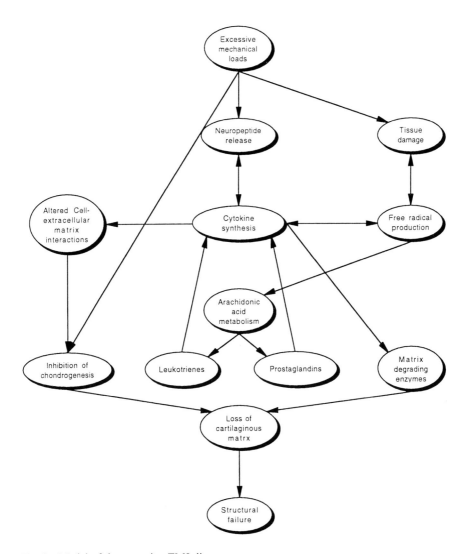

Fig. 2. Model of degenerative TMJ disease.

(i.e., articular disk displacement). Alternatively, other persons, given a similar insult, can apparently mount an adaptive response and not exhibit signs of significant TMJ disease.

Future studies of the TMJ are required to provide specific criteria that can reliably distinguish between adaptation and disease. Animal models of degenerative TMJ disease may provide some information, but these models have significant limitations. However, with the recent developments in molecular biology, it may be possible to conduct sophisticated clinical studies. For example, reverse transcription polymerase chain reaction (Chen and Klebe 1993) and immuno-polymerase chain reaction (Sano et al. 1992) methods allow for the quantitation of mRNA and protein, respectively, from extremely small tissue samples. In fact, these methods are so sensitive that they allow for the quantitation of moderately expressed proteins produced by a single cell. Samples obtained by arthrocentesis, for example, could be examined for the expression of molecules that could be used as markers for disease or for response to therapeutic intervention.

It is likely that nonsurgical approaches to the management of temporomandibular disorders will develop as a result of our understanding of the molecular events that underlie disease processes affecting the TMJ. Agents will probably be developed that will positively influence both catabolic and anabolic processes. However, defining those conditions that require intervention therapy will undoubtedly be the greatest challenge facing future researchers in the field.

REFERENCES

Abubaker, A.O., Raslan, W.F. and Sotereanos, G.C., Estrogen and progesterone receptors in temporomandibular joint discs of symptomatic and asymptomatic persons: a preliminary study, J. Oral Maxillofac. Surg., 51 (1993) 1096–1100.

Adams, C.D., Meikle, M.C., Norwick, K.W. and Turpin, D.L., Dentofacial remodeling produced by intermaxillary forces in *Macaca mulatta*, Arch. Oral Biol., 17 (1972) 1519–1535.

Ala, Y., Palluy, O., Favero, J., Bonne, C., Modat, G. and Dornand, J., Hypoxia/reoxygenation stimulates endothelial cells to promote interleukin-1 and interleukin-6 production: effects of free radical scavengers, Agents Actions, 37 (1992) 134–139.

Annandale, T., On displacement of the interarticular cartilage of the lower jaw and its treatment by operation, Lancet, 1 (1887) 411.

Aufdemorte, T.B., Van Sickels, J.E., Dolwick, M.F., Sheridan, P.J., Holt, G.R., Aragon, S.B. and Gates, G.A., Estrogen receptors in the temporomandibular joint of the baboon (*Papio cynocephalus*): an autoradiographic study, Oral Surg. Oral Med. Oral Pathol., 61 (1986) 307–314.

Axelsson, S., Human and experimental osteoarthrosis of the temporomandibular joint: morphological and biochemical studies, Swed. Dent. J., 92 (1993) 1–45.

Axelsson, S., Fitins, D., Hellsing, G. and Holmlund, A., Arthrotic changes and deviation in form of the temporomandibular joint: an autopsy study, Swed. Dent. J., 11 (1987) 195–200.

Axelsson, S., Holmlund, A. and Hjerpe, A., An experimental model of osteoarthrosis in the temporomandibular joint of the rabbit, Acta Odontol. Scand., 50 (1992) 273–280.

Ben, A.Y., von der Mark, K, Franzen, A., de Bernard, B., Lunazzi, G.C. and Silbermann, M., Immunohistochemical studies of the extracellular matrix in the condylar cartilage of the human fetal mandible: collagens and noncollagenous proteins, Am. J. Anat., 190 (1991) 157–166.

Ben, A.Y., Lewinson, D. and Silbermann, M., Structural characterization of the mandibular condyle in human fetuses: light and electron microscopy studies, Acta Anat., 145 (1992) 79–87.

Bender, S., Haubeck, H.D., Van de Leur, E., Dufhues, G., Schiel, X., Lauwerijns, J., Greiling, H. and Heinrich, P.C., Interleukin-1 beta induces synthesis and secretion of interleukin-6 in human chondrocytes, FEBS Lett., 263 (1990) 321–324.

Bissell, M.J., Hall, H.G. and Parry, G., How does the extracellular matrix direct gene expression? J. Theor. Biol., 99 (1982) 31–68.

Blackwood, H.J.J., Cellular remodeling in articular tissue, J. Dent. Res., 45 (1966) 480–489.

Blake, D.R., Unsworth, J., Outhwaite, J.M., Morris, C.J., Merry, P., Kidd, B.L., Ballard, R., Gray, L. and Lunec, J., Hypoxic-reperfusion injury in the inflammed human joint, Lancet, 1 (1989) 288–293.0

Blaustein, D.I. and Scapino, R.P., Remodeling of the temporomandibular joint disk and posterior attachment in disk displacement specimens in relation to glycosaminoglycans content, Plast. Reconstr. Surg., 78 (1986) 756–764.

Block, M.S. and Bouvier, M., Adaptive remodeling of the rabbit temporomandibular joint following discectomy and dietary variations, J. Oral Maxillofac. Surg., 48 (1990) 482–486.

Boyd, R.L., Gibbs, C.H., Mahan, P.E., Richmond, A.F. and Laskin, J.L., Temporomandibular joint forces measured at the condyle of *Macaca arctoides*, Am. J. Orthod. Dentofacial Orthop., 97 (1990) 472–479.

Brandt, K.D. and Radin, E., The physiology of articular stress: osteoarthrosis, Hosp. Pract., Jan. 15 (1987) 103–126.

Breitner, C., Bone changes resulting from experimental orthodontic treatment, Am. J. Orthod., 26 (1940) 521–547.

Breitner, C., Further investigations of bone changes resulting from experimental orthodontic treatment, Am. J. Orthod., 27 (1941) 605–632.

Burkhardt, H., Schwingel, M., Meninger, H., McCartney, H. W. and Tschesche, H., Oxygen radicals as effectors of cartilage destruction: direct degradative effect on matrix components and indirect action via activation of latent collagenase from polymorphonuclear leukocytes, Arthritis Rheum., 29 (1986) 379–387.

Buttle, D.J. and Saklatvala, J., Lysosomal cysteine endopeptidases mediate interleukin-1 stimulated cartilage proteoglycan degradation, Biochem. J., 287 (1992) 657–661.

Campbell, I.K., Piccoli, D.S., Butler, D.M., Singleton, D.K. and Hamilton, J.A., Recombinant human interleukin-1 stimulates human articular cartilage to undergo resorption and human chondrocytes to produce both tissue and urokinase-type plasminogen activator, Biochim. Biophys. Acta, 967 (1988) 183–194.

Campbell, I.K., Piccoli, D.S. and Hamilton, J.A., Stimulation of human chondrocyte prostaglandin E2 production by recombinant human interleukin-1 and tumour necrosis factor, Biochim. Biophys. Acta, 1051 (1990a) 310–318.

Campbell, I.K., Piccoli, D.S., Roberts, M.J., Muirden, K.D. and Hamilton, J.A., Effects of tumor necrosis factor alpha and beta on resorption of human articular cartilage and production of plasminogen activator by human articular chondrocytes, Arthritis Rheum., 33 (1990b) 542–552.

Campbell, I.K., Waring, P., Novak, U. and Hamilton, J.A., Production of leukemia inhibitory factor by human articular chondrocytes and cartilage in response to interleukin-1 and tumor necrosis factor alpha, Arthritis Rheum., 36 (1993) 790–794.

Carlson, D.S., McNamara, J.A. and Jaul, D.H., Histological analysis of the growth of the mandibular condyle in the rhesus monkey (*Macaca mulatta*), Am. J. Anat., 151 (1978) 103–118.

Castelli, W.A., Nasjleti, C.E., Diaz, P.R. and Caffesse, R.G., Histopathologic findings in temporomandibular joints of aged individuals, J. Prosthet. Dent., 53 (1985) 415–419.

Chandra, H. and Symons, M.C.R., Sulphur radicals formed by cutting α-keratin, Nature, 328 (1987) 833–834.

Chang, J., Gilman, S.C. and Lewis, A.J., Interleukin 1 activates phospholipase A2 in rabbit chondrocytes: a possible signal for IL-1 action, J. Immunol., 136 (1986) 1283–1287.

Chang, J.S., Quinn, J.M., Demaziere, A., Bulstrode, C.J., Francis, M.J., Duthie, R.B. and Athanasou, N.A., Bone resorption by cells isolated from rheumatoid synovium, Ann. Rheum. Dis., 51 (1992) 1223–1229.

Charlier, J.-P., Petrovic, A. and Hermann-Stuzmann, J., Effects of mandibular hyperpropulsion on the prechondroblastic zone of young rat condyle, Am. J. Orthod., 55 (1969) 71–74.

Chen, D. and Klebe, R.J., Controls for validation of relative reverse transcription polymerase chain reaction assays, PCR Methods Appl., 3 (1993) 127–129.

Chevalier, X., Fibronectin, cartilage, and osteoarthritis, Semin. Arthritis Rheum., 22 (1993) 307–318.

Copray, J.C., Brouwer, N., Prins, A.P. and Jansen, H.W., Effects of polypeptide growth factors on mandibular condylar cartilage of the rat in vitro, J. Biol. Buccale., 16 (1988a) 109–117.

Copray, J.C., Dibbets, J.M. and Kantomaa, T., The role of condylar cartilage in the development of the temporomandibular joint, Angle Orthod., 58 (1988b) 369–380.

Corbett, J.A., Wang, J.L., Sweetland, M.A., Lancaster, J.J. and McDaniel, M.L., Interleukin 1 beta induces the formation of nitric oxide by beta-cells purified from rodent islets of Langerhans. Evidence for the beta-cell as a source and site of action of nitric oxide, J. Clin. Invest., 90 (1992) 2384–2391.

Cruz, T.F., Kandel, R.A. and Brown, I.R., Interleukin 1 induces the expression of a heat-shock gene in chondrocytes, Biochem. J., 277 (1991) 327–330.

Cutolo, M., Accardo, S., Villaggio, B., Clerico, P., Bagnasco, M., Coviello, D.A., Carruba, G., Lo Casto, M. and Castagnetta, L., Presence of estrogen-binding sites on macrophage-like synoviocytes and CD8+, CD29+, CD45RO+ T lymphocytes in normal and rheumatoid synovium, Arthritis Rheum., 36 (1993) 1087–1097.

Davies, M.E., Horner, A., Franz, B. and Schuberth, H.J., Detection of cytokine activated chondrocytes in arthritic joints from pigs infected with *Erysipelothrix rhusiopathiae*, Ann. Rheum. Dis., 51 (1992) 978–982.

Dean, D.D., Martel-Pelletier, J., Pelletier, J.-P., Howell, D.S. and Woessner, J.F.J., Evidence for metalloproteinase and metalloproteinase inhibitor imbalance in human osteoarthritic cartilage, J. Clin. Invest., 84 (1989) 678–685.

de Bont, L.G.M. and Stegenga, B., Pathology of temporomandibular joint internal derangement and osteoarthrosis., Int. J. Oral Maxillofac. Surg., 22 (1993) 71–74.

de Bont, L.G.B., Boering, G., Liem, R.S.B., Eulderink, F. and Westesson, P.-L., Osteoarthritis and internal derangement of the temporomandibular joint: a light microscopic study, J. Oral Maxillofac. Surg., 44 (1986) 634–643.

Dedhar, S., Regulation of expression of the cell adhesion receptors, integrins, by recombinant human interleukin-1beta in human osteosarcoma cells: inhibition of cell proliferation and stimulation of alkaline phosphatase activity, J. Cell. Physiol., 138 (1989) 291–299.

DeMarco, D., Kunkel, S.L., Strieter, R.M., Basha, M. and Zurier, R.B., Interleukin-1 induced gene expression of neutrophil activating protein (interleukin-8) and monocyte chemotactic peptide in human synovial cells, Biochem. Biophys. Res. Commun., 174 (1991) 411–416.

Elford, P.R. and Cooper, P.H., Induction of neutrophil-mediated cartilage degradation by interleukin-8, Arthritis Rheum., 34 (1991) 325–332.

Farrar, W.B. and McCarty, W.J., Inferior joint space arthrography and characteristics of condylar paths in internal derangements of the TMJ, J. Prosthet. Dent., 41 (1979) 548–555.

Faulkner, M.G., Hatcher, D.C. and Hay, A., A three-dimensional investigation of temporomandibular joint loading, J. Biomech., 20 (1987) 997–1002.

Freidin, M. and Kessler, J.A., Cytokine regulation of substance P expression in sympathetic neurons, Proc. Natl. Acad. Sci. USA, 88 (1991) 3200–3203.

Fritton Jackson, S., Enviromental control of macromolecular synthesis in cartilage and bone, Proc. R. Soc. Lond. (Biol.), Series B, 175 (1970) 131–133.

Gay, T., Bertolami, C.N., Donoff, R.B., Keith, D.A. and Kelly, J.P., The acoustical characteristics of the normal and abnormal temporomandibular joint, J. Oral Maxillofac. Surg., 45 (1987) 397–407.

Georgopoulos, C. and Welch, W.J., Role of the major heat shock proteins as molecular chaperones, Ann. Rev. Cell. Biol., 9 (1993) 601–634.

Gilman, S.C., Chang, J., Zeigler, P.R., Uhl, J. and Mochan, E., Interleukin-1 activates phospholipase A2 in human synovial cells, Arthritis Rheum., 31 (1988) 126–130.

Glukhova, M.A. and Thiery, J.P., Fibronectin and integrins in development, Semin. Cancer Biol., 4 (1993) 241–249.

Goldring, M.B., Birkhead, J., Sandell, L.J., Kimura, T. and Krane, S.M., Interleukin 1 suppresses expression of cartilage-specific types II and IX collagens and increases type I and III collagens in human chondrocytes, J. Clin. Invest., 82 (1988) 2026–2037.

Goldring, M.B., Sohbat, E., Elwell, J.M. and Chang, J.Y., Etodolac preserves cartilage-specific phenotype in human chondrocytes: effects on type II collagen synthesis and associated mRNA levels, Eur. J. Rheumatol. Inflamm., 10 (1990) 10–21.

Hamerman, D., The biology of osteoarthritis, N. Engl. J. Med., 320 (1989) 1322–1330.

Hamilton, J.A., Waring, P.M. and Filonzi, E.L., Induction of leukemia inhibitory factor in human synovial fibroblasts by IL-1 and tumor necrosis factor-alpha, J. Immunol., 150 (1993) 1496–1502.

Hart, R.P., Shadiack, A.M. and Jonakait, G.M., Substance P gene expression is regulated by interleukin-1 in cultured sympathetic ganglia, J. Neurosci. Res., 29 (1991) 282–291.

Haskell, B., Day, M. and Tetz, J., Computer-aided modeling in the assessment of the biomechanical determinants of diverse skeletal patterns, Amer. J. Orthod., 89 (1986) 363–382.

Haskin, C.L., Athanasiou, K.A., Klebe, R. and Cameron, I.L., A heat-shock-like response with cytoskeletal disruption occurs following hydrostatic pressure in MG-63 osteosarcoma cells, Biochem. Cell. Biol., 71 (1993) 361–371.

Heinegard, D. and Hascall, V.C., Aggregation of cartilage proteoglycans. III. Characteristics of the proteins isolated from trypsin digests of aggregates, J. Biol. Chem., 249 (1974) 4250–4257.

Heinegard, D. and Saxne, T., Macromolecular markers in joint disease, J. Rheumatol., 27 (1991) 27–29.

Helmy, E., Bays, R. and Sharawy, M., Osteoarthrosis of the temporomandibular joint following experimental disc perforation in *Macaca fascicularis*, J. Oral Maxillofac. Surg., 46 (1988) 979–990.

Helmy, E.S., Bays, R.A. and Sharawy, M.M., Histopathological study of human TMJ perforated discs with emphasis on synovial membrane response, J. Oral Maxillofac. Surg., 47 (1989) 1048–1052.

Hinton, R.J., Effect of condylotomy on DNA synthesis in cells of the mandibular condylar cartilage in the rat, Arch. Oral Biol., 32 (1987) 865–872.

Hinton, R.J., Effect of condylotomy on matrix synthesis and mineralization in the rat mandibular condylar cartilage, Arch. Oral Biol., 34 (1989) 1003–1009.

Hinton, R.J., Jaw protruder muscles and condylar cartilage growth in the rat, Amer. J. Orthod. Dentofacial Orthop., 100 (1991) 436–442.

Hinton, R.J., Alterations in rat condylar cartilage following discectomy, J. Dent. Res., 71 (1992) 1292–1297.

Holmlund, A., Ekblom, A., Hansson, P., Lind, J., Lundeberg, T. and Theodorsson, E., Concentrations of neuropeptides substance P, neurokinin A, calcitonin gene-related peptide, neuropeptide Y and vasoactive intestinal polypeptide in synovial fluid of the human temporomandibular joint: a correlation with symptoms, signs and arthroscopic findings, Int. J. Oral Maxillofac. Surg., 20 (1991) 228–231.

Hylander, W. L., Functional anatomy. In: B.G. Sarnat and D.M. Laskin (Eds.), The Temporomandibular Joint: A Biological Basis for Clinical Practice, 4th ed. W.B. Saunders, Philadelphia, 1992, pp. 60–92.

Ichikawa, H., Wakisaka, S., Matsuo, S. and Akai, M., Peptidergic innervation of the temporomandibular disk in the rat, Experientia, 45 (1989) 303–304.

Isacsson, G., Isberg, A. and Persson, A., Loss of directional orientation control of lower jaw movements in persons with internal derangement of the temporomandibular joint, Oral Surg. Oral Med. Oral Pathol., 66 (1988) 8–12.

Isberg, A., Widmalm, S.E. and Ivarsson, R., Clinical, radiographic, and electromyographic study of patients with internal derangement of the temporomandibular joint, Am. J. Orthod., 88 (1985) 453–460.

Johansson, A.-S., Isacson, G., Isberg, A. and Granholm, A.-C., Distribution of substance P-like immunoreactive nerve fibers in temporomandibular joint soft tissues of monkey, Scand. J. Dent. Res., 94 (1986) 225–230.

Joho, J.-P., The effects of extraoral low-pull traction to the mandibular dentition of *Macaca mulatta*, Am. J. Orthod., 64 (1973) 555–577.

Jonakait, G.M. and Schotland, S., Conditioned medium from activated splenocytes increases substance P in sympathetic ganglia, J. Neurosci. Res., 26 (1990) 24–30.

Jonakait, G.M., Schotland, S. and Hart, R.P., Interleukin-1 specifically increases substance P in injured sympathetic ganglia, Ann. N.Y. Acad. Sci., 594 (1990) 222–230.

Jonakait, G.M., Schotland, S. and Hart, R.P., Effects of lymphokines on substance P in injured ganglia of the peripheral nervous system, Ann. N.Y. Acad. Sci., 632 (1991) 19–30.

Kawamura, H., Qujada, J.G., Throckmorton, G.S. and Bell, W.H., Temporomandibular joint adaptation following inferior repositioning of the maxilla in adult monkeys, Cranio, 10 (1992) 51–58.

Kempson, G.E., Muir, H., Swanson, S.A.V. and Freeman, M.A.R., Correlations between the compressive stiffness and chemical constituents of human articular cartilage, Biochim. Biophys. Acta, 215 (1970) 70–76.

Kido, M.A., Kiyoshima, T., Kondo, T., Ayasaka, N., Moroi, R., Terada, Y. and Tanaka, T., Distribution of substance P and calcitonin gene-related peptide–like immunoreactive nerve fibers in the rat temporomandibular joint, J. Dent. Res., 72 (1993) 592–598.

Kimball, E.S., Substance P, cytokines, and arthritis, Ann. N.Y. Acad. Sci., 594 (1990) 293–308.

Kimball, E.S., Persico, F.J. and Vaught, J.L., Substance P, neurokinin A, and neurokinin B induce generation of IL-1-like activity in P388D1 cells. Possible relevance to arthritic disease, J. Immunol., 141 (1988) 3564–3569.

Kurita, K., Bronstein, S.L., Westesson, P.-L. and Sternby, N.H., Arthroscopic diagnosis of perforation and adhesions of the temporomandibular joint: correlation with postmortem morphology, Oral Surg. Oral Med. Oral Pathol., 68 (1989a) 130–134.

Kurita, K., Westesson, P.-L., Sternby, N.H., Eriksson, L., Carlsson, L.E., Lundh, H. and Toremalm, N.G., Histologic features of the temporomandibular joint disk and posterior disk attachment: comparison of symptom-free persons with normally positioned disks and patients with internal derangement, Oral Surg. Oral Med. Oral Pathol., 67 (1989b) 635–643.

Lang, T.C., Zimny, M.L. and Vijayagopal, P., Experimental temporomandibular joint disc perforation in the rabbit: a gross morphologic, biochemical, and ultrastructural analysis, J. Oral. Maxillofac. Surg., 51 (1993) 1115–1128.

Lanz, W., Discitis mandibularis, Zentralbl. Chir., 36 (1909) 289–291.

Laurenzi, M.A., Persson, M.A., Dalsgaard, C.J. and Haegerstrand, A., The neuropeptide substance P stimulates production of interleukin 1 in human blood monocytes: activated cells are preferentially influenced by the neuropeptide, Scand. J. Immunol., 31 (1990) 529–533.

Levine, J.D., Goetzl, E.J. and Basbaum, A.I., Contribution of the nervous system to the pathophysiology of rheumatoid arthritis and other polyarthritides, Rheum. Dis. Clin. North Am., 13 (1987) 369–381.

Li, Z.G., Danis, V.A. and Brooks, P.M., Effect of gonadal steroids on the production of IL-1 and IL-6 by blood mononuclear cells in vitro, Clin. Exp. Rheumatol., 11 (1993) 157–162.

Liedberg, J. and Westesson, P.-L., Sideways position of the temporomandibular joint disk: coronal cryosectioning of fresh autopsy specimens, Oral Surg. Oral Med. Oral Pathol., 66 (1988) 644–649.

Liedberg, J., Westesson, P.-L. and Kurita, K., Sideways and rotational displacement of the temporomandibular joint disk: diagnosis by arthrography and correlation to cryosectional morphology, Oral Surg. Oral Med. Oral Pathol., 69 (1990) 757–763.

Livne, E., von der Mark, K. and Silbermann, M., Morphological and cytological changes in maturing and osteoarthritic articular cartilage in the temporomandibular joint of mice, Arthritis Rheum., 28 (1985) 1027–1038.

Livne, E., Weiss, A. and Silbermann, M., Articular chondrocytes lose their proliferative activity with aging yet can be restimulated by PTH-(1-84), PGE1, and dexamethasone, J. Bone Miner. Res., 4 (1989) 539–548.

Lohmander, L.S., Neame, P.J. and Sandy, J.D., The structure of aggrecan fragments in human synovial fluid: evidence that aggrecanase mediates cartilage degradation in inflammatory joint disease, joint injury, and osteoarthritis, Arthritis Rheum., 36 (1993) 1214–1222.

Lotz, M., Vaughan, J.H. and Carson, D.A., Effect of neuropeptides on production of inflammatory cytokines by human monocytes, Science, 241 (1988) 1218–1221.

Macher, D.J., Westesson, P.-L., Brooks, S.L., Hicks, D.G. and Tallents, R.H., Temporomandibular joint: surgically created disk displacement causes arthrosis in the rabbit, Oral Surg. Oral Med. Oral Pathol., 73 (1992) 645–649.

Mankin, H.J. and Lippiello, L., The glycosaminoglycans of normal and arthritic cartilage, J. Clin. Invest., 50 (1971) 1712–1719.

McCachren, S.S., Expression of metalloproteinases and metalloproteinase inhibitor in human arthritic synovium, Arthritis Rheum., 34 (1991) 1085–1093.

McCord, J.M., Free radicals and inflammation: protection of synovial fluid by superoxide dismutase, Science, 185 (1974) 529–531.

McCord, J.M., Oxygen-derived free radicals in postischemic tissue injury, N. Engl. J. Med., 312 (1985) 159–163.

McCord, J.M. and Fridovich, I., The reduction of cytochrome c by milk xanthine oxidase, J. Biol. Chem., 243 (1968) 5753–5760.

McNamara, J.J. and Carlson, D.S., Quantitative analysis of temporomandibular joint adaptations to protrusive function, Am. J. Orthod., 76 (1979) 593–611.

Meikle, M.C., Remodeling, In: B.G. Sarnat and D.M. Laskin (Eds.), The Temporomandibular Joint: A Biological Basis for Clinical Practice, 4th ed., W.B. Saunders, Philadelphia, 1992, pp. 93–107.

Miao, F.J., Benowitz, N.L., Basbaum, A.I. and Levine, J.D., Sympathoadrenal contribution to nicotinic and muscarinic modulation of bradykinin-induced plasma extravasation in the knee joint of the rat, J. Pharmacol. Exp. Ther., 262 (1992) 889–895.

Milam, S.B., Cell-extracellular matrix interactions with special emphasis on the primate temporomandibular joint, Ph.D. diss., University of Texas Health Science Center, 1990.

Milam, S.B., Aufdemorte, T.B., Sheridan, P.J., Triplett, R.G., Van Sickels, J.E. and Holt, G.R., Sexual dimorphism in the distribution of estrogen receptors in the temporomandibular joint complex of the baboon, Oral Surg. Oral Med. Oral Pathol., 64 (1987) 527–532.

Milam, S.B., Haskin, C., Zardeneta, G., Chen, D., Magnuson, V.L., Klebe, R.J. and Steffenson, B., Cell adhesion proteins in oral biology, Crit. Rev. Oral Biol. Med., 2 (1991a) 451–491.

Milam, S.B., Klebe, R. J., Triplett, R.G.and Herbert, D., Characterization of the extracellular matrix of the primate temporomandibular joint, J. Oral Maxillofac. Surg., 49 (1991b) 381–391.

Milam, S.B., Magnuson, V.L., Steffensen, B., Chen, D. and Klebe, R.J., IL-1 beta and prostaglandins regulate integrin mRNA expression, J. Cell Physiol., 149 (1991c) 173–183.

Moffett, B.C., Johnson, L.C., McCabe, J.B. and Askew, H.C., Articular remodeling in the adult human temporomandibular joint, Am. J. Anat., 115 (1964) 119–142.

Muir, H., Maroudas, A. and Wingham, J., The correlation of fixed negative charge with glycosaminoglycan content of human articular cartilage, Biochim. Biophys. Acta, 177 (1969) 494–499.

Nannmark, U., Sennerby, L. and Haraldson, T., Macroscopic, microscopic and radiologic assessment of the condylar part of the TMJ in elderly subjects: an autopsy study, Swed. Dent. J., 14 (1990) 163–169.

Nitzan, D.W., Intraarticular pressure in the functioning human temporomandibular joint and its alteration by uniform elevation of the occlusal plane, J. Oral Maxillofac. Surg., 52 (1994) 671–679.

O'Byrne, E.M., Blancuzzi, V.J., Wilson, D.E., Wong, M., Peppard, J., Simke, J.P. and Jeng, A.Y., Increased intra-articular substance P and prostaglandin E2 following injection of interleukin-1 in rabbits, Int. J. Tissue React., 12 (1990) 11–14.

Pennypacker, J. P., Modulation of chondrogenic expression in cell culture by fibronectin, Vision Res., 21 (1981) 65–69.

Pennypacker, J. P., Hassell, J. R., Yamada, K. M. and Pratt, R. M., The influence of an adhesive cell surface protein on chondrogenic expression in vitro, Exp. Cell Res., 121 (1979) 411–415.

Petrovic, A., Mechanisms and regulation of mandibular condylar growth, Acta Morph. Neerl. Scand., 10 (1972) 25–34.

Pickvance, E.A., Oegema, T.J. and Thompson, R.J., Immunolocalization of selected cytokines and proteases in canine articular cartilage after transarticular loading, J. Orthop. Res., 11 (1993) 313–323.

Pirttiniemi, P., Kantomaa, T., Tuominen, M. and Salo, L., Articular disc and eminence modeling after experimental relocation of the glenoid fossa in growing rabbits, J. Dent. Res., 73 (1994) 536–543.

Poole, A.R., Rizkalla, G., Ionescu, M., Reiner, A., Brooks, E., Rorabeck, C., Bourne, R. and Bogoch, E., Osteoarthritis in the human knee: a dynamic process of cartilage matrix degradation, synthesis and reorganization, Agents Actions, 39 (1993) 3–13.

Pringle, J.H., Displacement of the mandibular meniscus and its treatment, Br. J. Surg., 6 (1918) 385–389.

Quinn, J.H., Pain mediators and chondromalacia in internally deranged temporomandibular joints. In: W. Bell (Ed.), Modern Practice in Orthognathic and Reconstructive Surgery, W.B. Saunders, Philadelphia, 1992, pp. 471–481.

Rohlin, M., Westesson, P.L. and Eriksson, L., The correlation of temporomandibular joint sounds with joint morphology in fifty-five autopsy specimens, J. Oral Maxillofac. Surg., 43 (1985) 194–200.

Rosner, I.A., Goldberg, V.M., Getzy, L. and Moskowitz, R.W., Effects of estrogen on cartilage and experimentally induced osteoarthritis, Arthritis Rheum., 22 (1979) 52–58.

Rossomando, E.F., White, L.B., Hadjimichael, J. and Shafer, D., Immunomagnetic separation of tumor necrosis factor alpha. I. Batch procedure for human temporomandibular fluid, J. Chromatogr., 583 (1992) 11–18.

Ruoslahti, E., Integrins, J. Clin. Invest., 87 (1991) 1–5.

Salo, L. and Kantomaa, T., Type II collagen expression in the mandibular condyle during growth adaptation: an experimental study in the rabbit, Calcif. Tissue Int. 52 (1993) 465–469.

Sandy, J.D., Barrach, H.-J., Flannery, C.R. and Plaas, A.H.S., The biosynthetic response of the mature chondrocyte in early osteoarthritis, J. Rheum., 14 (1987) 16–19.

Sano, T., Smith, C.L. and Cantor, C.R., Immuno-PCR: very sensitive antigen detection by means of specific antibody-DNA conjugates, Science, 258 (1992) 120–122.

Saxne, T., Glennas, A., Kvien, T.K., Melby, K. and Heinegard, D., Release of cartilage macromolecules into the synovial fluid in patients with acute and prolonged phases of reactive arthritis, Arthritis Rheum., 36 (1993) 20–25.

Scapino, R.P., The posterior attachment: its structure, function, and appearance in TMJ imaging studies, Part 1, J. Craniomand. Dis., 5 (1991) 83–95.

Shadiack, A.M., Hart, R.P., Carlson, C.D. and Jonakait, G.M., Interleukin-1 induces substance P in sympathetic ganglia through the induction of leukemia inhibitory factor (LIF), J. Neurosci., 13 (1993) 2601–2609.

Shafer, D., Rossomando, E., White, L., Assael, L. and Rogerson, K., Clinical implications of TNF-alpha in synovial fluid from TMJs, J. Dent. Res., 71 (1992) 621.

Silbermann, M. and Frommer, J., Dynamic changes in acid mucopolysaccharides during mineralization of the mandibular condylar cartilage, Histochemistry, 36 (1973) 185–192.

Silbermann, M. and von der Mark, K., An immunohistochemical study of the distribution of matrical proteins in the mandibular condyle of neonatal mice. I. Collagens, J. Anat., 170 (1990) 11–22.

Silbermann, M., Reddi, A.H., Hand, A.R., Leapman, R.D., Von, der, Mark, K. and Franzen, A., Further characterisation of the extracellular matrix in the mandibular condyle in neonatal mice, J. Anat., 151 (1987) 169–188.

Solberg, W.K., Hansson, T.L. and Nordström, B., The temporomandibular joint in young adults at autopsy: a morphologic classification and evaluation, J. Oral Rehabil., 12 (1985) 303–321.

Stegenga, B., de Bont, L.G.M. and Boering, G., Osteoarthrosis as the cause of craniomandibular pain and dysfunction: a unifying concept, J. Oral Maxillofac. Surg., 47 (1989) 249–256.

Stegenga, B., Dijkstra, P.U., de Bont, L.G.M. and Boering, G., Temporomandibular joint osteoarthrosis and internal derangement. Part II: Additional treatment options, Int. Dent. J., 40 (1990) 347–353.

Stegenga, B., de Bont, L.G.M., Boering, G. and van Willigen, J.D., Tissue responses to degenerative changes in the temporomandibular joint: a review, J. Oral Maxillofac. Surg., 49 (1991) 1079–1088.

Stegenga, B., de Bont, L.G.M., van der Kuijl, B and Boering, G., Classification of temporomandibular joint osteoarthrosis and internal derangement. 1. Diagnostic significance of clinical and radiographic symptoms and signs, Cranio, 10 (1992) 96–106.

Strauss, P.G., Closs, E.I., Schmidt, J. and Erfle, V., Gene expression during osteogenic differentiation in mandibular condyles in vitro, J. Cell. Biol., 110 (1990) 1369–1378.

Sutton, D.I., Sadowsky, P.L., Bernreuter, W.K., McCutcheon, M.J. and Lakshminarayanan, A.V., Temporomandibular joint sounds and condyle/disk relations on magnetic resonance images, Amer. J. Orthod. Dentofacial Orthop., 101 (1992) 70–78.

Suzuki, K., Shimizu, K., Hamamoto, T., Nakagawa, Y., Murachi, T. and Yamamoro, T., Characterization of proteoglycan degradation by calpain, Biochem. J., 285 (1992) 857–862.

Symons, N.B., A histochemical study of the secondary cartilage of the mandibular condyle in the rat, Arch. Oral Biol., 10 (1965) 579–584.

Takano-Yamamoto, T., Soma, S., Nakagawa, K., Kobayashi, Y., Kawakami, M. and Sakuda, M., Comparison of the effects of hydrostatic compressive force on glycosaminoglycan synthesis and proliferation in rabbit chondrocytes from mandibular condylar cartilage, nasal septum, and spheno-occipital synchondrosis in vitro, Am. J. Orthod. Dentofacial Orthop., 99 (1991) 448–455.

Throckmorton, G.S., Groshan, G.J. and Boyd, S.B., Muscle activity patterns and control of temporomandibular joint loads, J. Prosthet. Dent., 63 (1990) 685–695.

Tuominen, M., Kantomaa, T. and Pirttiniemi, P., Effect of food consistency on the shape of the articular eminence and the mandible: an experimental study on the rabbit, Acta Odontol. Scand., 51 (1993) 65–72.

Verschure, P.J. and Van, N.C., The effects of interleukin–1 on articular cartilage destruction as observed in arthritic diseases, and its therapeutic control, Clin. Exp. Rheumatol., 8 (1990) 303–313.

Vilamitjana, A.J. and Harmand, M.F., Biochemical analysis of normal and osteoarthritic human cartilage, Clin. Physiol. Biochem., 8 (1990) 221–230.

Vincent, F., Corral-Debrinski, M. and Adolphe, M., Transient mitochondrial transcript level decay in oxidative stressed chondrocytes, J. Cell. Physiol., 158 (1994) 128–132.

Ward, D. M., Behrents, R.G. and Goldberg, J.S., Temporomandibular synovial fluid pressure response to altered mandibular positions, Am. J. Orthod. Dentofacial Orthop., 98 (1990) 22–28.

Werb, Z., Tremble, P.M., Behrendtsen, O., Crowley, E. and Damsky, C.H., Signal transduction through the fibronectin receptor induces collagenase and stromelysin gene expression, J. Cell. Biol., 109 (1989) 877–889.

Westesson, P.-L., Structural hard-tissue changes in temporomandibular joints with internal derangement, Oral Surg. Oral Med. Oral Pathol., 59 (1985) 220–224.

Westesson, P.-L. and Brooks, S.L., Temporomandibular joint: relationship between MR evidence of effusion and the presence of pain and disk displacement, Am. J. Roentgenol., 159 (1992) 559–563.

Westesson, P.-L. and Rohlin, M., Internal derangement related to osteoarthrosis in temporomandibular joint autopsy specimens, Oral Surg. Oral Med. Oral Pathol., 57 (1984) 17–22.

Westesson, P.-L., Bronstein, S.L. and Liedberg, J., Internal derangement of the temporomandibular joint: morphologic description with correlation to joint function, Oral Surg. Oral Med. Oral Pathol., 59 (1985) 323–331.

Whyte, A. and Williams, R.O., Bromocriptine suppresses postpartum exacerbation of collagen-induced arthritis, Arthritis Rheum., 31 (1988) 927–928.

Widmalm, S.E., Westesson, P.-L., Brooks, S.L., Hatala, M.P. and Paesani, D., Temporomandibular joint sounds: correlation to joint structure in fresh autopsy specimens, Am. J. Orthod. Dentofacial Orthop., 101 (1992) 60–69.

Xie, D.L., Meyers, R. and Homandberg, G.A., Fibronectin fragments in osteoarthritic synovial fluid, J. Rheumatol., 19 (1992) 1448–1452.

Yaillen, D.M., Shapiro, P.A., Luschei, E.S. and Feldman, G.R., Temporomandibular joint meniscectomy: effects on joint structure and masticatory function in *Macaca fascicularis*, J. Maxillofac. Surg., 7 (1979) 255–64.

Correspondence to: Stephen B. Milam, DDS, PhD, University of Texas Health Science Center, 7703 Floyd Curl Dr., San Antonio, TX 78284-7908, USA. Tel: 210-567-3465; Fax: 210-567-3493.

Temporomandibular Disorders and Related Pain Conditions, Progress in Pain Research and Management, Vol. 4, edited by B.J. Sessle, P.S. Bryant, and R.A. Dionne, IASP Press, Seattle, © 1995.

Reaction Paper to Chapters 5 and 6

Daniel M. Laskin

Department of Oral and Maxillofacial Surgery, Medical College of Virginia, Richmond, Virginia, USA

Dolwick (this volume) stresses several important concepts regarding internal derangements that merit additional emphasis. Moreover, he also raises several questions that should be addressed. Perhaps the most important issue is the need to know the etiology of internal derangements to understand their pathogenesis. Much remains to be learned in this regard, which Milam (this volume) emphasizes by providing a detailed hypothesis concerning how biomechanical alterations can lead to destructive biochemical changes. However, certain causative factors are well established, even though the precise details of how they change the anatomy and biochemistry of the articular structures are not.

The first factor is acute macrotrauma. Depending on the severity of the injury and the direction of the force, there can be damage to the articular surfaces, the discal attachments, or both. When there is articular damage, the resultant degenerative changes can produce an increase in the frictional properties of the joint that eventually leads to an internal derangement. If the trauma results in damage to the discal attachments, patients can also develop alterations in the disk-condyle relationship that lead to immediate clicking and locking. Thus, acute macrotrauma can produce an internal derangement either directly, or indirectly by first inducing degenerative joint changes. Patients with primary myofascial pain and dysfunction can also develop secondary internal derangements. In such cases, the alterations in the articular surfaces produced by chronic clenching and grinding habits (microtrauma) gradually change the frictional properties of the joint and ultimately lead to disk displacement.

An understanding of the effects of micro- and macrotrauma on the temporomandibular joint (TMJ) helps to answer the "chicken and egg" question posed by Dolwick regarding the relationship of degenerative joint disease and internal derangements. Clearly, it depends on what is the "chicken." If it is the degenerative joint disease, the derangement occurs secondarily. If it is the internal derangement (as a result of macrotrauma), then the degenerative joint disease occurs secondarily. In both instances, however, the end result is the same—varying degrees of internal derangement and degenerative disease occur together.

An understanding of the concept of primary and secondary forms of internal derangement makes it easier to explain why some patients with disk displacement have no pain while others have severe pain. If the derangement develops slowly, there is often sufficient time for adaptive changes to occur in the synovium and retrodiscal tissues, and the patient will experience little or no pain. However, an acute change in the disk-condyle relationship usually will be extremely painful due to the lack of time for such adaptations. Other factors influencing the presence or absence of pain, or the degree of severity, are the amount of disk displacement, the direction of displacement, and the extent of parafunctional activity in which the patient engages. As pointed out by Milam, the degree of biochemical change accompanying the derangement also influences the severity of the pain.

Another interesting question raised by Dolwick is whether disk displacement can cause a growth disturbance. Although TMJ clicking and popping are relatively common in children, the incidence of facial deformity is very low and there is limited evidence that these two conditions are associated. When an occasional internal derangement is found in a person with facial asymmetry, the severity of the changes seen in the condyle would suggest traumatic injury rather than altered disk position as the cause, which would more readily explain the associated growth disturbance.

In his review, Dolwick refers to the phenomenon of reciprocal clicking as the first stage of disk displacement, yet clinically, clicks are rarely heard during mouth closure. However, if the patient's joint clicks each time the mouth is opened, the disk must again slip off the condyle during closure. Thus, it is evident that the same changes in disk-condyle relationship occur whether or not a sound is heard. Therefore, use of the term *reciprocal clicking* is confusing, because it appears to imply a clinical significance that does not exist. It would be much better merely to say that clicking on opening is pathognomic of the first stage of disk displacement and that sometimes a closing click can be heard.

Dolwick makes several points that need reemphasis. First, although some patients may progress from one stage of disk derangement to the next, this is not a common occurrence, even in patients who go untreated. Moreover, it is now clear that disk mobility, with its associated effect on joint lubrication, function, and repair, is more important than disk position, and that the structures of the TMJ have an excellent adaptive capacity. It is also evident, as he points out, that anterior disk displacement without reduction is not the only derangement causing locking. Limitation of mouth opening can also be produced by adhesion of the disk to the fossa, resulting in an inability of the condyle to translate, and thereby reducing opening to a hinge movement.

Finally, Dolwick raises the question of what constitutes anterior disk displacement. The presence of the posterior band anterior to the traditional 12 o'clock position in TMJs free of signs and symptoms may represent an early preclinical phase of internal derangement or it may merely be a variation of normal. Longitudinal studies need to be done on such patients to determine which explanation is correct. Until then, however, we need to remember that we treat patients and not radiographic or magnetic resonance images, and that the clinical findings should be the final determinant of therapy.

Correspondence to: Daniel M. Laskin, DDS, MS, Department of Oral and Maxillofacial Surgery, Medical College of Virginia, P.O. Box 980566 MCV Station, Richmond, VA 23298. Tel: 804-828-0602; Fax: 804-828-1753.

Part III

Degenerative and Inflammatory Temporomandibular Joint Disorders

Temporomandibular Disorders and Related Pain Conditions, Progress in Pain Research and Management, Vol. 4, edited by B.J. Sessle, P.S. Bryant, and R.A. Dionne, IASP Press, Seattle, © 1995.

7

Degenerative and Inflammatory Temporomandibular Joint Disorders: Clinical Perspectives

Sigvard Kopp

Department of Clinical Oral Science, Section of Clinical Oral Physiology, School of Dentistry, Karolinska Institutet, Huddinge, Sweden

This chapter reviews inflammatory temporomandibular joint (TMJ) disorders and related pain with clinical perspectives on their pathophysiology. Rheumatoid arthritis (RA) will be dealt with as a representative of the inflammatory joint diseases. The TMJ may be involved with both systemic and local inflammatory joint disorders (IJD) as well as degenerative joint disorders (DJD). RA is the most frequent systemic inflammatory disease that involves the TMJ, but others include psoriatic arthritis, systemic lupus erythematosus, ankylosing spondylitis, and gout. The local inflammatory conditions may be of traumatic or nonspecific origin and the demarcation line toward DJD is not absolutely clear. The severity of TMJ disorders varies considerably between patients, from short periods of slight pain to severe, long-term chronic pain and dysfunction. In some patients with RA (about 10%), permanent damage to the TMJ and dental occlusion also occur.

The first therapeutic goal in DJD as well as IJD of the TMJ is to achieve the best possible control of local pain and inflammation. This is the primary objective in the early acute phase of the diseases, so it is important that the patient be referred to a dental specialist at this stage. The second goal is to prevent the development of permanent destruction of the TMJ and occlusion. This is yet an unsolved problem because there are no effective local treatments. A third goal in the late or chronic phase of the TMJ disorders is to restore permanently damaged occlusion, to restore and maintain mandibular mobility, as well as to restore muscle strength and performance. The inflammatory process in RA and similar systemic diseases often follows a slow, chronic course with progressive destruction of cartilage, bone, and other joint tissues as well as reduced strength of the nearby muscles.

The occurrence of TMJ pain caused by RA involvement depends on the severity of the systemic disease, and according to several clinical investigations, it can be expected that about one-third to one-half of patients with RA will experience pain sometime from this joint (Tegelberg and Kopp 1987). The development of TMJ involvement varies in relation to the progression of the general disease. For more than one-third of the RA patients the TMJ symptoms develop less than one year after the onset of the general disease (Uotila 1964). However, about 40% of patients report TMJ involvement five years or more after the start of the general disease. Bilateral involvement of the TMJ is common, i.e., about 60% of patients with TMJ involvement have bilateral chronic pain condition. Severe forms of the disease with great general functional disability occur in about 10–15% of patients. A similar proportion of patients with TMJ involvement experience severe pain as well as occlusal and functional disability of the masticatory system.

ETIOLOGY

The etiology of RA is still largely unknown, but there is substantial evidence that immunological and neural mechanisms cooperate and play an important role. The development of immune (antigen/antibody) complexes in the joint elicits synovitis, which is considered an immunological disease. The etiology is complex, however, and several other factors, among them genetic, microbial, hormonal, and environmental, participate and modulate the progression of the disease.

PATHOPHYSIOLOGY

RA is a chronic inflammatory disease that may affect the heart, blood vessels, lungs, eyes, skin, muscles, and peripheral nerves as well as joints (arthritis). The progression of arthritis is often relatively slow and episodes of both acute and chronic inflammation occur. The rheumatoid process starts as an inflammatory reaction in the synovial membrane (synovitis) and surrounding connective tissue (capsulitis). Stimulation of T lymphocytes by presentation of an unknown antigen is probably a key event in the initiation of RA. The synovial membrane later becomes hyperplastic and granulomatous owing to release of lymphokines, grows to extend over the articular surfaces, and may destroy the cartilage down to the bone surface and then also the bone.

Interleukin 1 (IL-1) as well as tumor necrosis factor (TNF) directly promote proteoglycan degradation in the synovial joint and production of prostaglandins (PG). PGE_2 increases the sensitivity of the nociceptive receptors (hyperalgesia) in the synovial membrane of the joint. Bone resorption is stimulated by TNF and PGE_2, which are osteoclast-activating. The inflammatory process in RA is not only confined to the joint tissues, but also to the tendons, ligaments, and nearby muscle attachments, which impairs function and weakens the muscles. Healing of the joint inflammation often results in partial and sometimes in complete ankylosis of the joint surfaces and contraction of the joint capsule with deleterious effects on joint mobility.

The progression of the disease in the TMJ follows this general scheme with exudation, cellular infiltration, and pannus formation. The articular surfaces of the temporal and condylar components are destroyed and the disk becomes grossly perforated and the subchondral bone is resorbed. Complete ankylosis of the TMJ seldom occurs, although most persons have reduced mandibular mobility. The progression of RA in the TMJ is slow in most patients, although a few experience severe joint destruction within a few months. The presence of a high erythrocyte sedimentation rate is a negative prognostic factor (Tegelberg et al. 1987).

We have little knowledge about the factors that influence the development of the local inflammatory process, i.e., the development of pain, microcirculatory disturbances, and tissue destruction. However, there is reason to assume that neuropeptides contribute to the local development of joint inflammation and that they might be useful as markers of joint disorder.

NEUROGENIC MECHANISMS

There is now evidence that peripheral terminals of primary afferent nociceptors not only respond to noxious stimuli and produce pain, but also that inflammatory mediators are released from them (Buck et al. 1982). Likewise, the sympathetic nerves of the peripheral nervous system contribute to joint inflammation by increased activity of the postganglionic sympathetic fibers (Koizumi et al. 1970; also see Hargreaves et al., this volume).

Substance P (SP) has a well-documented effect in modulating pain and inflammation and elicits long-lasting hyperalgesia. SP is released from peripheral C-fiber terminals as a result of noxious stimuli. The ensuing neurogenic inflammation that it induces can be interpreted as a defense reaction to remove the causative agent. Receptors for SP are found on many cells, e.g., smooth muscle cells of blood vessels, macrophages, and lymphocytes. SP amplifies experimental adjuvant arthritis in rats (Levine et al. 1984) and activates synoviocytes to secrete PGE_2 (Lotz et al. 1987), which sensitizes the nerve fibers. It also stimulates pannus formation and transformation of muscle into fibrous connective tissue. SP has local effects causing vasodilatation, increased capillary permeability, release of bradykinin, release of histamine from mast cells (Juan and Sametz 1980), secretion by exocrine glands, and interaction with leukocyte function. The concentration of SP is significantly higher in high-risk joints than in low-risk joints prior to onset of experimental arthritis (Levine et al. 1987). Some SP-immunoreactive nerve fibers have been demonstrated in the TMJ capsule, disk attachment, fascia, adjacent periosteum, and in the interfascicular connective tissue of the lateral pterygoid muscle of the monkey (Johansson et al. 1986).

   Calcitonin gene-related peptide (CGRP) also is found in C-fibers (Lundberg et al. 1985) and interacts with SP in mediating pain and local reflex reactions due to sensory nerve activation. It has a vasodilatory effect in joints and muscles, which is several-fold stronger and more long-lasting than that of SP. CGRP does not increase vascular permeability to a similar degree as SP. It has been found in the anterior margin of the TMJ disk, the fibrous tissue around the condyle, and the capsule of the TMJ in the young rat (Ichikawa et al. 1989). Some of the CGRP-containing nerve fibers accompany blood vessels and some branch as free nerve endings. Both CGRP and SP have profound stimulatory effects on mast cells and lymphocytes as well as other types of leukocytes and are thereby able to modulate the immunologic and inflammatory responses (Payan et al. 1986). They also are involved in the regulation of tissue repair by stimulating the proliferation of smooth muscle cells and fibroblasts (Nilsson et al. 1985).

   Sensory nerve endings associated with C-fibers in several organs contain the tachykinin *neurokinin A (NKA)*, which is chemically related to SP and has similar physiologic properties, i.e., vasodilatation and increased vascular permeability. This neuropeptide is found together with SP and CGRP and amplifies nociception. It is also a most potent constrictor of smooth muscle. The effects of NKA in the local development of arthritis are largely unknown and warrant further investigation, but it is known to be released into the spinal cord in cats upon induction of experimental knee joint arthritis (Hope et al. 1990).

   Neuropeptide Y (NPY) is produced together with norepinephrine in certain peripheral sympathetic nerve fibers (Lundberg et al. 1982) and has strong and longstanding vasoconstrictive effect on both arteries and veins. It activates both alpha and beta receptors in the tissues. In adjuvant-induced arthritis of rats, NPY plays , together with SP, an important role as a regulator of the severity of joint inflammation. Increased activity in peripheral nerves of the sympathetic system has thereby been associated with increase in joint pain, inflammation, and destruction (Levine et al. 1986). NPY is located predominantly in perivascular sympathetic nerves of the human synovial membrane (Mapp et al. 1990). In the TMJ of the rat it has been found around blood vessels in the capsule but not in the disk (Ichikawa et al. 1989). NPY has been found in significantly higher concentrations in the synovial fluid of patients with arthritis of the knee than in controls with traumatic or degenerative joint disease (Larsson et al. 1989). It has been found in the TMJ of patients with RA at concentrations well above plasma level (Appelgren et al. 1991). The clinical findings suggest that this neuropeptide also acts as a modulator of pain and inflammatory joint disease in humans.

Mapp and colleagues (1990) investigated the sensory and sympathetic nerve distribution of normal and inflamed human synovial tissue. They did not find immunostaining for NPY, SP, and CGRP in the superficial tissues in synovial membranes during RA, but found it to be weaker in the diseased deeper joint tissues compared with healthy control tissues. The reduced immunostaining might be caused by increased release of the neuropeptides, reducing the stores in the nerves.

TMJ PAIN AND DYSFUNCTION

The subjective symptoms in RA of the TMJ are dominated by pain, both at rest and upon chewing. There is also stiffness in the morning, difficulty in opening the mouth, and sometimes a sensation of swelling. In our laboratory, we found two of the peptides, CGRP and NPY, in high concentrations in the joint fluid of arthritic TMJs with pain (Figs. 1 and 2) and in joints with restricted mobility. SP is probably also involved because its presence is strongly correlated with the presence of both CGRP and NPY.

CIRCULATORY DISTURBANCES

The microcirculation in chronic arthritis is frequently decreased. Acidosis has been found in severely destructed knee joints of persons with RA, which indicates an impairment of the synovial microcirculation in severe forms of this disease (Geborek et al. 1989). The exact mechanisms behind these circulatory changes are unknown, although factors such as inflammation, disuse atrophy (Oka et al. 1971), chronic muscle tension, and vasoconstriction (Håkanson et al. 1986) take part. Recent results indicate that a significant part of the decrease in intra-articular temperature (IAT), and thereby synovial microcirculation in the arthritic TMJ, can be explained by release of NPY in the synovial membrane (Appelgren et al. 1993a). Decrease in IAT combined with increase in joint fluid NPY occurs relatively early in the disease. The mechanisms behind NPY release in joints are unknown, but pain is known to

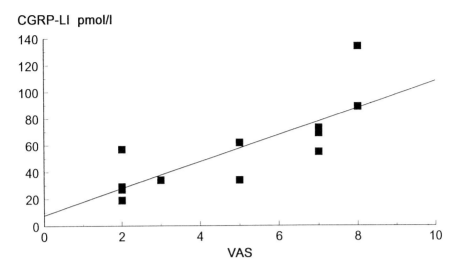

Fig. 1. Relation between CGRP in TMJ fluid and TMJ pain in 13 patients with rheumatoid arthritis ($r = 0.78$, $P < 0.001$); based on visual analog scale (VAS).

activate the sympathetic nervous system. The presence of CGRP in the joint fluid is associated with increased IAT and long duration of the disease (Appelgren et al. 1993b).

TISSUE BREAKDOWN

A feature of severe RA and other inflammatory disorders in the TMJ is a progressive anterior bite opening due to bilateral destruction of the mandibular condyles. The mandible is thereby rotated postero-superiorly around the molar teeth. The destruction of the joints is caused by the inflammation, and is usually, but not always, associated with pain. The open bite may be created in a period of months during an acute episode of the general disease or develop gradually during a chronic course. The amount of joint destruction and the degree of anterior bite opening depend on the severity of the systemic disease and vary considerably between patients. At our clinic we found anterior bite opening to be associated with high concentrations of CGRP and NPY in the joint fluid, but SP is probably also involved given a strong correlation between presence of all three peptides. Both the degree and the extension of radiographic signs of TMJ destruction are associated with high concentrations of SP, NKA, CGRP, and NPY in the joint fluid.

NPY-LI pmol/l

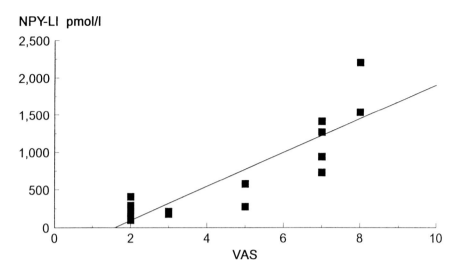

Fig. 2. Relation between NPY in TMJ fluid and TMJ pain (VAS) in 15 patients with rheumatoid arthritis ($r = 0.76$, $P < 0.001$).

DIAGNOSTIC PERSPECTIVES

CLINICAL SIGNS

The most characteristic clinical signs of RA in the TMJ are palpatory tenderness of the joint (laterally or posteriorly) and crepitus (palpable or audible) from the joint. Both these signs, however, may occur in degenerative joint disease and other joint disorders and thus are not specific. Pain confined to the joint during mandibular movements such as chewing is also a valuable sign, although it is more dependent on the patients' subjective judgment than are the other two. Swelling of the TMJ occurs occasionally. A characteristic, but not specific, feature of severe RA in the TMJ is the progressive anterior bite opening due to bilateral destruction of the mandibular condyles. Further nonspecific findings, such as tenderness to palpation of the masticatory muscles, reduced mandibular mobility, and irregular mandibular movement patterns, complete the clinical picture. Diagnosis on clinical grounds only is difficult, but the response to local anesthesia is of great importance for the determination of articular origin of pain.

RADIOGRAPHIC SIGNS

Radiography has long been an important tool for diagnosing and assessing mineralized tissue destruction of the TMJ. The most characteristic radio-

graphic signs of RA and other inflammatory disorders in the TMJ are erosions
of the cortical outline and reduced joint space (Åkerman et al. 1988). The
radiographic sign of cortical erosion of the TMJ is correlated to the severity of
the TMJ condition and to the duration and extension of the general disease.
Subchondral cystic destruction and severe destruction of the bone, which eventually may lead to a complete loss of the condyle, are later findings and are
relatively rare. The reduced joint space is caused by destruction of the articular cartilage, which results in a narrowing of the mineralized joint surfaces.
Reduced joint space is associated with joint crepitus as well as a higher
overall frequency of radiographic changes. Bone sclerosis and bony outgrowths
(osteophytes) also may appear, but are more characteristic of degenerative
joint disease. The radiographic diagnosis of RA in the TMJ is difficult to
establish with certainty, especially in the early phase, due to a time lag in the
development of radiographic changes as compared with clinical symptoms.
Absence of radiographic changes of the TMJ does not exclude the possibility
of early degenerative or inflammatory joint disorder.

TEMPERATURE-RELATED SIGNS

Infrared thermography or thermocouples allow measurement of temperature on the skin surface overlying joints with inflammation and intra-articular
temperature (IAT). Such temperature measurements indirectly assess the vascular changes in the synovial membrane and capsule of the TMJ associated
with arthritis. IAT measurement provides the most valid results with respect
to correlation with signs and symptoms (Åkerman and Kopp 1988).

The IAT of the TMJ in patients with RA is variable. High or low IAT and
ensuing temperature asymmetry is a consequence of microcirculatory or metabolic changes in the synovial membrane or nearby muscles. In a patient population with seropositive RA and TMJ involvement, 30% of the patients had
increased (> 36°C) and 18% decreased IAT (< 35.7°C) compared with healthy
persons. High IAT and skin surface temperature of the TMJ occur in patients
with extensive and severe RA. The TMJs with high IAT contain joint fluid
with a high concentration of CGRP (Appelgren et al. 1993b). Low IAT correlated with joint and muscle pain as well as palpatory tenderness. Furthermore,
temperature reduction was associated with joint crepitus, and thus destructive
arthritis. This temperature reduction in combination with crepitus has been
found in patients with a relatively short duration of disease (1–5 years). The
decrease in IAT is probably caused by sympathetic vasoconstriction because
it is associated with increase in joint fluid content of NPY (Appelgren et al.
1993a). The skin surface temperature over the TMJ and the IAT seems to
return toward normal levels with progression of RA. Present knowledge indi-

cates that increased as well as decreased IAT are early signs of pathophysiology in the TMJ.

SYNOVIAL FLUID ANALYSIS

Diagnostic aspiration of the TMJ is a valuable procedure in diagnosing organic diseases of the joint. It is possible to aspirate joint fluid/exudate in one-quarter to one-third of RA patients. In the remaining cases the joints can be washed with 1–2 ml saline. In both instances the fluid can be examined for presence of cells and substances associated with inflammation. Normally, blood cells and large plasma proteins do not enter the articular cavity. No molecules with a radius larger than 100 ångstroms enter into the joint space, which means that such substances as fibrinogen and immunoglobulins are excluded from the synovial fluid in healthy joints. The volume and viscosity of fluid aspirated and the presence of blood are also parameters of interest.

In patients with IJD involvement of the TMJ, cellular findings (polymorphonuclear and mononuclear cells) and abnormalities of plasma protein content (fibrinogen/fibrin, haptoglobin, IgG, IgM) in the synovial fluid indicate an inflammatory process. Furthermore, fibrocartilage debris and corresponding high amounts of chondroitin/dermatan sulfate, i.e., markers of fibrocartilage breakdown, can be detected by chemical or cytochemical analysis. Recently the synovial fluid of the TMJ in cases with RA has been examined for neuroendocrine peptides (Appelgren et al. 1991), which may be of diagnostic and prognostic interest.

TREATMENT PERSPECTIVES

Treatment aims to alleviate pain, reduce inflammation, restore function and, if possible, to prevent further destruction of the joints. The pain in the acute phase is associated with inflammation, and analgesics with anti-inflammatory effects should be prescribed, if necessary. If the pain and suffering are severe, an intra-articular injection of a glucocorticoid often gives efficient relief, although in many cases the effect is only temporary. Early and effective pain control are important aspects of treatment, because evidence shows that pain per se aggravates arthritis and joint destruction. Activation of nociceptive afferents elicits spinal cord reflexes that increase the activity of postganglionic sympathetic nerves (Koizumi et al. 1970), which in turn is believed to augment the joint pain and inflammation (Levine et al. 1987) as well as vasoconstriction. Furthermore, the degree of pain reported by patients with RA is strongly associated with both physical and mental disability and with the amount of medication required (Kazis et al. 1983). The current pain level of patients with RA is also reported to be a good predictor of future physical and mental disability (Pearson 1963).

PHARMACOLOGIC THERAPY

Nonsteroidal anti-inflammatory drugs (NSAIDs) can be used to reduce TMJ arthritis and associated pain. However, these drugs do not provide any long-term remedy for IJD or DJD in the TMJ. The NSAIDs are indicated as an initial temporary treatment in patients with painful exacerbations of TMJ involvement with arthritis. Effort should be made immediately, however, to find means for further local treatment.

Intra-articular injections of *glucocorticoids* into the TMJ are advocated in patients with acute exacerbations of IJD and DJD. Their use can only be recommended when the TMJ is the primary site of inflammation and pain.

Saxne et al. (1985) have shown that intra-articular glucocorticoid injected into arthritic knees shows release of proteoglycans into the joint fluid, and that relapse of pain and inflammation coincides with an increase of proteoglycan release. A trial of methylprednisolone acetate (Depo-Medrol) in patients with RA of the TMJ showed that this drug had a significant short-term (four weeks) effect on both subjective symptoms and clinical signs that exceeded that of hyaluronate and saline (Kopp et al. 1991). Glucocorticoids adminis-tered intra-articularly seem in the short term to cause a decrease in joint fluid content of NPY upon puncture and aspiration of TMJs with IJD. The cause of this decrease is at present unknown, but it occurs in parallel with a decrease in joint pain and tenderness as well as an improvement in joint mobility.

PHYSICAL TREATMENT

When the acute pain has subsided, or when patients have low-grade symp-toms, physical exercises are of great importance to improve joint-muscle func-tion and strength. Restricted mouth opening capacity is a frequent finding associated with acute degenerative and inflammatory conditions of the TMJ due to painful synovitis and intra-articular effusion (edema) of the joint. Heal-ing of the joint involves a risk for development of fibrous adhesions between the joint components. The jaw muscles are always affected by TMJ arthritis and may develop tension due to the articular pain or may be more directly involved in the inflammatory process. Muscular weakness and atrophy are early and prominent features in RA. Comparison of the short-term effects of a self-administered physical training program for TMJ dysfunction in RA ver-sus no training resulted in all patients reporting reduced severity of TMJ disorder (Tegelberg and Kopp 1988). Clinically, however, only those training showed a decreased degree of dysfunction.

OCCLUSAL TREATMENT

The condition of the dental occlusion is important, and occlusal interferences are related to muscular tenderness/pain and decreased intra-articular temperature of the TMJ with RA (Åkerman and Kopp 1988). The occlusion should be stable and free from interferences to exclude the possibility of aggravating the condition in the joint. Anterior bite opening caused by RA is an occlusal problem that should be solved according to the principles of selective grinding and prosthetic rehabilitation. However, the patient's physician should be consulted to obtain information about the general inflammatory activity before any irreversible prosthetic treatment begins. It is not advisable to make any permanent prosthetic treatment on a patient with active RA. High erythrocyte sedimentation rate is a risk factor for anterior bite opening (Tegelberg et al. 1987). From a general point of view, loss of occlusal supporting zones has a negative effect on both muscle and joint function. In the late stages of IJD in the TMJ, occlusal dysfunction might be the primary problem and a significant part of the clinical dysfunction is caused by mandibular muscle pain and tenderness.

REFERENCES

Åkerman, S. and Kopp, S., Intra-articular and skin surface temperature of the temporomandibular joint in patients with rheumatoid arthritis, Acta. Odontol. Scand., 46 (1988) 41–48.

Åkerman, S., Kopp, S., Nilner, M., Peterson, A. and Rohlin, M., Relationship between clinical and radiologic findings of the temporomandibular joint in rheumatoid arthritis, Oral Surg. Oral Med. Oral Path., 66 (1988) 639–643.

Appelgren, A., Appelgren, B., Eriksson, S., Kopp, S., Lundeberg, T., Nylander, M. and Theodorsson, E., Neuropeptides in temporomandibular joints with rheumatoid arthritis: a clinical study, Scand. J. Dent. Res., 99 (1991) 519–521.

Appelgren, A., Appelgren, B., Kopp, S., Lundeberg, T. and Theodorsson, E., Relation between the intra-articular temperature of the temporomandibular joint and the presence of neuropeptide Y-like immunoreactivity in the joint fluid: a clinical study, Acta. Odontol. Scand., 51 (1993a) 1–8.

Appelgren, A., Appelgren, B., Kopp, S., Lundeberg, T. and Theodorsson, E., Relation between intra-articular temperature of the arthritic temporomandibular joint and presence of calcitonin gene-related peptide in the joint fluid: a clinical study, Acta Odontol. Scand., 51 (1993b) 285–291.

Buck, S.H., Walsh, J.H. and Yamamura, H.T., Neuropeptides in sensory neurons, Life Sci., 30 (1982) 1857–1866.

Geborek, P., Saxne, T., Pettersson, H. and Wollheim, F.A., Synovial fluid acidosis correlates with radiological joint destruction in rheumatoid knees, J. Rheumatol., 16 (1989) 468–472.

Håkanson, R., Wahlestedt, C., Ekblad, E. and Sundler, F., Neuropeptide Y: coexistence with noradrenaline, functional implications, Prog. Brain Res., 68 (1986) 279–287.

Hope, P.J., Jarrott, B., Schaible, H.G., Clarke, R.W. and Duggan, A.W., Release and spread of immunoreactive neurokinin A in the cat spinal cord in a model of acute arthritis, Brain Res., 19 (1990) 292–299.

Ichikawa, H., Wakisaka, S., Matsuo, S., and Akai, M., Peptidergic innervation of the temporomandibular disk in the rat, Experientia, 45 (1989) 303–304.

Johansson, A.-S., Isacsson, G., Isberg, A. and Granholm, A.-C., Distribution of substance P–like immunoreactive nerve fibers in temporomandibular joint soft tissues of monkey, Scand. J. Dent. Res., 94 (1986) 225–230.

Juan, H. and Sametz, W., Histamine-induced release of arachidonic acid and prostaglandins in the peripheral vascular bed, Arch. Pharm., 314 (1980) 183–190.

Kazis, L.E., Meenan, R.F. and Anderson, J.J., Pain in the rheumatic diseases: investigation of a key health status component, Arthritis Rheum., 26 (1983) 1017–1022.

Koizumi, K., Collier, R. and Kaufman, A., Contribution of unmyelinated afferent excitation to sympathetic reflexes, Brain Res, 20 (1970) 99–106.

Kopp, S., Åkerman, S. and Nilner, M., Short-term effects of intra-articular sodium hyaluronate, glucocorticoid, and saline injections on rheumatoid arthritis of the temporomandibular joint, J. Craniomandib. Disord. Facial Oral Pain, 5 (1991) 231–238.

Larsson, J., Ekblom, A., Henriksson, K., Lundeberg, T. and Theodorsson, E., Immunoreactive tachykinins, calcitonin gene-related peptide and neuropeptide Y in human synovial fluid from inflamed joints, Neuroscience Lett., 100 (1989) 326–330.

Levine, J.D., Clark, R., Devor, M., Helms, C., Moskowitz, M.A. and Basbaum, I.A., Intraneuronal substance P contributes to the severity of experimental arthritis, Science, 226 (1984) 547–549.

Levine, J.D., Dardick, S.J., Roizen, M.F., Helms, C. and Basbaum, A.I., Contribution of sensory afferents and sympathetic efferent to joint injury in experimental arthritis, J. Neurosci., 6 (1986) 3423–3429.

Levine, J.D., Goetzl, M.D. and Basbaum, A.I., Contribution of the nervous system to the pathophysiology of rheumatoid arthritis and other polyarthritides, Rheumatic Dis. Clin. North Am., 13 (1987) 369–383.

Lotz, M., Carson, D.A. and Vaughan, J.H., Substance P activation of rheumatoid synoviocytes: neural pathway in pathogenesis of arthritis, Science, 235 (1987) 893–895.

Lundberg, J.M., Terenius, L., Hökfelt, T., Martling, C.-R., Tatemoto, K., Mutt, V., Polak, J., Bloom, S. and Goldstein, M., Neuropeptide Y (NPY)–like immunoreactivity in peripheral noradrenergic neurons and effects of NPY on sympathetic function, Acta Physiol. Scand., 116 (1982) 477–480.

Lundberg, J.M., Franco-Cereceda, A., Hua, X.-Y., Hökfelt, T. and Fischer, J.A., Co-existence of substance P and calcitonin gene-related peptide–like immunoreactivities in sensory nerves in relation to cardiovascular and bronchoconstrictor effects of capsaicin, Eur. J. Pharmacol., 108 (1985) 315–319.

Mapp, P.I., Kidd, B.L., Gibson, S.J., Terry, J.M., Revell, P.A., Ibrahim, B.N., Blake, D.R. and Polak, J.M., Substance P-, calcitonin gene-related peptide- and C-flanking peptide of neuropeptide Y-immunoreactive fibres are present in normal synovium but depleted in patients with rheumatoid arthritis, Neuroscience, 37 (1990) 143–153.

Nilsson, J., von Euler, A.M. and Dalsgaard, C.J., Stimulation of connective tissue cell growth by substance P and substance K, Nature, 315 (1985) 61–63.

Oka, M., Rekonen, A. and Elomaa, A., Muscle blood flow in rheumatoid arthritis, Acta. Rheum. Scand., 17 (1971) 205–208.

Payan, D.G., McGillis, J.P. and Organist, M.L., Binding characteristic and affinity labeling of protein constituents of the human IM-9 lymphoblast receptor for substance P, J. Biol. Chem., 261 (1986) 14321–14329.

Pearson, C.M., Experimental joint disease, J. Chronic. Dis., 16 (1963) 863–874.

Saxne, T., Heinegård, D. and Wollheim, F.A., Proteoglycans in synovial fluid: the effect of intra-articular corticosteroid injections, Br. J. Rheumatol., 24 (1985) 221.

Tegelberg, Å. and Kopp, S., Subjective symptoms from the stomatognathic system in individuals with rheumatoid arthritis and osteoarthrosis, Swed. Dent. J., 11 (1987) 11–22.

Tegelberg, Å. and Kopp, S., Short-term effect of physical training on temporomandibular joint disorders in individuals with rheumatoid arthritis and ankylosing spondylitis, Acta. Odontol. Scand., 46 (1988) 49–56.

Tegelberg, Å., Kopp, S., Huddenius, K. and Forssman, L., Relationship between disorder in the stomatognathic system and general joint involvement in individuals with rheumatoid arthritis, Acta. Odontol. Scand., 45 (1987) 391–398.

Uotila, E., The temporomandibular joint in adult rheumatoid arthritis. A clinical and roentgenological study, Acta. Odontol. Scand., Suppl. 39 (1964).

Correspondence to: Sigvard Kopp, DDS, PhD, Department of Clinical Oral Science, Section of Clinical Oral Physiology, School of Dentistry, Karolinska Institutet, Box 4064, S-141 04 Huddinge, Sweden. Tel: 46-8-608-82-81; Fax: 46-8-779-40-57 or 46-8-608-08-81.

Temporomandibular Disorders and Related Pain Conditions, Progress in Pain Research and Management, Vol. 4, edited by B.J. Sessle, P.S. Bryant, and R.A. Dionne, IASP Press, Seattle, © 1995.

8

Degenerative and Inflammatory Temporomandibular Joint Disorders: Basic Science Perspectives

Lambert G.M. de Bont

Department of Oral and Maxillofacial Surgery, University Hospital Groningen, Groningen, The Netherlands

Degenerative and inflammatory temporomandibular joint (TMJ) disorders include noninflammatory chondro-osteoarthropathies (e.g., osteoarthrosis and internal derangement), primary arthritides (e.g., rheumatoid arthritis, psoriatic arthritis), and secondary arthritides (e.g., osteoarthritis, crystal-induced arthropathies) (de Bont and Stegenga 1993a). Many authors emphasize the relationship between osteoarthrosis (OA) and internal derangement (ID) of the TMJ. Although OA may develop without disk displacement, ID is highly correlated with OA of the TMJ (de Bont et al. 1986). The pathologic state in the TMJ is similar to other synovial joints (de Bont et al. 1985) and should be described with terminology used for other synovial joints (de Bont and Stegenga 1993b).

Research of OA was initially confined to histopathologic and electron microscopic changes in human osteoarthritic cartilage; over the last decade it has focused on the biochemical and metabolic changes in osteoarthritic cartilage. OA results from an imbalance between anabolic and catabolic processes (predominantly chondrocyte controlled) characterized by progressive degradation of components of the extracellular matrix (ECM) of articular cartilage, with secondary inflammatory components (Mankin and Brandt 1992).

A whole network of interacting enzymes and cytokines are involved in the cartilage degradation process, and undoubtedly more factors will be discovered in the future. Due to the scarce availability of human cartilage, especially in the early stage of the disease, many data confirming these changes derive from studies of animal models and in vitro cartilage explant studies.

Articular cartilage, synovial membrane, and synovial fluid are the basic elements in a synovial joint. Articular cartilage is composed of chondrocyte cells and ECM. The ECM is composed of collagen fibrils, proteoglycans, and glycoproteins. Chondrocytes are active cells that produce the ECM components and enzymes. The collagen fibrils in TMJ articular cartilage are organized in a three-dimensional network of layers and bundles of fibrils (de Bont et al. 1984). The proteoglycan aggregates, which are hydrophilic and form a gel that can swell, are situated between and interact with the collagen fibrils and occupy all the interstitial spaces. The collagen network prevents the complete swelling of the proteoglycan aggregates. During normal functioning, the external pressure from loading will be in equilibrium with the internal cartilage pressure (de Bont et al. 1991a).

Proteases, cytokines, growth factors, and arachidonic acid metabolites are involved in the biochemistry and metabolism of normal and osteoarthritic cartilage. Proteases or proteolytic enzymes play an important role both in maintaining normal tissue turnover and in the degradation of ECM components of articular cartilage in the osteoarthritic process. Proteases are capable of cleaving internal peptide bonds of proteins (Werb 1989). Normal articular cartilage contains large amounts of protease inhibitors, e.g., tissue inhibitor of metalloprotease (TIMP). An imbalance between protease and protease inhibitor levels has been postulated as a possible pathogenic pathway of OA (Dean et al. 1989). Cytokines and growth factors are soluble polypeptides, capable of regulating growth, differentiation, and metabolic activity of cells (Pelletier et al. 1991; Howell et al. 1992). In articular cartilage, cytokines (including IL-1 to IL-12, tumor necrosis factor, and interferon) generally exert a catabolic effect, whereas growth factors including insulin-like growth factor, transforming growth factor, and fibroblast growth factor exert an anabolic effect. Cytokines induce protease production resulting in proteoglycan depletion in cartilage and subsequent increase in the rate of cartilage degradation and decrease in the rate of proteoglycan synthesis and of other ECM components.

Arachidonic acid metabolites are mediators of inflammation. In response to specific stimuli, arachidonic acid is released from cell membrane phospholipids. Subsequently, the arachidonic acid is converted to several prostaglandins and thromboxanes by the cyclo-oxygenase pathway, and to several leukotrienes by the lipoxygenase pathway (Goetzl 1989). Arachidonic acid metabolites can be synthesized by synovial cells, mediated by cytokines. Prostaglandin E_2 (PGE_2), for example, is a major mediator of inflammation, and its synthesis is induced by IL-1 (Lewis 1989).

DEGENERATIVE SYNOVIAL JOINT DISORDERS

If a primary insult, whether (bio)mechanical, biochemical, inflammatory, or immunologic in character, disturbs the chondrocyte controlled balance between synthesis and degradation of ECM components, cartilage degradation ensues. Initially cartilage degradation will be counteracted by attempts at repair (Howell 1989). Mechanical forces to which articular cartilage is normally exposed are insufficient to destroy the tissue directly. Direct mechanical damage only becomes possible if the biochemical integrity of the matrix has been compromised. However, both overloading as well as underloading may result in loss of biochemical integrity of the ECM.

In the early stage of OA the increased synthesis of ECM components is exceeded by their degradation due to increased synthesis and activity of proteases, resulting in an initially focal net degradation and loss of articular cartilage. The hyaline articular cartilage swells and softens due to increased volume of the proteoglycan-water gel, which presumably results from localized breakdown of collagen fibrils within the matrix, as a result of proteolytic activity. Besides an increased water content and collagen fibril fragmentation, a proteoglycan depletion and a clustering of the chondrocytes occur. The cells proliferate and become very active in an attempt to repair the lost matrix (Freeman and Meachim 1979). Nevertheless, the ratio of proteases and their inhibitors (e.g., TIMPs) may increase, resulting in more proteolytic activity such as cleavage of collagen and proteoglycans. Once cartilage degradation has begun, the breakdown products released into synovial fluid are phagocytosed by the synovial membrane, producing an inflammatory reaction. Consequently, the synovial fluid composition and the synovial membrane will change. When the cartilage degradation continues, the tissue loses its integrity, resulting in blistering, fibrillation, horizontal splitting, adhesion formation, cartilage thinning, and responses in adjacent tissues.

Hypotheses regarding the pathogenesis of OA include the relationship between loading and cartilage degradation: is there a biomechanical failure of the articular cartilage, or, is there a chondrocyte injury or a failing chondrocyte response involving both degradation and repair? In both mechanisms, degenerative changes will result due to an imbalance between the anabolic and catabolic activity of the articular cartilage or an imbalance between repair and degradation processes inside the tissue. Modern definitions of OA (Howell et al. 1992) include this mechanism: OA is a disruption of a steady-state balance in a complex of interacting degradative and repair processes in cartilage, bone, and synovium with secondary inflammatory components.

In the etiopathology of OA we are probably dealing with a biochemically induced cascade of events in cartilage breakdown. Extensive in vitro studies with cartilage explant cultures have proven the significant role of degradative enzymes in cartilage breakdown. Animal models with artificially induced OA have shown the same mechanisms. Cartilage breakdown and cartilage repair are dual processes, always continuously present. The breakdown is caused by proteolytic enzymes, the repair is expressed by chondrocyte proliferation and increased synthesis of collagen and proteoglycans. In both processes, the chondrocytes seem to have a key position and control homeostasis.

The cell is surrounded by numerous peptide factors that modulate the growth and differentiation of cartilage cells. There is increasing evidence that these factors interact such that one factor may influence the production and also the biological effects of others. Consequently, we are dealing with a complicated and interactive system. The involved biochemical factors are now categorized in cytokines, growth factors, metalloproteases, and TIMPs; all seem to play a critical role in the regulation of cartilage degradation and repair during normal and pathological turnover of the cartilage matrix. Various hypotheses about the role of cytokines, growth factors, metalloproteases, and TIMPs in the etiopathogenesis of OA suggest an imbalance between the amount of proteases and their inhibitors (e.g., metalloproteases and TIMPs), corresponding to a relative deficit of the inhibitors (Dean et al. 1989).

Stromelysin, collagenase, and gelatinase are the major metalloproteases. Their synthesis and secretion by the chondrocytes may be influenced by the presence of IL-1, which is one of the major cytokines produced by the synovial lining cells and is responsible for increasing the synthesis of proteases by the synovial lining cells in the osteoarthritic joint.

The intermediate stage of OA is characterized biochemically by a failing synthesis of ECM components, whereas the synthesis of proteases remains increased, mediated by the network of interacting cytokines. The late stage of OA may be characterized biochemically by a continued increased synthesis of proteases or by a decreased synthesis of proteases in the case of residual OA. The content of several ECM components, however, is further reduced. Thus, the TMJ obeys the same biologic laws as do other synovial joints in the body.

TMJ OSTEOARTHROSIS

OA affects all synovial joint components, not only the articular cartilage but also the subchondral bone, the synovial lining cells, the synovial fluid, and the capsular ligaments (Stegenga et al. 1991). Because osteoarthritis is OA with synovitis, it includes an inflammatory component caused by waste products and inflammatory mediators.

Our concept of OA of the TMJ (Stegenga et al. 1989a) describes the different conditions of the articular cartilage from a normal variation to initial degenerative changes, from initial degenerative changes to advanced changes, and finally to destroyed cartilage. Throughout life, the TMJ articular cartilage and the underlying bone display shifting equilibria between changes in form and function by tissue remodeling, just as do all other joints. The tissues will adapt to applied stresses. When the stress or loading is beyond the limits of the system, compensatory responses may lead to new steady states.

Increased loading may stimulate remodeling, involving increased synthesis of proteoglycans and collagen fibrils. An overloading may disturb the equilibrium between form and function and give rise to tissue breakdown. Only severe overloading will cause irreversible changes and damage. Remodeling, both progressive and regressive, takes place continuously. Features of progressive and regressive remodeling have been found in OA of the TMJ (de Bont et al. 1991b). When regressive remodeling dominates, it will result in a shortening of the mandibular ascending ramus. In this way, the relationship among the adaptive capacity of articular cartilage, joint loading, and degenerative cartilage breakdown can be explained.

Chondromalacia is a term used rather loosely by the medical profession to describe a clinically distinctive posttraumatic softening of the articular cartilage of the patella in young persons. The term is now also applied to the TMJ. The anatomic lesions are microscopically indistinguishable from those of early OA (de Bont et al. 1991b). OA starts focally in a joint; clinical symptoms occur when it is present to a certain degree or when a certain area is affected.

Light microscopy characteristics of osteoarthritic articular cartilage include fibrillation, splitting and thinning, and clustering of the chondrocytes, while the interface between subchondral bone and calcified cartilage may be irregular. The TMJ articular zone, the superficial cartilage layer at the articular surface, often seems unaffected, while the degenerative changes such as horizontal splitting, fibrosis of the bone marrow, and clustering of the chondrocytes are clearly present in the deeper layers of the tissue (de Bont et al. 1991b).

The macroscopically detectable degenerative changes of the TMJ on radiographs include lipping caused by osteophyte formation, sclerosis, surface erosions, subchondral cysts, and deformation.

DISCUSSION

Articular cartilage was once considered an inert tissue because of its relative isolation from factors normally carried by the circulation, due to the absence of capillaries and the abundance of proteoglycans, which limit the diffusion of these factors (Howell 1989). Now, however, it is recognized that articular cartilage is a dynamic system that is capable of remodeling under functional demands and of turnover of ECM components. Presumably, the chondrocytes are involved in an enzymatically mediated "internal remodeling system." The chondrocytes produce precisely regulated amounts of proteases and protease inhibitors to induce normal turnover of ECM components. Under normal conditions, the chondrocytes maintain a balanced ECM by equating anabolic and catabolic processes, i.e., synthesis and degradation. However, when this balance is disturbed, either by local or systemic factors, cartilage degradation ensues (Schwartz 1989).

Many proteases, cytokines, growth factors, and arachidonic acid metabolites play a role in the pathogenesis of OA. A unique initiating factor, if any indeed exists, has not yet been identified. The finding of one or more of these factors in the synovial fluid or cartilage is not pathognomic for OA, because all these factors also can be found in several other pathologic conditions including inflammation, trauma, and allergy. Therefore, the mere presence of one or more of these factors in the osteoarthritic TMJ has little clinical value.

Classification of TMJ signs and symptoms has until now been based on the stage of internal derangement (Wilkes 1989). However, in many cases TMJ signs and symptoms are attributable to OA. In our classification of TMJ disorders, we distinguish primary OA with disk displacement from primary OA without disk displacement (Stegenga et al. 1989a). Further, the posterior band of the disk in a twelve o'clock position is no longer considered a prescription of nature, because asymptomatic normal subjects showed TMJ disk malposition and deformity in a significant portion of the studied population (Kircos et al. 1987). Therefore, in studies of proteases, cytokines, growth factors, and arachidonic acid metabolites, as well as in studies of cartilage degradation products present in the synovial fluid, findings should be related to the grade of degradation of articular cartilage and to the grade of synovitis, rather than to the stage of internal derangement. Consequently, a classification of OA of the TMJ should be based on the grade of degradation of articular cartilage and the grade of synovitis. The stage of internal derangement should be diagnosed as a separate entity.

CONCLUSIONS

Primary OA will result in degenerative changes, disk displacement, and finally changes in joint morphology. All signs and symptoms seem to be the result of this primary, idiopathic OA process.

Secondary OA shows degenerative changes due to joint afflictions such as rheumatoid arthritis, but also may be due to disk displacement. For OA of the TMJ, we are dealing with synovial joint pathology, primarily with a connective tissue disease.

Cartilage matrix degradation is the subject of extensive biochemical research. Several proteases, protease inhibitors, cytokines, and growth factors are involved in the cartilage matrix degradative and repair processes. It is becoming increasingly obvious that enzymatic pathways, in addition to mechanical factors, are involved in OA cartilage matrix degradation. Clearly, to establish an effective regimen of therapy to decrease the extent of joint destruction, it is important to understand how matrix degradation develops and what enzymes mediate the process. Therefore, future research will focus on the biochemical aspects of OA of the TMJ.

ACKNOWLEDGMENT

The author thanks Dr. Leonore Dijkgraaf, research associate, for support in the preparation of this chapter.

REFERENCES

Dean, D.D., Martel-Pelletier, J., Pelletier J.-P., et al., Evidence for metalloproteinase and metalloproteinase inhibitor (TIMP) imbalance in human osteoarthritic cartilage, J. Clin. Invest., 84 (1989) 678–685.

de Bont, L.G.M. and Stegenga, B., Pathology of temporomandibular joint internal derangement and osteoarthrosis, Int. J. Oral Maxillofac. Surg., 22 (1993a) 71–74.

de Bont, L.G.M. and Stegenga, B., Terminology for normal findings. In: G.T. Clark, B. Sanders and C. Bertolami (Eds.), Advances in Diagnostic and Surgical Arthroscopy of the Temporomandibular Joint, W.B. Saunders, Philadelphia, 1993b, pp. 3–4.

de Bont, L.G.M., Boering, G., Havinga, P. and Liem, R.S.B., Spatial arrangement of collagen fibrils in the articular cartilage of the mandibular condyle: a LM and SEM study, J. Oral Maxillofac. Surg., 42 (1984) 306–313.

de Bont, L.G.M., Liem, R.S.B. and Boering, G., Ultrastructure of the articular cartilage of the mandibular condyle: ageing and degeneration, Oral Surg. Oral Med. Oral Pathol., 60 (1985) 631–641.

de Bont, L.G.M., Liem, R.S.B., Boering, G., Eulderink, F. and Westesson, P.L., Osteoarthritis and internal derangement of the temporomandibular joint: a light microscopic study, J. Oral Maxillofac. Surg., 44 (1986) 634–643.

de Bont, L.G.M., Stegenga, B. and Boering, G., Normal physiology of synovial joints: articular cartilage. In: M. Thomas and S.L. Bronstein (Eds.), Arthroscopy of the Temporomandibular Joint, W.B. Saunders, Philadelphia, 1991a, pp. 28–35.

de Bont, L.G.M., Stegenga, B. and Boering G., Hard tissue pathology: osteoarthrosis. In: M. Thomas and S.L. Bronstein (Eds.), Arthroscopy of the Temporomandibular Joint, W.B. Saunders, Philadelphia, 1991b, pp. 258–269.

Freeman, M.A.R. and Meachim, G., Ageing and degeneration. In: M.A.R. Freeman (Ed.), Adult Articular Cartilage, 2nd ed., Pitman Medical, London, 1979, pp. 487–540.

Goetzl, E.J. and Goldstein, I.M., Arachidonic acid metabolites. In: D.J. McCarty (Ed.), Arthritis and Allied Conditions: A Textbook of Rheumatology, 11th ed., Lea & Febiger, Philadelphia, 1989, pp. 409–425.

Howell, D.S., Etiopathogenesis of osteoarthritis. In: D.J. McCarty (Ed.), Arthritis and Allied Conditions: A Textbook of Rheumatology, 11th ed., Lea & Febiger, Philadelphia, 1989, pp. 1595–1604

Howell, D.S., Treadwell, B.V. and Trippel, S.B., Etiopathogenesis of osteoarthritis. In: R.W. Moskowitz, D.S. Howell, V.M. Goldberg and H.J. Mankin (Eds.), Osteoarthritis: Diagnosis and Medical/Surgical Management, 2nd ed., W.B. Saunders, Philadelphia, 1992, pp. 233–252.

Kircos, L.T., Ortendahl, D.A., Mark, A.S. and Arakawa, M., Magnetic resonance imaging of the TMJ disc in asymptomatic volunteers, J. Oral Maxillofac. Surg., 45 (1987) 852–854.

Lewis, R.A., Prostaglandins and leukotrienes. In: W.N. Kelley, E.D. Harris, S. Ruddy and C.B. Sledge (Eds.), Textbook of Rheumatology, 3rd ed., W.B. Saunders, Philadelphia, 1989, pp. 253–265.

Mankin, H.J. and Brandt, K.D., Biochemistry and metabolism of articular cartilage in osteoarthritis. In: R.W. Moskowitz, D.S. Howell, V.M. Goldberg and H.J. Mankin (Eds.), Osteoarthritis: Diagnosis and Medical/Surgical Management, 2nd ed., W.B. Saunders, Philadelphia, 1992, pp. 109–154.

Pelletier, J.P., Roughley, P.J., DiBattista, J.A., McCollum, R. and Martel-Pelletier, J., Are cytokines involved in osteoarthritic pathophysiology? Semin. Arthritis Rheum., 20 (1991) 12–25.

Schwartz, E.R., Chondrocyte structure and function. In: D.J. McCarty (Ed.), Arthritis and Allied Conditions: A Textbook of Rheumatology, 11th ed., Lea & Febiger, Philadelphia, 1989, pp. 289–295.

Stegenga, B., de Bont, L.G.M. and Boering, G., A proposed classification of temporomandibular disorders based on synovial joint pathology, Craniomandib. Pract., 7 (1989a) 107–118.

Stegenga, B., de Bont, L.G.M. and Boering, G., Osteoarthrosis as the cause of craniomandibular pain and dysfunction: a unifying concept, J. Oral Maxillofac. Surg., 47 (1989b) 249–256.

Stegenga, B., de Bont, L.G.M., Boering, G. and Van Willigen, J.D., Tissue responses to degenerative changes in the temporomandibular joint: a review, J. Oral Maxillofac. Surg. 49 (1991) 1079–1088.

Werb, Z., Proteinases and matrix degradation. In: W.N. Kelley, E.D. Harris, S. Ruddy and C.B. Sledge (Eds.), Textbook of Rheumatology, 3rd ed, W.B. Saunders, Philadelphia, 1989, pp. 300–321.

Wilkes, C.H., Internal derangement of the temporomandibular joint: pathologic variations, Arch. Otolaryngol. Head Neck Surg., 115 (1989) 469–477.

Correspondence to: Lambert G.M. de Bont, DDS, PhD, Department of Oral and Maxillofacial Surgery, University Hospital Groningen, P.O. Box 30.001, 9700 RB Groningen, The Netherlands. Tel: 31-50613840; Fax: 31-50696724.

Temporomandibular Disorders and Related Pain Conditions, Progress in Pain Research and Management, Vol. 4, edited by B.J. Sessle, P.S. Bryant, and R.A. Dionne, IASP Press, Seattle, © 1995.

9

Proteoglycan Components of Articular Cartilage in Synovial Fluids as Potential Markers of Osteoarthritis of the Temporomandibular Joint

Anthony Ratcliffe[a] and Howard A. Israel[b]

[a]Department of Orthopaedic Surgery and [b]Division of Oral and Maxillofacial Surgery, Columbia University, New York, New York, USA

Recent studies have emphasized the importance of osteoarthritis (OA) in the pathogenesis of temporomandibular joint (TMJ) disorders (Holmlund and Hellsing 1988; Stegenga et al. 1989; Israel et al. 1991). Characteristics of OA include progressive degeneration and loss of articular cartilage and subchondral bone accompanied by proliferation of new bone and soft tissue, and often involves synovial inflammation (synovitis). The morphologic changes observed in OA of the TMJ include degeneration of the articular cartilage that results in fibrillation, erosion, and eventual loss of cartilage from the joint. Clinical signs and symptoms reported to be associated with OA of the TMJ include joint pain and stiffness, tenderness to palpation, crepitus, and limited motion (Stegenga et al. 1989). Radiographic signs of OA include sclerosis, osteolytic cysts, flattening of the condyle, loss of condylar height, and osteophytic lipping. OA is a disease associated with advancing age, although it does occur in younger persons (Israel et al. 1991).

Studies on the incidence of OA show little agreement. Clinical diagnosis of TMJ lesions shows OA to be present in less than 10% of cases examined, although examination of cadaveric TMJ specimens indicates OA in up to 40% (Westesson and Rohlin 1984). This finding suggests that the diagnosis of OA by clinical and radiological examination is difficult and may identify OA only at the late stage of the disease process. TMJ arthroscopy allows a more exact diagnosis of cartilage degeneration (Murakami and Ito 1986; Holmlund and Hellsing 1988; Israel et al. 1991; Israel 1992) and permits the diagnosis of

OA at an earlier stage than previously possible. Recent studies (Holmlund and Hellsing 1988; Israel et al. 1991) have now shown that OA occurs in approximately 70% of patients who undergo arthroscopy for TMJ disorders, and that radiographic and clinical signs are not sufficiently sensitive to diagnose early OA. Indeed, these observations are consistent with the proposed theory that osteoarthritis is a major cause of temporomandibular pain and dysfunction (Stegenga et al. 1989).

ARTICULAR CARTILAGE: COMPOSITION, METABOLISM, AND CHANGES IN OA

Normal TMJ cartilage, like other cartilage, is composed of a large extracellular matrix with a sparse population of specialized cells, the chondrocytes, distributed throughout the tissue (Mow et al. 1992; Mankin et al. 1994). However, the articular surface of the TMJ consists of fibrocartilage, whereas most synovial joints are covered with hyaline cartilage. The matrix consists mainly of water (60–80%), collagen, the large proteoglycan aggrecan, and other quantitatively minor proteoglycans, glycoproteins, and proteins. The collagen forms a dense meshwork of fibrils that are embedded in a highly concentrated solution of proteoglycans, and together they provide the unique mechanical properties of the tissue: the proteoglycans supply compressive stiffness and resiliency, and the collagen provides the tensile properties (Fig. 1; for a review, see Mow et al. 1992). The primary proteoglycan of cartilage is aggrecan, a complex glycoprotein with an approximate molecular weight of 2×10^6 daltons, which consists of an extended protein core to which many keratan sulfate and chondroitin sulfate glycosaminoglycan chains are attached (Fig. 2) (Heinegard and Oldberg 1989). The protein core comprises several

Fig. 1. The collagen network interacting with the aggrecan aggregates in the extracellular matrix of cartilage. (Mow et al. 1992)

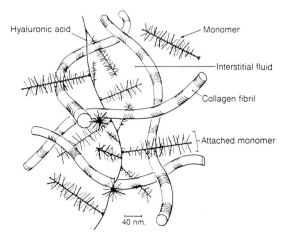

Hyaluronic acid

Monomer

Interstitial fluid

Collagen fibril

Attached monomer

40 nm.

distinct domains, one of which, the N-terminal G1 domain, has sites that are specifically involved in aggregation. These proteoglycans form large aggregates by binding to a chain of hyaluronan, with binding stabilized by a separate link protein. The principal function of aggregation is considered to be immobilization of the proteoglycans within the collagen network.

Articular cartilage is a metabolically active tissue involved in maintenance and repair. Matrix components are continuously synthesized by the chondrocytes, secreted from the cells, and incorporated into the extracellular matrix. At the same time, the matrix components are continuously catabolized, and the degradation products are released into the synovial fluid (Saxne et al. 1985; Ratcliffe et al. 1988; Lohmander et al. 1989; Ratcliffe et al. 1992). The normal maintenance of the extracellular matrix depends on a balance between the events of anabolism and catabolism, usually controlled by the chondrocytes (Fig. 3). In degenerative joint disease, whatever the underlying cause, an imbalance between synthesis, incorporation into the matrix, and breakdown occurs; degradation of the matrix is the result.

Experimental evidence suggests that OA develops as a result of definable alterations in biochemical composition and structure and biomechanical properties of articular cartilage and the associated tissues. Osteoarthritis-associated morphological and biochemical changes in cartilage include surface fibrillation,

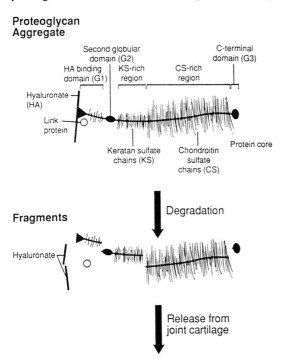

Proteoglycan Aggregate

Second globular domain (G2)
C-terminal domain (G3)
HA binding domain (G1)
KS-rich region
CS-rich region
Hyaluronate (HA)
Link protein
Keratan sulfate chains (KS)
Chondroitin sulfate chains (CS)
Protein core

Fragments

Hyaluronate

Degradation

Release from joint cartilage

Fig. 2. A schematic diagram of an aggrecan molecule bound to hyaluronan, and the representation of the mechanism of its degradation in articular cartilage. The protein core of aggrecan has several globular domains and other extended regions containing the keratan sulfate and chondroitin sulfate glycosaminoglycan chains. The N-terminal G1 domain binds to hyaluronan, and is stabilized by a separate globular link protein. The major cleavage site is between the G1 and G2 domains, making the glycosaminoglycan-containing portion of the aggrecan molecule nonaggregating. This fragment is then released from the cartilage. Other proteolytic events can result in the G1 domain and link protein also leaving the cartilage. (Mankin et al. 1994)

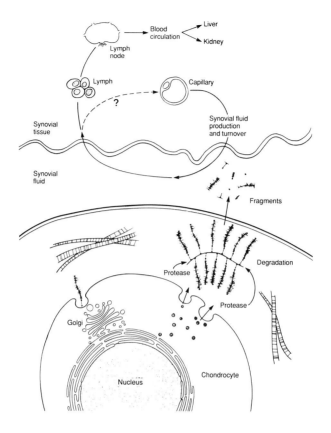

Fig. 3. Metabolic events controlling the proteoglycans in articular cartilage of a synovial joint. The chondrocytes synthesize the aggrecan molecules and release them into the extracellular matrix where they are incorporated. At the same time, proteolytic events result in the aggrecan molecules becoming nonaggregating and being released from the cartilage into the synovial fluid. They are then cleared through the synovium and lymphatics into the blood. (Mankin et al. 1994)

fissuring, and erosion, as well as chondrocytic, biosynthetic, compositional, and biomechanical changes. In early osteoarthritis, major changes have been observed in the organization, composition, and content of the upper region of the articular cartilage (Guilak et al. 1994). The mechanisms responsible for this increase are not well defined but may be the result of a weakening or loosening of the collagen network that eventually impairs its ability to restrain the swelling pressure exerted by the proteoglycans. This hypothesis is consistent with the observed reduction in the tensile properties of OA cartilage (Guilak et al. 1994). Changes in the chondrocytes may include localized areas of increased cellularity, cloning, and cell activity. Proteoglycan and collagen degradation rates are increased (Stegenga et al. 1989; Ratcliffe et al. 1992), as are synthesis rates, apparently representing an attempt at repair. Changes in the fundamental composition and structure of the proteoglycans have been observed with OA; these include increased extractability, decreased aggregate size, decreased ratio of aggregate, and increased size of the glycosamino-glycan chains. Recent studies now add some exciting new insights into our characterization of OA. Monoclonal antibodies to specific chondroitin sulfate structures recognize native chondroitin sulfate in OA cartilage but not in non-OA cartilage (Caterson et al. 1990; Ratcliffe et al. 1993). This epitope may therefore be indicative of reparative mechanisms that ultimately fail, with degeneration of articular cartilage as the result.

The cause of degeneration of the articular cartilage in OA remains un-known. Chondrocytes are able to respond to their mechanical environment in vitro, resulting in changed rates of synthesis and breakdown of cartilage ma-trix components. In vivo, experimental changes in the mechanical stability of a joint elicit changes in the cartilage remarkably similar to those of natural OA. Inflammatory mediators also can generate cartilage degradation. How-ever, it has been proposed that the resultant changes in the mechanical (com-pressive and tensile) properties of the cartilage impair TMJ movement, result-ing in the common signs and symptoms of craniomandibular pain and dysfunction (Stegenga et al. 1989).

THE CATABOLISM OF AGGRECAN AND LINK PROTEIN IN CARTILAGE

A major event of proteoglycan aggregate metabolism in articular cartilage is its breakdown and release from the tissue. This occurs in normal articular cartilage as part of maintenance, and it occurs at an accelerated rate in carti-lage pathology. An important step in this procedure is the cleavage of the aggrecan protein core to produce nonaggregating proteoglycan fragments and G1 domain and link protein with reduced functionality. These fragments leave the cartilage and can be detected in the synovial fluid. A major site of cleav-age in the aggrecan protein core has been identified in the interglobular do-main between the G1 and G2 domains at a glutamate-alanine bond (residues 373–374) (Sandy et al. 1992). Analysis of synovial fluids from patients with injury and with OA show that this aggrecan cleavage product is the major fragment in all samples, suggesting that the mechanism of aggrecan cleavage occurs during all stages of OA and probably in normal cartilage as well (Sandy et al. 1992). Other sites within aggrecan that are susceptible to cleav-age include bonds between residues 1714–1715, 1819–1820, and 1919–1920. The amino acid sequences around all these cleavage sites show significant similarities, suggesting that a single enzyme may be responsible for these cleavage products. However, this enzyme has yet to be identified; it has tentatively been termed "aggrecanase."

Link protein is present in mature human articular cartilage in three forms of molecular weight (M_r) 48,000, 44,000, and 41,000 (LP1, LP2, LP3). All are derived from the same protein core. LP1 differs from LP2 by the presence of an N-linked oligosaccharide at residue 6, and LP3 has a shorter protein core due to a cleavage at residue 16. Levels of LP3 increase with age, as does a cleavage within its globular region. The N-terminal regions of LP1 and LP2 are prone to proteolytic attack, and analysis of the N-terminal sequences of LP3 from human articular cartilage shows identity with three different enzymatic events, caused by stromelysin, cathepsin G, and cathepsin B.

MATRIX COMPONENTS IN SYNOVIAL FLUIDS AS INDICATORS OF CARTILAGE CATABOLISM

The determination of cartilage extracellular matrix components in synovial fluids as well as their use as specific biochemical markers in joint disease is based on two hypotheses involving catabolism and anabolism (Fig. 3). First, increased rates of cartilage degeneration produce increased concentrations of extracellular matrix components in the synovial fluids, reflecting changes in the rates of cartilage catabolism. Second, cartilage degeneration in OA induces a change in the type or structure of molecules synthesized by the chondrocytes: the presence of these novel molecules or structures may therefore be a marker of degenerative events in the tissues. Experimental and clinical (Saxne et al. 1985, 1986; Ratcliffe et al. 1988) studies (including longitudinal studies [Saxne et al. 1986; Ratcliffe et al. 1988]) of knee joints with acute inflammatory conditions show high levels of proteoglycan in the synovial fluids, reflecting a depletion of proteoglycan from cartilage. In patients with advanced joint disease, low concentrations of synovial proteoglycan may be observed that correspond to the amount of cartilage in the joint, irrespective of other parameters of disease activity. Such observations support the premise that levels of matrix components in the synovial fluids may indicate cartilage catabolism. A recent study of post-traumatic knee joint lesions (diagnosed by arthroscopy) of varying duration (Lohmander et al. 1989) demonstrated that, particularly in post-traumatic cruciate ligament injuries, synovial fluid proteoglycan levels were greatly elevated compared with those found in a control population.

Experimental studies in animals have allowed investigation of the early events in OA. They have shown elevated levels of cartilage matrix components (keratan sulfate epitope, link protein, G1 domain) in the synovial fluids of affected joints, corresponding to increased rates of release of these matrix components from the OA cartilage (Ratcliffe et al. 1992, 1994). Interestingly, it was possible to use levels of keratan sulfate epitope and link protein to distinguish between two different types of cartilage pathology (Ratcliffe et al. 1994). Thus, matrix component levels in the synovial fluids appeared to reflect the catabolic rate of those components in cartilage.

Use of a newly developed immunoassay with the monoclonal antibody 3B3 has yielded exciting data. This epitope was first detected in canine experimental OA cartilage (Caterson et al. 1990; Ratcliffe et al. 1993); it has now also been detected in the synovial fluids of experimental OA joints (Ratcliffe et al. 1993), but not in fluids from non-OA joints. More recently, studies of human knee cartilage and synovial fluids indicate the presence of the 3B3 native epitope in OA samples but not in non-OA samples (Ratcliffe et al., unpublished data, 1994), and appears before arthroscopic evidence of OA.

Studies of TMJ synovial fluids have been limited, likely due to the difficulties of aspirating such a small joint, and they have been restricted primarily to examples of inflammation (Kopp et al. 1983). In our laboratory we recently performed a study to determine the prevalence of OA (diagnosed by arthroscopy) in a patient population with severe TMJ disorders (Israel et al. 1991). Inclusion into the study required significant pain and dysfunction of the TMJ and failure of conservative reversible treatment to alleviate symptoms (Israel 1992). Levels of immunoreactive keratan sulfate (an important component of cartilage proteoglycans) in TMJ synovial fluid aspirates were compared with the arthroscopic diagnosis (OA and non-OA).

TMJ arthroscopy was performed on 25 joints in 20 patients (mean age 33.2; female to male ratio 5.7:1) with symptoms of pain and dysfunction that did not resolve after nonsurgical treatment. The preoperative diagnosis was based on clinical examination and diagnostic imaging (panoramic radiograph and magnetic resonance imaging). Synovial fluid aspirates were obtained just prior to the insertion of cannulas into the joint. Arthroscopy of the superior joint space was performed with a 1.7-mm arthroscope using the inferolateral approach (Murakami and Ito 1986; Israel 1992). The diagnosis of OA was based on the presence of fibrillation or more extensive degeneration of the articular surfaces. A preoperative diagnosis of OA was made in only 3 of the 25 joints (12%) (Fig. 4). Additional clinical diagnoses included internal derangement (24 joints) and fibrosis (2 joints). Arthroscopic examination showed 17 of the 25 joints (68%) with OA, including the 3 joints clinically diagnosed with OA (Fig. 4). Analysis of the synovial fluids from these joints showed that keratan sulfate epitope levels in the synovial fluids from the OA joints were significantly elevated compared with those from the non-OA joints (Fig. 4).

Fig. 4. (a) Preoperative clinical diagnosis of TMJ OA in a population of patients with severe TMJ disorders. (b) Arthroscopic diagnosis of TMJ OA in the same patient population. (c) Levels of keratan sulfate epitope in the synovial fluids of those patients diagnosed as OA and non-OA. (Adapted from Israel et al. 1991)

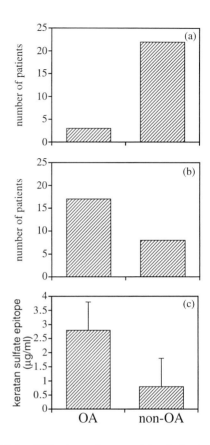

In summary, the data indicate that OA is difficult to detect with clinical and radiographic methods, and that arthroscopic investigation and synovial fluid analysis may indicate OA in joints at earlier stages than previously possible. In the future, the determination of a combination of several markers, or indicators, in the synovial fluids may become particularly valuable in establishing a diagnosis of OA, and monitoring progression and treatment of the disease.

CLINICAL RELEVANCE OF THESE STUDIES

TMD symptoms are prevalent among the general population. Within the group whose symptoms are severe enough for them to seek treatment, the accurate diagnosis of OA is difficult. When based on conventional clinical indicators, the diagnosis of OA of the TMJ is not predominant in patients with severe, persistent symptoms. However, recent arthroscopic diagnostic findings indicate that OA is a major condition in patients with severe, persistent TMJ symptoms who undergo TMJ arthroscopy (Holmlund and Hellsing 1988; Israel et al. 1991). Thus, the limited accuracy in the clinical diagnosis of TMJ OA may be improved by arthroscopy, which has potential for a more accurate approach to the diagnosis and characterization of TMJ disorders.

Little is known about TMJ OA and the underlying biochemical events in the TMJ articular cartilage and disk. New biochemical advances have resulted in attempts to define markers of cartilage metabolism that may be applied to synovial fluids. Our initial studies indicate that TMJ OA has some features in common with OA of other synovial joints: catabolic rates of cartilage proteoglycans are increased. The analysis of the synovial fluids of patients with severe, persistent TMJ symptoms who undergo arthroscopy will provide new insight into the biochemical events in TMJ OA. Determination of the levels of specific matrix components in the synovial fluids of a joint may serve to indicate degenerative events taking place in the cartilage of that joint. However, the potential clinical usefulness of TMJ synovial fluid analysis for following the course of the disease is uncertain, due to the invasive nature of synovial fluid aspiration, which may prevent its use in patients whose symptoms improve with treatment.

The combination of arthroscopic diagnosis of TMJ disorders and biochemical analysis of TMJ synovial fluids provides an excellent model for studying the disease process. This model may improve our ability to diagnose TMJ OA and enable us to acquire new insight into the relationship between the biochemical events associated with proteoglycan degradation and the morphologic appearance of osteoarthritic cartilage, which in turn may result in the future development of useful models for studying the prevention and management of TMJ OA.

ACKNOWLEDGMENT

This work was supported in part by National Institutes of Health grants DE10493 and RR00645.

REFERENCES

Caterson, B., Mahmoodian, F., Sorrell, J.M., Hardingham, T.E., Bayliss, M.T., Carney, S.L., Ratcliffe, A. and Muir, H., Modulation of native chondroitin sulphate structure in tissue development and in disease, J. Cell Sci., 97 (1990) 411–417.
Guilak, F., Ratcliffe, A., Lane, N., Rosenwasser, M.P. and Mow, V.C., Mechanical and biochemical changes in the superficial zone articular cartilage of canine experimental osteoarthritis, J. Orthop. Res., 12 (1994) 474–484.
Heinegard, D. and Oldberg, A., Structure and biology of cartilage and bone noncollagenous macromolecules, FASEB J., 3 (1989) 2042–2051.

Holmlund, A. and Hellsing, G., Arthroscopy of the temporomandibular joint: occurrence and location of osteoarthrosis and synovitis in a patient material, Int. J. Oral Maxillofac. Surg., 17 (1988) 36–40.

Israel, H.A., Temporomandibular joint arthroscopy. In: L. Peterson (Ed.), Principles of Oral and Maxillofacial Surgery, J.B. Lippincott, Philadelphia, 1992, pp. 2015–2042.

Israel, H.A., Saed-Nejad, F. and Ratcliffe, A., Early diagnosis of osteoarthrosis of the temporomandibular joint: correlation between arthroscopic diagnosis and keratan sulfate levels in the synovial fluid, J. Oral Maxillofac. Surg., 49 (1991) 708–711.

Kopp, S., Wenneberg, B. and Clemensson, E., Clinical, microscopical and biochemical investigation of synovial fluid from temporomandibular joints, Scand. J. Dent. Res., 91 (1983) 33.

Lohmander, S.L., Dahlberg, L., Ryd, L. and Heinegard, D., Increased levels of proteoglycan fragments in knee joint fluid after injury, Arthritis Rheum., 32 (1989) 1434–1442.

Mankin, H.J., Mow, V.C., Buckwalter, J.A., Iannotti, J.P. and Ratcliffe, A., Form and function of articular cartilage. In: S.R. Simon (Ed.), Orthopaedic Basic Science, AAOS, Park Ridge, Ill., 1994, pp. 1–44.

Mow, V.C., Ratcliffe, A. and Poole, A.R., Cartilage and diarthrodial joints as paradigms for hierarchical materials and structures, Biomaterials, 13 (1992) 67–97.

Murakami, K. and Ito, K., Arthroscopy of the temporomandibular joint. In: E. Watanabe (Ed.), Arthroscopy of Small Joints, Tokyo, Igaku Shon, 1986, pp. 128–139.

Ratcliffe, A., Doherty, M., Maini, R.N. and Hardingham, T.E., Increased concentrations of proteoglycan components in the synovial fluids of patients with acute but not chronic joint disease, Ann. Rheum. Dis., 47 (1988) 826–832.

Ratcliffe, A., Billingham, M.E.J., Saed-Nejad, F., Muir, H. and Hardingham, T.E., Increased release of matrix components from articular cartilage in experimental canine osteoarthritis, J. Orthop. Res., 10 (1992) 350–358.

Ratcliffe, A., Shurety, W. and Caterson, B., The quantitation of a native chondroitin sulfate epitope in synovial fluid and articular cartilage from canine experimental osteoathritis and disuse atrophy, Arth. Rheum., 36 (1993) 543–551.

Ratcliffe, A., Beauvais, P.J. and Saed-Nejad, F., Differential levels of synovial fluid aggrecan aggregate components in experimental osteoarthritis and joint disuse; J. Orthop. Res., 12 (1994) 464–473.

Sandy, J.D., Flannery, C.R., Neame, P.J. and Lohmander, S.L., The structure of aggrecan fragments in human synovial fluid: evidence for the involvement in osteoarthritis of a novel proteinase which cleaves the Glu 373-Ala 374 bond of the interglobulin domain, J. Clin. Invest., 89 (1992) 1512–1516.

Saxne, T., Heinegard, D., Wollheim, F.A. and Pettersson, H., Difference in cartilage proteoglycan level in synovial fluid in early rheumatoid arthritis and reactive arthritis, Lancet, 2 (1985) 127–128.

Saxne, R., Heinegard, D. and Wolheim, F.A., Therapeutic effects on cartilage metabolism in arthritis as measured by release of proteoglycan structures into the synovial fluid, Ann. Rheum. Dis., 45 (1986) 491–497.

Stegenga, B., DeBont, L.G.M. and Boering, G., Osteoarthrosis as the cause of craniomandibular pain and dysfunction, J. Oral. Maxillofac. Surg., 47 (1989) 249–256.

Westesson, P. and Rohlin, M., Internal derangement related to osteoarthrosis in temporomandibular joint autopsy specimens, Oral Surg. Oral Med. Oral Pathol., 57 (1984) 17–22.

Correspondence to: Anthony Ratcliffe, PhD, Orthopedic Research Laboratory, Department of Orthopedic Surgery, Columbia Presbyterian Medical Center, 630 West 168th St., New York, NY 10032, USA; Tel: 212-305-3707; Fax: 212-305-2741; E-mail: ratcliffe@cuorma.orl.columbia.edu

Temporomandibular Disorders and Related Pain Conditions, Progress in Pain Research and Management, Vol. 4, edited by B.J. Sessle, P.S. Bryant, and R.A. Dionne, IASP Press, Seattle, © 1995.

Reaction Papers to Chapters 7–9

David A. Keith and Jon D. Levine

David A. Keith

Department of Oral and Maxillofacial Surgery, Massachusetts General Hospital, and Harvard Center for Orofacial Pain and Temporomandibular Disorders, Harvard School of Dental Medicine, Boston, Massachusetts, USA

Because of an accident of anatomy and professional delineation, temporomandibular joint (TMJ) problems historically have been treated by professionals with little or no understanding of other joint pathologies and mechanics. This situation has led to a somewhat narrow view of TMJ problems. However, the mechanical forces under which the TMJ operates may well have characteristics unique to this joint system, and we need to pay attention to the biomechanical influences of joint function and dysfunction. A greater understanding of the interactive enzymes and cytokines and how they participate in the degradation of the extracellular matrix of articular cartilage and adjacent bone will lead to some innovative approaches to managing destructive change of the TMJ.

The highly complex world of nociception in the masticatory system also is an area of great interest. Kopp's observation that two peptides, neuropeptide Y (NPY) and calcitonin gene-related peptide (CGRP), occur in high concentrations in joint fluid of arthritic TMJs with pain and joints with restricted mobility is of great interest and may lead to significant clinical applications in the relief of pain (Kopp, this volume).

Of specific interest is the process of remodeling, which has the capacity to alter the form of the components of the TMJ in response to biomechanical forces. The ability of the joint to adapt to these forces is crucial to many of the nonsurgical interventions. Clinical results have frequently demonstrated that the osseous components of the joint, namely the condyle and the eminence, can adapt to changes in occlusion and position of the meniscus.

The chief feature of progressive or regressive remodeling (Blackwood 1966; Moffett et al. 1964; Meikle 1994) appears to be the activation of chondrocytes, which lie between the surface articular layer of the subchondral plate of bone and the mature condyle. Much of our research information is concerned with growing condyles where this layer is quite apparent, but in the mature person, these cells are the residue of cells creating growth in this area, and they appear to be a constant feature of adult specimens. They also appear to retain the capacity to respond to biomechanical forces in several ways. The stimulus will cause the chondrocyte zone to increase in size and lay down a cartilaginous matrix, which appears to be accompanied by an increase in the vascularity of the area. The cartilage becomes calcified, and subsequently, new bone is formed. The result is that the articular surface layer, which does not appear to have been active in the process, is advanced. Regressive remodeling is the reverse process; the cellular zone is activated and osteoclasts resorb the subchondral bone. Again, this change is associated with an increase in vascularity. As a result of this resorption, the articular layer is moved away from the joint space.

In both these types of remodeling the process involves the subarticular tissues while the articular layer appears to remain unaffected. Both processes can occur concurrently, and they also can be associated with subsequent degenerative changes.

While many persons can adapt quite readily to increased biomechanical loads and marked changes in their occlusion, in others apparently normal tissue breaks down and degeneration occurs under normal loading conditions. In many cases of internal derangement, the "correct" anatomic position of the meniscus within the joint is by no means a prerequisite for a full range of pain-free motion. As we concentrate on the details of joint breakdown and degradation, we also should pay attention to the normal processes of adaption, which in the long run could protect the joint from the various biomechanical, biochemical, and inflammatory insults.

While the progressive destruction of condylar structure is well demonstrated in severe forms of rheumatoid and other types of degenerative arthritis, extensive loss of condylar tissue also can be seen in other conditions. Resorption of the mandibular condyle has been reported in progressive systemic sclerosis (scleroderma) (Osial et al. 1981). This condition may be associated with bone resorption at the angle of the mandible, and it has been suggested that the resorption is due either to ischemia or to the excessive force applied to the joint by the tight soft tissues. Similarly, patients who wear the Milwaukee brace may show condylar change, and condylar bone loss is seen in patients with renal osteodystrophy or who are undergoing hemodialysis for chronic renal disease (Sellers et al. 1973).

Other recognizable causes of condylysis are trauma and previous orthognathic or TMJ surgery (Vallerand and Dolwick 1990). In some patients the loss of condylar structure and the development of malocclusion is unassociated with obvious local trauma or any recognizable systemic condition. This condition, idiopathic condylysis, should be distinguished from prenatal condylar aplasia or hypoplasia, as it is probably a postnatal local disturbance of unknown etiology (Rabey 1977). The development of condylysis and an anterior open bite in the teenage years or in young adult life may coincide but not necessarily be associated with orthodontic treatment or treatment for temporomandibular dysfunctions with splint therapy.

Massive condylar destruction can occur in the failed implant patient (Ryan 1989; Yih and Merrill 1989). It is now well recognized that the Proplast Teflon implant and, to a lesser extent, the Silastic implant, can fragment and particulate and lead to serious systemic and local consequences. The foreign-body granuloma can produce extensive bone loss in the condyle, eminence, and glenoid fossa, leading to discontinuities in the posterior aspect of the zygomatic arch and perforation into the middle cranial fossa.

After implantation, the patient remains well for a variable amount of time but eventually may develop a flulike illness characterized by intermittent fatigue, malaise, and fever. There is a demonstrable leukocytosis, increase in sedimentation rate, and fever. This condition may be associated with local swelling and local or distant adenopathy. The assumption is that this illness complex is associated with the fragmentation and dissemination of particulate matter. Locally, the destructive change may proceed with or without pain but with occlusal changes and instability of the mandible.

Many questions need to be asked about this process. Why do patients behave differently? Are there any genetically based factors that can modulate the host response to fragmented implant materials? Is there a host-specific hypersensitivity reaction? What are the cellular and biochemical mechanisms involved in the tissue response?

The orthopedic literature contains a useful model system for evaluating peri-implant osteolysis, which will help to conceptualize this process. Goldring's model suggests that the breakdown of the implant releases particles into the local environment (Fig. 1; Wang et al. 1993; Wang and Goldring 1993). The quality and rate of delivery of particles may be important. If a person rapidly breaks down the implant, possibly because of bruxism habits, the large quantity of rapidly produced particles may exceed the clearance capacity of local tissues and form a local granuloma. A slower rate of breakdown may allow clearance from the local site and widespread dissemination.

Once in the tissues, the particles, which may be of varying size, shape, and surface characteristics, attach to cells of the monocyte and macrophage

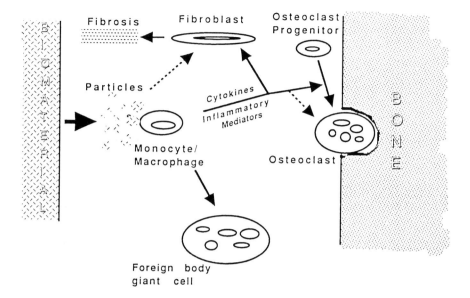

Fig. 1. Suggested model for bone resorption associated with implant breakdown. (Wang et al. 1993)

series, and are internalized by a process of phagocytosis. They then will be processed in the lysosomal system, causing a release of soluble factors, which may include cytokines, proteinases, and prostaglandins. These products in turn will act on bone cells (osteoclasts and/or osteoblasts) to directly or indirectly enhance focal bone resorption. These same products also may stimulate fibroblasts to produce increased extracellular matrix and enhance fibrous tissue deposition.

We need to further investigate the cellular mechanisms leading to bone loss in the TMJ, and also the cellular and molecular events involved in physiologic adaptation and healing.

REFERENCES

Blackwood, H.J., Adaptive changes in mandibular joints with function, Dent. Clin. North Am., 10 (1966) 559–566.
Meikle, M.C., The temporomandibular joint: a biological basis for clinical practice. In: B.G. Sarnat and D.M. Laskin (Eds.), Remodelling, 4th Edition, W.B. Saunders, Philadelphia, 1992.
Moffett, B.C., Jr., Lent, C.J., McCabe J.B., et al., Articular remodeling in the adult human temporomandibular joint, Am. J. Anat., 115 (1964) 119–142.
Osial, T.A., Avakian, A., Sassoun, V., Agarwal, A., Medsger, T.A. and Rodnan, G.P., Resorption of the mandibular condyles and coronoid processes in progressive systemic sclerosis (scleroderma), Arthritis Rheum., 24 (1981) 729–733.

Rabey, G.P., Bilateral condylysis: a morphoanalytic diagnosis, Br. J. Oral Maxillofac. Surg., 15 (1977–78) 121–134.

Ryan, D.E., Alloplastic implants in the temporomandibular joint, Oral and Maxillofacial Surgery Clinics of North America, 1 (1989) 427–441.

Sellers, A., Winfield, A.C., and Massry, S.G., Resorption of condyloid process of mandible, Arch. Intern. Med., 131 (1973) 727–728.

Vallerand, W.P. and Dolwick M.F., Complications of temporomandibular joint surgery, Oral and Maxillofacial Surgery Clinics of North America, 2 (1990) 481–488.

Wang, J.-T. and Goldring, S.R., The role of particulate orthopaedic implant materials in peri-implant osteolysis: mechanisms of granuloma formation and particle-induced osteolysis. In: B.F. Morrey (Ed.), Biological Material and Mechanical Considerations of Joint Replacement, Raven Press, New York, 1993, pp. 119–126.

Wang, J.-T., Harada, Y. and Goldring, S.R., Biological mechanisms involved in the pathogenesis of aseptic loosening after total joint replacement, Seminars in. Arthroplasty, 4 (1993) 215–222.

Yih, W.Y. and Merrill, R.G., Pathology of alloplastic interpositional implants in the temporomandibular joint, Oral and Maxillofacial Surgery Clinics of North America, 1 (1989) 415–426.

Correspondence to: David A. Keith, DMD, Department of Oral and Maxillofacial Surgery, Wang Ambulatory Care Center 230, Massachusetts General Hospital, 15 Parkman St., Boston, MA 02114-3139. Tel: 617-724-1640; Fax: 617-726-6195.

Jon D. Levine

Department of Medicine and Oral Surgery, University of California, San Francisco, California, USA

It is important to consider the individual physiological components of the inflammatory response. The inflammatory process has evolved primarily to respond to injury and foreign substances so as to *protect* the organism and *repair* tissue. In any disease process involving inflammation, some of the numerous components may be major contributors to the tissue injury observed while others may actually ameliorate the disease process. For example, plasma extravasation may play a protective role. Therefore, it is important for researchers and clinicians alike to sort out these individual contributions so that the most appropriate anti-inflammatory therapies may be employed.

The role of the nervous system in inflammatory diseases may be pertinent to the temporomandibular disorders. Examples of neurogenic inflammation include the well-described axon reflex. It is worthwhile mentioning some of the more recent concepts regarding the role of the neural contribution to inflammation because these processes probably are active in TMJ inflammation. Investigations of mechanisms underlying the axon reflex have revealed that this phenomenon may represent a purely peripheral interaction rather than a true reflex; that is, action potentials to and from the central nervous system may not be required. Rather, local action on peripheral nerve terminals, at receptors for signaling molecules from the immune system, may then result in the production as well as release of stores of proinflammatory mediators. Similar peripheral actions may occur at receptors on terminals of the postganglionic sympathetics, which can produce or release numerous proinflammatory mediators including prostaglandins, purines, catecholamines, and neuropeptides; the postganglionic sympathetics contribute significantly to inflammation in experimental arthritis. These peripheral neural actions affecting inflammation are modulated through neuroendocrine controls and, in particular, by activity in the sympathoadrenal and hypothalamic-pituitary-adrenal axes. Finally, because these neural and endocrine influences can promote ongoing inflammation or suppress it, in any disease state characterized by inflammation it is important to ascertain the specific contributions of these mechanisms.

Kopp and de Bont (this volume) discuss differences between "inflammatory" and "degenerative" diseases, a classical terminology, for example, for such conditions as rheumatoid versus osteoarthritis. While the differences in the common presentations of these processes are very important clinically, and historically led to the term "degenerative" joint disease, we should rethink this concept in view of current knowledge. For example, the processes activated and leading to tissue injury in osteoarthritis appear to involve similar mechanisms to those in inflammatory arthritides, albeit in most patients to a significantly less severe degree. In other words, the distinction may be quantitative rather than qualitative, and the use of two distinct descriptions thus could be misleading. Charcot joint, for example, which is categorized pathologically as a degenerative process, actually involves extensive activation of the inflammatory process. Viewing diseases of the TMJ as a spectrum involving different degrees of activation of different components of the inflammatory response is probably more consistent with our current understanding of the mechanisms involved than is a categorization into inflammatory or degenerative processes.

These authors and Ratcliffe and Israel also discussed biochemical findings as specific disease markers. Certainly many markers are employed clinically and reliably indicate a statistically greater likelihood that a certain disease process is present. However, the time variation in occurrence of the marker, correlation with disease severity, and the not uncommon phenomenon of patients with a classical presentation who never develop the appropriate marker should serve as caveats. We should not attribute a causal relationship to the abnormal biochemical process that results in the marker. Similarly, markers representing activation of specific aspects of the inflammatory response, while important for a general characterization, are unlikely to provide substantial clues to the specific expressions of injury.

Finally, while the description of a disease category and entity is indispensable in clinical practice, such a description can be a handicap to understanding disease mechanisms. In general, human diseases are expressed by abnormal function (either hypo- or hyperfunction). While the expressions may vary in different diseases, underlying pathologies may have elements in common. For example, many diseases with different presentations, such as diabetes, the various arthritides, the collagen vascular diseases, neurologic disorders, and malignancies, may manifest quite similar local aberrations in the inflammatory response and its modulation. Looking across diseases may provide heretofore undiscovered patterns that may help explain the clinical manifestations of many common afflictions characterized, to a varying degrees, by inflammation.

Correspondence to: Jon D. Levine, MD, PhD, Department of Medicine and Oral Surgery, University of California, San Francisco, 513 Parnassus Ave., Campus Box 0452A, Rm. S-1334, San Francisco, CA 94143, USA. Tel: 415-476-5108; Fax: 415-476-4845.

Part IV

Diagnosis and Assessment of Temporomandibular Disorders

Temporomandibular Disorders and Related Pain Conditions, Progress in Pain Research and Management, Vol. 4, edited by B.J. Sessle, P.S. Bryant, and R.A. Dionne, IASP Press, Seattle, © 1995.

10

Physical Characteristics Associated with Temporomandibular Disorders

Charles G. Widmer

Department of Oral and Maxillofacial Surgery, University of Florida, Gainesville, Florida, USA

Identification of specific characteristics that are uniquely associated with a disease or dysfunctional condition is prerequisite for an accurate diagnosis. In addition, this enables clinicians to separate patients who are disease-positive from other patients with similar conditions but without the disease, as well as from nonpatient, asymptomatic persons. In the field of orofacial pain it is important to develop and validate positive diagnostic criteria for each orofacial pain condition and not rely on diagnosis by exclusion (i.e., ruling out all other pain conditions and defaulting to a diagnosis such as musculoskeletal disorders). This approach is especially important because of the multiple potential sources of orofacial pain such as odontogenic, vascular, neurologic, neoplastic, otologic, and various headaches, to name a few. Given so many conditions and their overlapping characteristics of pain, development of criteria specific for each diagnostic category becomes imperative for both research studies and for clinical diagnosis.

For temporomandibular disorders (TMDs), physical characteristics have been identified that have served as a basis for case definitions specifically related to these painful masticatory musculoskeletal system disorders. In addition, assessment techniques have been developed to identify and grade the presence of these characteristics. For a positive diagnosis of a TMD, patients must have a positive history of facial pain combined with positive physical evaluation findings supplemented by radiographic or imaging when appropriate (McNeill et al. 1990). However, it is important to understand the relative merit of each component of physical assessment and how it can reliably contribute to the formulation of the TMD diagnosis. There is also a need to develop specific criteria sets diagnostic for subtypes of TMDs to identify research patient populations with similar characteristics. Toward this end, research diagnostic criteria (RDC) have been developed for TMDs, allowing researchers to reliably classify patients into specific, well-defined categories based on assessment of physical findings (Axis I) and assessment of psychosocial status (Axis II) (Dworkin and LeResche 1992). Eventually, after refinement and validation of the diagnostic ability of the criteria set, these definitions may be used for clinical diagnosis. However, the need for subtypes would imply that different treatment regimens have been identified that are effective for each specific condition.

This chapter will focus on our current ability to use reliably and accurately the physical measures proposed in Axis I of the research diagnostic criteria and to examine their relative contribution to diagnosis of TMDs. In addition, it will discuss alternative techniques that have been suggested as replacement or adjunctive measures.

MEASUREMENT RELIABILITY AND VALIDITY

Determining the ability to discriminate subtypes of TMD patients on a physical basis (Axis I) requires an evaluation of the physical assessment techniques that provide measures used as part of the diagnostic criteria. Physical assessment parameters used in the RDC Axis I include manual palpation of muscle and temporomandibular joint (TMJ), mandibular range of motion studies, determination of TMJ sounds and, when indicated and available, TMJ tomography, arthrography, or magnetic resonance imaging. These individual parameters are characterized using a standardized protocol and form criteria for the diagnostic subtypes. Measurement reliability and validity of each physical assessment technique is determined to permit comparison of techniques.

Measurement reliability refers to the ability to obtain the same measure over sequential measures and reflects intraexaminer and interexaminer variability in making the measures as well as normal variation of the phenomenon that is measured. Some clinical variables for TMDs are not stable for long- nor short-term intervals, which confounds the ability to evaluate test-retest reliability. Examples include muscle palpation and joint sound assessment.

Measurement validity is the ability to determine the truthfulness of the technique and requires a comparison to another measure that has been accepted as "true." This aspect of clinical measures is extremely important for diagnosis because measures may be reliable for a particular variable, but if they do not accurately reflect the phenomenon of interest then there is no usefulness for diagnosis. Studies of reliability and validity of clinical measures for TMDs have been reported for all the basic TMD physical assessment techniques. However, as pointed out by Dworkin et al. (1988), many studies failed to examine a population sample with a full range of symptom severity. In general population studies where symptoms were mainly mild or absent, reliability of scores were reported to be higher than in studies assessing both asymptomatic and symptomatic patients. Tables I-III summarize measurement reliability and validity for pertinent physical assessment techniques. These parameters were taken only from studies that examined the full range of symptoms from asymptomatic and symptomatic patients to reflect a more accurate representation of the reliability and validity.

MUSCLE AND TMJ PALPATION

Evaluation of measures used for muscle and temporomandibular joint manual palpation techniques has been reported in a few studies and generally shows good reliability. Both extraoral muscle and TMJ palpation reliability fall in the acceptable agreement range (kappa = 0.4–0.6) (Dworkin et al. 1988; Goulet and Clark 1990). In addition, Dworkin et al. (1988, 1990b) found that retraining examiners improved the reliability of extraoral muscle palpation scores from acceptable (kappa = 0.47) to good (0.65) levels and slightly elevated the TMJ palpation scores within the acceptable (0.47–0.54) level. Intraoral palpation (kappa = 0.27) was lower in reliability than extraoral or TMJ palpation but also improved to good (0.61) levels after retraining. These reliability outcomes are promising considering that they reflect variability of the examiner for test-retest, variation of the phenomenon of muscle or joint tenderness over time, and variable reliability of the patient report used to score the palpation tenderness.

Pressure algometers also have been examined for their reliability in measuring muscle and joint tenderness. It has been suggested that algometers might improve reliability due to their constant area of skin contact and the ability to control the rate and direction of pressure application. Although higher values of reliability were reported for extraoral muscle using algometry (0.61–0.71), the reliability level remained within the acceptable range.

MANDIBULAR KINESIOLOGY

Mandibular range of motion studies for vertical and horizontal movements, pain assessment during movement, and the mandibular opening pattern are parameters used to distinguish the major diagnostic classifications of muscle, disk displacement, and arthralgia/arthritis. Vertical mandibular openings are measured using a millimeter ruler to assess pain-free opening, maximum unassisted and maximum assisted openings, as well as lateral and protrusive excursions; these measures are highly reliable and valid (Table I). Opening patterns such as corrected or uncorrected deviation upon opening are less

Table I
Reliability and validity of mandibular kinesiology

Assessment Technique	Reliability	Validity
Vertical mandibular movements		
Maximum pain-free opening		
Untrained examiners	ICC = 0.72[a,b]	high with calibrated ruler
Trained examiners	ICC = 0.90[a,b]	
Trained examiners	$r = 0.89$[c]	
Maximum unassisted opening		
Untrained examiners	ICC = 0.90[a,b]	high with calibrated ruler
Trained examiners	ICC = 0.96[a,b]	
Maximum assisted opening		
Untrained examiners	ICC = 0.92[a,b]	high with calibrated ruler
Trained examiners	ICC = 0.96[a,b]	
Trained examiners	$r = 0.95$[c]	
Opening movement pattern		
Trained examiners	kappa = 0.70[b]	n/a
Horizontal mandibular movements		
Lateral	ICC = 0.70[b]	high with calibrated ruler
Protrusive	ICC = 0.68[b]	
Electronic kinesiology		
Vertical movement	good[d]	poor—error up to 15%[d,e]
Lateral movement	poor[d]	poor—error up to 30%[d,e]

Sources: [a]Dworkin et al. 1988; [b]Dworkin et al. 1990b; [c]Goulet and Clark 1990; [d]Throckmorton et al. 1992; [e]Tsolka et al. 1992.
Note: ICC = intraclass correlation coefficient.

reliable and there are no available validity data.

Suggested alternative measures include electronic kinesiologic instruments. However, these instruments are unreliable in lateral measures and demonstrate significant error in both vertical and lateral measures (Balkhi and Tallents 1991; Throckmorton et al. 1992; Tsolka et al. 1992). The recordings from these instruments underrepresent the actual movement so that a 40-mm vertical movement, which is within the normal range of motion, would be measured as 34 mm by the instrument and interpreted as limited. This error in measurement will inevitably lead to an underestimation of the velocity of opening and closing and distortions could be interpreted as deviations. Therefore, these unreliable and invalid electronic measures should not be used to acquire information for diagnosis of TMDs.

Table II
Reliability and validity of TMJ sounds

Assessment Technique	Reliability	Validity
Manual palpation		
Presence or absence and type of sound		
Uncalibrated examiner	kappa = 0.30[a,b]	15% silent joints had
Calibrated examiner	kappa = 0.62[a,b]	disk displacement[c]
Stethoscope		
Presence or absence and type of sound		
Uncalibrated examiner	kappa = 0.35[a,b]	14% silent joints had
Calibrated examiner	kappa = 0.61[a,b]	disk displacement[d]
Tape recordings		
Presence or absence and type of sound*	14.0%[e]	n/a
	49.8%[f]	
Sonography	n/a	n/a
Electrovibratography	ICC = 0.75–1.0[g]	n/a

Sources: [a]Dworkin et al. 1988; [b]Dworkin et al. 1990b; [c]Westesson et al. 1989; [d]Schiffman et al. 1989; [e]Eriksson et al. 1987; [f]Milner et al. 1991; [g]Christensen and Orloff 1992.
* Percentage agreement of examiners.

TMJ SOUNDS

TMJ sounds are used to subclassify disk displacements from degenerative bony changes within the joint. The reliability of assessing TMJ sounds by manual palpation or stethoscope is poor with uncalibrated examiners and improves to acceptable levels after calibration (Table II). Westesson et al. (1989) evaluated the validity of using TMJ sounds to classify intracapsular conditions. Arthrographic examination of a group of 40 asymptomatic subjects showed that 15% of clinically silent joints had some form of disk displacement. In a similar arthrotomographic study of symptomatic patients, Schiffman et al. (1989) found that 14% of clinically silent temporomandibular joints had some form of internal derangement. These studies emphasize that absence of joint sounds does not indicate absence of disk displacement. Validation of joint sounds/vibrations includes a verification that the sound/vibration truly originates from an intracapsular source rather than ligament, skin, or other sources of potential contamination (Widmer 1989).

TMJ IMAGING

Imaging can be used as an optional source of information for assessing disk and bony morphology in the RDC. Arthrographic reliability information

Table III
Reliability and validity of TMJ imaging

Assessment Technique	Reliability	Validity
Arthrography		
Disk displacement		
Inferior joint space	n/a	84% true correlation to anatomy[a]
Magnetic resonance imaging (MRI)		
Disk displacement		
Sagittal view	kappa = 0.59[b]	73–85% true correlation to anatomy[c,d]
Tomography		
Degenerative changes	kappa = 0.47–0.80[e]	63–85% true correlation to anatomy[f–h]

Sources: [a]Westesson et al. 1986; [b]van der Kuijl et al. 1992; [c]Drace et al. 1990; [d]Hansson et al. 1989; [e]Cholitgul et al. 1990; [f]Bean et al. 1977; [g]Rohlin et al. 1986; [h]Tanimoto et al. 1990.

is not available but MRI and tomography both have good to very good reliabilities (Table III), especially when trained examiners and reference films are used (Rohlin and Petersson 1989). Validation of the imaged structures has been performed using cryosections of human TMJs and correlations up to 85% have been reported.

SUMMARY

The goal of the researcher (or clinician) involved in TMD diagnosis is to have a set of measuring tools that are reliable and can accurately measure physical attributes that are used as criteria for case ascertainment. The tools that are used as part of the RDC for TMDs have sufficient reliability and validity to allow classification of discrete subtypes of TMDs. Although some clinicians may suggest that tools with more precision (i.e., measuring vertical range of opening to the nearest hundredth millimeter or recording joint sounds with higher amplification) should be used to evaluate certain physical attributes, it is important to understand that higher precision may not be necessary. Physical attributes associated with TMDs certainly vary, which probably contributes to the inability to attain higher reliability scores for many of the physical measures. Until the need for higher precision is demonstrated, using physical evaluation techniques such as those used in the TMD/RDC with appropriate training and retraining is the most reliable and valid approach that we can use for diagnosing TMDs.

DIAGNOSTIC RELIABILITY AND VALIDITY

Research diagnostic criteria for TMDs form boundary conditions under which a specific disorder can be evaluated as present or absent. Diagnostic reliability and validity may be assessed by using these criteria for classification. Diagnostic reliability, or the ability to consistently classify persons as having or not having the disease, can indicate the repeatability of the diagnostic classifications. One study has assessed diagnostic reliability of the RDC and reported good to excellent reliability scores for all of the categories except osteoarthrosis (Zaki et al. 1994). This important information helps to support the ability to acquire the physical measures by different investigators and to apply their results to the formulation of a consistent diagnosis.

Diagnostic validity is the extent that diagnostic criteria can be used to classify persons regarding presence or absence of a disorder and is consistent with the "gold standard" classification. Although ideally a biological assay would be used as the standard for comparison, such an assay does not exist for musculoskeletal conditions. Given this dilemma (not unlike other medical specialties such as psychiatry where no biological assay exists), Feighner-like criteria can be used to determine the validity of diagnostic criteria by examining cross-sectional and longitudinal evidence to determine homogeneity of diagnostic groups (Feighner and Herbstein 1987). Evidence may include examining risk factors for developing the disorder, evaluation of the natural history of the disorder, monitoring how different treatments will affect the disorder, and evaluating potential genetic factors that may be used to predict the susceptibility to the disorder. In the area of TMDs, there are few well-designed studies that have addressed these issues.

At present, there are no data to assess the validity of various physical assessment techniques for each diagnostic subgroup of the RDC. Therefore, to gain a general impression of the diagnostic abilities of each measure, diagnosis will consist of TMD or non-TMD as assessed from various studies of asymptomatic and TMD-positive groups. Parameters such as sensitivity, specificity, and positive predictive values have been compiled and calculated (Tables IV–VI) to allow a relative comparison of the various techniques. Sensitivity refers to the ability to successfully identify TMD patients in a TMD-positive group while specificity is the ability to successfully identify non-TMD subjects in a non-TMD group. Positive predictive value (PPV) refers to the ability to correctly identify a TMD patient when the diagnostic test is positive and incorporates the prevalence of the disease in the general population. For comparison purposes, random selection was calculated as a standard for comparing the abilities of each of the physical measures for TMD diagnosis.

Table IV
Sensitivity, specificity, and positive predictive values of random selection
and palpable tenderness assessment techniques for TMD

Assessment Technique	Cutoff	Sensitivity	Specificity	PPV*
Random selection (tossing a coin)	Heads = TMD Tails = normal	0.50	0.50	0.12
Muscle/TMJ palpation *Manual palpation*				
Muscle tenderness	Males: 2/16 sites	0.69	0.59	0.19
	Females: 2/16 sites	0.75	0.50	0.17
	Males: 3/16 sites	0.62	0.73	0.24
	Females: 3/16 sites	0.64	0.61	0.18
	Males: 4/16 sites	0.45	0.80	0.23
	Females: 4/16 sites	0.52	0.71	0.20
	Males: 5/16 sites	0.31	0.89	0.28
	Females: 5/16 sites	0.40	0.87	0.30
TMJ tenderness	Males: lateral	0.28	0.96	0.46
	Females: lateral	0.37	0.87	0.29
	Males: EAM†	0.14	0.96	0.30
	Females: EAM	0.17	0.93	0.26
	Males: lateral/EAM	0.35	0.93	0.41
	Females: lateral/EAM	0.45	0.86	0.30
Pressure algometer	—	n/a	n/a	n/a

Source: Data on muscle/TMJ palpation from personal communication, Dworkin and
LeResche, 1994.
* PPV calculated from sensitivity and specificity using TMD prevalence of 12%.
† EAM = external auditory meatus.

Prior to discussing physical assessment techniques, it is important to recognize the impact that a positive history for orofacial pain can have on identifying TMD patients. In a cross-sectional study of patients enrolled in a health
care group, patients were classified as community controls or community
cases based on their response to a question of "facial ache or pain in the jaw
muscles, the joint in front of the ear, or inside the ear in the previous six
months" (Truelove et al. 1992). The community cases with a positive history
of pain were then classified as TMD patients using operationalized criteria
developed from TMD clinical experts. For the community cases, 82% were
positively identified as TMD patients. This finding suggests that the patient
history by itself can identify a significant number of TMD patients based on

Table V
Sensitivity, specificity, and positive predictive values of manual
and electronic kinesiology assessment techniques for TMD

Assessment Technique	Cutoff	Sensitivity	Specificity	PPV*
Mandibular kinesiology				
Maximum opening				
Pain-free opening (part of	Males: 40 mm	0.14[a]	0.99[a]	0.66
myofascial pain diagnosis)	Females: 40 mm	0.26[a]	0.89[a]	0.24
Maximum opening with pain (part	Males: 35 mm	0.00[a]	0.99[b]	0.00
of disk displacement diagnosis)	Females: 35 mm	0.012[a]	1.00[a]	1.00
Opening movement pattern	> 3 mm	n/a	n/a	n/a
Horizontal mandibular movement	Males: < 7 mm	0.28[a]	0.73[a]	0.12
	Females: < 7 mm	0.24[a]	0.75[a]	0.12
Electronic kinesiology				
Movement speed	300 mm/sec	n/a	0.24[c]	n/a
	250 mm/sec	1.00[d]	0.20[d]	0.15
	250 mm/sec	0.75[e]	0.48[e]	0.16
Anterior/vertical ratio	1:2	0.86[d]	0.30[d]	0.14
Chewing motion	descriptive	0.26[d]	0.70[d]	0.11
Crossover pattern	sagittal plane	0.26[e]	0.65[e]	0.09
		0.57[d]	0.40[d]	0.11
Deviated pattern	frontal plane	1.00[e]	0.00[e]	0.12
Deviated pattern	sagittal plane	0.83[e]	0.42[e]	0.16

Sources: [a]Personal communication, Dworkin and LeResche 1994; [b]Dworkin et al.
1990a; [c]Cooper and Rabuzzi 1984; [d]Feine et al. 1988; [e]Tsolka et al. 1994.
* PPV calculated from sensitivity and specificity using a TMD prevalence of 12%.

awareness of pain in the region of the masticatory musculoskeletal system. For the community controls, nonpain diagnoses were found in 0.5% of the group and included disk displacement and osteoarthrosis. Based on these findings, it is important to consider the history as providing a substantial portion of the TMD diagnosis.

MUSCLE/TMJ PALPATION

Although there are no published studies reporting palpation of the same muscle sites as described in the research diagnostic criteria, the cross-sectional study by Dworkin et al. (1990a) evaluated 16 of 20 sites used in the RDC. As an approximation, the sensitivity, specificity, and PPV were calculated using the data set from Dworkin et al. (Table IV) using cutoff levels from two sites or more up to five sites or more for comparison purposes. For all cutoff levels,

Table VI
Sensitivity, specificity, and positive preditive values of TMJ sounds
and TMJ imaging for assessment of TMD

	Cutoff	Sensi-tivity	Speci-ficity	PPV*
TMJ sounds				
Manual palpation				
Click	single sound	0.43[a]	0.75[a]	0.19
Crepitus	soft multiple sound	0.08[a]	0.92[a]	0.12
Grating	hard multiple sound	0.06[a]	0.98[a]	0.45
Any sound	all types	0.57[a]	0.66[a]	0.19
Electrovibratography				
Click†	I(T) = 2.9	0.75[b]	0.77[b]	0.31
Imaging				
Arthrography				
Disk displacement†	inferior joint space	0.95[c]	0.76[c]	0.35
Magnetic resonance imaging (MRI)				
Disk displacement†	sagittal view	0.86[d]	0.63[d]	0.24
	sagittal and coronal views	0.90[e]	1.0[e]	1.0
Tomography				
Degenerative changes	sagittal view	0.47[f]	0.94[f]	0.52

Sources: [a]Dworkin et al. 1990a; [b]Ishigaki et al. 1993; [c]Westesson et al. 1986; [d]Westesson et al. 1987; [e]Tasaki and Westesson 1993; [f]Tanimoto et al. 1990.
* PPV calculated from sensitivity and specificity using a TMJ prevalence of 12% (Dworkin et al. 1990a).
† Sensitivity and specificity determined from a known disk displacement TMD population and a normal group without TMJ sounds, not from a random sampling of the population.

females consistently showed higher sensitivity and lower specificity values when compared to males. This finding suggests that females may have an elevated response to muscle palpation and that establishing optimal cutoff levels may require consideration of gender effects.

Palpable lateral TMJ or external auditory meatus (EAM) tenderness has a modest sensitivity but high specificity. This finding probably reflects a hetero-geneous population of TMD patients who have either muscle or joint related tenderness. Comparing lateral joint tenderness or EAM tenderness as positive discriminators of TMD patients shows that both criteria have nearly the same specificity but different abilities to identify TMD patients (sensitivity). Lateral tenderness has approximately double the sensitivity of EAM tenderness in both sexes. When criteria are used that incorporate either lateral tenderness or EAM tenderness, there is little improvement in the classification of TMD and non-TMD patients over lateral tenderness alone.

Both muscle tenderness and joint tenderness along with maximum vertical opening comprise measures that have the highest positive predictive value, probably because of the larger numbers of patients with these signs. However, the PPV rarely exceeds 0.66 for any criterion used to identify TMD patients from non-TMD patients. In the one case where PPV was perfect (35-mm cutoff for a female with a diagnosis of displaced disk), the sensitivity was poor (0.012).

MANDIBULAR KINESIOLOGY

In general, maximum opening values do not adequately separate asymptomatic subjects from TMD patients (Table V). The two cutoffs for maximum opening that are used for myofascial pain and displaced disk diagnoses are not corrected for gender in the RDC and it is apparent that there are sex differences for sensitivity, specificity, and PPV. Therefore, establishing gender-related maximum opening cutoffs should be a parameter to examine in future studies. Horizontal movement ranges of less than 7 mm do not predict a substantial portion of the TMD population (sensitivity of 0.12) and probably represent a small number patients with disk displacement without reduction found in the TMD group.

The use of electronic instruments to evaluate various parameters of jaw movement such as mandibular velocity, anterior/vertical ratio, chewing motion, crossover pattern, or deviated pattern does not improve the ability to detect TMD from non-TMD patients and, in fact, have no better diagnostic ability than chance (PPV are nearly equal to random selection). These values are substantially lower than manual techniques that are used in research and clinical studies for evaluation of mandibular range of motion. Therefore, the use of electronic kinesiology is contraindicated given the unacceptable measurement reliability and validity as well as diagnostic reliability and validity.

TMJ SOUNDS

Due to the high prevalence of sounds in the general population, the use of this criteria to correctly identify a TMD patient is low no matter how the joint sound is identified (Table VI). This situation is reflected in the low PPV values representing the various sounds used in the RDC. Other studies that have proposed alternative techniques have not examined a normal population, but instead selected subjects without joint sounds as control (normal) subjects. One such electrovibratography study of clicks in the TMD population was designed to test the ability to detect clicks in patients with arthrographically identified disk displacement. Even using this modified population of normals, this technique of recording vibrations using accelerometers over each TMJ does not substantially improve the ability to predict TMD patients and would be substantially lower in a random sample of subjects.

IMAGING

The sensitivity and specificity of imaging data were calculated using a modified TMD group of known disk displacement patients and nonclicking, asymptomatic subjects. These data, therefore, do not incorporate the other categories that are more commonly found, such as muscle disorders. The low PPVs of arthrography and tomography reflect the low prevalence of disk disorders in the general population (Table VI). The specificity of 1.0 found with sagittal and coronal MRI views reflects the preselected "normals" under study and, if a general population were used, would have a much lower PPV.

SUMMARY

It was not unexpected to find low positive predictive values for each of the measurement techniques because TMDs comprised of multiple subgroups. The higher specificity values are more important in diseases or disorders that are not life-threatening and, in addition, would help to exclude persons without TMD from pursuing expensive and irrelevant treatment modalities. A more extensive discussion of this topic has been made elsewhere (Widmer 1992).

Physical assessment parameters incorporated in the RDC classification for subtypes of temporomandibular disorders have relatively good reliability and validity. In addition, the RDC measures show good to excellent diagnostic reliability, suggesting their potential for classifying patients into consistent RDC-defined subgroups. Lacking, however, are data evaluating diagnostic validity for various TMD subtypes. This information would be necessary to ascertain the specific parameters required to define each TMD subtype. Additionally, there is a lack of data evaluating the ability of the RDC to accurately identify TMDs from other orofacial pain diagnoses. Obtaining such data would involve evaluating other orofacial pain groups in addition to TMD patients to determine the RDC diagnostic capability. This information also will be crucial in validating and refining a positive diagnostic criteria set specifically for TMDs.

ACKNOWLEDGMENT

This work was supported in part by USPHS Grants DE00333 (CGW) and DE10130 (CGW). The data and the specific analyses for sensitivity and specificity calculations were supported in part by USPHS Grants DE07197 (Samuel F. Dworkin) and DE08773 (SFD). Constructive comments provided by Drs. Samuel Dworkin and Linda LeResche were greatly appreciated.

REFERENCES

Balkhi, K.M and Tallents, R.H., Error analysis of a magnetic jaw-tracking device, J. Craniomandib. Disord. Facial Oral Pain, 5 (1991) 51–56.

Cholitgul, W., Petersson, A., Rohlin, M., Tanimoto, K. and Åkerman, S., Diagnostic outcome and observer performance in sagittal tomography of the temporomandibular joint, Dentomaxillofac. Radiol., 19 (1990) 1–6.

Christensen, L.V. and Orloff, J., Reproducibility of temporomandibular joint vibrations (electrovibratography), J. Oral Rehabil., 19 (1992) 253–263.

Cooper, B.C. and Rabuzzi, D.D., Myofacial [sic] pain dysfunction syndrome: a clinical study of asymptomatic subjects, Laryngoscope, 94 (1984) 68–75.

Drace, J.E., Young, S.W. and Enzmann, D.R., TMJ meniscus and bilaminar zone: MR imaging of the substructure-diagnostic landmarks and pitfalls of interpretation, Radiology, 177 (1990) 73–76.

Dworkin, S.F. and LeResche, L., Research diagnostic criteria for temporomandibular disorders: review, criteria, examination and specifications, critique, J. Craniomandib. Disord. Facial. Oral Pain, 6 (1992) 301–355.

Dworkin, S.F., Le Resche, L. and Derouen, T., Reliability of clinical measurement in temporomandibular disorders, Clin. J. Pain, 4 (1988) 88–99.

Dworkin, S.F., Huggins, K.H., Le Resche, L., Von Korff, M.R., Howard, J., Truelove, E. and Sommers, E., Epidemiology of signs and symptoms in temporomandiublar disorders: clinical signs in cases and controls, J. Am. Dent. Assoc., 120 (1990a) 273–281.

Dworkin, S.F., LeResche, L., Derouen, T. and Von Korff, M.R., Assessing clinical signs of temporomandibular disorders: reliability of clinical examiners, J. Prosthet. Dent., 63 (1990b) 574–579.

Eriksson, L., Westesson, P.-L. and Sjoberg, H., Observer performance in describing temporomandibular joint sounds, J. Craniomandib. Pract., 5 (1987) 32–35.

Feighner, J.P. and Herbstein, J., Diagnostic validity. In: C.G. Last and M. Hersen (eds.), Issues in Diagnostic Research, Plenum Press, New York, 1987, pp. 121–140.

Feine, J.S., Hutchins, M.O. and Lund, J.P., An evaluation of the criteria used to diagnose mandibular dysfunction with the mandibular kinesiograph, J. Prosthet. Dent., 60 (1988) 374–380.

Goulet, J. and Clark, G.T., Clinical TMJ examination methods, J. Calif. Dent. Assoc., 18 (1990) 25–33.

Hansson, L.-G., Westesson, P.-L., Katzberg, R.W., Tallents, R.H., Kurita, K., Holtas, S., Svensson, S.A., Eriksson, L. and Johansen, C.C., MR imaging of the temporomandibular joint: comparisons of images of autopsy specimens made at 0.3 T and 1.5 T with anatomic cryosections, Am. J. Roentgenol., 152 (1989) 1241–1244.

Ishigaki, S., Bessette, R.W. and Maruyama, T., A clinical study of temporomandibular joint (TMJ) vibrations in TMJ dysfunction patients, J. Craniomandib. Pract., 11 (1993) 7–13.

McNeill, C., Mohl, N.D., Rugh, J.D. and Tanaka, T., Temporomandibular disorders: diagnosis, management, education, and research, J. Am. Dent. Assoc., 120 (1990) 253–263.

Milner, D., LeResche, L., Dworkin, S.F. and Hammen, V., TMJ sounds: characteristics and examiner reliability (abstract), J. Dent. Res., 70 (1991) 371.

Rohlin, M. and Petersson, A., Rheumatoid arthritis of the temporomandibular joint: radiologic evaluation based on standard reference films, Oral Surg. Oral Med. Oral Pathol., 67 (1989) 594–599.

Rohlin, M., Akerman, S. and Kopp, S., Tomography as an aid to detect microscopic changes of the temporomandibular joint, Acta Odontol. Scand., 44 (1986) 131–140.

Schiffman, E., Anderson, G.C., Fricton, J., Burton, K. and Schellhas, K., Diagnostic criteria for intraarticular TM disorders, Community Dent. Oral Epidemiol., 17 (1989) 252–257.

Tanimoto, K., Petersson, A., Rohlin, M., Hansson, L.-G. and Johansen, C.C., Comparison of computed with conventional tomography in the evaluation of temporomandibular joint disease: a study of autopsy specimens, Dentomaxillofac. Radiol., 19 (1990) 21–27.

Tasaki, M.M. and Westesson, P., Temporomandibular joint: diagnostic accuracy with sagittal and coronal MR imaging, Radiology, 186 (1993) 723–729.

Throckmorton, G.S., Teenier, T.J. and Ellis, E., Reproducibility of mandibular motion and muscle activity levels using a commercial computer recording system, J. Prosthet. Dent., 68 (1992) 348–354.

Truelove, E., Sommers, E.E., LeResche, L., Dworkin, S.F. and Von Korff, M.R., Clinical diagnostic criteria for TMD: new classification permits multiple diagnoses, J. Am. Dent. Assoc., 123 (1992) 47–54.

Tsolka, P., Woelfel, J.B., Man, W.K. and Preiskel, H.W., A laboratory assessment of recording reliability and analysis of the K6 diagnostic system, J. Craniomandib. Disord. Facial Oral Pain, 6 (1992) 273–280.

Tsolka, P., Fenlon, M.R., McCullock, A.J. and Preiskel, H.W., A controlled clinical, electromyographic, and kinesiographic assessment of craniomandibular disorders in women, J. Orofacial Pain, 8 (1994) 80–89.

van der Kuijl, B., Schellhas, K.P., Mooyaart, E.L., de Bont, L.G.M. and Boering, G., Temporomandibular joint magnetic resonance imaging: reliability of articular disk visualization. In: Temporomandibular Joint: Evaluation of Imaging Techniques, University of Groningen, Groningen, The Netherlands, 1992, pp. 57–67.

Westesson, P.-L., Bronstein, S.L. and Liedberg, J., Temporomandibular joint: correlation between single-contrast videoarthrography and postmortem morphology, Radiology, 160 (1986) 767–771.

Westesson, P.-L., Katzberg, R.W., Tallents, R.H., Sanchez-Woodworth, R.E., Svensson, S.A. and Espeland, M.A., Temporomandibular joint: comparison of MR images with cryosectional anatomy, Radiology, 164 (1987) 59–64.

Westesson, P.-L., Eriksson, L. and Kurita, K., Reliability of a negative clinical temporomandibular joint examination: prevalence of disk displacement in asymptomatic temporomandibular joints, Oral Surg. Oral Med. Oral Pathol., 68 (1989) 551–554.

Widmer, C.G., Temporomandibular joint sounds: a critique of techniques for recording and analysis, J. Craniomandib. Disord. Facial Oral Pain, 3 (1989) 213–217.

Widmer, C.G., Reliability and validation of examination methods, J. Craniomandib. Disord. Facial Oral Pain, 6 (1992) 318–326.

Zaki, H.S., Rudy, T.E., Turk, D.C. and Capirano, M., Reliability of axis I research diagnostic criteria for TMD (abstract), J. Dent. Res., 73 (1994) 186.

Correspondence to: Charles G. Widmer, DDS, MS, Dept. of Oral and Maxillofacial Surgery, Box 100416, JHMHSC, University of Florida, Gainesville, FL 32610-0416, USA. Tel: 904-392-8964; Fax: 904-392-7609.

Temporomandibular Disorders and Related Pain Conditions, Progress in Pain Research and Management, Vol. 4, edited by B.J. Sessle, P.S. Bryant, and R.A. Dionne, IASP Press, Seattle, © 1995.

11

Behavioral Characteristics of Chronic Temporomandibular Disorders: Diagnosis and Assessment

Samuel F. Dworkin

Department of Oral Medicine, School of Dentistry, University of Washington, Seattle, Washington, USA

Current research findings make clear that patients with suspected temporomandibular disorders (TMDs) should be assessed for behavioral characteristics along with the expected assessment of physical signs necessary to determine a muscle and/or joint TMD diagnosis. This chapter reviews representative scientific evidence to support the utility of conducting such behavioral assessments, includes a brief review of how behavioral assessments have led some investigators to offer schemes for classifying TMD patients according to level of psychosocial function, and describes the more common methods used to accomplish behavioral assessment and psychosocial classification of TMDs, as well as other chronic pain disorders.

Behavioral assessment, in its narrowest sense, is the measurement of observable behavior only, to the exclusion of emotional and mental states such as depression, anxiety, beliefs, and expectations. The first application of psychological concepts to the management of chronic pain, introduced at the University of Washington Pain Clinic by Fordyce (1976), stressed almost exclusively this behavioral approach. These notions had a tremendous impact, radically altering the management of chronic pain, reinforcing the multidisciplinary focus on treatment that was already emerging, and compelling a predominate focus on behaviorally based treatment methods.

OVERVIEW OF BEHAVIORAL ASSESSMENT

Most clinical pain researchers strongly advocate use of the term *behavioral assessment,* but with the broader definition it has acquired over the past

25 years (Turk and Flor 1987). It now encompasses assessment of the patient's cognitive and emotional status as well as the current level of psychosocial functioning, which includes assessment of pain coping and treatment seeking behaviors. For persistent TMD pain, assessment should emphasize the extent to which it disrupts or interferes with socially adaptive behavior at home, work, or school, and the association between pain course and treatment.

Undeniably, a compelling reason to incorporate behavioral assessment is that the most important, almost universal feature of TMDs is chronic pain. About 97% of TMD patients seek treatment for pain predominantly in the preauricular area of the temporomandibular joint (TMJ) and/or in the muscles of mastication, sometimes radiating to the temples and sometimes to the back of the head and neck, and which is frequently aggravated by mandibular function. The remaining few patients seek treatment in the absence of pain, largely because of joint sounds that bother them or someone else or, even rarer, because they feel something is wrong in the way their jaws work (Dworkin et al. 1990a).

The ultimate objective for research on TMDs is to provide long-lasting and effective treatment for this clinical disorder. Thus, the principal reason for conducting a behavioral assessment of a TMD patient—indeed any chronic pain patient—is that it opens up additional treatment possibilities. There would be no reason to be concerned with behavioral assessment if it did not make a difference in how these patients can be treated (Table I).

The most common chronic pain conditions, including back pain, headache, and TMDs, each have unique features and those they share in common. The features unique to each chronic pain condition relate, of course, to the physical structures involved and the pathophysiologic processes that may affect those structures; assessment of these physical dimensions leads to the familiar clinical diagnoses such as migraine headache, sciatica, or TMJ disk displacement without reduction. In contrast, the features that all chronic pain

Table I
The rationale and objectives of TMD
behavioral assessment

Behavioral assessment seeks to identify:
Psychosocial factors affecting
pain perception
pain behavior
functional impairment
Individualized treatment goals
Effective treatment interventions
Biomedical treatment
Biobehavioral interventions

conditions have in common fall in the behavioral or psychosocial domain and cannot be assessed with the same methods and measuring instruments used to assess pathologic physical change. The most important of these chronic pain behavioral characteristics are:

1. Poor correspondence between the nature or extent of pathophysiologic change and global severity of pain and suffering;

2. Transient psychological distress;

3. The potential for clinically meaningful depression, anxiety, and somatization—the tendency to become preoccupied with physical symptoms;

4. Interference with ability to perform usual activities at home, work, or school;

5. Dysfunctional behaviors that directly affect the pain condition, such as oral parafunctional habits; and

6. Frequent use of the health care system, with potential for excessive treatment seeking and abuse of medications.

Are TMDs chronic pain conditions that share characteristics in common with other common chronic pain conditions? Data from many studies confirm this point, including studies of Turk and Rudy (Rudy et al. 1989), Keefe (Keefe et al. 1992), Gatchel (Gatchel and Baum 1993a), Marbach (Marbach et al. 1990) and Dohrenwend (Lennon et al. 1990), and their respective colleagues.

Table II compares behavioral assessment of patients reporting chronic

Table II

Comparison of pain, psychological, and behavior variables for chronic pain conditions in primary care patients

	TMD	Headache	Back Pain
Pain variables (means)			
Average pain intensity (VAS)	5.0	6.0	4.7
Disability days	10.4	10.1	19.8
Days in pain	91.7	55.2	78.5
Years since onset	6.0	17.5	12.3
Selected variables (% of subjects)			
Elevated depression	25.6	28.4	22.0
Health rated fair to poor	12.8	13.7	9.9
Frequent pain visits	7.5	9.2	8.1
High pain impact	23.8	35.4	32.8

headache, back pain, and TMD pain on several important psychological, behavioral, and psychosocial dimensions along which chronic pain is commonly
assessed. These data clearly show that TMDs do indeed pose a significant
chronic pain problem for many persons. Its severity, persistence, and associated psychological or behavioral dysfunction appear at least as problematic,
and for some parameters—for example, number of days with pain—more
problematic than for those suffering chronic back pain and headache. The data
cited here and similar findings from the numerous investigators already mentioned lend construct validity to the concept that TMDs are chronic pain
conditions, justifying research into etiology and treatment that is not limited to
the pathophysiologic domain but extends into the multidimensional
biopsychosocial sphere.

To help our understanding of how biologic and psychosocial dimensions
of chronic pain are related, an integrated biopsychosocial model for chronic
pain (Dworkin et al. 1992) provides both a clinical and theoretical framework
for generating specific, behaviorally based treatment interventions (Fig. 1).
These biobehavioral interventions do not target *pathophysiology* as the direct
object of change. Nevertheless, they may be used not only to control pain, but
to control disability, depression, somatization, and inappropriate health care
behavior. The proposed model helps to pinpoint at which level to make those
behavioral interventions.

Nested schematically at the base of the model is the presumption of
physical pathology, or at least physical changes in muscle, joints, and nerves
that generate signals that make their way to the brain via the nociceptive
transmission system, which is reviewed elsewhere in this volume. These signals are called nociception at the physiologic or pathophysiologic level of
analysis because they are not yet pain; the nociceptive information has not yet
been subjected to higher order psychological or mental processes performed
by the brain process to determine the following:

1. How the information is *perceived*—whether the information is described
   as pain, and if so, what type of pain—aching, sharp, well-localized or
   diffuse, of brief or long duration, etc.

2. The next level involves one of the most crucial determinations—the
   perception is *appraised*. Patients given cognitive and emotional meaning
   to the buzzing signals: this pain will kill me; it's nothing, I can live with it;
   I'd better get to the doctor right now; I'm worried to death over this; I'm
   so down, nothing will help.

3. Next comes *behavior*. Several terms describe a behavioral response to
   persistent pain that exceeds adaptive limits: Fordyce (1976) called it
   chronic pain behavior; others label it chronic pain syndrome or dysfunc-

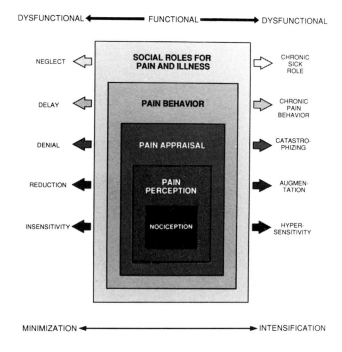

DYSFUNCTIONAL ◄──────── FUNCTIONAL ────────► DYSFUNCTIONAL

NEGLECT	SOCIAL ROLES FOR PAIN AND ILLNESS	CHRONIC SICK ROLE
DELAY	PAIN BEHAVIOR	CHRONIC PAIN BEHAVIOR
DENIAL	PAIN APPRAISAL	CATASTRO-PHIZING
REDUCTION	PAIN PERCEPTION	AUGMEN-TATION
INSENSITIVITY	NOCICEPTION	HYPER-SENSITIVITY

MINIMIZATION ◄──────────────────────────► INTENSIFICATION

Fig 1. An integrated biopsychosocial model for chronic pain.

tional chronic pain, which is the label we prefer. Dysfunctional chronic pain implies two types of behavioral excess related to the sick role that are now thought worthy of assessment:

a. An *avoidance* excess associated with avoiding personal and social responsibilities, including avoidance of responsibilities for *self-manage-ment* of the disorder.

b. An *approach* excess associated with undue reliance on the health care system—an *other-oriented* approach that relies on drugs and doctors for management of the disorder.

By recognizing that all these processes are occurring simultaneously in TMD patients, as they would to some extent in each of us, and by assessing behavioral components in addition to physical ones, the clinician can determine the need for biobehavioral interventions, using a decision-making process analogous to that invoked to arrive at physical diagnoses and treatment plans. Many of these biobehavioral interventions, such as relaxation training, biofeedback, modifying inappropriate beliefs, and developing behavioral coping strategies, could be competently delivered by dentists and physicians. These biobehavioral interventions to facilitate coping with pain and its fre-

quent concomitants—stress, anxiety, depression, dysfunctional chronic pain—
are never conceived by behavioral scientists as alternatives to biomedically
based therapies, but as complements. Abundant research opportunities abound
to investigate clinical decision-making processes that establish the relative
emphasis to be placed on biomedical and biobehavioral treatments. Obviously, such integrated clinical research is possible only through inclusion, in
the TMD diagnostic workup, of a dependable behavioral assessment.

METHODS FOR CONDUCTING BEHAVIORAL ASSESSMENT

Many methods have evolved for the behavioral assessment of patients
with chronic pain conditions. The two most important methods are observational and self-report.

OBSERVATIONAL METHODS

Keefe and his colleagues first developed direct observations of behavior
for back pain (Rosenstiel and Keefe 1983). The coding of facial expression
for pain has been developed by LeResche (LeResche and Dworkin 1988) and
others, including Craig (1984) and Prkachin and Mercer (1990). Direct
behavioral measures of TMD patients are not as well developed as are the
self-report measures available for assessing TMDs. However, the assessment
of facial expressions of chronic pain does indicate a potential use for this
measure in clinical research. For example, LeResche and colleagues (1992)
have shown that patients with recent onset TMDs show few facial expressions
of pain but these expressions increase in frequency as a function of chronicity
of the disorder, implying that facial expressions become an increasingly important means for communicating pain and suffering for the chronic TMD
patient. At present, the coding and analysis of facial expression data for pain
and other emotions remains a relatively specialized and labor-intensive task
probably limiting its widespread availability as a method for direct observation of TMD pain-related behavior.

SELF-REPORT METHODS

Typically, self-report measures take the form of symptom checklists, psychological and behavioral rating scales, and psychological tests assessing mental
and emotional status, psychosocial adaptation, coping behaviors, and health
care utilization. Several worthwhile measures have received at least some
attention from biobehaviorally oriented TMD clinical researchers. Gatchel
and others (Butterworth and Deardorff 1987) incorporate criteria from the

DSM-III-R (the diagnostic and statistical manual of the American Psychiatric Association), which indicate that clinical psychopathology is present in an appreciable number of chronic TMD patients. Pain coping measures developed by Keefe and colleagues (1992) indicate that coping strategies such as catastrophizing and praying may be common among less psychosocially functional pain patients. Active versus passive pain coping styles can be assessed by the coping measure developed by Brown and Nicassio (1987).

Measures of coping with stress not specific to chronic pain also have been employed successfully. These include the Ways of Coping Checklist and the measures of daily stress, which Dohrenwend, Marbach, and their colleagues (Lennon et al. 1990) used to study psychosocial adaptation of TMD patients. These studies also confirm the extent to which TMDs can be disabling for an appreciable segment of TMD sufferers. Measures developed by Pilowsky (1986) and by Bergner and colleagues (1981), including the Sickness Impact Profile and the Illness Behavior Questionnaire, assess the impact of illness and illness beliefs. These measures have provided useful information about behavioral adaptation to chronic pain, including disability associated with chronic pain conditions, notably back pain and differences in beliefs and expectations between pain clinic populations and chronic pain patients seeking treatment elsewhere.

Numerous additional measures assess diverse dimensions of the chronic pain experience. Those that seem to warrant attention from biobehavioral TMD researchers include the Millon Behavioral Health Inventory, Chronic Illness Problem Inventory, the Psychosocial Pain Inventory, and the Pain Beliefs Questionnaire (Bradley et al. 1992; Gatchel and Baum 1993). Self-report measures that have received attention in the TMD literature include the MMPI and the SCL-90R, widely used psychological scales; the TMJ Scale and the IMPATH Scale, which are specific to TMDs; and the Multidimensional Pain Inventory and the Graded Chronic Pain Scale, which are useful for any chronic pain condition.

Use of the MMPI for TMDs

The MMPI, or Minnesota Multiphasic Personality Inventory, is perhaps the best known and most widely used instrument for assessing psychological status. It is not a diagnostic instrument, but rather gives a profile of psychological function. The test is long and requires highly specialized training to interpret, hence many researchers do not consider it suitable for use. MMPI findings remain somewhat controversial. Several independent studies report that standardization samples used for MMPI scale construction are not appropriate for chronic pain patients. However, clustering methods have proven somewhat more useful for identifying MMPI scale profiles that characterize how the person is functioning cognitively and emotionally. Generally, for both the MMPI or the more recently revised and restandardized MMPI-2, elevations on Scales 1, 2, and 3—Hypochondriasis, Depression, and Hysteria—were associated with perceptions of severe pain, affective disturbance, and maladaptive patterns of psychosocial functioning. Not surprisingly, when elevations on the Psychopathic Deviancy and Schizophrenia scales accompanied elevations in Scales 1, 2, and 3, clinicians observed higher levels of psychopathology and resistance to modification of pain behavior (Bradley et al. 1992).

Although it was originally anticipated that distinct MMPI profiles would be confirmed for chronic pain patients, such profiles have not emerged clearly, and the use of the MMPI for predicting pain clinic treatment outcome, for example, remains problematic. Using the MMPI in a study predicting response to treatment for TMDs, McCreary et al. (1992) found that somatization was related to jaw function problems at long-term follow-up, but not at early follow-ups, and that "somatization was a significant predictor of outcome" for chronic TMD patients. McCreary concluded "if treatment does not address this somatization process, there is an increased risk there will be no improvement." Somatization appears to be a critical issue requiring attention in the management of dysfunctional chronic pain.

Use of the SCL-90R for TMDs

The Symptom Checklist-90 revised (SLC-90R; Derogatis 1983) is a 90-item symptom checklist that yields several scales, of which the most relevant for TMDs are those assessing depression, anxiety, and somatization. Although the SCL-90R is much briefer than the MMPI, its overall usefulness with chronic pain patients has not been unequivocally established. The SCL-90R has been used extensively to study all types of chronic pain populations, but problems have emerged. For example, those using the entire SCL-90R have encountered difficulty in replicating the original 10-factor structure obtained by Derogatis (Bradley et al. 1992). Interestingly, when comparing responses of chronic pain and psychiatric populations, Buckelew and colleagues (1986) found that the chronic pain population was distinguished by reports of psychological distress limited to somatic, as opposed to emotional or cognitive, symptoms of anxiety and depression.

We have used SCL-90R scales in our own research, taking care to develop our own population norms for the scales, and have reported extensively on findings with TMD and other chronic pain patients (Dworkin et al. 1990b, 1992, 1994). As an example, using SCL-90R data to examine the relationship between depression and somatization in TMD patients, we observed that when TMDs were accompanied by multiple somatic pain complaints, the likelihood of an SCL-90R algorithm diagnosis of major depression increased dramatically (Dworkin et al. 1990b). The risk for depression, in fact, increased by more than five- and eight-fold, respectively, depending on whether the TMD was accompanied by one or more than one coexisting self-reported pain condition, such as headache, back pain, chest, or stomach pain.

TMJ Scale

The TMJ Scale (Levitt et al. 1988, 1994; Levitt 1991) has been developed for use in the home or office and assesses three domains: physical, psychosocial, and global. The physical domain includes assessment of pain while the psychosocial domain assesses psychological factors and stress. The scale, which requires scoring and interpretation by its developers, seems to yield information that may be useful to guide clinicians treating TMDs, although Rugh et al. (1993), Deardorff (1994), and others (Glaros and Glass 1993) have raised some questions about its validity as a psychological assessment.

Levitt and McKinney (1994) have demonstrated the kinds of information that can be obtained with the TMJ scale when it is used in research; for example, that "joint dysfunction and range of motion limitation symptoms demonstrate significant trend of lower severity as age increases," and "psychological factors and stress do not show continuous increase in severity or prevalence in older age groups." Additionally, findings from the TMJ Scale indicate that women with TMDs report a higher level higher level of severity of all physical and psychological symptoms compared with men, and point to a relation between severity of psychological problems and chronicity of TMDs. As these authors readily acknowledge, the TMJ Scale has not been the subject of longitudinal studies; rather, the long-term data available reflect cross-sectional data collection over several years—specifically, cohorts of patients have not been repeatedly assessed with the TMJ Scale over time.

The IMPATH Scale for TMDs

The IMPATH Scale for TMDs is an interactive computer-based assessment instrument developed at the University of Minnesota by Fricton and colleagues (1987) for use as a screening and personal history instrument. It has the advantage of instantaneous feedback, but unfortunately the psychometric characteristics of its illness behavior components are not yet well established. Like the TMJ Scale, it may serve as a useful guide to clinicians wishing to obtain a clinical impression of how their patients are doing psychologically and behaviorally.

The Multidimensional Pain Inventory

Turk and colleagues have developed a widely used pain measure, the Multidimensional Pain Inventory (MPI), to assess psychosocial function in chronic pain patients (Turk and Rudy 1988; Rudy et al. 1989). The measure was developed with pain clinic populations and yields consistent profiles of pain patients across different chronic pain conditions, such as headache, back pain, and TMDs. The chronic pain groups distinguished by the MPI are labeled adaptive copers (AC), who maintain adequate psychosocial functioning despite their chronic pain; interpersonally distressed (ID), persons experiencing stress which impacts interpersonal relationships; and dysfunctional (DYS), representing persons rendered psychosocially dysfunctional due to chronic pain. The three types reflect a continuum of increasing disability and pain-related psychosocial dysfunction. Rudy and Turk (1989) have demonstrated that TMD patients characterized as dysfunctional show significantly elevated depression and reported significantly more physical symptoms than do TMD patients the MPI categorizes as adaptive copers (Table III). By contrast, dysfunctional TMD patients and adaptive copers are not significantly different along physical parameters (e.g., proportion of positive computerized tomography (CT) scan findings, objective findings from a TMD clinical exam).

Table III
Multidimensional pain inventory (MPI) results for TMD patients classified as
psychosocially dysfunctional (DYS), interpersonally
distressed (ID), and adaptive copers (AC)

	DYS	ID	AC	P
Psychological findings				
Pain rating (mean)	1.8	1.4	1.1	.001
Pain behaviors	5.0	3.3	2.8	.001
CES depression	21.7	14.5	9.5	.001
POMS (total)	48.4	29.1	5.0	.001
Daily hassles	73.6	51.7	44.7	.001
Wahler physical symptoms	1.6	1.3	1.1	.001
Physical findings				
Age	32.2	33.5	30.7	n.s.
Pain duration (years)	4.7	5.9	6.0	n.s.
Number of TMJ exam signs	1.2	1.2	1.4	n.s.
Maximum assisted open (mm)	30.2	30.3	32.0	n.s.
Percentage of positive CT findings	0.4	0.5	0.5	n.s.

Source: Rudy et al. 1989.
Note: CES = Center for Epidemiologic Studies; POMS = Profile of Mood States.

More recently, Rudy and colleagues have used the MPI to assess that relative efficacy of a cognitive-behavioral treatment intervention compared to a physical treatment that involved use of an intra-oral occlusal splint. They presented evidence indicating that dysfunctional versus adaptive copers and interpersonally stressed patients responded differentially to these treatments, supporting their conclusion that clinical treatment decisions for TMDs include not only assessment of behavioral status but assignment of TMD patients to treatment interventions specifically designed according to the assessed level of psychosocial function (Rudy et al. 1994). It appears that the MPI is one of the most carefully designed and well-studied self-report measure for assessing behavioral and psychosocial functioning in chronic pain patients.

RDC DUAL AXIS SCHEMATIC

An international team of clinical researchers has developed a research diagnostic criteria (RDC) dual axis system for diagnosing and classifying TMD patients (Dworkin and LeResche 1992). Axis I is reserved for physical diagnoses of muscle and/or joint disorders (see Widmer, this volume).

Axis II is used to accommodate classification of chronic pain grade, psychological distress reflected specifically as depression, the presence of non-specific physical symptoms to assess somatization tendencies, and also includes a measure of orofacial disability. RDC/TMD operationally defined criteria for Axes I and II are now available for researchers who wish to conduct studies assessing their reliability, validity, and clinical usefulness.

GRADED CHRONIC PAIN SCALE

An easy-to-use graded chronic pain scale, ranging from Grade 0 to Grade IV, has been developed from population-based data gathered in extensive longitudinal studies of chronic pain (Von Korff et al. 1992). The graded chronic pain scale was derived from population-based studies of chronic pain in the community and not from a pain clinic populations, so it can be used for data collection under a variety of research designs, ranging from random sample surveys to clinical intervention studies.

The graded chronic pain scale was created to provide a meaningful quantitative index of the extent to which pain is perceived not only as mild or severe in intensity, but simultaneously, to capture in the same quantitative index the extent to which pain is disabling (Table IV). Disability is measured by extent of pain-related interference with daily activities and number of lost activity days (e.g., days unable to go to work or school, attend to household

S.F. DWORKIN

Table IV
Definitions and prevalence of grades in the
graded chronic pain scale

Grade	Definition	Prevalence in Clinic Cases (%)	
		1986 (N = 261)	1992 (N = 148)
Functional chronic pain			
I	Low disability Low-intensity pain	39	43
II	Low disability High-intensity pain	42	35
Dysfunctional chronic pain			
III	High disability Moderate limitation	15	17
IV	High disability Severe limitation	4	5

responsibilities, etc.) attributed to TMD pain. Grades I and II include persons who report TMD pain of low or high intensity, respectively, but which, in either case, is associated with low disability, while Grades III and IV are associated with increasing levels of pain-related psychosocial disability regardless of pain level. Grades III and IV are, in fact, rarely associated with low levels of pain intensity. Functional TMD patients, i.e., those not significantly disabled by their TMD condition, are classified as Grades I and II. By contrast, dysfunctional chronic pain is defined as Grades III and IV on the Graded Chronic Pain Scale.

Although these demarcations of functional and dysfunctional have some empirical support (Von Korff et al. 1992), they have not been subjected to cross-validation of their clinical utility. Similarly, despite widespread agreement regarding the public health, research, and treatment implications, the concept of dysfunctional chronic pain has only minimally been extended to clinical research concerning TMDs.

The distribution of TMD patients by chronic pain grade was assessed in two samples: consecutive clinic cases referred to a large health maintenance organization (HMO) for TMD treatment in 1986 (N = 261), and clinic cases referred for treatment to both a large HMO and the University of Washington Orofacial Pain and Dysfunction Clinic about six years later (N = 148). More recent data (not shown) indicate an estimated 25–30% prevalence of dysfunctional TMD patients (Grades III/IV) in a more highly specialized and tertiary care TMD clinic at the University of Washington during 1992.

Important distinctions emerge when we attempt to relate the grade of

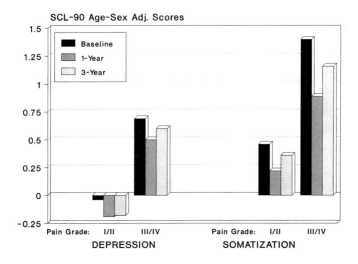

Fig. 2. Depression/somatization scores (SCL-90) compared with graded chronic pain status: baseline and one- and three-year follow-ups. Chronic pain grades I and II = functional; III and IV = dysfunctional.

TMD pain dysfunction to presumed underlying physical and psychological factors, using data from our longitudinal studies of TMD cases and controls. Fig. 2 compares chronic pain grade to depression and somatization scores using items from the SCL-90R scales for the same group of TMD cases over three years. Depression scores reflect the extent of self-reported subdued mood, feeling blue and sad, psychomotor and thought retardation, as well as loss of interest in social activities, work, appetite, and libido. Somatization as a psychiatric construct is generally described as having three components: (1) the predisposition to report numerous nonspecific physical symptoms (e.g., pounding heart, sweating, trembling, as well as reporting the presence of pain complaints, such as headache, back pain, stomach upset), (2) the tendency to seek medical treatment, and (3) emotional disturbance. Both depression and somatization have been heavily implicated in chronic pain, including TMDs (Dworkin et al. 1994; Wilson et al. 1994).

Functional patients, that is Grades I and II, show scores for both depression and somatization that are at or near the population mean for these measures. Dysfunctional TMD patients, Grades III and IV, score significantly higher, in the top 15–25% of scores on measures of depression and of the presence of nonspecific physical symptoms, including other pains. These values are age-sex adjusted and the population mean is zero for these scales.

In marked contrast, Fig. 3 depicts the relationship of chronic pain grade to unassisted vertical jaw opening. Dysfunctional TMD patients, who report high pain intensity together with frequently occurring pain that appreciably limits

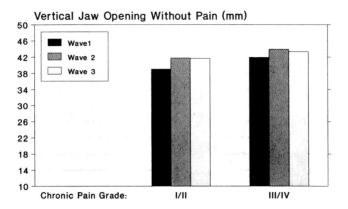

Fig. 3. Range of vertical jaw opening (mm) without pain compared with graded chronic pain status: baseline and one- and two-year follow-ups. Chronic pain grades I and II = functional; III and IV = dysfunctional.

their daily activities, nevertheless are indistinguishable from functional (Grades I and II) TMD patients in unassisted vertical range of jaw motion (or the total number of joint sounds detected; not shown in Fig. 3) on both vertical and lateral excursions of the jaw. These data indicate that TMD pain dysfunction is not significantly associated with these commonly assessed TMD signs.

Treatment history data also present challenges to evaluating how best to clinically manage TMDs. The graded chronic pain scale also differentiates TMD patients by treatment seeking behavior. Only about 11% of functional TMD patients sought treatment from five or more providers while significantly more—about half—of dysfunctional TMD patients had seen five or more TMD health care providers. Remember that presently available data indicate that clinical signs appear comparable for functional and dysfunctional cases. A parallel finding is observed with regard to somatization score: about half of those scoring in the top quartile for somatization also have seen as many as five or more TMD providers, while only about 18% of those in the lowest quartile have sought care from so many providers.

The RDC/TMD Axis II also includes a measure of jaw disability, whose psychometric properties have not been studied extensively. Since publication of this Axis II measure, other investigators have produced comparable scales of the behavioral impact on jaw function associated with TMDs. These scales have better-known psychometric properties and suggest the need to compare reliability, validity, and clinical utility of the Axis II jaw dysfunction scale to comparable measures recently reported in the TMD clinical literature.

SEMISTRUCTURED INTERVIEW FOR BEHAVIORAL
ASSESSMENT OF TMDs

The available clinical literature as well as the current consensus that has emerged from the shared clinical experiences of behavioral medicine clinicians working in this area yields guidelines for gathering relevant behavioral information about TMD patients. The following outline for a semistructured interview, adapted from a review by Bradley et al. (1992), is divided into four major domains of behavioral information, summarized without regard to assessment methods:

1. The *cognitive* domain, or what patients think, believe, and expect with regard to their TMD condition.

2. The *affective* domain, or the emotion state accompanying their TMD problem.

3. The *behavioral* domain, or what actions they take in response to TMDs.

4. Finally, an inquiry into specific pain coping strategies.

The purpose of such a behavioral inquiry is to gather clinical evidence about the current behavioral status of TMD patients to develop a more rational clinical treatment decision process.

In the *cognitive* domain, inquiry is directed to the patient's understanding of TMDs and the physical structures involved: what they believe went wrong (their theory about their problem), their understanding of the nature of chronic pain, their motivation for different kinds of treatment, and the extent to which they believe they have some control over how they are doing versus placing responsibility on the clinician—is the "cure" going to come entirely from the doctor?

In the *affective*, or emotional, domain, it is essential to evaluate whether the patient is significantly depressed or anxious or whether their current emotional status reflects a reasonable adaptation to a painful condition whose significance and future is uncertain.

In the *behavioral* domain, emphasis is given to evaluating how much the TMD is interfering with usual daily activities at home, work, school, and socially, and how much the TMD is preventing patients from continuing to discharge their personal, work, and social responsibilities. The second behavioral aspect relates to the use of health care. Is it reasonable or excessive? Are patients using or seeking many drugs or using or abusing street or recreational drugs to cope with their TMD problem?

We suggest this approach to clinical interviewing because it represents reinforcement—a kind of construct validity—to the concept that behavioral assessment is an integral part of chronic pain assessment. It also reinforces the widespread agreement regarding domains of inquiry that are most relevant to the eventual well-being of patients. It is clear that a wide variety of measures are available to researchers. Admittedly, the measures are in different stages of development and evaluation, some requiring further assessment of their reliability and validity, others requiring assessment of their clinical utility. Regardless, behavioral assessment of TMDs is possible through systematic approaches applicable to large-scale population-based studies and to randomized clinical trials of biobehavioral interventions.

SUMMARY OF RESEARCH QUESTIONS

This review suggests questions that researchers should address to shed light on this too often enigmatic condition.

1. Establish the validity and clinical utility of simultaneously classifying TMD patients according to their level of psychosocial function as well as their level of physical function.

2. Derive and confirm methods for integrating physical findings and psychosocial data into clinical diagnoses that yield differential treatment decisions based on effective integration of biomedical and biobehavioral treatments.

3. Identify dependable predictors of the long-term course of TMD signs and symptoms. Are the determinants of getting better or getting worse more heavily loaded with physical factors or are recurrent and longstanding TMD conditions more heavily associated with such factors as depression and somatization?

4. Ascertain under what conditions a TMD is a self-limiting and reversible condition and when it is a condition characterized by progressive deterioration of the physical structures and/or of quality of life.

5. Longitudinal data are needed concerning realistic outcomes for TMD patients. We need to develop an empirically derived basis for short- and long-term expectations we can offer TMD patients with regard to pain, jaw function, and psychosocial adaptation.

In summary, this chapter has discussed behavioral assessment of TMD through a biopsychosocial model. This model suggests that understanding the etiology, prevention, and course of TMDs requires attending to assessment of broadly defined behavioral factors, including emotional status and level of psychosocial adaptation, as well as assessment of physical factors. It is only natural that the choice of instruments to assess behavioral status be determined by specific research interests, but it is encouraging to note that a fair number of useful and reasonably well-studied measures are available for such purposes. Both clinical research and treatment for TMDs must encompass inquiry into the full range of biologic, psychologic, and social factors known to influence all chronic pain conditions.

REFERENCES

Bergner, M., Bobbitt, R.A., Carter, W.B. and Gilson, B.S., The sickness impact profile: development and final revision of a health status model, Med. Care, 19 (1981) 787–805.

Bradley, L.A., McDonald Haile, J. and Jaworski, T.M., Assessment of psychological status using interviews and self-report instruments. In: D.C. Turk and R. Melzack (Eds.), Handbook of Pain Assessment, The Guilford Press, New York, 1992, pp. 193–213.

Brown, G.K. and Nicassio, P.M., Development of a questionnaire for the assessment of active and passive coping strategies in chronic pain patients, Pain, 31 (1987) 53–64.

Buckelew, S.P., DeGood, D.E., Schwartz, D.P. and Kern, R., Cognitive and somatic item response pattern of chronic pain patients, psychiatric patients, and hospital employees, J. Clin. Psychol., 42 (1986) 852–860.

Butterworth, J.C. and Deardorff, W.W., Psychometric profiles of craniomandibular pain patients: identifying specific subgroups, J. Craniomandib. Pract., 5 (1987) 225–232.

Christiansen, E.L., Thompson, J.R., Hasso, A.N. and Hinshaw, D.B., Correlative thin section temporomandibular joint anatomy and computed tomography, Radiographics, 6 (1986) 703–723.

Craig, K., Emotional aspects of pain. In: P.D. Wall and R. Melzack (Eds.), Textbook of Pain, Churchill Livingstone, Edinburgh, 1984.

Deardorff, W.W., Reliability of the TMJ scale, The Mental Measurements Yearbook, Buros Institute of Mental Measurements, University of Nebraska, Lincoln, Nebr., in press.

Derogatis, L.R., SCL-90-R: Administration, Scoring and Procedures Manual - II, for the Revised Version, Clinical Psychometric Research, Towson, Md., 1983,

Dworkin, S.F. and LeResche, L., Research diagnostic criteria for temporomandibular disorders, J. Craniomandib. Disord. Facial Oral Pain, 6 (1992) 301–355.

Dworkin, S.F., Huggins, K.H., LeResche, L., Von Korff, M., Howard, J., Truelove, E. and Sommers, E., Epidemiology of signs and symptoms in temporomandibular disorders: clinical signs in cases and controls, J. Am. Dent. Assoc., 120 (1990a) 273–281.

Dworkin, S.F., Von Korff, M.R. and LeResche, L., Multiple pains and psychiatric disturbance: an epidemiologic investigation, Arch. Gen. Psychiatry, 47 (1990b) 239–244.

Dworkin, S.F., Von Korff, M. and LeResche, L., Epidemiologic studies of chronic pain: a dynamic-ecologic perspective, Ann. Behav. Med., 14 (1992) 3–11.

Dworkin, S.F., Wilson, L. and Massoth, D.L., Somatizing as a risk factor for chronic pain. In: R. Grzesiak and D. Ciccone (Eds.), Psychologic Vulnerability to Chronic Pain, Springer Pub., New York, 1994.

Fordyce, W.E., Behavioral Methods in Chronic Pain and Illness, C.V. Mosby, St. Louis, 1976.

Fricton, J.R. and Schiffman, E.L., The craniomandibular index: validity, J. Prosthet. Dent., 58 (1987) 222–228.

Gatchel, R.J. and Baum, A., Overview. In: An Introduction to Health Psychology, McGraw-Hill, New York, 1993a.

Gatchel, R.J. and Baum, A., An introduction to health psychology. In: An Introduction to Health Psychology, McGraw-Hill, New York, 1993b.

Glaros, A.G. and Glass, E.G., Temporomandibular disorders. In: R.J. Gatchel and E.B. Blanchard

(Eds.), Psychophysiological Disorders, American Psychological Association, Washington, D.C., 1993, pp. 299–356.

Keefe, F.J., Dunsmore, J. and Burnett, R., Behavioral and cognitive-behavioral approaches to chronic pain: recent advances and future directions, J. Consult. Clin. Psychol., 60 (1992) 528–536.

Lennon, M.C., Dohrenwend, B.P., Zautra, A.J. and Marbach, J.J., Coping and adaptation to facial pain in contrast to other stressful life events, J. Pers. Soc. Psychol., 59 (1990) 1040–1050.

LeResche, L. and Dworkin, S.F., Facial expressions of pain and emotions in chronic TMD patients, Pain, 35 (1988) 71–78.

LeResche, L., Dworkin, S.F., Wilson, L. and Ehrlich, K.J., Effect of temporomandibular disorder pain duration on facial expressions and verbal report of pain, Pain, 51 (1992) 289–295.

Levitt, S.R., Predictive value: a model for dentists to evaluate the accuracy of diagnostic tests for temporomandibular disorders as applied to the TMJ scale, J. Prosthet. Dent., 66 (1991) 385–390.

Levitt, S.R. and McKinney, M.W., Validating the TMJ scale in a national sample of 10,000 patients: demographic and epidemiologic characteristics, J. Orofacial Pain, 8 (1994) 25–35.

Levitt, S.R., Lundeen, T.F. and McKinney, M.W., Initial studies of a new assessment method for temporomandibular joint disorders, J. Prosthet. Dent., 59 (1988) 490–495.

Levitt, S.R., Lundeen, T.F. and McKinney, M.W., The TMJ Scale Manual, Pain Resource Center, Durham, N.C., 1994.

Linton, S.J., Bradley, L.A., Jensen, I., Spangfort, E. and Sundell, L., The secondary prevention of low back pain: a controlled study with follow-up, Pain, 36 (1989) 197–207.

Marbach, J.J., Schleifer, S.J. and Keller, S.E., Facial pain, distress and immune function, Brain, Behavior and Immunity, 4 (1990) 243–254.

McCreary, C.P., Clark, G.T., Oakley, M.E. and Flack, V., Predicting response to treatment for temporomandibular disorders, J. Craniomandib. Disord. Facial Oral Pain, 6 (1992) 161–169.

Pilowsky, I., Abnormal illness behaviour: a review of the concept and its implications. In: S. McHugh and T.M. Vallis (Eds.), Illness Behavior: A Multidisciplinary Model, Plenum Press, New York, 1986.

Prkachin, K. and Mercer, S.R., Pain expression in patients with shoulder pathology: validity, properties and relationship to sickness impact, Pain, 39 (1990) 257–265.

Rosenstiel, A.K. and Keefe, F.J., The use of coping strategies in chronic low back pain patients: relationship to patient characteristics and current adjustment, Pain, 17 (1983) 33–44.

Rudy, T.E., Turk, D.C., Zaki, H.S. and Curtin, H.D., An empirical taxometric alternative to traditional classification of temporomandibular disorders, Pain, 36 (1989) 311–320.

Rudy, T., Turk, D., Kubinski, J. and Zaki, H., Efficacy of tailoring treatment for dysfunctional TMD patients, J. Dent. Res., 73 (spec. iss.) (1994) 439.

Rugh, J.D., Woods, B.J. and Dahlstrom, L., Temporomandibular disorders: assessment of psychosocial factors, Adv. Dent. Res., 7 (1993) 127–136.

Turk, D. and Flor, H., Pain pain behaviors: the utility of the pain behavior construct, Pain, 31 (1987) 277–295.

Turk, D.C. and Rudy, T.E., Toward an empirically derived taxonomy of chronic pain patients: integration of psychological assessment data, J. Consult. Clin. Psychol., 56 (1988) 1–6.

Von Korff, M., Ormel, J., Keefe, F.J. and Dworkin, S.F., Grading the severity of chronic pain, Pain, 50 (1992) 133–149.

Wilson, L., Dworkin, S.F., Whitney, C. and LeResche, L., Somatization and pain dispersion in chronic temporomandibular disorder pain, Pain, 57 (1994) 55–61.

Correspondence to: Samuel F. Dworkin, DDS, PhD, Department of Oral Medicine SC-63, School of Dentistry, University of Washington, Seattle, WA 98195, USA. Tel: 206-543-5912; Fax: 206-685-8024.

Temporomandibular Disorders and Related Pain Conditions, Progress in Pain Research and Management, Vol. 4, edited by B.J. Sessle, P.S. Bryant, and R.A. Dionne, IASP Press, Seattle, © 1995.

Reaction Papers to Chapters 10 and 11

Rigmor Jensen and Jes Olesen, Norman D. Mohl, and Robert J. Gatchel

Rigmor Jensen[a] and Jes Olesen[b]

[a]Department of Neurology, Rigshospitalet, and [b]Department of Neurology, Glostrup Hospital, University of Copenhagen, Copenhagen, Denmark

THE IDEAL CLASSIFICATION SYSTEM

The prevalence of temporomandibular disorders (TMDs) varies considerably from series to series (Rugh and Solberg 1985; Schiffman and Fricton 1988; Jensen et al. 1993a), probably due to lack of a universally accepted classification scheme with specific diagnostic criteria. The suggested research diagnostic criteria (RDC) for TMDs (outlined by Dworkin in this volume and in Dworkin 1992) have not yet been used in prospective studies.

Several demands must be fulfilled for the perfect disease classification system. It must be:

1. valid—must reflect a true biological disturbance;

2. reliable—permits different clinicians seeing the same patient to assign the same diagnosis;

3. comprehensive—includes all TMDs and other facial pain disorders;

4. generalizable—applies to a broad range of settings including primary care, specialty centers, and population-based studies;

5. hierarchical—constructed so that it is possible to use it at different levels of sophistication;

6. operational—with explicit definitions instead of vague descriptions;

7. exclusive—any TMD must fit one set of criteria and only one at a given time (but patients may have more than one disorder).

Such a list of demands for the ideal classification system is difficult to fulfill, but they should be kept in mind when discussing the classification of TMDs and related pain disorders. Future research of prevalence, social impact, pathogenetic mechanisms, and treatment are highly dependent on a valid diagnostic classification system. Although the necessary data for creating such a system are not available at present, we must try to create a classification system that combines as high a sensitivity and specificity as possible, knowing that the best solution always represents a compromise between sensitivity and specificity.

An example of a classification system of chronic pain is the International Headache Classification (IHS 1988) created by the International Headache Society in 1988. This system has been widely accepted and is used worldwide. Most of its major diagnostic categories have been included in the most recent disease classification system from the World Health Organization (ICD 10). All studies on epidemiology, social impact, pathogenetic mechanisms, and treatment in recent years refer to this classification system.

ASSESSMENT OF MYOFASCIAL PAIN

Can myofascial pain originate from the masticatory system? Simple co-occurrence of TMDs and muscle tenderness is frequent but could occur by chance because both disorders are extremely prevalent (Jensen et al. 1993a,b). Given that tenderness may be a part of a generalized myofascial syndrome, the question is whether temporomandibular joint problems are the cause of tenderness or vice versa, and this question remains largely unanswered. The possible causal relation between myofascial tenderness and TMDs is difficult to elucidate further as long as muscle tenderness is included in the RDC. We thus suggest subdivision of the diagnostic criteria to TMDs—one with increased tenderness of the jaw muscles, and one subform without muscle tenderness.

In addition, assessment of myofascial tenderness is highly controversial, and a precise quantification of tenderness is difficult. The data presented by Widmer (this volume) leave the impression that recording of myofascial tenderness is reliable and valid. Nevertheless, systematic studies of suggested RDC methods have not yet been performed, and much more work to assess their consistency is needed. The quantification of tenderness depends on the given instructions, the exerted pressure, and the observer. Among these factors, the intensity of the exerted pressure is probably the most important. The exact relation between pressure and pain remains unclear. The RDC recommend a 2-lb pressure for palpation of the extraoral and 1-lb pressure on the intraoral muscles. Are these pressures the best choice? A 4-kg pressure is recommended in the diagnostic criteria for fibromyalgia (Wolfe 1990), but again the recommendation is not based on studies of sensitivity and specificity. Until recently, it has not been possible to record the exact pressure intensity during the palpation procedure. A recently developed device, called a palpometer, attempts to control palpation pressure (Bendtsen et al. 1994).

Although several pain rating systems have been developed, none have been properly tested in TMD patients. The Copenhagen Headache Center has developed a combined verbal and behavioral pain scoring system where the observer scores tenderness according to the verbal and facial expression of the patient, the so-called total tenderness score system (Langemark et al. 1987). In a study using the palpometer, Bendtsen and colleagues (unpublished data,1994) found this system to be reproducible and reliable.

A detailed analysis of the masseter, temporal, and pterygoid muscles is recommended in the RDC, but it is questionable if these muscles are the most relevant for TMDs. Also, the suggested subdivisions of these muscles are very detailed and not practical for daily clinical use. The number of tender points is the most important determinant of both sensitivity and specificity of fibromyalgia, and a cut-off limit at 11 tender points out of 18 locations is required (Wolfe 1990). In the RDC, 3 tender spots out of 20 locations are required to fulfill the criteria of muscle tenderness. We recently evaluated pericranial tenderness in 14 pairs of pericranial muscles and tendon insertions in 735 randomly selected Danish adults (Jensen et al. 1993b) The majority of these subjects had more than three tender spots, indicating that the specificity of the RDC criteria is likely to be very low. Subjects with TMDs or frequent tension-type headaches had significantly more tender spots than did healthy subjects. Further clarification of the exact cut-off limits is thus needed.

QUANTIFICATION OF TMDs

The quantitative aspects of TMDs also should be taken into account. It is frequently claimed that TMDs represent a chronic disorder, and little is known about the episodic, acute form. We suggest, therefore, that a chronic and an episodic subform of these disorders should be defined. It can be difficult to assess the quantitative aspects of these disorders at the first consultation. At the Copenhagen Headache Center, patients are asked prospectively to use a headache diary based on the operational criteria of the International Headache Society. It is our experience that this diary is a valuable aid in the diagnosis of headache patients, who often have difficulties in recalling symptoms and medications during retrospective clinical interviews. A diagnostic diary in which the quantity, the intensity, and the quality of TMDs are recorded daily should be demanded in clinical research studies of TMDs.

BEHAVIORAL CHARACTERISTICS

It is a popular and common belief that chronic pain patients in general, and TMD and headache patients in particular, have severe psychosocial problems as a primary causative factor to their pain disorder. However, most of the referred studies have been carried out in highly selected patients with severe and chronic TMDs. A recent population-based study noted that anxiety and neuroticism are no more frequent in migraine sufferers than in headache-free subjects (Rasmussen et al. 1992). The main reason for the former belief is probably a considerable referral bias. Those patients who are anxious, depressive, or neurotic can not cope with their pain and seek highly specialized pain clinics much more often than do those subjects who tolerate their pain disorder. According to many recent pain studies the majority of the suspected psychosocial and personality factors may be results of specific coping strategies for recurrent pain rather than specific reactions leading to the pain, and may gradually disappear after effective treatment (Bech et al. 1993).

These secondary reactions are, however, important because chronic pain often appears to cause a vicious cycle of increased muscle tension/depression and more pain. The International Headache Classification uses the fourth digit in the code to identify the most likely causative factors in tension-type headache. Although TMDs in some ways differ from tension-type headache, these factors also may modify and identify some of the clinical and psychological features, as well as the therapeutic approach to TMDs. Additional factors capable of inducing the onset and/or the worsening of TMDs may be identified, but the scientific documentation for these factors is limited. We suggest that Axis II in the RDC should be combined with these possible aggravating and causative factors until further evidence about the behavioral characteristics is available. Axis II is highly valuable when the individual patient is diagnosed and a treatment program is planned. Nevertheless, the different syndromes must be diagnosed by their specific symptoms and signs. The diagnosis of any underlying psychological factors is of secondary importance, and the treatment of such factors is largely independent of the primary RDC diagnosis.

RECOMMENDATIONS FOR FUTURE RESEARCH

Although the suggested RDC are extremely important and indispensable for future studies of TMDs, they are too complex for clinical use. A simpler, but hierarchical and operational classification system is needed. We suggest development of a new TMD classification along the lines used in the International Headache Classification, for the following reasons: the IHC system has

Table I

Suggestions for a future operational diagnostic classification system for temporomandibular disorders (TMDs)

First and Second Digits

1.1   *TMDs*

A. At least five episodes with mild to moderate pain located around the temporomandibular joint.

B. At least two of the following four clinical signs should be fulfilled:
   1. increased myofascial tenderness
   2. restricted opening
   3. disc displacement
   4. signs of arthritis or arthrosis
   1–4 defined as in the present research diagnostic criteria (RDC)

1.2   *TMDs not fulfilling above criteria*

A. Pain as above

B. One of the four clinical signs listed above

Third Digit

1.1.1   *Episodic TMDs*

Average pain frequency < 180 days per year or < 15 days per month for at least six months

1.1.2   *Chronic TMDs*

Average pain frequency ≥ 180 days per year or ≥ 15 days per month for at least six months

1.1.3   *Chronicity undetermined*

Pain as above but with a duration less than six months

Fourth Digit

Most important causative/aggravating factor:

0   No identifiable causative factor
1   More than one of the factors 2–6 (list in order of importance)
2   Axis II (psychosocial stress, anxiety, depression)
3   TMD as a delusion or an idea
4   Muscular stress (bruxism, clenching)
5   Drug overuse
6   Other factors

proved its utility, has a low interobserver variability, and has gained world-wide use, and finally, headache disorders and TMDs overlap considerably. Table I gives suggestions for operationalized RDC criteria. Such criteria likely will be improved further as more research data become available. It is a great challenge to refine the present RDC and to develop a valid classification system for future epidemiological, clinical, and scientific work in the TMD area.

REFERENCES

Bech, P., Langemark, M., Loldrup, D., Rasmussen, B.K. and Krabbe, A., Tension-type headache: psychiatric aspects. In: J. Olesen and J. Schoenen (Eds.), Tension-Type Headache: Classification, Mechanisms, and Treatment. Raven Press, New York, 1993, pp. 143–146.

Bendtsen, L., Jensen, R., Jensen, N.K. and Olesen, J., Muscle palpation with controlled finger pressure: a new equipment for the study of tender myofascial tissues, Pain 59 (1994) 235–239.

Dworkin, S.F. and LeResche, L., Research diagnostic criteria for temporomandibular disorders: review, criteria, examinations and specifications, critique, J Craniomandib. Disord. Facial Oral Pain, 6 (1992) 301–355.

IHS. Headache Classification Committee of the International Headache Society. Classification and diagnostic criteria for headache disorders, cranial neuralgias and facial pain, Cephalalgia, 8, suppl. 7 (1988) 1–96.

Jensen, K., Quantification of tenderness by palpation and use of pressure algometer, Adv. Pain Res. Ther., 17 (1990) 165–181.

Jensen, R., Rasmussen, B.K., Pedersen, B., Lous, I. and Olesen, J., Cephalic muscle tenderness and pressure pain threshold in a general population, Pain, 48 (1992) 197–203.

Jensen, R., Rasmussen, B.K., Pedersen, B., Lous, I. and Olesen, J., Prevalence of temporomandibular dysfunctions in a general population, J. Orofacial Pain, 7 (1993a) 175–182.

Jensen, R., Rasmussen, B.K., Pedersen, B. and Olesen, J., Cephalic muscle tenderness and pressure pain threshold in headache, Pain, 52 (1993b) 193–199.

Langemark, M. and Olesen, J., Pericranial tenderness in tension headache, Cephalalgia, 7 (1987) 249–255.

Rasmussen, B.K., Jensen, R., Schroll, M. and Olesen, J., Epidemiology of headache in a general population: a prevalence study, J. Clin. Epidemiol. 44 (1991) 1147–1157.

Rasmussen, B.K., Migraine and tension-type headache in a general population: psychosocial factors, Int. J. Epidemiol., 21 (1992) 1138–1143.

Rugh, J.D. and Solberg, W.K., Oral health status in the United States: temporomandibular disorders, J. Dent. Educ. 49 (1985) 398–404.

Russel, M., Rasmussen, B.K., Brennum, J., Iversen, H., Jensen, R. and Olesen, J., Presentation of a new instrument: the diagnostic headache diary, Cephalalgia, 12 (1992) 369–374.

Schiffmann, E. and Fricton, J.R., Epidemiology of TMJ and craniofascial pain. In: J.R. Fricton, R.J. Kroening and K.M. Hathaway (Eds.), TMJ and Craniofacial Pain: Diagnosis and Management, IEA Publishers, St. Louis, 1988, pp. 1–10.

Wolfe, F., Methodological and statistical problems in the epidemiology of fibromyalgia. In: J.R. Fricton and E. Awad (Eds.), Advances in Pain Research and Therapy, Vol. 17, Raven Press, New York, 1990, 147–162.

Correspondence to: Rigmor Jensen, MD, Department of Neurology, Rigshospitalet, Copenhagen University Hospital, DK-2100 Copenhagen Ö, Denmark. Tel: 45-3-545-2082; Fax: 45-4-583-1089.

Norman D. Mohl

Department of Oral Diagnostic Sciences, State University of New York, Buffalo, New York, USA

The diagnosis of presumptive temporomandibular disorders (TMDs) in patients who seek advice or care for a TMD or for any other orofacial pain condition should not be prematurely categorized as a specific disorder or disease. Patients should be seen as having one or more signs and symptoms, and only after the relatively structured process of *differential* diagnosis should the clinician arrive at a working diagnosis that adheres to some acceptable taxonomic system. To do otherwise could reinforce the clinician's predetermined theoretical bias, which can strongly influence the outcome of the diagnostic process, not to mention its therapeutic consequences. Thus, the process of differential diagnosis requires that the clinician be able to discriminate the presumptive disorder from normal anatomical and functional variability, from benign and unimportant conditions, and, very importantly, from other diseases or disorders whose physical and/or behavioral characteristics may be similar to the actual conditions from which the patient is suffering. Furthermore, because any given orofacial pain patient may have signs and symptoms reflecting one or more overlapping TMDs, another orofacial pain condition, or a concomitant TMD and non-TMD, the process of differential diagnosis should be conducted in a manner that will increase the probability that the resulting working diagnosis will be as accurate as possible.

To deal with and reconcile all these diagnostic possibilities, the clinician should use a clinical reasoning process that involves the sequential consideration of every diagnostic option that may appear to account for the signs and symptoms. Thus, diagnostic information is obtained, refined, and interpreted to eliminate inappropriate options until the most likely diagnostic conclusions can be reached. In this manner, the level of uncertainty can be reduced, giving the clinician more confidence that a correct working diagnosis has been achieved. Thus, a differential diagnosis actually involves the process of ruling *out* diagnostic choices that do *not* apply to a given patient instead of ruling *in* the clinician's preconceived choice or choices. When seen in this context, the process of differential diagnosis may be regarded as a diagnosis by exclusion.

However, this does not imply that such a process is in any way incompatible with the importance of validated inclusion criteria for identification of the presumptive disorder. The rationale for this type of critical reasoning process in differential diagnosis and the need for a classification system based upon such criteria are not mutually exclusive. A so-called diagnosis by exclusion does not mean that the clinician ends the process with a basketful of unrelated signs and symptoms that do not fit any known taxonomy. In fact, a taxonomy based on validated diagnostic criteria better enables the clinician to make the discriminatory judgments that are such a necessary part of the differential diagnostic process. Therefore, I completely agree with Widmer (this volume) that the development of criteria specific for each TMD diagnostic category is imperative for research studies and for clinical diagnosis and that the field would be greatly enhanced if we also had data that would permit the development of operationalized and validated inclusion criteria for all of the non-TMD conditions that must be considered when conducting a differential diagnosis.

The issue of physical characteristics in the diagnosis and assessment of TMDs and related orofacial pain conditions is, even without the addition of a second axis, extremely important given that so many clinicians base their diagnoses, etiological hypotheses, and treatment regimens almost entirely on an assessment of the physical characteristics of a particular patient. It would be comforting to know that the procedures and tests used to evaluate the physical characteristics of a presumptive TMD patient had a high degree of reliability, validity, and clinical utility. It is worth noting that the clinical assessment of these physical factors, along with the patient's history, forms the basis of the traditional diagnostic "gold standard" for TMDs.

Some have claimed that TMDs have no gold standard because they cannot be diagnosed by some objective test or assay. The term *gold standard* is meant to represent the best currently available evidence or indicator of the true state of the patient. However, in medicine, dentistry, or psychology, the true state of the patient is frequently determined from the clinical assessment of the patient's signs and symptoms without the use of a so-called objective test. For example, neurological, psychiatric, and musculoskeletal disorders are commonly identified and categorized through an assessment of their clinical characteristics. The same is true for many painful conditions such as trigeminal neuralgia, cluster headache, and low back pain, to name a few. The important point is that the patient's report of pain, accompanied by information about its onset, location, characteristics, severity, modifying factors and degree of incapacitation, is a significant indicator of the problem, even if the information is derived from a patient's subjective responses. That information, coupled with an assessment of the information derived from the clinical examination, is essential and provides the best means now available to arrive at a differential diagnosis of TMDs.

Widmer notes that, although there appears to be acceptable to good interexaminer reliability for muscle palpation, temporomandibular joint (TMJ) palpation, and joint sounds, particularly after training, the instability of muscle tenderness and joint sounds can reduce the overall reliability of these procedures in those clinical studies that require repeated measurements. If this is indeed a genuine measurement problem, as it appears to be, its solution may lie in adding a time-based multiple examination protocol to the research diagnostic criteria (RDC). Also, Widmer's comment about the failure of patient study samples to include a spectrum of symptom severities raises an important issue in future epidemiological research, in RDC and other diagnostic validation studies, and in treatment efficacy studies.

We should also be reminded that the clinical significance of joint sounds, particularly clicking, is still equivocal, even if the measurement of this phenomenon met all of the appropriate assessment criteria. In addition, most structural factors, including those identified with TMJ imaging, seem to correlate poorly with TMJ and masticatory muscle pain. For example, joint pain, although certainly clinically significant, does not correlate with condylar position, disk position, or with the degree of degenerative joint disease. Also, there is no clear and direct correlation between muscle pain and the relative amount of muscle activity. Thus, TMD pain seems to be produced by other pathophysiologic phenomena, the exact identification and underlying nociceptive mechanisms of which should continue to be intensively investigated. It would be helpful, for example, if, in addition to our current dependence on the methods of and responses to palpation, physical diagnosis could include tests that could reliably and accurately identify those underlying pathophysiological factors that account for the nociceptive input. In this regard, techniques such as magnetic resonance imaging (MRI) spectroscopy may have the potential to be of great diagnostic value in the future.

Past reports on the use of electronic devices in the diagnosis of TMDs have often confused measurement validity with diagnostic validity and have often involved comparisons against their own internal standard instead of blinded comparisons against the clinical gold standard. Thus, the absence of replicable studies that clearly establish satisfactory levels of reliability, measurement and diagnostic validity, and clinical utility, including cost-effectiveness, clearly diminish the value of these devices as aids in TMD diagnosis or as techniques to monitor the results of treatment. In addition, there is no evidence showing that these devices can help to discriminate TMDs from other orofacial pain conditions, an imperative in differential diagnosis. Furthermore, the biological phenomena that supposedly underlie some of these devices are equivocal at best. Therefore, the clinical use of electronic devices for patients with presumptive or actual TMDs should, at least at present, be considered experimental.

Despite Widmer's concerns about some of the issues regarding physical characteristics, I agree with his conclusions that physical evaluation parameters have levels of reliability and validity that are sufficiently high to permit their continued use in identifying and classifying TMD patients. Nonetheless, I do believe that the almost total reliance by clinicians on Axis I physical characteristics, as previously noted, probably accounts for the large amount of disparity among clinicians regarding who is and who is not a TMD patient. Thus, I would hope that the Axis II behavioral characteristics, in addition to their own intrinsic value, would help to resolve this problem over time.

Dworkin's assessment of the RDC Axis II characteristics left no doubts, if any still exist, of the value of including behavioral characteristics in a TMD classification system (Dworkin, this volume). Dworkin also makes an important distinction between acute and chronic pain. However, considering the relatively arbitrary six-month time frame for defining the onset of chronic pain, the questions may be asked: Do we really know when and why pain becomes chronic and, with regard to the biopsychosocial model, the specific biological components of chronicity? For example, have the tissue injury, edema, ischemia, inflammation, or other pathophysiologic processes eliciting the original nociception been resolved when chronicity begins to dominate the clinical picture? If they have been resolved, why does the original pain site often still hurt? If they have not been resolved, should not treatment continue to be directed toward their resolution? My point is that the underlying mechanisms that account for the pathophysiology and resultant nociception, e.g., the bio-part of the biopsychosocial model, still require intense study. This position in no way implies that behavioral and psychosocial factors that may cause, contribute to, or maintain the signs and symptoms are not extremely important factors in TMDs and related pain conditions.

A good example of the integration of the biopsychosocial model is reflected in Dr. Dworkin's discussion of the differences between dysfunctional TMD patients and adaptive copers, as defined by the Multidimensional Pain Inventory (MPI) for chronic pain patients. If the dysfunctional patients have significantly more physical symptoms, as characterized by multiple pain sites, than do the adaptive copers, and if there is a differential response to treatment between these groups, it would seem valuable to study the possibility of developing operationalized criteria for the identification of these multiple pain sites, of combining Axis I and Axis II characteristics, and of using the resulting new diagnostic category as a predictor of treatment outcome. Should this scenario be sustained by additional research data, it would go a long way to satisfy Feinstein's injunction that an ideal taxonomy should include objective information on cause, prognosis, and treatment implications.

In summary, relationships between the Axis I physical characteristics and the Axis II behavioral characteristics already exist and are consistent with the so-called biopsychosocial model. It appears certain that these relationships will increasingly overlap as new research is conducted and additional data are obtained. It would be advantageous, therefore, if more studies were developed around research hypotheses and protocols that involved the use and integration of both sets of characteristics.

Correspondence to: Norman D. Mohl, DDS, PhD, Department of Oral Diagnostic Sciences, 355 Squire Hall, 3435 Main St., SUNY Buffalo, Buffalo, NY 14214, USA. Tel: 716-829-3558; Fax: 716-829-3554.

Robert J. Gatchel

Department of Psychiatry, Division of Psychology, University of Texas Southwestern Medical Center at Dallas, Texas, USA

The intent of the research diagnostic criteria (RDC) for temporomandibular disorders (TMDs) is to encourage standardization and replication of clinical research on TMDs by providing reliable and valid diagnostic criteria that will be reproducible across clinicians and researchers (Dworkin and LeResche 1992). The inclusion of both an Axis I, which delineates physical characteristics of the disorder, and an Axis II, which assesses pain-related disability and psychosocial status, provides a more comprehensive evaluation of psychophysiological factors involved in TMDs. My reactions to the previous chapters will focus on two major issues: (1) the difficulties inherent in differentiating among physical impairment, disability, and pain issues; and (2) the potential importance of a conceptual model of the development of TMDs for planning the most comprehensive treatment strategy.

IMPAIRMENT, DISABILITY, AND PAIN

Dworkin (this volume) is quite correct in pointing out that prevalent chronic pain conditions, including back pain, headache, and TMDs, not only have unique features, but also have features they share in common. One of the most significant common characteristics they share is the poor correspondence among the pathophysiologic change, global severity of pain and suffering, and degree of disability displayed by the patient. Indeed, there is frequently *discordance* found among the levels of impairment, pain, and disability. Such discordance often creates major problems for treatment personnel in selecting the best goal for indexing therapeutic progress. Indeed, Waddell (1987) has indicated that, although correlations are found among impairment, pain, and disability (usually in the range of 0.3–0.6), overlap among these categories is not perfect. Fig. 1 depicts his categorization of their relationship in low back pain. As can be seen, although these factors are all logically and clinically related, there is usually not a 1:1:1 relation among them. What makes this imperfect correlation even more complex is the wide range of individual differences in such discordance from one patient to the next. Therefore, treatment personnel need to be aware of the varying relationships among these concepts.

Clinicians also should be aware of the definitions of these three categories or concepts, because they are fundamentally different. These terms have been discussed in the medical impairment and disability evaluation literature. *Impairment* is a physical/medical term that refers to an alteration of the patient's usual health status (i.e., some objective anatomical or pathological abnormality) that is evaluated by physical or medical means. The evaluation of impairment has traditionally been a medical/dental responsibility in which there is an attempt to objectively evaluate structural limitations. This is the role of RDC Axis I, which focuses on physical diagnoses of muscle and/or joint disorders. Unfortunately, as we have seen in both the medical and dental literature, the current technology does not allow totally accurate or objective physical impairment evaluation; it relies upon methods that are not completely reliable, that are sometimes subject to examiner bias, and that are not yet associated with good diagnostic validity.

Disability has traditionally been an administrative term that refers to the diminished capacity or inability to perform certain activities of everyday living; it is the resulting loss of function due to impairment. Disability evaluations, too, are often not totally reliable and are subject to various examiner and patient response biases. The assessment of disability is usually based upon subjective self-report measures of restrictions of activities such as walking,

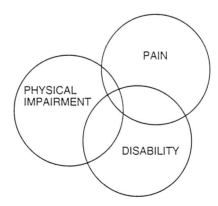

Fig. 1. Relation among pain, disability, and physical impairment, according to Waddell (1987).

chewing, sleep, and sex. Axis II of the RDC attempts to assess this dimension.

Finally, *pain* is a psychophysiologic concept based primarily upon experiential or subjective evaluation. It is also quite often difficult to quantify objectively in a reliable manner. Axis II of the RDC also evaluates this dimension.

Although physical impairment, disability, and pain can be separately assessed, they are not highly correlated. One patient may verbally report a significant amount of pain but show little impairment that can be objectively evaluated, with disability perhaps lying somewhere between the two in severity. Another patient may report little pain but display great disability and some impairment. Dworkin also has highlighted the possibility of low correlations; i.e., patients who are classified as either Grade I or Grade II may be indistinguishable from patients who are at Grade III or IV in terms of physical signs such as unassisted vertical jaw opening and total number of joint sounds. Consequently, it is important to assess all three constructs in specific situations whenever possible, with the expectation that there may be complex interactions among them that may differ from one patient to the next, as well as from one time to the next. The advantage of the RDC is that they provide the ability to evaluate all three simultaneously.

RDC AXIS II ASSESSMENT OF PAIN AND DISABILITY

The major measure of pain and disability in Axis II is the Graded Chronic Pain Scale originally developed by Von Korff et al. (1992). Both pain measures and disability measures are combined to classify patients into one of four graded levels. As Dworkin notes, what he refers to as functional TMD patients (Grades I and II) usually are associated with low disability and either low or high pain intensity. Dysfunctional chronic pain patients (Grades III and IV) are associated with increasing levels of disability and rarely with low levels of pain intensity. Thus, a composite score is used that combines both pain and disability constructs. An important question is whether combining the two measures is the most heuristic approach, especially when planning treatment. It has both positive and negative features. On the positive side, combining the two does not give greater relevance to either pain or disability measures. This approach may be appropriate with TMDs because of the absence of workers' compensation and other disability-related economic issues and incentives. On the negative side, there are often instances where the two need to be separated, for example, in the area of low back pain. That is to say, the initial primary goal of treatment may be to decrease disability by increasing function, without much focus on pain reduction per se. In fact, pain may actually increase at first during attempts to restore function, so if self-reported pain is used to determine the pace of treatment, therapeutic progress may appear to be impeded.

DYSFUNCTIONAL CHRONIC PAIN: A CONCEPTUAL MODEL OF ITS DEVELOPMENT

Dworkin appropriately notes that the primary reason for conducting a psychosocial assessment of a TMD patient is that it opens up the possibility of additional treatment options. His biopsychosocial model is important in its conceptualization of the need for an integrated assessment/treatment approach. Along with this biopsychosocial model that delineates the important variables involved, the development of a conceptual model of how the disorder evolves also may prove to be fruitful for refining the most effective assessment and treatment approach. A conceptual model of how chronic low back pain develops has implications for the degree or magnitude of assessment and treatment that may be needed (Gatchel 1991). I have proposed that patients pass through several stages of pain from acute to more chronic. Stage 1 is associated with emotional reactions such as fear, anxiety, and worry as a consequence of the perception of pain during the acute phase. Pain or hurt is usually associated with harm, so there is a natural emotional reaction to the potential for physical harm. Pain that persists past a reasonable acute period (a few months) can progress to stage 2, or the subacute stage. This stage is associated with a wider array of behavioral/psychological reactions and problems, such as learned helplessness, depression, anger, distress, and somatization, which are the result of suffering from the now more chronic pain and disability. I hypothesize that the form these problems take primarily depends upon the *premorbid* or preexisting personality/psychological characteristics of the person, as well as current economic/environmental conditions. Thus, a person with a premorbid problem with depression who is seriously affected interpersonally by the pain and disability will experience greatly exacerbated depressive symptomatology during this stage. Similarly, a person who has premorbid hypochondriacal characteristics and receives significant secondary gain in the form of attention and sympathy for the pain and disability symptoms most likely will display a great deal of somatization and symptom magnification.

This model does not propose that there is one primary, preexisting "pain personality," but assumes a general *nonspecificity* in the relationship between personality/psychological problems and pain. This approach concerns the significant body of research that has not found any such consistent personality syndrome (Mayer and Gatchel 1988). Moreover, even though a relationship usually is found between pain and certain psychological problems such as depression (Romano and Turner 1985), the nature of the relationship between the two variables remains inconclusive. Some, but not all patients develop depression secondary to chronic pain. Others show depression as a primary syndrome, of which pain is a symptom.

Finally, this conceptual model proposes that persistent behavioral/psychological problems lead to progression into stage 3, which can be reviewed as the acceptance or adoption of a sick role or abnormal illness behavior during which patients are excused from their normal responsibilities and social obligations. The medical and psychological "disabilities" or abnormal illness behaviors are consolidated during this phase. More persistent forms of psychopathology also are frequent during this chronic and subchronic stage.

Superimposed on these above stages is what is known as the physical deconditioning syndrome, a significant decrease in physical capacity due to disuse and resultant atrophy of the injured area. A two-way path usually develops between the physical deconditioning and the above psychosocial stages of mental deconditioning. For example, research has demonstrated that physical deconditioning can negatively affect emotional well-being and self-esteem and lead to further psychological sequelae. Conversely, negative emotional reactions such as depression can significantly impair physical functioning by, for example, decreasing the motivation to get involved in work or recreational activities, and thereby further contribute to physical deconditioning.

Thus, this model suggests that, besides the potential development of physical deconditioning, specific patients who later become chronic have certain premorbid or predisposing psychological/personality characteristics or disorders (a *diathesis*) that are exacerbated by the stress of attempting to cope with pain and disability. Other factors within this diathesis-stress model also can lead to chronicity (socioeconomic and environmental variables). These predisposed patients, however, are more likely to subsequently become the difficult-to-treat chronic patients, especially when significant physical deconditioning is occurring. Finally, this does not imply that these predisposing factors lead chronic pain patients to develop "functional" disorders and that it is "all in the patient's head." The chronic problem represents a complex interaction between physical and psychosocioeconomic variables.

Our research team is beginning to document the degree of psychopathology during the various stages of chronic pain and to evaluate whether it is a major predictor of who develops chronicity or who remains chronic following treatment attempts. Kinney et al. (1992) administered the Structured Clinical Interview for DSM-III-R Diagnosis (SCID) to a group of chronic TMD patients to evaluate the prevalence of DSM-III-R disorders. Results of this investigation demonstrated that chronic TMD patients had rates of psychopathology that far exceeded the base rates for the general population. An important question raised by these data is the degree to which the psychopathology must be directly treated to produce some decrease in impairment, pain, and disability. Although many studies have investigated and discussed physical and psychological treatment approaches to TMDs, few studies have investigated treatment efficacy using a combined physical and psychological approach. Almost all studies to date have looked at either physical treatments exclusively or psychological treatments exclusively. Rudy, Turk, and colleagues are evaluating the relative efficacy of cognitive-behavior treatment versus physical treatment, while taking into account psychosocial differences in patients based upon the Multidimensional Pain Inventory. More studies such as this are needed.

Thus, it is apparent that systematic studies incorporating both physical and psychological treatments for TMDs while taking into account the psychosocial status of the patient are greatly needed. According to the literature, routine nonsurgical care is, at least initially, the standard treatment for TMDs. However, patients who are unresponsive to this conservative care and who do *not* have symptoms of psychopathology (as assessed by DSM-IV and RDC/TMD criteria) might find it helpful to receive other physically based treatment such as relaxation-biofeedback, with the goal of more directly relaxing jaw muscles and thereby addressing the physical underpinnings of their TMDs. In contrast, TMD patients who are also, for example, depressed may benefit from behavioral-cognitive therapy, which addresses the psychopathological concomitants of their TMDs. Finally, for those patients who have both significant physical and psychological symptoms, a combined treatment approach may be needed.

REFERENCES

Dworkin, S.F. and LeResche, L., Research diagnostic criteria for temporomandibular disorders, J. Craniomandib. Disord. Facial Oral Pain, 6 (1992) 301–355.
Gatchel, R.J., Early development of physical and mental deconditioning in painful spinal disorders. In: T.G. Mayer, V. Mooney and R.J. Gatchel (Eds.), Contemporary Conservative Care for Painful Spinal Disorders, Lea & Febiger, Philadelphia, 1991, pp. 278–289.
Kinney, R.K., Gatchel, R.J., Ellis, E. and Holt, C., Major psychological disorders in chronic TMD patients: management implications, J. Am. Dent. Assoc., 123 (1992) 49–54.
Mayer, T.G. and Gatchel, R.J., Functional Restoration for Spinal Disorders: The Sports Medicine Approach, Lea & Febiger, Philadelphia, 1988.
Romano, J.M. and Turner, J.A., Chronic pain and depression: does the evidence support a relationship? Psychological Bull., 97 (1985) 18–34.
Von Korff, M., Ormel, J., Keefe, F.J. and Dworkin, S.F., Grading the severity of chronic pain, Pain, 50 (1992) 133–149.
Waddell, G., Clinical assessment of lumbar impairment, Clin. Orthop., 221 (1987) 110–120.

Correspondence to: Robert J. Gatchel, PhD, Department of Psychiatry/Division of Psychology, University of Texas Southwestern Medical Center at Dallas, 5323 Harry Hines Blvd., Dallas, TX 75235-9044, USA. Tel: 214-648-5277; Fax: 214 -648-5297.

Part V

Epidemiology and Health Services Research Related to Temporomandibular Disorders

Temporomandibular Disorders and Related Pain Conditions, Progress in Pain Research and Management, Vol. 4, edited by B.J. Sessle, P.S. Bryant, and R.A. Dionne, IASP Press, Seattle, © 1995.

12

Epidemiology of Temporomandibular Disorders

Gunnar E. Carlsson[a] and Linda LeResche[b]

[a]Department of Prosthetic Dentistry, Faculty of Odontology, Göteborg University, Göteborg, Sweden, and [b]Department of Oral Medicine, University of Washington, Seattle, Washington, USA

The primary concerns of epidemiology are generally considered to be the description of health status and prevalence of disease in a population. In a broader context, however, the aims of epidemiology are to provide a scientific basis for analysis of etiological factors, for efforts to prevent and control disease, and for assessment of needs and potential demand for treatment of a disease (Rothman 1986). Morris (1975) suggests that the uses of epidemiology also include identifying and defining syndromes and diseases, describing the full clinical spectrum of specific syndromes, diseases, and conditions, describing the natural history of disease in terms of onset, duration, recurrence, complications, disability, and mortality, and identifying factors that influence or predict clinical course. Thus, investigation in epidemiology can follow many avenues. However, in the field of temporomandibular disorders (TMDs), most research has concentrated on estimation of prevalence rates and description of characteristics of cases vs. controls.

The cardinal signs and symptoms of TMDs are pain in the temporomandibular region, pain and tenderness of masticatory muscles and the temporomandibular joints (TMJs), sounds in the joints, and limitation or disturbance of mandibular movement. These signs and symptoms can be present in a wide variety of different TMDs. Epidemiological studies of TMDs have concentrated almost exclusively on such signs and symptoms of pain and dysfunction rather than on the various disorders that constitute TMDs. A serious problem in evaluating the prevalence of signs and symptoms has been the lack of consensus on diagnostic criteria among investigators (Dworkin and LeResche 1992).

211

Interest in the epidemiology of TMDs was first aroused in Scandinavia and Northern Europe and all but one of the 11 studies in the early review by Helkimo (1979) were from that part of the world. These studies showed varying and often surprisingly high prevalences of signs and symptoms of TMDs. Helkimo's review concluded: "Symptoms of dysfunction of the masticatory system are more common in unselected material than hitherto assumed. This implies that dentists in the future must interest themselves more than before for diagnosis and treatment of functional disturbances of the masticatory system in general practice." In retrospect, 15 years later, it is easy to see that Helkimo's hope has been realized. Interest in TMD epidemiology, as well as diagnosis and treatment, has increased rapidly, reaching an almost explosive force during the late 1980s, at least in North America.

EPIDEMIOLOGICAL STUDIES OF TMDs

TERMINOLOGY AND DEFINITIONS

The basic units of analysis in descriptive epidemiologic studies are prevalence and incidence. Although these concepts are simple, the terms are sometimes misused; to avoid confusion they will be defined here. *Prevalence* indicates the proportion of the population with the disease or condition at a given time. Prevalence is formally calculated as the number of persons in a defined population with the disease or condition divided by the total number of persons in the population. The term prevalence is usually used to signify "point" prevalence, i.e., the proportion of the population with the condition at a single point in time, although prevalence rates for other time periods (e.g., one month, six months) or the proportion of the population affected over the lifetime (lifetime prevalence) may be specified. *Incidence* is the rate of onset of the condition over time (conventionally, one year). The formula for incidence is the number of new cases beginning in the specified interval divided by the number of persons in the population at risk of onset. Those at risk include persons in the population who are capable of developing the condition (e.g., women who have had hysterectomies are not at risk for uterine cancer) and who do not already have the condition. A more thorough discussion of incidence and prevalence measures can be found in many textbooks of epidemiology (e.g., Lilienfeld and Lilienfeld 1980; Kleinbaum et al. 1982).

Prevalence and incidence are related such that prevalence equals incidence multiplied by average duration of the disease or disorder (Kleinbaum et al. 1982). For an acute disease with short duration, prevalence and incidence are approximately equal. However, for chronic conditions, a high prevalence rate may reflect the many long-standing cases in the population; under these circumstances, the incidence rate of the condition may even be relatively low. For chronic episodic conditions, including chronic pain conditions such as TMDs, the prevalence is approximated by the product of the incidence rate, the average duration of episodes, and the average number of episodes over the course of the illness (Von Korff and Parker 1980).

EPIDEMIOLOGIC METHODS

Five study designs are commonly used in epidemiologic research:

1. Cross-sectional studies assess the prevalence of a condition or its signs and symptoms in a defined population or populations.

2. Longitudinal studies follow persons with the condition over time.

3. Prospective or cohort studies begin by assessing potential risk factors in persons initially free of the disorder of interest, then follow those persons over time to see who develops the condition.

4. Case-control, or retrospective, study designs compare persons with the condition to those without, in an attempt to identify putative risk factors that are more prevalent in the cases than in the controls.

5. Experimental studies, or intervention trials, compare persons randomly assigned to one treatment condition to those assigned to a different treatment or control condition.

Experimental studies aimed at preventing a condition in persons at risk are called preventive trials. Perhaps the most well-known preventive trial ever undertaken involved a comparison of the rates of onset of caries in a community with a fluoridated water supply versus a control community without fluoridated water (Dean et al. 1942). Clinical trials are experimental studies aimed at testing the efficacy of treatments in persons already experiencing a disease or condition.

Each of these study designs has its own advantages and disadvantages. For example, case-control studies are fairly inexpensive to carry out but rely on subject self-report of risk factors, which may be biased among persons experiencing a condition. Prospective or cohort studies can produce estimates of incidence rates and can accurately identify risk factors present before the onset of the condition; however, such studies are relatively expensive to conduct because they require identification and repeated examination or interview of many subjects. With the exception of preventive trials, TMD epidemiology has employed each of the methodologic approaches mentioned above. Cross-sectional study designs are common and some longitudinal studies of TMD cases have been carried out. A few cohort studies of adolescents have been reported as have the initial results of one prospective study of adults without TMD pain. Numerous case-control investigations have compared persons seeking treatment for TMDs to various control groups, including general dental patients. Finally, although a few well-designed clinical trials have been conducted, "action-oriented" or intervention research has not been tried to any great extent (Carlsson 1984; Dworkin et al. 1990a).

RESULTS OF EPIDEMIOLOGICAL STUDIES OF TMD SIGNS AND SYMPTOMS

CROSS-SECTIONAL STUDIES

In the five years after the publication of Helkimo's review at least 18 epidemiologic studies were published (Carlsson 1984). Although the majority were Scandinavian, a worldwide distribution of studies was found. The methodology of these studies showed considerable variability but the prevalence figures reported were similar to those in Helkimo's review (1979). The prevalences ranged from 16% to 59% for reported symptoms and from 33% to 86% for clinical signs. The median values were 32% for subjective and 61% for clinical dysfunction. The 18 papers presented great ranges of prevalence figures for single reported symptoms and clinical signs. For example, the range for reported TMJ sounds was 6–48% with a median value of 19%, while the corresponding values for clinically recorded TMJ sounds were 9–50% and 26%, respectively. Even if we focus on the median values of these studies it must be concluded that signs and symptoms of TMDs, according to the criteria applied in these studies, are common in nonpatient populations.

In a recent publication De Kanter and co-workers (1993) performed a meta-analysis on 51 TMD prevalence studies selected from the MEDLINE database for 1974 and later. This analysis, using compound samples of randomly selected subjects, revealed (1) a perceived dysfunction rate of 30%, based on more than 15,000 subjects (23 studies), and (2) a clinically assessed dysfunction rate of 44% based on more than 16,000 subjects (22 studies). Several deficiencies were noted in study design for the literature reviewed, including the lack of accepted definitions. State of the dentition was seldom reported, and reports of examiner reliability and observer variation were rare. The prevalences also varied extremely: 6–93% based on subjects' reports, and 0–93% according to clinical assessment.

It is obvious upon more thorough reading of these papers that the interpretation of the results is difficult, if not impossible, because of the lack of generally accepted standards for definitions, methods of investigation, and presentation of results. These factors probably explain more of the variation than do any real differences between samples.

Thus, over the past few decades several epidemiological studies using cross-sectional designs have been conducted. An evaluation of their quality rather than quantity probably prompted an American research group (Dworkin et al. 1990a) to conclude that "there is a paucity of data regarding descriptive epidemiology of chronic pain conditions in general, and of TMDs in particular."

As an addition to the papers reviewed above, this chapter will briefly report a few of the most extensive of recent studies. Salonen et al. (1990) studied more than 900 persons selected according to epidemiological principles from the population of a Swedish county; the response rate was 95%. The proportion of subjects who did not report any symptoms increased from about 50% in the lower age groups (20–40 years) to more than 70% at age 60 and above, with similar patterns in men and women. The mean frequency of persons with severe symptoms including pain on function was about 10%, and did not differ much in the various age groups. The clinical examination revealed an increase with age of subjects with one or more clinical signs of TMDs. Severe signs were, however, extremely rare. The prevalence of general diseases and regular medication use in the same sample increased markedly with age. One explanation for the weak correlation between reported symptoms and clinical signs in the elderly might be the growing impact that generally impaired health may have on the salience of symptoms of TMDs.

As part of a nationwide epidemiological survey of oral health in the adult Dutch population, De Kanter (1990) investigated the prevalence and need for treatment of TMDs. About one fifth of the respondents reported one or more symptoms of dysfunction. The prevalence was slightly higher in women than in men and most of the reported symptoms were mild. In contrast to the low levels of symptom report, about half of the population had one or more clinical signs of dysfunction, mainly mild and not considered inconvenient. Transformation of the data on signs and symptoms into the Helkimo indices (Helkimo 1974) showed that about 4% of the men and 6% of the women had severe symptoms according to the anamnestic index. The prevalence of subjects with moderate or severe signs and symptoms on the clinical dysfunction index was around 5% for the Dutch population. When the distribution of the index values was presented according to dentition, the figures were remarkably similar for those with natural dentition and those with complete dentures.

In an extensive epidemiologic study in the United States, Dworkin and co-workers (1990a) used a two-stage study design. In a questionnaire screening survey completed by 80% of the age-stratified sample, 12% were identified as cases of TMD pain, defined as those who reported "facial ache or pain in the jaw muscles, the joint in front of the ear, or inside the ear (other than infection)" in the previous six months (Von Korff et al. 1988). This group was clinically examined and interviewed and compared with another group selected at random from those who did not report pain in the past six months. A third group, comprising a consecutive series of clinical cases referred for treatment of TMDs from the same population, also was included. As in most other clinical series, the clinic cases had a great preponderance of women (84%); about three-quarters of the community group with TMD pain were women. The clinic cases reported pain more frequently on jaw movements and in response to muscle palpation. They had less vertical opening capacity but did not differ from the other groups with respect to horizontal jaw movements. They also more frequently had deviation of the mandible on opening and joint clicking. There were no significant differences between the three groups with respect to occlusal or other dental factors.

Lipton et al. (1993) recently reported data on several different oral and facial pains from a national survey of the U.S. population comprising more than 42,000 households. After adjusting for the complex sampling design, prevalence rate estimates were derived for the civilian population over the age of 18. An estimated 6% of the population reported experiencing a symptom pattern involving pain in the jaw joint and/or face. Women reported these symptoms about twice as frequently as did men. Estimated prevalence rates decreased with age for jaw joint pain. Face pain showed its lowest prevalence in the 55–74 year-old age group, with a somewhat higher rate in the 75 and older age group. However, it is difficult to interpret this finding because of the complex sampling method and the possible low sample size in the very oldest group.

In all these studies, with the possible exception of the last, TMD symptoms were reported less frequently by the older subjects than by younger ones. One reasonable interpretation of these findings is that TMDs in general do not progress to a further deterioration of masticatory function and TMD pain often seems to disappear with advancing age. This finding has been corroborated in clinical material. In samples of more than 10,000 patients with TMDs, Levitt and McKinney (1994) found that severity and prevalence of symptoms of joint dysfunction and range of motion limitation were lower in older age groups than in younger ones.

TMD signs and symptoms in children and adolescents

Several epidemiologic investigations have focused on the prevalence of signs and symptoms of TMDs in children and adolescents (for reviews see Nilner 1985; Tallents et al. 1991). The prevalence figures reported in these studies have varied greatly, but apparently a substantial proportion of each of these young samples demonstrated positive findings. However, most of the signs and symptoms were characterized as mild, and TMJ clicking and muscle pain on palpation were the most frequent findings. When comparing the results of these studies with those of adults we can conclude that the prevalences of signs and symptoms of TMDs were lower in children than in adults and decreased with decreasing age in the children. For example, in children aged 3–6 years, signs of dysfunction were found in only 3.5% (De Vis et al. 1984; De Boever and van den Berghe 1987).

Thus, epidemiologic studies suggest that the clinician also should be prepared to find signs and symptoms characteristic of TMDs in young patients. Whether these signs represent a condition warranting treatment is questionable, because more severe dysfunctional pain occurs only in a small segment of this young population (Wänman 1987; Tallents et al. 1991).

Gender differences in TMD signs and symptoms

A strong female predominance has been observed in practically all series of patients in TMD clinics. A recent study of more than 10,000 TMD patients also showed that women reported a higher level of severity of all physical and psychological symptoms than did men (Levitt and McKinney 1994). These observations have been interpreted in different ways, some emphasizing hormonal or constitutional factors, others behavioral, compliance, or psychosocial differences between the sexes. The early epidemiological studies found no great differences in prevalence of signs and symptoms of TMDs between men and women in the general population. It was thus believed that the gender distribution among the patients could be explained mainly in psychosocial terms and by sex-role behavior. Gender differences in tolerance to pain and other physical symptoms are common, with men showing more tolerance to a wide range of painful stimuli and seeking medical and dental care less often than do women (DeLeeuw 1993; Lipton et al. 1993). However, at least one study has shown no significant gender difference in rates of seeking care for TMDs (Von Korff et al. 1991) and more recent epidemiological data indicate that women really have more problems related to joints and musculoskeletal structures (De Kanter 1990; Dworkin et al. 1990a; Salonen et al. 1990; DeLeeuw 1993). Whether men and women differ in the presence of estrogen receptors in the TMJ remains uncertain (Abubaker et al. 1993; Campbell et al. 1993). However, recent research has suggested the existence of an estrogen-mediated pain modulation system in mice (Mogil et al. 1993), and epidemiologic studies have demonstrated a possible role for exogenous hormones (e.g., oral contraceptives) in TMDs (LeResche et al. 1993, 1994). In addition, many hypotheses remain to be explored at the psychological and social level, so the issue of gender differences in TMDs remains a puzzle and warrants further investigation.

Because chronic pain and pain-related behavior may be viewed as arising from the interaction of biological, psychological, and social processes, potential reasons for the observed age and gender differences might be sought in the pathophysiology of TMDs, in neurophysiologic changes with age, in different perceptual processes related to age or sex, in differing social roles that might influence risks of onset and continuation of specific pain conditions, or in the expectations of individuals and society regarding the expression of certain pains in relation to age and/or sex. Moreover, several of these factors might be operating simultaneously (Dworkin et al. 1992). Cross-sectional studies of TMDs most likely will not provide needed data on how age and gender are related to onset, episode duration, remission, and relapse rates. It has been hoped that longitudinal studies of population samples would give such data to determine how age and gender can influence critical features of the natural history of TMDs.

LONGITUDINAL STUDIES

The majority of epidemiologic research up to the late 1980s comprised cross-sectional studies. Since that time, a few longitudinal and prospective studies have been presented (Magnusson et al. 1985, 1986, 1993; De Boever and van den Berghe 1987; Wänman and Agerberg 1987; Österberg et al 1992; Rafael and Marbach 1992; Von Korff et al. 1993). These studies have provided the first prospective estimates of incidence rates for TMD pain in adults (Von Korff et al. 1993) and have documented the great variability in intensity of myofascial pain over time, even in chronic patients (Rafael and Marbach 1992).

The longitudinal epidemiologic studies of children and young adolescents have mainly confirmed results from cross-sectional studies, with slightly increasing prevalences of signs and symptoms as children grow older. However, a still more interesting finding is the great fluctuation of signs and symptoms of TMDs over time. Table I gives an example of the fluctuation of TMJ clicking. Almost half of the subjects with TMJ clicking at age 15 had no clicking at age 20, while half of those who had TMJ clicking at age 20 had not had clicking at age 15. In the clinical literature on TMDs it has often been stated that the natural history of internal derangement of the TMJ starts with clicking, continues with locking to a closed lock, and eventually develops into degenerative joint disease. Clicking did not progress to locking in any of the subjects in a five-year follow-up (Magnusson et al. 1986). At the 10-year follow-up of the same material only one of 293 subjects reported intermittent

Table I
Cross-tabulation of TMJ clicking in 119 subjects
on two occasions

TMJ Clicking at 20 Years	TMJ Clicking at 15 Years			
	None	Grade 1	Grade 2	Total
None	65	13	3	81
Grade 1*	15	7	4	26
Grade 2†	4	2	6	12
Total	84	22	13	119

Source: Magnusson et al. 1985.
* Palpable.
† Evidently audible.

locking (Magnusson et al. 1993). It thus seems as if the purported development of TMJ clicking to locking and degenerative joint disease is extremely rare from an epidemiological perspective.

Despite these interesting results, longitudinal studies have not yet fulfilled the expectation that they would solve many of the questions unanswered by cross-sectional research. Longitudinal research presents many difficulties in design and analysis, and careful attention to methodologic detail is necessary if results are to be of value. With careful methodologic approaches, longitudinal studies, especially prospective studies of young adult populations where incidence rates of TMDs appear to be high, continue to hold promise for identification of risk factors for these conditions.

TMD signs and symptoms in older adults

Findings from a longitudinal population study of elderly persons indicate that signs and symptoms of TMDs decrease with increasing age (Österberg et al. 1992). This trend was especially obvious for reported symptoms. For example, difficulty in opening the mouth widely was reported in about 12% of respondents at age 70 but decreased to only a few percent at age 80 (0% for men at that age). TMJ sounds fluctuated over time, which might indicate that the wide fluctuations of TMJ sounds in young people also hold true for the elderly. The conclusion drawn from this study is that there is no increased risk of developing symptoms of TMDs with increasing age. On the contrary, the general awareness of those symptoms decreased with age. A study of patients followed up 30 years after nonsurgical treatment of TMJ osteoarthrosis or internal derangement (mean age at follow-up approximately 59 years) also found that clinical signs generally subsided over time (DeLeeuw et al. 1994). In this respect the findings corroborate the results of the extensive cross-sectional studies referred to previously (Von Korff et al. 1988; De Kanter 1990; Salonen et al. 1990).

EPIDEMIOLOGY OF SPECIFIC TMDs

Assessing the prevalence of specific TMDs in the population requires reliable diagnostic definitions of those individual disorders. In an initial approach to this problem, Truelove et al. (1992) applied operational clinical decision criteria in a post hoc manner to data from standardized clinical examinations and reported prevalences of specific muscle disorders, internal derangements, and degenerative joint disease in clinic and community cases with TMD pain as well as pain-free population controls. Further studies using standardized diagnostic criteria such as the Research Diagnostic Criteria for TMDs (Dworkin and LeResche 1992) are needed to develop an understanding of the prevalence of and risk factors for specific temporomandibular disorders—as opposed to signs and symptoms—in populations.

Many diseases can produce symptoms related to the masticatory system (Carlsson et al. 1979). The most prevalent of such disorders is degenerative joint disease or osteoarthrosis/osteoarthritis (OA). The prevalence of OA increases with age but differs in different joints. The knees and hips especially are commonly affected and in the oldest age groups most persons have signs or symptoms indicating OA in these joints. After about age 50 OA is more common in women than in men.

The prevalence of OA of the TMJ is also common according to a series of reports (Zarb and Carlsson 1994) but it differs widely depending on methods of examination and criteria for diagnosis, age and selection of samples. In clinical studies of nonpatient groups, crepitation, which is considered a clinical sign of OA, has been reported with frequencies ranging from 1% to 24%. Radiographic changes have been observed in 14–44%, macroscopic degenerative changes have been found at autopsy in prevalences varying from 22% to 84%, and similar figures have been reported for microscopic changes (Zarb and Carlsson 1994). Interestingly, Åkerman (1987) observed disk perforation in 36% of an elderly group. In different series of TMD patients, OA of the TMJ has been diagnosed in 8–16%. With other diagnostic criteria, such as those suggested by Stegenga (1991), higher prevalences probably would have been found.

The prevalence of OA of the TMJ is thus appreciable, but the great variation found in the literature indicates the necessity for a clearer definition of diagnostic criteria in future studies. Among the polyarthritides that can affect the TMJ, rheumatoid arthritis is most common. A very great variation (2–88%) has been reported in the literature for the frequency of involvement of the TMJ in this systemic disease (Carlsson et al. 1979). It can be concluded, however, that the more severe the general disease, the more common is the involvement of the TMJ in rheumatoid arthritis. Signs and symptoms of TMDs have been reported to be more common in subjects with rheumatoid arthritis, ankylosing spondylitis, and psoriatic arthritis than in healthy controls, and the number of signs and symptoms has been correlated with the extent and severity of the systemic disease (Könönen et al. 1992).

Several studies have recently reported that persons with general joint hypermobility have more signs and symptoms of TMDs—especially of the TMJ—than do controls (Westling 1992). Although these results have not consistently been replicated (e.g., Dijkstra et al. 1992), this is an interesting finding. Together with other previously reported observations, it indicates the need to consider general health factors in the diagnosis and management of TMDs.

The associations found between TMDs and other disorders such as headaches and neck pain, and the fact that the severity of these problems can be alleviated after TMD treatment, suggest that TMDs may represent a more general health problem. Persons with pain at multiple sites also are more likely to be depressed than are persons with only a single pain (Dworkin et al. 1990b), and the presence of an initial pain at baseline was found to increase the risk of onset of additional pains at three-year follow-up (Von Korff et al. 1993). The finding that the length of sick leave both in TMD patients and in population samples was correlated with the severity of signs and symptoms also suggests that TMDs may be of greater importance in the general health care system than is usually assumed (Wedel 1988; Kirveskari 1991). This issue deserves further epidemiologic study.

SEVERITY OF TMDs AND INDICES OF DYSFUNCTION

The ratio between reported symptoms and clinical findings of TMDs in a group of subjects is usually about 1:2 according to the median values of several studies (Carlsson 1984). This observation means that the subjects examined are not aware of many of the clinically recorded signs. An interesting question, of course, is how relevant are such findings? One way of quantifying the severity of a disorder is to use an index system. Although a detailed discussion of the reliability and validity of specific indices is beyond the scope of this chapter, we will review population-based findings for the most commonly used severity indices.

Helkimo's indices (1974) for anamnestic and clinical dysfunction were the first developed and are still the most frequently used. These indices were developed to facilitate a standardized classification and evaluation of signs and symptoms, especially for epidemiological research. The anamnestic dysfunction index, based on information furnished by the person examined, is divided into three groups: 0 = subjectively symptom free, 1 = mild (TMJ sounds, fatigue/stiffness of the jaws), and 2 = severe (pain, difficulty in jaw movements, locking, luxation) symptoms. The clinical dysfunction index, based on observations by the dentist at clinical examinations, is divided into four groups: 0 = clinically free of signs, 1 = mild, 2 = moderate, and 3 = severe signs. The basis of the evaluation of the degree of clinical dysfunction is dependent on signs, each judged according to a three-grade scale of severity. The signs are: impaired range of mandibular movement, impaired TMJ function, muscle pain/tenderness on palpation, TMJ pain on palpation, and pain on movement of the mandible.

Population-based studies using the Helkimo indices have found prevalence rates of severe symptoms, based on the anamnestic index of 5–26% for adult populations. Severe dysfunction based on the clinical dysfunction index ranges from 1% to 22% of the general population. The higher figures were reported in Helkimo's studies of a Lapp population in Northern Finland and appear higher than those recorded in other population samples using the same indices.

In the last few years attempts have been made to present other indices (for surveys see Levitt et al. 1988; Pullinger and Monteiro 1988; Widmer 1992). Some of these new index systems seem promising but none have yet become so widely used in population-based studies as the Helkimo index so the possibility of evaluating them is still limited. A recent study (Schiffman et al. 1992) compared Helkimo's clinical dysfunction index and the Craniomandibular Index (CMI). The correlation between these two indices was as high as $r = 0.9$, but the authors nevertheless concluded that numerous differences exist between the two indices.

It is complex and probably impossible to construct an ideal index for TMDs that can encompass their many specific disorders. It is generally acknowledged that all indices are deficient because they are not diagnosis-specific and cannot assess the multidimensional problems involved. Even if there is only a modest hope of finding an ideal index for TMDs, the work must continue to further develop and improve methods to classify these disorders and assess severity of signs and symptoms that can be of value to both clinical and epidemiological studies.

GEOGRAPHIC DISTRIBUTION OF TMDs

Interest in the epidemiology of TMDs started and has been strongest in Northern Europe. This interest spread to many other countries in Europe and to North America (both the United States and Canada). Results of epidemiological studies also have been published from, among other countries, Egypt, India, Israel, Japan, New Zealand, Saudi Arabia, and Singapore. These studies from outside Europe and North America give no indication that the prevalences of signs and symptoms of TMDs differ markedly from those reviewed earlier in this chapter. It must be remembered, however, that the ranges of prevalences reported have been wide. This situation might be due more to variations in methodology (e.g., sampling, definitions, examinations) than to differences in prevalences in the studied populations. This uncertainty cannot be resolved until more standardized investigational criteria have been employed. An important step in this process has been the recent publication of research diagnostic criteria for the major TMDs (Dworkin and LeResche 1992).

During a visit to Czechoslovakia (spring 1992), the senior author noted that the interest in and knowledge of TMDs was minimal. No studies of TMDs could be identified. It is remarkable that TMD or "TMJ" was termed an "in-malady" in the United States at the end of the 1980s while it was a practically unknown disorder in Czechoslovakia. Probably a scrutiny of the "geography" of TMDs and use of modern epidemiological methods internationally will increase our understanding of the disorder. Based on Payer's description of the impact of culture on medical treatment in some Western countries (1989), it is tempting to suggest that cultural influences are probably also great in the field of TMDs.

CONCLUSIONS

It is easy to say, in interpreting of the results of the epidemiologic studies, that dental practitioners should know how to diagnose and treat signs and symptoms of TMDs. It is, however, also evident that the work must continue to provide a better definition of criteria and principles of diagnosis and need for treatment. Epidemiological research will continue to have great utility in the field of TMDs given the still numerous controversies. In addition to descriptive and cross-sectional surveys, it is necessary to include more longitudinal designs, case-control, cohort, intervention, and experimental studies as approaches in epidemiological research on TMDs. Epidemiology should not be isolated from basic and clinical research. Rather, epidemiologic findings should provide hypotheses to be tested by basic and clinical research, and the results of basic and clinical investigations should influence our epidemiologic hypotheses and research designs. In this way epidemiology can further improve our understanding of TMDs.

ACKNOWLEDGMENT

During preparation of this chapter, Dr. LeResche was supported by NIH Grant P01 DE08773.

REFERENCES

Abubaker, A.O., Raslan, W.F. and Sotereanos, G.C., Estrogen and progesterone receptors in temporomandibular joint discs of symptomatic and asymptomatic persons: a preliminary study, J. Oral Maxillofac. Surg., 51 (1993) 1096–1100.

Åkerman, S., Morphologic, radiographic and thermometric assessment of degenerative and inflammatory temporomandibular joint disease. An autopsy and clinical study, Swed. Dent. J., Suppl. 52 (1987).

Campbell, J.H., Courey, M.S., Bourne, P. and Odziemiec, C., Estrogen receptor analysis of human temporomandibular disc, J. Oral Maxillofac. Surg., 51 (1993) 1101–1105.

Carlsson, G.E., Epidemiological studies of signs and symptoms of temporomandibular joint-pain-dysfunction, A literature review, Austr. Prosthodont. Soc. Bull., 14 (1984) 7–12.

Carlsson, G.E., Kopp, S. and Öberg, T., Arthritis and allied diseases of the temporomandibular joint. In: G.A. Zarb and G.E. Carlsson (Eds.), Temporomandibular Joint: Function and Dysfunction, Munksgaard, Copenhagen, 1979, pp. 269–320.

Dean, H.T., Arnold, F.A., Jr. and Elvove, E., Domestic water and dental caries, Publ. Health Rep., 57 (1942) 1155–1179.

De Boever, J.A. and van den Berghe, L., Longitudinal study of functional conditions in the masticatory system in Flemish children, Community Dent. Oral Epidemiol., 15 (1987) 100–103.

De Kanter, R.J., Prevalence and etiology of craniomandibular dysfuuction: an epidemiologic study of the Dutch adult population, Thesis, University of Nijmegen, 1990.

De Kanter, R., Käyser, A., Battistuzzi, P., Truin, G. and Van't Hof, M., Demand and need for treatment of craniomandibular dysfunction in the Dutch adult population, J. Dent. Res., 71 (1992) 1607–1612.

De Kanter, R., Truin, G.J., Burgersdijk, R., Van't Hof, M., Battistuzzi, P., Halsbeek, H. and Käyser, A., Prevalence in the Dutch adult population and a meta-analysis of signs and symptoms of temporomandibular disorder, J. Dent. Res., 72 (1993) 1509–1518.

DeLeeuw, J.R.J., Psychosocial aspects and symptom characteristics of craniomandibular dysfunction, Thesis, University of Utrecht, 1993.

DeLeeuw, R., Boering, G., Stegenga, B. and de Bont, L.G.M., Clinical signs of TMJ osteoarthrosis and internal derangement 30 years after nonsurgical treatment, J. Orofac. Pain, 8 (1994) 18–24.

De Vis, H., De Boever, J.A. and van Cauwenberghe, P., Epidemiologic survey of functional conditions of the masticatory system in Belgian children aged 3–6 years, Community Dent. Oral Epidemiol., 12 (1984) 203–207.

Dijkstra, P.U., de Bont, L.G., Stegenga, B. and Boering, G., Temporomandibular joint osteoarthrosis and generalized joint hypermobility, Cranio, 10 (1992) 221–227.

Dworkin, S.F.and LeResche, L. (Eds.), Research diagnostic criteria for temporomandibular disorders: review, criteria, examinations and specifications, critique, J. Craniomandib. Disord. Facial Oral Pain, 6 (1992) 301–355.

Dworkin, S.F., Huggins, K.H., LeResche, L., Von Korff, M., Howard. J., Truelove, E. and Sommers, E., Epidemiology of signs and symptoms in temporomandibular disorders: clinical signs in cases and controls, J. Am. Dent. Assoc., 120 (1990a) 273–281.

Dworkin, S.F., Von Korff, M. and LeResche, L., Multiple pains and psychiatric disturbance: an epidemiologic investigation, Arch. Gen. Psychiatry, 47 (1990b) 239–244.

Dworkin, S.F., Von Korff, M.R. and LeResche, L., Epidemiologic studies of chronic pain: a dynamic-ecologic perspective, Ann. Behav. Med., 14 (1992) 3–11.

Greene, C.S. and Marbach, J.J., Epidemiologic studies of mandibular dysfunction: a critical review, J. Prosthet. Dent., 48 (1982) 184–190.

Helkimo, M., Studies on function and dysfunction of the masticatory system. II. Index for anamnestic and clinical dysfunction and occlusal state, Swed. Dent. J., 67 (1974) 101–121.

Helkimo, M., Epidemiological surveys of dysfunction of the masticatory system. In: G.A. Zarb and G.E. Carlsson (Eds.), Temporomandibular Joint: Function and Dysfunction, Munksgaard, Copenhagen, 1979, pp. 175–192.

Holland, W., Detels, R. and Knox, O. (Eds.), Oxford Textbook of Public Health, 2nd ed., Vol. 2, Oxford University Press, Oxford, 1991.

Jagger, R.G. and Wood, C., Signs and symptoms of temporomandibular joint dysfunction in a Saudi Arabian population, J. Oral Rehabil., 19 (1992) 353–359.

Kirveskari, P., Are craniomandibular disorders a general health problem? Proc. Finn. Dent. Soc., 87 (1991) 309–313.

Kleinbaum, D.G., Kupper, L.L. and Morgenstern, H., Epidemiologic Research: Principles and Quantitative Methods, Lifetime Learning Publications, Belmont, 1982.

Könönen, M., Wenneberg, B. and Kallenberg, A., Craniomandibular disorders in rheumatoid arthritis, psoriatic arthritis and ankylosing spondylitis: a clinical study, Acta Odontol. Scand., 50 (1992) 281–287.

Kopp, S. and Wenneberg, B., Intra- and interobserver variability in the assessment of signs of disorder in the stomatognathic system, Swed. Dent. J., 7 (1983) 239–246.

LeResche., L., Saunders. K., Barlow, W., Von Korff, M. and Dworkin, S.F., Does oral contraceptive use increase the risk of temporomandibular disorder pain? Abstracts: 7th World Congress on Pain, IASP Publications, Seattle, 1993, pp. 294–295.

LeResche, L., Dworkin, S.F., Saunders, K., Von Korff. M. and Barlow, W., Is postmenopausal hormone use a risk factor for TMD? J. Dent. Res. 73 (spec. iss.), Abs. no. 675 (1994) 186.

Levitt, S.R., Lundeen. T.F.and McKinney, M.W., Initial studies of a new assessment method for temporomandibular joint disorders, J. Prosthet. Dent., 59 (1988) 490–495.

Levitt, S.R. and McKinney, M.W., Validating the TMJ scale in a national sample of 10,000 patients: demographic and epidemiologic characteristics, J. Orofac. Pain, 8 (1994) 25–35.

Lilienfeld, A.M and Lilienfeld, D.E., Foundations of Epidemiology, 2nd ed., Oxford University Press, New York, 1980.

Lipton, J.A., Ship, J.A. and Larach-Robinson, D., Estimated prevalence and distribution of reported orofacial pain in the United States, J. Am. Dent. Assoc., 124 (1993) 115–121.

Magnusson, T., Egermark-Eriksson, I. and Carlsson, G.E., Four-year longitudinal study of mandibular dysfunction in children, Community Dent. Oral Epidemiol., 13 (1985) 117–120.

Magnusson, T., Egermark-Eriksson, I. and Carlsson, G.E., Five year longitudinal study of signs and symptoms of mandibular dysfunction in adolescents, J. Craniomandib. Pract., 4 (1986) 338–344.

Magnusson, T., Carlsson, G.E, and Egermark-Eriksson, I., An evaluation of the need and demand for treatment of craniomandibular disorders in a young Swedish population, J. Craniomandib. Disord. Facial Oral Pain 5 (1991) 57–63.

Magnusson, T., Egermark, I. and Carlsson, G.E., Changes in subjective symptoms of craniomandibular disorders in children and adolescents during a ten-year period, J. Orofacial Pain, 7 (1993) 76–82.

Mogil, J.S., Sternberg, W.F., Kest, B., Marek, P. and Liebeskind, J.C., Sex differences in the antagonism of swim stress–induced analgesia: effects of gonadectomy and estrogen replacement, Pain 53 (1993) 17–25.

Morris, J.N., Uses of Epidemiology, 3rd ed., Churchill Livingstone, Edinburgh, 1975.

Nilner, M., Functional disturbances and diseases in the stomotognathic system among 7- to 18-year olds, Cranio, 3 (1985) 350–367.

Ohrbach, R. and Stohler, C., Current diagnostic systems. In: S.F.Dworkin and L.LeResche (Eds.), Research diagnostic criteria for temporomandibular disorders: review, criteria, examinations and specifications, critique, J. Craniomandib. Disord. Facial Oral Pain, 6 (1992), pp. 307–317.

Österberg, T., Carlsson, G.E., Wedel, A. and Johansson, U., A cross-sectional and longitudinal study of craniomandibular dysfunction in an elderly population, J. Craniomandib. Disord. Facial Oral Pain, 6 (1992) 237–246.

Payer, L., Medicine and Culture, Penguin, New York, 1989.

Pullinger, A.G. and Monteiro, A.A., Functional impairment in TMJ patient and nonpatient groups according to a disability index and symptom profile, J. Craniomandib. Pract., 6 (1988) 156–164.

Rafael, K.G. and Marbach, J.J., A year of chronic TMPDS: evaluating patients' pain patterns, J. Am. Dent. Assoc., 123 (1992) 53–58.

Rothman, K., Modern Epidemiology, Little, Brown, Boston, 1986.

Rugh, J.D. and Solberg, W.L., Oral health status in the United States: temporomandibular disorders, J. Dent. Educ., 49 (1985) 398–405.

Salonen, L., Hellden, L. and Carlsson, G.E., Prevalence of signs and symptoms of dysfunction in the masticatory system. an epidemiological study in an adult Swedish population, J. Craniomandib. Disord., 4 (1990) 241–250.

Schiffman, E.L., Fricton, J.R. and Haley, D., The relationship of occlusion, parafunctional habits and recent life events to mandibular dysfunction in a non-patient population, J. Oral Rehabil., 19 (1992) 201–223.

Stegenga, R., Temporomandibular joint osteoarthrosis and internal derangement: diagnostic and therapeutic outcome assessment, Thesis, University of Groningen, 1991.

Tallents, R.H., Catania, J. and Sommers, E., Temporomandibular joint findings in pediatric populations and young adults: a critical review, Angle Orthod., 61 (1991) 7–16.

Truelove, E.E., Sommers, E., LeResche, L., Dworkin, S.F. and Von Korff, M., Clinical diagnostic criteria for TMD: new classification permits multiple diagnoses, J. Am. Dent. Assoc., 123 (1992) 47–54.

Von Korff, M. and Parker, R.D., The dynamics of the prevalence of chronic episodic disease, J. Chron. Dis., 33 (1980) 79–85.

Von Korff, M., Dworkin, S.F., LeResche, L. and Kruger, A., An epidemiologic comparison of pain complaints, Pain, 32 (1988) 173–183.

Von Korff, M., Wagner, E.H., Dworkin, S.F. and Saunders, K.W., Chronic pain and use of ambulatory health care, Psychosom. Med., 53 (1991) 61–79.

Von Korff, M., LeResche, L. and Dworkin, S.F., First onset of common pain symptoms: a prospective study of depression as a risk factor, Pain, 55 (1993) 251–258.

Wänman, A., Craniomandibular disorders in adolescents, Swed. Dent. J., Suppl. 44 (1987).

Wänman, A. and Agerberg, G., Recurrent headache and craniomandibular disorders in adolescents: a longitudinal study, J. Craniomandib. Disord., 1 (1987) 229–236.

Wedel, A., Heterogeneity of patients with craniomandibular disorders. a longitudinal study, Swed. Dent. J., Suppl. 55 (1988).

van der Weele, L.T. and Dibbets, J.M.H., Helkimo's index: a scale or just a set of symptoms? J. Oral Rehabil., 14 (1987) 229–237.

Westling, L., Temporomandibular joint dysfunction and systemic joint laxity, Swed. Dent. J., Suppl. 81 (1992).

Widmer, C., Review of the literature: reliability and validation of examination methods. In: S.F. Dworkin and L. LeResche (Eds.), Research Diagnostic criteria for temporomandibular disorders: review, criteria, examinations and specifications, critique, J. Craniomand. Disord. Facial Oral Pain, 6 (1992), pp. 318–326.

Zarb, G.A. and Carlsson, G.E., Osteoarthrosis/osteoarthritis. In: G.A. Zarb, G.E. Carlsson, B. Sessle and N.D. Mohl (Eds.), Temporomandibular Joint and Masticatory Muscle Disorders, Munksgaard, Copenhagen, 1994, pp. 298–314.

Correspondence to: Linda LeResche, Department of Oral Medicine, SC-63, University of Washington, Seattle, WA 98195 USA. Tel: 206-543-5912; Fax: 206-685-8412.

Temporomandibular Disorders and Related Pain Conditions, Progress in Pain Research and Management, Vol. 4, edited by B.J. Sessle, P.S. Bryant, and R.A. Dionne, IASP Press, Seattle, © 1995.

13

Health Services Research and Temporomandibular Pain

Michael Von Korff

Center for Health Studies, Group Health Cooperative of Puget Sound, Seattle, Washington, USA

Pain in the temporomandibular region is a common symptom affecting more than 10% of adults at any one time, and one in three adults over their life span (Von Korff et al. 1988a). The course of temporomandibular pain is typically recurrent and often chronic. The severity of pain and related behavioral dysfunction is highly variable both between patients and for individual patients over time. However, it is unusual for patients to experience progressive deterioration in either mandibular or in behavioral function. Disability associated with back pain and headache is typically greater than that observed among patients with temporomandibular pain (Keefe and Dolan 1986; Turk and Rudy 1990), but some patients with temporomandibular pain report substantial interference with work, family, and social activities (Von Korff et al. 1992). Thus, temporomandibular pain can be characterized as a chronic-recurrent, nonprogressive pain condition, typically associated with low to moderate impact on social role function.

Like back pain, temporomandibular pain might be thought of as "an illness in search of a disease" (Williams and Hadler 1983). Although standardized and reliable diagnostic criteria for temporomandibular disorders (TMDs) have been recently developed (Dworkin and LeResche 1992), the validity of these criteria and how specific diagnoses relate to either etiology or response to specific treatments is largely unknown. Temporomandibular pain is rarely associated with a well-defined disease. Evidence is lacking that dental, medical, or behavioral treatments produce appreciably better outcomes than can be achieved without treatment.

Given this uncertain state of affairs, developing rational strategies for provision of health care for persons with temporomandibular pain is a difficult task indeed. Efforts to define guidelines for diagnosis and treatment of patients with temporomandibular disorders, and for insuring such services, are likely to be controversial. Differing views about appropriate diagnosis and treatment are held by providers who treat patients in different ways, patients with various treatment preferences, and insurers of health care. Efforts to promulgate treatment guidelines could be expected to generate conflict among providers with an economic and professional interest in providing particular services. Such conflict is nurtured by the lack of rigorous scientific data concerning what kinds of treatments are effective and how to provide cost-effective therapeutic services.

In the United States, hundreds of millions of dollars are spent annually on diagnostic and therapeutic services for persons with temporomandibular pain. Despite this resource expenditure, little research has examined the magnitude of treatment services provided, where patients are cared for, what kinds of services they receive, cost of services, the short-term and long-term outcomes of treated and untreated patients, and whether the services provided are effective and cost-effective. Applying health services research to the provision of services for persons with temporomandibular pain is needed to identify how to provide effective care at a cost that individual patients and society can afford. It is now recognized that health care dollars are limited and that care for patients with temporomandibular pain consumes resources that might be used for other potentially beneficial health services or to achieve other societal goals. To the extent that there is social provision for health insurance, there is a societal interest in ensuring that health care dollars are spent on services that are cost-effective relative to competing uses of those resources.

Within this context, the objective of this chapter is to identify key research issues needed to provide a scientific basis for the provision of health care services for patients with temporomandibular pain. This paper draws on epidemiologic and health services data on the care of persons with temporomandibular pain in a single health maintenance organization (Group Health Cooperative of Puget Sound) to identify critical issues and to suggest how health services research might contribute to their resolution.

ALTERNATIVE VIEWS OF SERVICE REQUIREMENTS

At present, a scientific basis is lacking for consensus regarding the kinds of services likely to benefit the typical patient with temporomandibular pain. Three alternative strategies for the care of such a patient may be characterized as follows:

- Specialty care: The patient requires a comprehensive diagnostic evaluation followed by specialized treatment to address the underlying disorder.

- Generalist care: The patient requires a brief screening examination conducted by a generalist (primary care physician or general dentist) to assess whether significant disease may be present. Most patients are managed with nonspecific palliative care to control pain and inflammation. A small percentage of patients (less than 10%) are referred to a specialist for further evaluation and treatment.

- Self-care: Temporomandibular pain is a condition, like the common headache, that usually does not require diagnostic evaluation or medical management.

This chapter describes the issues to be considered in determining whether specialty care, generalist care, or self-care is likely to be the most cost-effective approach to managing the typical patient with temporomandibular pain.

As with other common pain symptoms, about one in four persons experiencing temporomandibular pain seek health care for their pain (Von Korff et al. 1988a; Linet et al. 1989). Those whose pain is more severe, more persistent, and of more recent onset are more likely to seek treatment (Von Korff et al. 1991). Among adults in Group Health Cooperative of Puget Sound who reported temporomandibular pain in the prior six months, men and women were equally likely to seek treatment, while there was a (nonsignificant) trend toward increased likelihood of seeking care among persons of higher income (Table I). Only 23.1% of all persons with temporomandibular pain were treated, suggesting that the remainder tolerated their symptoms or coped with self-care.

Although self-care is a common form of managing common pain symptoms, including temporomandibular pain, there has been remarkably little re-

Table I

Prevalence of temporomandibular pain and percentage treated among patients of the Group Health Cooperative of Puget Sound by gender and income (1986 data)

	Prevalence (%)	Cases Treated (%)
All persons	12.1	23.1
Men	8.3	22.9
Women	14.9	23.3
Annual income		
Less than $20,000	13.6	15.2
$20,000–$35,000	12.2	27.5
Greater than $35,000	12.4	26.7

Table II
Initial source of treatment for patients with temporomandibular
pain: patients eventually treated by TMD specialist and patients
identified in population survey (1986 data)

Initial Source	TMD Specialist (%; n = 240)	Survey (%; n = 53)
Physician	54.6	35.8
General dentist	36.7	50.9
Dental specialist	4.2	1.9
TMD specialist	0.0	1.9
Other	4.6	9.4

search studying how people self-manage pain or how that might be enhanced. Important exceptions are the growing body of research on minimal interventions for headache (Nash and Holroyd 1992) and on self-care of arthritis (Lorig and Holman 1993).

Insurance arrangements and the organization of health care affect the setting in which persons with a pain symptom are treated. At Group Health Cooperative, the large majority of persons with temporomandibular pain who sought care made their first contact with a primary care physician or with a general dentist (Table II). Less than 5% of treated cases made their initial contact with a specialist. However, of the 2235 patients who received services for temporomandibular pain from Group Health Cooperative in 1992, 40% were seen by a TMD specialist. In contrast, less than 10% of back pain and headache patients were seen by a specialist at Group Health Cooperative. Although temporomandibular pain has many features that make it appropriate for management by a primary care physician or general dentist, generalists often feel inadequately prepared to evaluate and manage these patients. As a result, there may be greater utilization of specialty care for this common pain symptom than would otherwise be warranted.

PATIENT OUTCOMES

The most essential criterion for evaluating the relative benefits of specialty care, generalist care, and self-care is their impact on patient outcomes. The two most critical patient outcomes are pain (intensity and persistence) and interference with activities. Rigorous comparison of the effects of specialty care, generalist care, and self-care on patient outcomes is likely to require randomization of patients to these different modalities of care.

PAIN AND INTERFERENCE WITH ACTIVITIES

Why are randomized controlled trials necessary to evaluate service effectiveness? Some of the reasons can be exemplified with observational data comparing the outcomes of care of TMD specialists to those of patients seen by a primary care physician. In a two-year follow-up of patients treated by a TMD specialist versus those seen only by a primary care physician at Group Health Cooperative, the two patient groups reported comparable pain intensity and levels of interference with activities at the initial interview (Fig. 1). Both sets of patients showed reduced pain levels and reduced interference with activities at one-year and at two-year follow-up. The patients seen only by a primary care physician showed greater reductions in pain intensity than did those treated by a specialist. While improvement after seeing a health care provider is often attributed by patients and providers to the effects of treatment, such improvement may be largely due to the natural history of the condition (Whitney and Von Korff 1992). For this reason, the expert opinions of clinicians regarding beneficial effects of therapeutic services may be an unreliable guide to their actual effectiveness. Randomized controlled trials, with appropriate control groups, are needed to determine whether before-after reductions in pain and disability are attributable to the effects of treatment or if they would have occurred in the absence of treatment.

The results in Fig. 1 also exemplify a difficulty in drawing conclusions about differences in effectiveness based on observational data alone. In Fig. 1, it appears that the patients of primary care physicians experienced greater

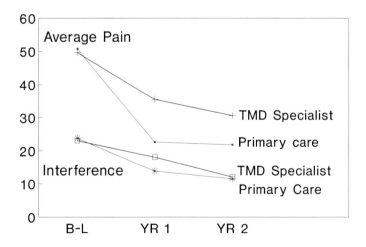

Fig. 1. Pain and interference outcomes over a two-year follow-up period for patients initially treated by a primary care physician or by a TMD specialist.

reductions in average pain intensity than did the patients of the TMD specialist. However, the explanation for this difference may be that the patients seen by a TMD specialist were more likely to have chronic temporomandibular pain at baseline (a mean of 101 pain days in prior six months) than were patients initially treated by a primary care physician (a mean of 50 days). In general, it is quite difficult to draw firm conclusions about treatment effectiveness based on a nonrandomized comparison because differences in outcomes may be due to pre-existing differences in prognosis that are unmeasured at baseline.

PATIENT SATISFACTION

A second criterion for evaluating health care services is their contribution to patient satisfaction. Patient preferences are increasingly recognized as important in deciding how services should be organized. In our research at Group Health Cooperative, we found that patients treated by a TMD specialist were significantly more satisfied with the diagnostic and treatment services provided and with the quality of patient education about care of their condition. Because the specialist was able to spend substantially more time with each patient (45–60 minutes versus 10–15 minutes) and was more knowledgeable and experienced in working with patients with temporomandibular pain, it is not surprising that satisfaction ratings were higher for specialty care than for primary care. An unresolved issue in the provision of health services is whether publicly subsidized insurance benefits should provide for services that are more satisfactory to patients irrespective of whether they produce more favorable outcomes. With the social provision of health insurance, the interests of business and of government in limiting insurance coverage to services that have health benefits commensurate with their cost may conflict with the desires of individual patients for care from a specialist who spends more time and who is more experienced in treating the patient's particular problem.

COSTS OF CARE

Differences in patient outcomes and satisfaction between specialist care, generalist care, and self-care need to be balanced against differences in the costs of care. At Group Health Cooperative, the annual cost to the insurance plan for TMD services was three times greater for patients seen by a TMD specialist ($304 per case) than for patients seen in primary care only ($93 per case). These cost estimates did not include patients' out-of-pocket costs for therapeutic appliances. The costs of specialty care for TMDs at Group Health also reflected substantial cost savings resulting from a negotiated per referral charge. Thus, differences in the total costs of specialty versus generalist care of temporomandibular pain would be substantially greater than shown here if patient costs were included and if service charges had not been negotiated by an insurance plan on behalf of a large population of patients.

SAFETY AND EFFICACY

A critical concern in the organization of health care services for patients with a poorly defined pain condition is that patients may be exposed to expensive treatments that are ineffective or that cause harm. At present, the safety and efficacy of nonconservative interventions for temporomandibular disorders have not been established by scientifically valid methods. This lack of scientific evaluation sometimes has deleterious results. In 1986, data from the National Hospital Discharge Survey indicated that 14,000 procedures performed on the temporomandibular joint involved implanting synthetic material. Over the 1970s and 1980s, tens of thousands of patients had surgical implants of Silastic or Teflon-Proplast replacements for the temporomandibular disk as a treatment for disk derangements. These surgical procedures were not preceded by adequate animal or experimental studies evaluating whether this procedure was safe or effective. After years of surgical experience with implants, it became apparent that Silastic and Teflon-Proplast implants were not safe (Ryan 1989).

PATIENT CAREERS

Patients with temporomandibular pain, like patients afflicted by other common pain problems, sometimes cycle through multiple providers and treatments over the course of a patient career. Consulting many providers may be harmful to some patients while wasting health care resources. For example, among patients with temporomandibular pain at Group Health Cooperative, 29% had seen at least three different providers and 12% had been to five or more different providers at the beginning of the treatment episode at which they were identified. These patients typically experience an unplanned succession of acute treatment episodes in which the problem is continually reevaluated and new treatments prescribed. Williams and Hadler (1983) characterized the distinction between management of acute and chronic illness as follows: "The quest to define the disease response for a patient's distress is important when the disease is acute or potentially remediable or both. . . . A disease-specific focus de-emphasizes the dominant issue in the management of chronic illness, which is the maximization of the patient's productivity, creativity, well-being and happiness. This goal of improving patient function and satisfaction to the utmost is usually achieved without curing the underlying disease." Surprisingly little research attention has been paid to determining how to organize services to prevent patients with chronic pain from developing an expensive and potentially harmful "chronic patient" career.

PRACTICE VARIATION

While extended patient careers may bring patients into contact with many different providers, patients exposed to multiple providers are likely to observe heterogeneous diagnostic and therapeutic practices across providers. Table III compares the assessments and treatments of providers at two different TMD specialty clinics referred comparable patients by Group Health Cooperative. The assessments and treatments were markedly different between the two clinics, while the long-term outcomes were remarkably similar (Von Korff et al. 1988b). Such variation in clinical methods across providers may not be a benign phenomenon. Because patients affected by chronic pain often seek care from multiple providers, they are likely to observe that providers diverge in their diagnostic assessments, tests ordered, and treatments prescribed. Such variation may contribute to patient uncertainty, and may encourage patients to seek care from different practitioners until they find a diagnostic explanation and a therapeutic regimen to their liking. The search for cure

Table III
Practice variation in assessment, treatment, and referral
between two TMD clinics treating comparable patients

	Clinic A (%)	Clinic B (%)
Assessment		
Myofascial pain	93.2	65.6
Derangement	37.0	51.6
Malocclusion	13.9	59.4
Treatment		
Bruxism appliance	64.4	4.7
Repositioning appliance	9.6	25.0
Stabilizing appliance	2.7	29.7
Referral for dental or orthodontic treatment	1.4	42.2

of a chronic pain condition may be both an expensive and a risky undertaking. An antidote to the costs and risks of doctor shopping may be greater uniformity in practice standards for diagnosis and treatment of chronic pain conditions such as temporomandibular disorders and greater scientific rigor in the evaluation of commonly prescribed treatments.

SUMMARY

Although hundreds of millions of dollars are being spent annually on services for patients with temporomandibular pain, there has been relatively little health services research assessing the effectiveness of these services, how satisfactory they are to patients, what forms of service are most cost-effective, or whether nonconservative interventions are safe. Health services research that rigorously evaluates the effectiveness, costs, patient satisfaction, and safety of services for patients with temporomandibular pain is urgently needed. In particular, it needs to be determined whether and under what circumstances patients with temporomandibular pain are best cared for by a specialist or a generalist, or when self-care is adequate.

ACKNOWLEDGMENT

This work was supported by grants from the National Institute of Dental Research P01 DE08773 and the Agency for Health Care Policy and Research R01 HS07759.

REFERENCES

Dworkin, S. and LeResche, L. (Eds.) Research Diagnostic Criteria for Temporomandibular Disorders, National Institute of Dental Research, Washington D.C., 1992.

Keefe, F. and Dolan, E., Pain behavior and pain coping strategies in low back pain and myofascial pain dysfunction syndrome patients, Pain, 24 (1986) 49–56.

Linet, M.S., Stewart, W.F., Celantano, D.D., Ziegler, D. and Sprecher, M., An epidemiologic study of headache among adolescents and young adults, JAMA, 261 (1989) 2211–2216.

Lorig, K. and Holman, H., Arthritis self-management studies: a twelve-year review, Health Educ. Q., 20 (1993) 17–28.

Nash, J. and Holroyd, K., Home-based behavioral treatment for recurrent headache: a cost-effective alternative? American Pain Society Bulletin, 2 (1992) 1–6.

Ryan, D., Alloplastic implants in the temporomandibular joint, Oral Maxillofacial Surg. Clin. North Am., 1 (1989) 427–441.

Turk, D.C. and Rudy, T.E., The robustness of an empirically derived taxonomy of chronic pain patients, Pain, 43 (1990) 27–35.

VonKorff, M., Dworkin, S.F., LeResche, L. and Kruger, A., An epidemiologic comparison of pain complaints, Pain, 32 (1988a) 173–183.

VonKorff, M., Howard, J.A., Truelove, E.L., Wagner, E. and Dworkin, S., Temporomandibular disorders: variation in clinical practice, Med. Care, 26 (1988b) 307–314.

VonKorff, M., Wagner, E.H., Dworkin, S.F. and Saunders, K.W., Chronic pain and use of ambulatory health care, Psychosom. Med., 53 (1991) 61–79.

VonKorff, M., Ormel, J., Keefe, F. and Dworkin, S., Grading the severity of chronic pain, Pain, 50 (1992) 133–149.

Whitney, C. and VonKorff, M., Magnitude of regression to the mean in before-after treatment comparisons of chronic pain, Pain, 50 (1992) 281–285.

Williams, M. and Hadler, N., The illness as the focus of geriatric medicine, N. Engl. J. Med., 308 (1983) 1357–1360.

Correspondence to: Michael Von Korff, ScD, Associate Director, Center for Health Studies, Group Health Cooperative of Puget Sound, 1730 Minor Ave., Suite 1600, Seattle, WA 98101, USA. Tel: 206-287-2874; Fax: 206-287-2871.

Temporomandibular Disorders and Related Pain Conditions, Progress in Pain Research and Management, Vol. 4, edited by B.J. Sessle, P.S. Bryant, and R.A. Dionne, IASP Press, Seattle, © 1995.

Reaction Papers to Chapters 12 and 13

Alexia Antczak-Bouckoms, Joseph J. Marbach, and Ernest G. Glass and Alan G. Glaros

Alexia Antczak-Bouckoms

Division of Clinical Care Research, New England Medical Center, Boston, Massachusetts, USA

Carlsson and LeResche (this volume) review some of the historical developments and problems associated with studies of the epidemiology of temporomandibular disorders (TMDs). Clearly the need for reliable and valid diagnostic criteria is paramount to moving forward in this area, and progress toward that end has been made with the research diagnostic criteria (Dworkin and LeResche 1992). Von Korff (this volume) makes forceful arguments for the need for randomized controlled trials of alternative treatments and care delivery systems. However, these studies will take time; meanwhile, clinical decisions are being made and patients are being treated in spite of a lack of consensus on diagnosis. I suggest we try to aid that decision-making process with the information that is currently available regarding therapy.

This paper will first describe a vision for the future of care of patients with TMDs when a diagnosis is agreed upon and randomized controlled trials abound; where we stand now will then be compared to that future. This vision is based on an approach proposed by the Evidence-Based Medicine Working Group at McMaster University (Guyatt 1992). The evidence-based medicine approach represents a paradigm shift in medical practice. Specifically, this approach stresses the examination of evidence from clinical research using an efficient literature search and the application of formal rules of evidence to evaluate that literature. It de-emphasizes the use of intuition, pathophysiologic rationales, individual expert opinion, and unsystematic clinical experience as the basis for clinical decision making.

The Evidence Based-Medicine Working Group describes this approach in a series of papers and guides the reader through methods to critically assess the information available in different types of clinical studies so that the quality, reliability, and relevance of the results can be judged (Guyatt 1992, 1993; Guyatt et al. 1993, 1994; Oxman et al. 1993; Jaeschke et al. 1994). To illustrate the benefits of the evidence-based approach they describe a junior medical resident admitting a patient who has experienced a first-time, witnessed grand mal seizure. The patient is worried about the likelihood of having another seizure and whether to take medication, drive a car, and so on. In the traditional approach of teaching the practice of medicine, the resident seeks the advice of the senior resident and the attending physician and then informs the patient that the risk of recurrence is high (but an exact probability can not be specified) and advises to continue taking the medication and not to drive. In contrast, following the new approach, the resident performs a computerized literature search, retrieves 25 relevant references, finds one that meets the criteria for a valid investigation of prognosis, and reports data useful to the patient's concerns. This study reports that the patient's risk of recurrence at one year is between 43% and 51%, and at three years between 51% and 60%. However, if the patient remains seizure-free for 18 months, the risk of recurrence would drop to 20%. This information provides the patient with a much better idea of the likely risks and what to expect.

Today what would a clinician find in the literature on TMDs? A meta-analysis was performed in response to a request by the National Institute of Dental Research for a systematic review of the state of the science regarding therapy for TMDs (Antczak-Bouckoms, unpublished data, 1994). The objective was to describe the literature on TMDs from 1980 to 1992 in terms of the total volume of citations, the proportion related to therapy, and the distribution according to study design with special emphasis on randomized controlled trials.

MEDLINE and hand-searching of bibliographies of articles and of selected journals produced a set of citations that was classified according to language, country of origin, and study design (Table I). More than 4000 references to TMDs were identified in the literature published from 1980 to 1992, with about 1200 of these focusing on therapy. Forty-five percent of the 1200 were classified as reviews and only 15% were clinical studies. Approximately 1% (n = 55) were randomized controlled trials (RCTs). Many of the RCTs were not identified by bibliographic searching but by hand-searching of journals. A clinician seeking information on therapy of TMDs thus encounters a substantial literature, which the average practitioner treating patients with TMDs, or most researchers in this area, might not be expected to assimilate readily. Thus, this resource may not be used to its maximum potential. The TMD literature consists primarily of uncontrolled observations of patients such as

Table I
Classifications of references to TMD therapy, 1980–1992

	1980–82	1983–85	1986–88	1989–92	Total	% *
Total papers	204	376	391	313	1284	
Non-English	85	109	114	101	409	32
Reviews	56	114	109	78	357	41
Reports of technique	22	34	41	35	132	15
Clinical studies	15	51	55	29	150	17
Case reports/series	7	24	36	20	87	10
Editorials	6	7	5	3	21	2
Letters	5	19	19	24	67	8
Management	3	4	5	9	21	2
Other	5	14	9	5	33	4

Note: The categories are not mutually exclusive; for example, some papers were reports of techniques followed by report of a case or series of cases.
* The percentage reported for non-English is the percentage of total references. For all other categories, it is the percentage of English-language references.

uncontrolled clinical trials, case series, case reports, and simple descriptions of techniques. It is generally agreed that such uncontrolled observations, while contributing to our knowledge about therapy of TMDs, are subject to considerable bias and thus are difficult to interpret. Emphasis should be placed on the results of the RCTs as this research design is the standard by which all other designs are judged. Limitations in indexing of MEDLINE, however, make it difficult to identify studies by design type.

The 55 randomized controlled trials identified in this review evaluated a variety of treatments, most of them reversible, conservative therapies. Some compared several different treatment modalities. Table II reports the number of trials and mean quality scores for each treatment including 26 RCTs of splint therapy, 12 of biofeedback or relaxation therapy, 6 of occlusal adjustment, 5 of pharmacologic agents, and 3 each of transcutaneous electrical nerve stimulation and intra-articular injections. The 26 trials that evaluated splint therapy included 15 different splint designs. Similarly, the trials of biofeedback and relaxation therapy considered several different approaches. The quality of each trial was assessed using the technique developed by Chalmers et al. (1981) that has been applied to several hundred RCTs in medicine and dentistry. The mean quality scores for these trials (out of a possible 1.0 points) were 0.28 ± 0.12 (SD) overall (range 0.05–0.59), 0.14 (SD) for study design, and 0.34 ± 0.16 (SD) for data analysis and presentation. Quality scores varied by the type of treatment being evaluated; studies of

Table II
Quality scores of randomized controlled trials by therapy, mean and (range)

Therapy	N	Study Design	Data Analysis	Overall Quality Score
Splint therapy	26	0.02 (0.03–0.48)	0.32 (0.03–0.70)	0.25 (0.12–0.53)
Biofeedback relaxation	12	0.16 (0.03–0.30)	0.32 (0.15–0.50)	0.22 (0.10–0.31)
Occlusal adjustment	6	0.26 (0.09–0.48)	0.31 (0.18–0.53)	0.28 (0.14–0.40)
Pharmacological agents	5	0.38 (0.08–0.60)	0.33 (0.09–0.47)	0.36 (0.10–0.54)
TENS	3	0.27 (0.17–0.39)	0.28 (0.07–0.50)	0.29 (0.26–0.31)
Intra-articular injections	3	0.45 (0.38–0.48)	0.63 (0.37–0.82)	0.51 (0.38–0.5)

Note: Quality scores derived using technique from Chalmers et al. 1981.
TENS = transcutaneous electrical nerve stimulation.

intra-articular injections had the highest mean scores (0.51 ± 0.11), and studies of biofeedback and relaxation therapy had the lowest (0.22 ± 0.06). Table III presents the number of trials and quality scores by year of publication. There does not appear to be a trend toward an increased number of trials over time, nor an increase in the quality scores.

Table IV provides a summary of the characteristics of the 26 trials of splint therapy to illustrate the difficulty a clinician might have upon consulting the literature regarding the effectiveness of one treatment approach for TMDs. Several different splint designs are evaluated, patient diagnosis is often poorly specified, and follow-up times and measures used to evaluate disease status and treatment outcome vary across the studies, making an overall conclusion elusive.

Although this systematic review found a large volume of literature on treatment of TMDs, only a small fraction were reports of randomized controlled trials. These 55 trials were published in 24 different journals, making it difficult for clinicians to identify and base therapy decisions on this gold standard of clinical research. All the RCTs evaluated conservative, nonsurgical approaches to the treatment of TMDs. Although surgery for TMDs, internal derangement, degenerative joint disease, and ankylosis is fairly common, there were no controlled trials of any surgical interventions. In addition, although many pharmacologic agents including nonsteroidal anti-inflammatory

Table III
Mean quality scores by year of publication

Year	Number of RCTs	Study Design	Data Analysis	Overall Quality Score
1971	1	0.32	0.09	0.24
1978	1	0.15	0.38	0.24
1979	1	0.08	0.38	0.19
1981	1	0.37	0.48	0.41
1982	2	0.34 ± 0.06	0.32 ± 0.15	0.34 ± 0.10
1983	5	0.24 ± 0.08	0.42 ± 0.19	0.31 ± 0.10
1984	5	0.19 ± 0.06	0.35 ± 0.10	0.25 ± 0.05
1985	9	0.26 ± 0.17	0.36 ± 0.21	0.30 ± 0.14
1986	5	0.16 ± 0.12	0.33 ± 0.14	0.23 ± 0.10
1987	5	0.25 ± 0.19	0.28 ± 0.25	0.26 ± 0.19
1988	8	0.20 ± 0.13	0.31 ± 0.15	0.24 ± 0.08
1989	3	0.24 ± 0.31	0.34 ± 0.10	0.26 ± 0.21
1990	2	0.26 ± 0.19	0.18 ± 0.15	0.24 ± 0.08
1991	7	0.29 ± 0.12	0.39 ± 0.17	0.33 ± 0.12

Note: Quality scores derived using technique from Chalmers et al. 1981.
RCTs = randomized controlled trials.

agents (NSAIDs), muscle relaxants, and anti-depressants are frequently pre-scribed for TMDs, there were virtually no trials of these agents. Although NSAIDs are commonly used for patients with temporomandibular joint pain, an abstract of one RCT evaluating NSAIDs reported no benefit for patients with myofacial pain dysfunction.

Where does this leave the clinician asking questions about prognosis and treatment effectiveness? Although the 55 RCTs identified indicate at least some controlled evaluation of TMD therapy, several weaknesses of these trials limit the inference that can be derived from them. First, they were not readily identified by routine bibliographic searching methods and thus are not easily accessible. Second, there is little or no consensus in these trials regard-ing descriptions of subjects and diagnoses. Third, there is wide variation in the outcome measures used to assess efficacy. Each study evaluates several outcome measures and often reports findings only for those measures demon-strating improvement. This lack of consensus with respect to diagnosis and outcomes makes comparison across these studies and between treatment meth-ods difficult or impossible. Thus, only general conclusions can be drawn regarding treatment effectiveness. The trials report improvement in signs and symptoms of TMJ dysfunction for almost all therapies considered. Many of

Table IV
Study characteristics of randomized controlled trials of splint therapy

Year	No. of Subjects	Age Range or Mean	% Female	Diagnosis	Timing	Therapies
1982	30	20–40	100	TMJD	Baseline 10 weeks	Occlusal splint Biofeedback
1983	190	14–60	NR	MPD	Baseline 0, 3, 6 months	Ultrasound Flat plane occlusal splint Biofeedback Relaxation training
1983	50	NR	NR	TMJD	Baseline 7 months	Spinal and occlusal adjustment No treatment controls
1983	24	30	87	TD	Baseline 4–6 weeks	Maxillary occlusal splint Relaxation therapy
1983	75	13–53	88	MPD/ Bruxism	Baseline 1, 3 days 1, 2, 3 weeks	Maxillary occlusal splint at three different vertical dimensions
1984	59	42	73	TMD	Baseline post	Occlusal adjustment and splint No treatment controls
1984	33	20–40	100	MD	Baseline 1, 12 months	Full coverage maxillary splint Biofeedback
1985	20	17–41	100	MD	Baseline 6 weeks	Bite plate with frontal plateau Stabilization splint
1985	20	14–39	95	ID	Baseline 3 weeks	Maxillary flat plane splint MORA/stabilization splint
1985	50	27	78	TMJD	Baseline 1 week 3 months	Stomatognathic treatment (including splint) Acupuncture

(continued)

Table IV (continued)

Year	No. of Subjects	Age Range or Mean	% Female	Diagnosis	Timing	Therapies
1985	96	30	100	Headache	Baseline 1 month	Occlusal adjustment ± splint Mock occlusal adjustment
1985	70	30	68	Reciprocal clicking	Baseline 6 weeks	Anterior repositioning splint Flat occlusal splint No treatment control
1985	60	13–52	85	TMD	Baseline 1, 3 days 1, 2, 3 weeks	Maxillary flat occlusal splints at three different vertical dimensions
1986	50	27	78	TMJD	Baseline 1 week 3 months	Stomatognathic Rx including splint Acupuncture
1986	21	NR	100	MPD	Baseline 8 weeks	Occlusal splint + physiotherapy Biofeedback TENS
1986	96	16–52	83	Headache	Baseline 4–8 months	Occlusal adjustment ± splint Mock occlusal adjustment
1987	5	15–25	60	MPDS	Baseline 6 weeks	Hard acrylic splint Soft resilient splint
1987	28	18–62	86	MPD	Baseline 2 weeks	Maxillary stabilization splint Nonoccluding splint (placebo)
1987	19	NR	NR	Headache	Baseline 6 months	Occlusal adjustment ± splint
1988	100	18–72	65	Bruxism	Baseline 2 weeks post	Diurnal biofeedback Nocturnal biofeedback Massed negative practice Flat plane occlusal splint No treatment controls

(continued)

Table IV (continued)

Year	No. of Subjects	Age Range or Mean	% Female	Diagnosis	Timing	Therapies
1988	63	13–74	86	DD-R	Baseline 6 months	Disk repositioning onlays Flat occlusal splint Control
1988	30	20–40	86	CMD	Baseline 2 months	Stomatognathic treatment with full coverage occlusal splint Occlusal adjustment
1989	20 20	28 33	55 80	Normal TM	Baseline 4 weeks	Movement feedback Occlusal stabilization splint
1989	10	23–46	80	Chronic bruxism	Baseline 7–14 days	Canine guidance splint Molar guidance splint
1991	55	16–50	85	TMJPDS	Baseline 1, 2, 3 months	Stabilization splint LOIS
1991	45	NR	NR	Chronic facial pain	Baseline 3 months	Acupuncture Full coverage maxillary splint No treatment controls

Note: NR = not reported; CMD = craniomandibular dysfunction; DD-R = disk displacement with reduction; ID = internal derangement; MD/MPD/MPDS = mandibular dysfunction; TM/TMD/TMJD = temporomandibular disorder; TMJPDS = temporomandibular joint pain-dysfunction syndrome; LOIS = localized occlusal interference splint; MORA = mandibular orthopedic repositioning appliance; TENS = transcutaneous electrical nerve stimulation.

the trials include a control or placebo group, and these groups also demonstrate considerable improvement. Although there appears to be benefit from most treatments, it is not clear whether these therapies evaluated provide any benefit over placebo alone.

ACKNOWLEDGMENT

This work was supported by a contract from the National Institute for Dental Research.

REFERENCES

Chalmers, T.C., Smith, H. Jr., Blackburn, B., Silverman, S., Schroeder, B., Reitman, D. and Ambroz, A., A method for assessing the quality of a randomized control trial, Controlled Clin. Trials, 2 (1981) 31–49.

Dworkin, S.F. and LeResche, L., Research diagnostic criteria for temporomandibular disorders, J. Craniomandib. Disord. Facial Oral Pain, 6 (1992) 301–355.

Guyatt, G., Evidence-based medicine: a new approach to teaching the practice of medicine, JAMA, 268 (1992) 2420–2425.

Guyatt, G., Users' guides to the medical literature, JAMA, 270 (1993) 2096–2097.

Guyatt, G.H., Sackett, D.L. and Cook, D.J., Users' guides to the medical literature. II. How to use an article about therapy or prevention. A. Are the results of the study valid? JAMA, 270 (1993) 2598–2601.

Guyatt, G.H., Sackett, D.L. and Cook, D.J., Users' guides to the medical literature. II. How to use an article about therapy or prevention. B. What were the results and will they help me in caring for my patients? JAMA, 271 (1994) 59–63.

Jaeschke, R., Guyatt, G.H. and Sackett, D.L., Users' guides to the medical literature. III. How to use an article about a diagnostic test. A. Are the results of the study valid?, JAMA, 271 (1994) 389–391.

Oxman, A.D., Sackett, D.L. and Guyatt, G.H., Users' guides to the medical literature. I. How to get started, JAMA, 270 (1993) 2093–2095.

Correspondence to: Alexia Antczak-Bouckoms, DMD, ScD, MPH, Division of Clinical Care Research, New England Medical Center #63, 750 Washington St., Boston, MA 02111, USA. Tel: 203-674-1927; Fax: 203-677-8700.

Joseph J. Marbach

School of Public Health and Department of Psychiatry, Columbia University, New York, New York, USA

Why have we learned so little about facial pain disorders from epidemiologic research? One problem is the terminology itself. Carlsson and LeResche (this volume) allude repeatedly to the term *TMDs* as a potential source of difficulty. Von Korff (this volume) more pointedly directs our attention to the same issue by rarely using the term. He writes of temporomandibular pain and principally reserves TMD as an adjective modifying "specialist." Carlsson and LeResche employ the term frequently, albeit carefully. They also quickly cut to the problem when they write that the lack of consensus on TMD diagnostic criteria is perhaps the most serious problem impeding progress. This statement is significant in that it comes from one of the authors of the new research diagnostic criteria (RDC) for TMDs (Dworkin and LeResche 1992). The RDC was expressly designed to provide standardized criteria to maximize reliability in research settings.

Carlsson and LeResche are well aware of the ambiguities inherent in use of the term. They, like many others, begin their chapter with statements acknowledging that TMDs represent signs and symptoms of "various disorders." Clearly there exists some confusion either with the term, its construct, or with both. Careful researchers such as Carlsson and LeResche have kept the confusion to a minimum, at least when they discuss their own work. The trouble begins when they try to interpret the work of others. In fact, their excellent review contains numerous examples of the problematic use of the term. How do we interpret, for example, the following: "longitudinal studies of TMDs . . . persons seeking treatment for TMDs . . . TMD prevalence studies . . . gender differences in TMDs." Certainly Carlsson and LeResche know that these phrases are not useful. Substitute Von Korff's term *temporomandibular pain* and these same phrases are transformed to research questions that lend themselves to investigation.

Currently (Dworkin et al. 1992), TMDs are divided into three groups: myofascial face pain, of which pain is the central feature; so-called disc displacements, in which for the vast majority of subjects, clicking noises associated with movement of the temporomandibular joint (TMJ) are the chief manifestation, and arthritis of the TMJ, specifically osteoarthritis, or degenerative joint disease. The term TMDs was originally conceived of as a much more ambitious list of diagnostic categories (Griffith 1983). Time and the inherent illogic of the term have taken their toll. The original list of "disorders" has atrophied to the three major groupings mentioned above. Recently, the term has been criticized both on anatomic and etiologic grounds. These critics, who helped develop the nosology, now comment that the term TMDs combines both disorders of the joints and muscle that are not anatomically or etiologically related under one rubric (see Marbach 1994). This situation has resulted in studies that are difficult or impossible to interpret.

Take, for example, the discussion by Carlsson and LeResche of TMD signs and symptoms in children and adolescents. Carlsson's own work demonstrates that osteoarthritis of the TMJ is rarely found in children and, indeed, the incidence appears to be positively correlated with age. How do we interpret, then, Carlsson and LeResche's conclusion that epidemiologic studies report that "apparently a substantial proportion of each of these young samples demonstrated positive [TMD] findings." Now skip to their discussion of TMD signs and symptoms in older adults, which states that signs and symptoms of TMDs have a tendency to decrease with increasing age. A little further on they note that "The prevalence of OA [osteoarthritis] increases with age." We need look no further to explain why various studies report prevalence rates for TMD symptoms that range from 6% to 93% or from 0% to 93% (De Kanter et al. 1993). Were researchers studying the same cluster of TMDs the rates should be somewhat similar. These rates likely suggest that different researchers are studying different TMDs.

The comprehensive review by Carlsson and LeResche of epidemiologic studies illustrates well the difficulties of using these data to achieve the goals set forth in their introduction. If several disorders that exhibit different natural histories, onset, duration, recurrence, clinical course, and treatment response are studied as a unit, important factors about these disorders will, in all likelihood, be obscured. For example, attempts to determine a prevalence rate for bruxism or, for that matter, gender in TMD cases, using the existing nomenclature, are bound to fail. These rates cannot be determined, either now or in the future. They do not exist. The participants of this workshop are in a position to evaluate whether the present taxonomic situation should continue or be replaced by one less likely to generate the confusion found with the TMD system. As can be shown, diagnostic labeling is not a trivial matter.

Taxonomy has an influence far beyond that of a mere words. As it was explained to Adam a long time ago, to name something is to obtain dominion over it (Genesis II, 19–20). This idea has not been lost in our era of political correctness. For example, what are the consequences of changing the label used to describe clicking noises to internal derangements (ID) of the TMJ and incorporating ID as a component of TMDs?

Carlsson and LeResche have chosen to include only one table. Give it careful attention. It shows that almost half the subjects with TMJ clicking at age 15 had none at age 20, while half who had clicking at 20 did not have it at 15. At a 10-year follow-up only one of the original 293 subjects reported intermittent locking. The authors question those who claim that clicking progresses to locking and eventually to OA. This conclusion is hardly news. Laszlo Schwartz, a pioneer in the clinical research of disorders of the TMJ, wrote nearly 50 years ago, "Clinical observations during the past 10 years stand in the way of the acceptance of the view that clicking [of the TMJ] is either a sign of degenerative changes or a precursor of them." (1959). Since Schwartz's death in 1966, the politically correct description for TMJ clicking has undergone a radical transformation. The process of labeling clicking as an ID and its inclusion as one of the TMD spectrum disorders has transformed ID into an example of what Illich (1976) calls "social iatrogenesis" or "the medicalization of life." "In this case, innocuous clicks and snapping noises in the TMJ found in many people, and for that matter most synovial joints, have been medicalized in spite of repeated studies that show no correlation of the sounds to pain or subsequent disease" (Marbach 1994). This position does not imply that clicking should not be studied. However, it should not be reified as a disease entity, or a potential surgical target, prior to adequate study.

Von Korff's paper makes an important statement by not regularly employing the term TMDs. He also surveys succinctly the "little health research assessing the effectiveness of these [facial pain disorders] services." In particular he singles out the importance of determining whether "nonconservative interventions are safe." Clearly, establishing safety must be determined before efficacy studies are undertaken. For example, clinical anecdotal data reported in Congressional hearings (U.S. Congress 1992) and elsewhere (Von Korff, this volume) indicate that TMJ surgery is associated with significant morbidity. Although emphasis has been placed on implants, the implants often represent the end product of other failed surgeries. Although epidemiologic evidence in support of high morbidity claims is difficult to obtain, some data suggest that factors other than clinical necessity influence the decision to perform TMJ surgery. Preliminary data from an ongoing study show that, for a given diagnosis, women are more likely to receive surgery than are men (Marbach, unpublished observations). The costs of such services, compared to nonsurgical treatment, also are noteworthy.

The findings presented here enable the reader to draw at least two conclusions. First, the construct TMDs should be reevaluated for usefulness. Second, Von Korff's recommendation for clinical trials should receive high funding priority. However, before clinical trials of treatments are undertaken to determine efficacy, the safety of the treatment must be established.

REFERENCES

De Kanter, R.J.A.M., Truin, G.J., Burgersdijk, R.C.W., Van 'T Hof, M.A., Battistuzzi, P.G.F.C.M., Kalsbeek, H. and Kayser, A.F., Prevalence in the Dutch adult population and a meta-analysis of signs and symptoms of temporomandibular disorder, J. Dent. Res., 72 (1993) 1509–1518.

Dworkin, S.F. and LeResche, L., Research diagnostic criteria for temporomandibular disorders: review, criteria, examinations and specifications, critique, J. Craniomandib. Disord. Facial Oral Pain, 6 (1992) 301–355.

Griffith, R.H., Report of the President's conferences on examination, diagnosis and management of temporomandibular disorders, J. Am. Dent. Assoc., 106 (1983) 75.

Illich, I., Medical Nemesis: The Expropriation of Health, Pantheon Books, New York, 1976.

Marbach, J.J., Coping with taxonomy, Clin. J. Pain, 10 (1994) 78–85.

Schwartz, L., Disorders of the Temporomandibular Joint, W.B. Saunders, Philadelphia, 1959.

U.S. Government, Are FDA and NIH ignoring the dangers of TMJ (jaw) implants? Committee on Government Operations, House of Representatives, 102nd Congress, June 4, 1992, U.S. Government Printing Office, Washington, D.C., 1993.

Correspondence to: Joseph J. Marbach, DDS, School of Public Health, Columbia University, c/o 600 West 168th St., New York, NY 10032, USA. Tel: 212-758-2215.

Ernest G. Glass and Alan G. Glaros

School of Dentistry, University of Missouri–Kansas City, Kansas City, Missouri, USA

HEALTH SERVICES RESEARCH ON TMDs

Because the symptomatology of patients with temporomandibular disorders (TMDs) can mimic a variety of disorders, patients seek care from a variety of health care providers. Von Korff (this volume) raises several issues based upon data on care-seeking patterns in health maintenance organization (HMO) patients. These findings are valuable but limited. We need to know how TMD patients seek care in the general community. We need to know more about the diagnostic procedures and treatment modalities used by medical and dental practitioners in the general community. And we need to know more about the efficacy of the treatments received by patients in the general community who complain of symptoms of TMDs.

Von Korff implies that physicians are an entry point into the health care system for patients who complain of symptoms of TMDs. For patients enrolled in an HMO, physicians may be the *only* entry point. Our data also suggest that patients who complain of TMD symptoms initially seek care from physicians (Glaros et al., in press): 40% of the patients we evaluated in our clinic had previously seen a physician. These data also indicate that a patient who consults a physician as part of his or her evaluation is more likely to seek a second opinion from another physician before entering our clinic.

The premise that physicians are qualified to diagnose and manage TMDs is, in our view, more problematic. In a patient sample we examined, we judged that nearly 90% had a TMD. A considerable proportion did not receive this diagnosis after examinations by other health care providers. More specifically, about 40% of our patients may have been misdiagnosed by physicians. In addition, the use of a physician as the entry point for the care of a TMD patient may increase total costs. Data from unpublished observations showed that the cost of an initial examination was nearly three times higher when provided by a physician than by a dentist. Approximately 20% of the patients seen by physicians incurred charges for CAT scans and MRIs that may not have been needed, but which certainly escalated the cost of care.

Von Korff also asks what the outcomes would be if patients were randomly assigned to self-care, generalist care, or specialty care. As stated by Von Korff, this question suggests that the TMDs are biological disorders that benefit from treatment by a biomedical professional, in spite of the fact that many current models of these disorders are more complex, and include psychosocial and behavioral aspects (cf. American Academy of Orofacial Pain 1993).

What Von Korff does not ask is: Who manages the psychosocial issues? Who intervenes with respect to behavior? Perhaps a more critical question would be: "Is biomedical care equivalent in outcome to care that incorporates psychosocial elements?" In our view, treatment protocols for TMDs that do not address psychosocial and behavioral issues fail to provide an adequate treatment for these patients.

Von Korff's chapter indicates that patients are more satisfied when they see a specialist. These findings lead to some interesting hypotheses. Research in medicine suggests that patient satisfaction is a proxy for quality of care (Hays et al. 1991). That is, patients who report satisfaction with their care tend to receive better, higher quality care than do dissatisfied patients. If we apply Von Korff's data to these findings, we can generate a provocative hypothesis—patients who see "TMD specialists" not only are more satisfied with their care, they also are receiving higher quality care than are patients who do not see specialists. Data from two surveys we conducted suggest that "TMD specialists" provide more intensive levels of service, not different levels, as compared to general dentists (Glass et al. 1991, 1993). These findings may imply that specialists generate high patient satisfaction ratings precisely because they are more attentive to the psychosocial needs of the patient.

Von Korff also addresses the issue of cost of care: Are differences in costs between self-care, generalist care, and specialty care justified by differences in patient outcomes or by differences in patient satisfaction?

Before we can answer this question, it is important to remember that patients may not go to physicians specifically complaining of TMD symptoms. We know that the symptoms of TMDs can mimic a variety of other disorders. For example, TMD patients can complain of ear problems, headache, or dizziness (Cooper and Cooper 1993; Haley et al. 1993). If a patient consults a physician for dizziness, the physician probably will follow a "dizziness protocol." This might include examining the ear and throat for infection, asking about other symptoms, and conducting cranial nerve tests or office-based tests of equilibrium. The physician also might order various laboratory tests or images (including skull X-rays, CAT scans, or MRIs).

In assessing the dizziness, the physician generates a differential diagnosis list, assesses each possibility until a definitive diagnosis is established, or refers the patient elsewhere. The patient, in turn, undergoes multiple tests or consults other providers (including dentists, internists and family practitioners, otolaryngologists, and rheumatologists). In short, before a person becomes a "TMD patient," she or he may have seen a variety of providers, had multiple diagnostic work-ups, and received several treatments.

Thus, the type of study that Von Korff proposes raises concern. If the definition of TMDs does not include all these other symptoms, one may inappropriately and prematurely conclude that self-care or general care is cost-efficacious as compared to specialist care. An examination of generalist care regimens for TMDs may inappropriately miss the patients who initially complain of, and seek care for, ear problems, headache, tinnitus, and so forth. We may find that specialty care for TMD costs less compared to general care that tests, and discards, hypotheses about infectious processes, neurological conditions, and rheumatological conditions.

Appropriately, Von Korff recommends research on the safety and effectiveness of nonconservative treatments. We think an equally important question is: Are conservative treatments effective? (cf. Dao et al. 1994). If they are, which ones work, either separately or together, for what types of TMDs? What are the costs involved in these treatments?

We also need to consider the possibility that many so-called placebo treatments are not necessarily inactive. All patients, including those in a placebo group likely receive a series of instructions that deal with behavior, such as "Don't eat chewy foods. Don't open wide. Don't chew gum or bite your fingernails. Try not to clench." These instructions may modify how patients think and behave and represent a therapeutic intervention, not a placebo treatment.

Von Korff also asks whether health care delivery systems can develop planned approaches to evaluating and managing patients with temporomandibular pain in ways that are consistent across providers and over the treatment career of individual patients. This question seems to suggest that a single, planned approach to the treatment of the TMDs is possible. Available data on this point suggest that accomplishing this goal would be difficult: patients who visit physicians get medical treatments, and not necessarily the correct ones. Not too surprisingly, patients who visit dentists get dental therapies, and not necessarily the recommended ones (Glass et al. 1991, 1993). Rarely do patients receive treatment involving comprehensive behavioral interventions.

If a patient has a clear-cut TMD and is fortunate to reside close to a treatment program that offers comprehensive care, this patient may receive effective, cost-conscious care. However, appropriately diagnosing TMD in a patient who complains of headache, ear pain, muscle soreness, or dizziness may well be difficult. A physician who is confronted with such symptoms will use diagnostic skills appropriate to his or her training. Similarly, a dentist who is confronted with these symptoms will think and act like a dentist (cf. Glaros et al., in press). These disparate professional biases and therapeutic approaches suggest that a single, planned approach to the care of a TMD patient cannot be established, nor is such a plan desirable.

EPIDEMIOLOGIC RESEARCH ON TMDs

Carlsson and LeResche propose epidemiological studies using well-operationalized diagnostic criteria such as those found in the research diagnostic criteria (Dworkin and LeResche 1992). They also recommend that these studies separate out the various subgroups of TMDs, including myalgia, internal derangement, and degenerative joint disorder. It would be helpful to know both the probability of each individual disorder and the conjunctive probabilities for persons with multiple disorders. Such data would add greater reliability and validity to our discussion on the prevalence and incidence of TMDs. Finally, studies about the long-term course of these problems would be particularly welcome.

When longitudinal studies are conducted, increased emphasis should be placed on behavioral and psychological components. The incidence of TMDs increases from childhood through early adulthood and then generally diminishes in the middle and older years. Possibly these data are telling us something about the psychosocial stresses people are experiencing at various stages of their lives (Kessler et al. 1994). For example, we know that late adolescence and early adulthood, a time when TMD incidence increases, is also a difficult transition phase for many persons. Leaving home, becoming financially independent, selecting a career, developing strong attachments to others outside the family, beginning one's own family—these too are occurring. If TMDs truly have both physical and psychological components, future epidemiological studies should include measures relevant to both of these components.

Carlsson and LeResche express concern regarding the number of studies that report on various signs and symptoms of TMDs without use of diagnostic categories. We do not share their concern. Until recently, the diagnostic systems for TMDs were imprecise, lacked operational definitions, and had unknown reliability (Ohrbach and Stohler 1992). An epidemiological study that uses such a poor system would ultimately fail to provide us with much information. Although many published papers did not use any diagnostic system, they did describe the signs and symptoms they assessed. Knowing these, we can interpret the data with reasonable accuracy.

Having complimented Carlsson and LeResche for their suggestions, we must now pose questions to them: What are we going to do with all these epidemiological data? Why do we want to know these data? How do they help us understand TMDs? Suppose that we obtain results consistent with prior research; that is, that the incidence of myalgia, internal derangement, and degenerative joint disease is fairly high in the population. Or, suppose that we find myalgia considerably more prevalent than internal derangement or degenerative joint disorder. Have we learned anything new?

We already have epidemiological data, summarized by Carlsson and LeResche, on many thousands of persons assessed for signs and symptoms of TMDs. The precise numbers reported by these studies rarely agree, but the general relationships among large data classes show remarkable consistency. For example, most studies show that the signs of TMDs occur more frequently than the symptoms. Perhaps if our epidemiological studies are more focused, as suggested by Carlsson and LeResche, or if they address smaller, more manageable issues, the data that result might be of higher quality.

The epidemiological data on TMDs tell us that these conditions are common. What they do not tell us is whether there is overlapping symptomatology between TMDs, broadly defined, and other medical disorders, including headache and neck and shoulder pain.

Health services research data tell us that multiple health care providers can diagnose and treat patients with symptoms of TMDs. Unfortunately, these data do not always convey the complex ways in which the problem presents itself, how providers diagnose and treat the condition, the efficacy of the treatment, or how costly the TMDs are.

We have data suggesting that behavioral and psychosocial factors affect TMDs. However, epidemiological and health services research rarely deal with behavioral and psychosocial issues. It is likely that behavioral and psychosocial issues contribute to the epidemiology of the disorder and that that they affect the ways in which patients seek care. It is also likely that they affect how patients respond to care; response to treatment may be improved if we consider these factors (Turk et al. 1993).

REFERENCES

American Academy of Orofacial Pain, Temporomandibular Disorders: Guidelines for Classification, Assessment, and Management, Quintessence, Chicago, 1993, 141 pp.

Cooper, B.C. and Cooper, D.L., Recognizing otolaryngologic symptoms in patients with temporomandibular disorders, J. Craniomandib. Pract., 11 (1993) 260–267.

Dao, T.T.T., Lavigne, G.J., Charbonneau, A., Feine, J.S. and Lund, J.P., The efficacy of oral splints in the treatment of myofascial pain of the jaw muscles: a controlled clinical trial, Pain, 56 (1994) 85–94.

Dworkin, S.F. and LeResche, L. (Eds.), Research diagnostic criteria for temporomandibular disorders: review, criteria, examinations and specifications, critique, J. Craniomandib. Disord: Facial Oral Pain, 6 (1992) 301–355.

Glaros, A.G. and Glass, E.G., Temporomandibular disorders. In: R.J. Gatchel and E.B. Blanchard (Eds.), Psychophysiological Disorders, American Psychological Association, Washington, D.C., 1993, pp. 299–356.

Glaros, A.G., Glass, E.G. and McLaughlin, L., Knowledge and beliefs of dentists regarding temporomandibular disorders and chronic pain, J. Orofacial Pain, 8 (1994) 216–221.

Glaros, A.G., Glass, E.G. and Hayden, W.J., History of treatment received by TMD patients: a preliminary investigation, J. Orofacial Pain, in press.

Glass, E.G., McGlynn, F.D. and Glaros, A. G., A survey of treatments for myofascial pain-dysfunction, J. Craniomandib. Pract., 9 (1991) 165–168.

Glass, E.G., Glaros, A.G. and McGlynn, F.D., Myofascial pain dysfunction: treatments used by ADA members, J. Craniomandib. Pract., 11 (1993) 25–29.

Haley, D., Schiffman, E., Baker, C. and Belgrade, M., The comparison of patients suffering from temporomandibular disorders and a general headache population, Headache, 33 (1993) 210–213.

Hays, R.D., Larson, C., Nelson, E.C. and Batalden, P.B., Hospital quality trends: a short-form patient-based measure, Med. Care, 29 (1991) 661–667.

Kessler, R.C., McGonagle, K.A., Zhao, S., Nelson, C.B., Hughes, M., Eshleman, S., Wittchen, H.-U. and Kendler, K.S., Lifetime and 12-month prevalence of DSM-III-R psychiatric disorders in the United States: results from the National Comorbidity Survey, Arch. Gen. Psychiatry, 51 (1994) 8–19.

Ohrbach, R. and Stohler, C., Review of the literature: current diagnostic systems, part IB. In: S. F. Dworkin and L. LeResche (Eds.), Research diagnostic criteria for temporomandibular disorders: review, criteria, examinations and specifications, critique, J. Craniomandib. Disord. Facial Oral Pain, 6 (1992) 301–355.

Turk, D.C., Zaki, H.S. and Rudy, T.E., Effects of intraoral appliance and biofeedback/stress management alone and in combination in treating pain and depression in patients with temporomandibular disorders, J. Prosthet. Dent., 70 (1993) 158–164.

Correspondence to: Ernest G. Glass, DDS, School of Dentistry, University of Missouri–Kansas City, 650 E. 25th St., Kansas City, MO 64108, USA. Tel: 816-235-2199; Fax: 816-235-2157.

Part VI

Temporomandibular Joint Structure, Function, and Repair

Temporomandibular Disorders and Related Pain Conditions, Progress in Pain Research and Management, Vol. 4, edited by B.J. Sessle, P.S. Bryant, and R.A. Dionne, IASP Press, Seattle, © 1995.

14

Biomechanical and Anatomical Aspects of the Temporomandibular Joint

Arthur Storey

Department of Orthodontics, School of Dentistry, University of Texas Health Science Center, San Antonio, Texas, USA

TMJ ANATOMY AND FUNCTION

Any review of temporomandibular joint (TMJ) anatomy and function cannot be meaningfully separated from a discussion of jaw and jaw muscle anatomy and function. Nevertheless, this chapter will focus on the TMJ and limit discussion of jaw and muscle anatomy and function to specific instances that require a broader perspective of joint anatomy and function. It will be assumed that the reader is familiar with the current traditional view of the human TMJ as presented by Mohl (1982, 1988) and Hylander (1992).

Two themes prominent for decades and that reappear in the literature on occlusion, temporomandibular disorders (TMDs), and TMJ function are stabilization and loading of the TMJ. Stabilization of joints is generally acknowledged to be a function of the muscles acting at the joint (Kornecki 1992). Kornecki postulates that joint stability is achieved by a complex feedback system controlling stiffness of muscles and estimates that about one quarter of the muscular work about limb joints is expended in stabilization. Jimenez (1987) arrived at a similar conclusion for stabilization of the TMJ when the dentition does not provide joint stabilization. This theme of an occlusal role for stabilization of the TMJ has prevailed in the occlusal literature as the need to "harmonize" occlusal position and condylar position in spite of differences in opinion as to location of the ideal condylar position. Muscle work to establish stability in the joint requires that the forces across the contact points be at right angles to the contacting surfaces and be regulated by a neural feedback system (Hylander 1979a). This author states that direction and magnitude of reaction forces acting on the TMJ are adjusted continuously by the muscles of mastication preventing jaw joint instability (Hylander 1979a). Both Osborn and Baragar (1985) and Jimenez (1987) present evidence for jaw muscle specialization for stabilization and biting. Given the muscle contribution to stabilizing the joint as well as executing a biting or clenching task, it is not surprising that some models of jaw function propose nonlinear relationships between muscle activity and biting force (Pruim et al. 1978; Sasaki et al. 1989). The receptors sensing joint stability or instability and their reflex connections are unknown and need to be explored. Physical and mathematical models addressing the issue of joint loading fail to consider the muscle contribution to joint stabilization.

TMJ loading impacts the growth and remodeling of the TMJ and when excessive leads to destruction of joint structures. It is widely accepted that the TMJ is variably loaded depending on the location of the bite force along the tooth row and on the jaw position. Speculation that the human TMJ is a loaded joint arose from the observation of thickening of the fibrous connective tissue overlying the articular eminence and the antero-superior surface of the condyle head (Moss 1959). This speculation was reinforced by the finding that these areas are highest in glycoproteins (Kopp 1976, 1978) and link proteins (Milam et al. 1991). Experiments in monkeys (Hylander 1979b) and mathematical modeling of the human TMJ (see Korioth and Hannam 1990 for list of studies) have established that the TMJ is variably loaded depending on the position of the mandible and the bolus (Fig. 1). As the bite force moves distally along the tooth row, the reaction force in the ipsilateral TMJ is reduced. In the monkey, biting on the third molar can actually unload the working side joint (Hylander 1979b).

This built-in protection of the TMJ against excessive loading is also manifest in the way in which the loading is shifted mediolaterally as well as anteroposteriorly on condylar translation. Due to the horizontal and vertical angulations of the condyle heads, the reaction forces across the translating condyle and disk are shifted forward and mediolaterally (Hylander 1979a;

Fig. 1. Schematic relationship of the working side TMJ loading to bolus location along the tooth row, derived from direct measurements in the primate and mathematical modeling in the human.

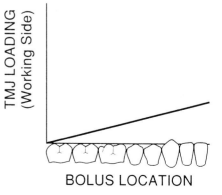

BOLUS LOCATION

Mohl 1982, 1988; Mack 1984). The fibrous connective tissue overlying the condyle and eminence is thought to better resist the shear loading of the TMJ than does articular cartilage (Mohl 1988). The glycosaminoglycans and their bound water in the disk and the articulating surfaces of the condyle and eminence cushion compressive loads. Shifting bearing points have yet to be documented for the TMJ as has been done for the hip, knee, and shoulder joints in humans and experimental animals. Techniques developed for other joints (see next section) would appear to be worth exploiting for study of the TMJ.

A much neglected aspect of TMJ loading and stability is the role of the disk. Mohl (1988) and others contend that the disk's role is to accommodate the incongruities between the articulating surfaces of the condyle and eminence. Osborn (1985) has argued that the disk protects the articular surface of the condyle from damage by preventing excessive indentation that would impede gliding movements. While Saizar (1971) has proposed a stabilization role for the disk, Osborn (1985) has advocated a destabilizing function. Interest in the disk and its role in TMDs is recent, beginning with the popularizing of disk imaging by Wilkes (1978) and the focus on disk displacement by Farrar and McCarty (1979). Several descriptive studies have documented the microscopic structure (Taguchi et al. 1980; de Bont et al. 1985) and chemical composition (Gage et al. 1990; Milam et al. 1991) of this structure in humans and in animals. Insights into the disk's functional role are few, and all published modeling studies have chosen to ignore it. The suggestion that the position of the disk is under the reflex regulation of the superior head of the lateral pterygoid must now be questioned (Hylander 1992; Dolwick, this volume).

BIOMECHANICS OF THE TMJ

Attempts to understand the mechanics of the TMJ are based on physical models, mathematical models, and direct measurement. The crudeness of physical models and the difficulties of direct measurement have fostered the current emphasis on mathematical modeling. Hatcher et al. (1986) measured joint and bite forces developed in a human skull in which synthetic muscle forces were generated by turnbuckles inserted into Kevlar strands with vectors oriented as in the muscles simulated. Mongini et al. (1981) recorded the stresses on the mandibular condyle of four dry human mandibles with loads applied to gonion and coronoid. Standlee et al. (1981) used plastic analogs of the mandible for three-dimensional photoelastic stress analysis to visualize the direction and magnitude of stresses within the modeled TMJ. These models suffer from oversimplified TMJ articulations, muscle vectors, and forces. The contribution of muscle work to stabilization has not been considered. It is surprising that physical modeling has not focused on the TMJ rather than the whole jaw as has been done for other joints such as the knee (Huson et al. 1989). Indeed, it is surprising the extent to which biomechanical analysis of the TMJ has developed independent of parallel investigations on other joints.

Insights on joint loading come from direct and indirect recording in primates and human cadavers. Hohl and Tucek (1982) used an instrumented strut in the condylar neck of a baboon, and Brehnan et al. (1981) and Boyd et al. (1990) used piezoelectric film inserted into the lower joint chamber of macaque monkeys. All studies found evidence for compressive loading in mastication. Hylander (1979b) used strain gauges cemented to the lateral subcondylar surface of the mandibular ramus in nine monkeys. Hylander inferred joint reaction forces from the principal strains in the condylar neck. He concluded that TMJ reaction forces were dependent on the ratio of ipsilateral to contralateral muscle forces: when the ratio is near 1:1 the contralateral joint forces are higher than the ipsilateral joint forces. Shortcomings of these studies are the suitability of the animal model, the inability to directly determine the magnitude and direction of joint reaction forces, and the extent to which the recording devices interfered with normal function. Although animal studies have shortcomings they do have the advantage of preserving the neural feedback systems.

While the above experiments were designed to measure the reaction forces across the articulating surface of the TMJ, other studies in the pig (Roth et al. 1984) and human (Dolwick, studies in progress) used catheters inserted into the upper joint chamber to measure chamber pressure. These studies shed useful light on disk and posterior band function and fluid accumulation in the joint but not on joint loading.

Takanashi (1979) and Ito et al. (1986) have attempted to estimate TMJ loading in human subjects by recording condylar displacements when biting forcibly in various jaw positions, with or without splints. Bilateral condylar intrusion occurred when biting on incisors, and contralateral condylar intrusion with minimal ipsilateral intrusion of the working side joint while biting on bicuspids.

While direct measurement of loading in the functioning, normal human TMJ appears unlikely in the near future, indirect techniques using current and emerging technologies offer exciting possibilities. Because magnetic resonance imaging is dependent on water content of the structures imaged it is possible to visualize changes in the size and signal intensity of the disk with and without clenching. Improved discrimination could lead to better resolution of the areas under stress. The technique of plastic casting within the excised joint with specific types of loading, as done by Walker and Hajek (1972) for

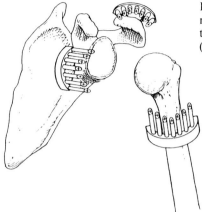

Fig. 2A. Noncontacting, optical stereophotogrammetry device used to quantitate contact areas in the glenohumeral joint of human cadavers. (Soslowsky et al. 1992)

the human knee joint, could be easily adapted to the human TMJ. Instrumented and optical linkages between two joint elements, as has been done in the dog (Kinzel et al. 1976; Scherrer et al. 1979) and human cadaver (Figs. 2A, 2B; Soslowsky et al. 1992) shoulder joint, offer the immediate possibility of studying the moving load-bearing points on the condyle or eminence. Measurement of the moving contact points between eminence and disk and disk and condyle offer a more difficult challenge. Force measurement at specific locations is likely to be elusive for the immediate future.

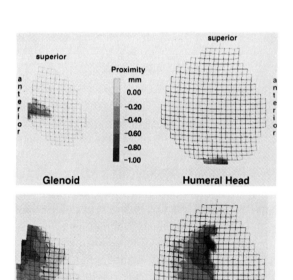

Fig. 2B. Glenohumeral contact patterns for a typical shoulder at 0° (top) and 120° (bottom) of arm elevation. The gray scale indicates the extent of cartilage compression for each contact area. (Soslowsky et al. 1992)

MATHEMATICAL MODELING

Because of shortcomings of the physical models and direct measurements, most of the research effort on TMJ loading over the past decade has focused on mathematical modeling and more recently on finite element analysis. In spite of numerous assumptions and simplifications used in this modeling, the results have been encouraging because they frequently support or confirm data collected from animals and humans. For example, the modeling results support the concept of a joint that is loaded more heavily on the balancing than the working side and more heavily on the working side as the bite location moves toward the incisor teeth. Static optimization can be used to estimate the muscle forces needed to generate specified bite and joint loads. Zajac and Gordon (1989) have used dynamic optimization techniques to estimate forces in multi-joint location tasks. The dynamic optimization algorithm uses inputs (e.g., electromyograms) and outputs (e.g., forces) that maximize "the performance" or "economy of movement" (Nelson 1983). All models have in common analysis based on the mandible as a rigid body assessed under conditions of static equilibrium, without the presence of a disk, and without any neural regulation. Muscle forces are usually represented by single vectors, and joint and bite loads at single points. Table I lists simplifications made in selected studies. Static muscle forces estimated from cross-sectional areas or electromyography (or both) are used to estimate bite and joint loading. Assumptions are sometimes made as to general principles such as minimization of energy expenditure of articular loading. Because all the simplifications and assumptions of these models can be challenged, inferences must be drawn with caution and subjected to subsequent testing in the animal.

All mathematical models based on static equilibrium must fulfill the requirement that the sum of all forces and moments equals zero. The variables that require quantification are magnitude, direction, and point of application of joint, muscle, and bite forces. The linear programming algorithm requires a sufficient number of givens to solve for a limited number of unknowns. There is no unique combination of givens to account for identical unknowns, so techniques of optimization and indeterminate constraint have been employed. The givens and unknowns for eight specific modeling studies assessing joint loading are summarized in Table II. While these studies have provided data that is in general agreement, cutting-edge modeling is now moving into static analyses with less limiting constraints, and into dynamic modeling and finite element analyses. The rigid body spring model of Kawai (1977) has been used by An and co-workers (1990) to study the pressure distribution on articular surfaces of an idealized joint and the consequences of this distribution on joint

Table I
Mathematical modeling of studies of TMJ loading

Assumptions	
Expenditure of energy is minimal	Osborn and Baragar 1985; Koolstra et al. 1988; Hannam and Wood 1989
Articular loading is minimal	Smith et al. 1986
Relation between muscle force and integrated EMG activity is linear	Pruim et al. 1980
Muscle force per cross sectional area is same for all jaw muscles	Pruim et al. 1980
Direction of joint forces is perpendicular to articular space at its most narrow site	Pruim et al. 1980

Simplifications	
Isometric muscle contraction	Applies to all models
Static equilibrium conditions	Applies to all models
Mandible a rigid body	Applies to all models
Single point origin and insertion of muscles	Applies to all models
Single vector for each muscle or group of muscles	Applies to all models except Baragar and Osborn 1987
Single point of joint loading	Applies to all models
Single point of bite loading	Applies to all models
Disk omitted	Applies to all models
No neural feedback	Applies to all models
Symmetrical bite	Van Eijden et al. 1988
No transverse bite forces	Van Eijden et al. 1988; Pruim et al. 1980; Throckmorton and Throckmorton 1985
Bite forces resolved to midline	Baragar and Osborn 1987; Van Eijden et al. 1988
Muscle forces proportional to muscle cross-sectional area	Faulkner et al. 1987; Korioth and Hannam 1990
Bite forces perpendicular to occlusal plane	Baragar and Osborn 1987
Symmetrical mediolateral joint loading	Pruim et al. 1980; Van Eijden et al. 1988; Throckmorton and Throckmorton 1985
No transverse joint forces	Faulkner et al. 1987
Single condylar fulcrum	Korioth and Hannam 1990
Jaw opening muscles excluded	Koolstra et al. 1988

Table II
Mathematical modeling of studies of TMJ loading

Given	Unknown	Source*
Bite force and muscle force magnitude (EMG activity)	Muscle forces and joint reaction forces	Pruim et al. 1980 (2D)
Bite force, magnitude, and direction of muscle forces Moment arms of bite and muscle forces	Direction and magnitude of summed joint reaction forces	Throckmorton and Throckmorton 1985 (2D)
Bite force and point application of bite force and joint force Location and direction of three muscle pairs	Joint force and direction Magnitude of muscle forces	Smith et al. 1986 (3D)
Muscle force magnitude and direction Bite force and direction	Joint reaction force	Baragar and Osborn 1987 (3D)
Muscle force magnitude and direction Unilateral bite force	Direction and magnitude of condylar loads	Faulkner, et al. 1987 (3D)
Bite force and direction	Muscle forces and joint reaction forces	Koolstra et al. 1988 (3D)
Muscle force direction and magnitude Point application of bite force and joint force	Bite force direction and magnitude and joint force magnitude	Van Eijden et al. 1988 (2D)
Muscle force magnitude and direction	Condylar loads and bite force	Korioth and Hannam 1990 (3D)

* 2D = two-dimensional analysis; 3D = three-dimensional analysis.

stability. This model could be adapted to the study of pressure distribution and stability in the TMJ. Ng et al. (1994) recently reported on dynamic modeling of the mandible and concluded that computer modeling with artificial intelligence to control muscle activation strategies may be the only way in the future to study this interaction in humans. New insights into how condylar loading is regulated reflexly will be needed to optimize the artificial intelligence directing these muscle activation strategies.

FINITE ELEMENT ANALYSIS

Finite element analysis (FEA) promises to be a useful tool in defining stress development in the condyle of the TMJ. FEA has been used in orthopedic biomechanics for two decades and in many artificial joint design and fixation studies. It also has been used to study stresses on the teeth, implants, and craniofacial skeleton (see Tanne et al. 1988 for list) and the mandible (see Korioth et al. 1992 for list). FEA analysis of the mandible, as in the modeling previously described, involves assumptions or simplifications needed to cope with the mathematical formulations and calculations. Initial FEA of the mandible was based on "gross simplifications" in mandible geometry or tissue properties. Hart et al. (1992) improved FEA modeling by grid refinement and assigning varying bone characteristics to different elements of the mesh. Their simplifications of muscle vectors and magnitudes and joint point and line of action were similar to those used in mathematical models discussed previously. Bite loads were imposed on a second premolar and on two incisors in a simulated dentate and partially edentate human mandible. The condylar reaction forces in simulated chewing were similar to those found in earlier modeling studies. This FEA model also points out that rapid and dramatic shifts occur in the magnitude and orientation of the principal strains and the importance of incorporating real-life bending into the model.

Korioth et al. (1992) have further improved the mandibular modeling by incorporating teeth and assigning different tissue characteristics to teeth, periodontium, bone, and condyle (Fig 3A). Displacements, stresses, strains, and element and reactive forces were estimated at each node position on simulating a clench. The condylar reaction forces in simulated clenching confirmed that the condyles are load bearing with heavier forces on the balancing side (Fig. 3B). This model predicts substantial shear stresses in the contralateral joint.

A recent abstract by Kikuchi et al. (1994) on mandibular forces generated during simulated clenching in the same FEA model predicts that the distribution of condylar loads is task dependent and that balancing side contacts (in contrast to interferences) decreases the balancing side condylar load. These observations support the concept of balancing side protection proposed by Minagi et al. (1990).

RESEARCH CHALLENGES

Hylander et al. (1992) have stated that muscle anatomy and function may be the key to better modeling studies. These authors conclude, however, that

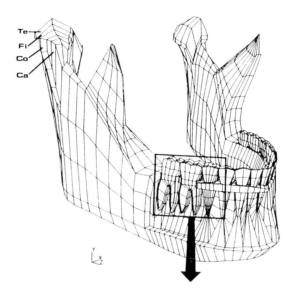

Fig. 3A. Wire frame model of the mandible used for three-dimensional function element analysis. The temporomandibular joints have been modeled as a condyle consisting of elements of cortical bone (Co) underlying cancellous bone (Ca), the disk as fibrocartilage (Fi), and the fossa or eminence as temporal cortical bone (Te). The dentition and its periodontal ligament and supporting bone have been fractionally modeled as well. (Korioth et al. 1992)

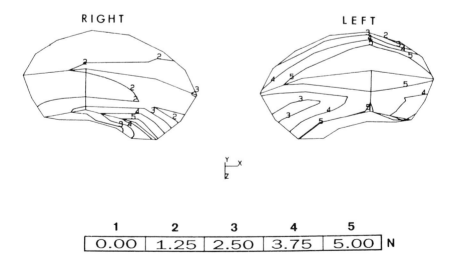

Fig. 3B. Element force distribution on the left (balancing side) and right (working side) condylar surfaces during isometric molar biting. Contour iso-force lines are given in newtons (N). (Korioth et al. 1992)

before more accurate modeling procedures can proceed, a considerable amount of research must be done on the biomechanics of jaw muscles during mastication. Throckmorton (1989) has estimated that for a TMJ force magnitude error of ± 4 kg and direction of ± 7°, muscle force magnitude must be specified to 1% and force direction to 1°. This precision may not be required of the jaw system if the efficiency is low or task execution strategies are highly variable. Hannam and Wood (1989) found no simple relationship between the tension-generating capacity of the muscles and their mechanical efficiency (as described by their spatial arrangement). Efficiencies appear to be independent of facial features (Hannam and Wood 1989; Isawaki 1992). Neural feedback may account for the disparities in these studies.

Following documentation by Herring et al. (1979, 1989) and McMillan and Hannam (1991, 1992) of the extent of anatomical and functional compartmentalization of the pig and human masseter, a vision is emerging of the multiple and changing muscle vectors in dynamic function. Adding these changing vectors to the complexities of dynamic modeling will be a challenge. The multichannel time-series myoprocessor of Triolo and Moskowitz (1989), which predicts both magnitude and direction of limb motion from the spectral content of the surface electromyogram, might be adapted to modeling of dynamic jaw function. Clearly there is much to be gained if those with interests in jaw biomechanics work closely with mechanical engineers and orthopedic investigators with biomechanical expertise.

In static modeling it is important to define the extent to which the muscle activity is divided between stabilization and synergistic functions before attempting to solve the static equilibrium equations relating joint load to bite load and muscle force. Defining the mix of stabilization and synergetic activity may help to better define clinical goals for occlusal therapy as well as conditions more likely to overload the joints. The mix of stabilizing and synergistic activity is determined by feedback mechanisms regulating TMJ stability and loading. The receptors, reflex pathways, and modulatory influences are unknown. Neurophysiological studies in this area are to be encouraged. Other biological principles besides loading or stability also may determine structural consequences. The extent to which efficiency, minimal joint loading, or condyle position dictate the final joint load needs to be explored.

All published modeling studies have assessed TMJ loading as punctate and without a disk. More information similar to that on limb joints needs to be collected on the manner in which loads are transmitted through the joint. Studies should investigate the locations (and areas) of pressure points and the dynamic shifting of these points in function and disease. In vitro studies of the physical properties of disk and articular fibrocartilage under various loading conditions need to be accelerated. These data, as well as those of the physical properties of compact and cancellous bone in the eminence and condyle, will be necessary to refine future mesh diagrams in FEA.

Finally, studies should address the question of the extent to which joint breakdown is due to overloading or inflammation. FEA modeling could include as variables differences in the properties of the mesh elements, reduction in range of shifting of bearing points, as well as magnitude of forces and area of loading under these conditions.

While all modeling frames the problem in mathematical terms, solves the mathematical problem, and then compares the results to those collected from the biological system, there is a challenge in selecting and justifying the assumptions and limitations imposed by mathematical and computational constraints. More thought should be given to the biological consequences of these simplifications and assumptions. Questions about the extent to which the jaw system is efficient or the extent to which function is randomized and loose need to be asked. How critical to prediction of TMJ loading is the precision of specifying jaw muscle forces and vectors? (Or is neural feedback the ultimate determinant?) How important is it to specify the vector of the active motor units, rather than the whole muscle? Osborn and Bagar (1985) contend that too much compartmentalization of muscle activity has led to predictions which cannot be supported. Throckmorton (1989) argues, on the other hand, that great precision in specification of muscle forces and vectors is necessary in estimating joint reaction forces (see above). While masticatory cycles have a recognizable pattern for side and subject, there is much randomization of occlusal contacts. Gnathologists are convinced of the importance of precision in tooth to tooth and tooth to joint relationships, while more biologically oriented clinicians acknowledge some play in the system. Answers to these types of questions would be helpful in determining reasonable assumptions and simplifications for future modeling. Perhaps the perspective could be reversed and modeling used to answer these long-standing controversies.

CONCLUSIONS

The theme of this session addresses the issues that cross the boundary between clinical practice and research. Given the long-standing sense among clinicians who treat TMDs that stability of the TMJ and adverse loading predispose or cause TMDs, this review has focused on the current knowledge on and research potential of these two issues. Both issues raise a question of the boundary between health and disease and the extent to which the compromised joint can heal itself. The lack of a well-defined definition of the healthy human TMJ at various ages handicaps decisions on whether to treat or not.

Those who review insurance claims for treatment report overtreatment as well as inappropriate treatment. Overtreatment can be attributed to a lack of agreement on what constitutes disease (or better health) of the human TMJ, a lack of knowledge of the impact of age on the health or disease of the TMJ, and a belief by some clinicians that internal derangements of the joint will get worse because adaptation or repair will not occur or will be inadequate. Inappropriate treatment can be attributed to inadequate or faulty diagnoses (especially with diagnostic criteria or instruments that generate excessive false positive diagnoses), overconfidence in the efficacy of treatment due to regression to the mean of TMDs of muscular origin, and unrealistic treatment objectives or estimates of success. A better understanding of the anatomy and biomechanics of the healthy TMJ could lead to a better definition of the structural and functional characteristics of a joint in need of, or not in need of, treatment.

REFERENCES

An, K.N., Himeno, S., Tsumura, H., Kawai, T. and Chao, E.Y.S., Pressure distribution on articular surfaces: application to joint stability evaluation, J. Biomech., 23 (1990) 1013–1020.

Baragar, F.A. and Osborn, J.W., Efficiency as a predictor of human jaw design in the sagittal plane, J. Biomech., 20 (1987) 447–457.

Boyd, R.L., Gibbs, C.H., Mahan, P.E., Richmond, A.F. and Laskin, J.L., Temporomandibular joint forces measured at the condyle of Macaca arctoides, Am. J. Orthod. Dentofacial Orthop., 97 (1990) 472–479.

Brehnan, K., Boyd, R.L., Laskin, J., Gibbs, C.H. and Mahan, P., Direct measurement of loads at the temporomandibular joint in *Macaca arctoides*, J. Dent. Res., 60 (1981) 1820–1824.

Farrar, W.B. and McCarty, W.L., Inferior joint space arthrography and characteristics of condylar paths in internal derangements of the TMJ, J. Prosthet. Dent., 41 (1979) 548–555.

Faulkner, M.G., Hatcher, D.C. and Hay, A., A three-dimensional investigation of temporomandibular joint loading, J. Biomech., 20 (1987) 997–1002.

Gage, J.P., Virdi, A.S., Triffitt, J.T., Howlett, C.R. and Francis, M.J.O., Presence of type III collagen in disc attachments of human temporomandibular joints, Arch. Oral Biol., 35 (1990) 283–288.

Hannam, A.G. and Wood, W.W., Relationships between the size and spatial morphology of human masseter and medial pterygoid muscles, the craniofacial skeleton and jaw biomechanics, Am. J. Phys. Anthropol., 80 (1989) 429–445.

Hart, R.T., Hennebel, V.V., Thongpreda, N., Van Buskirk, W.C. and Anderson, R.C., Modelling the biomechanics of the mandible: a three-dimensional finite element study, J. Biomech., 25 (1992) 261–286.

Hatcher, D.C., Faulker, M.G. and Hay, A., Development of mechanical and mathematic models to study temporomandibular joint loading, J. Prosthet. Dent., 55 (1986) 377–384.

Herring, S.W., Grimm, A.F. and Grimm, B.R., Functional heterogeneity in a multipinnate muscle, Am. J. Anat., 154 (1979) 563–576.

Herring, S.W., Wineski, L.E. and Anapol, F.C., Neural organization of the masseter muscle in the pig, J. Comp. Neurol., 280 (1989) 563–576.

Hohl, T.H. and Tucek, W.H., Measurement of condylar loading forces by instrumented prosthesis in the baboon, J. Max.-fac. Surg., 10 (1982) 1–7.

Huson, A., Spoor, C.W. and Verbout, A.J., A model of the human knee derived from kinematic principles and its relevance for endoprosthesis design, Acta Morphol. Neerl. Scand., 27 (1989) 45–62.

Hylander, W.L., Functional anatomy. In: B.G. Sarnatand D.M.Laskin (Eds.), The Temporomandibular Joint: A Biological Basis for Clinical Practice, 3rd ed., W.B. Saunders, Philadelphia, 1979a, pp. 85–113.

Hylander, W.L., An experimental analysis of temporomandibular joint reaction force in macaques, Am. J. Phys. Anthropol., 51 (1979b) 433–456.

Hylander, W.L., Functional anatomy. In: B.G.Sarnat and D.M.Laskin (eds.), The Temporomandibular Joint: A Biological Basis for Clinical Practice, 4th ed., W.B. Saunders, Philadelphia, 1992, pp 60–92.

Hylander, W.L., Johnson K.R. and Crompton A.W., Muscle force recruitment and biomechanical modeling: an analysis of masseter muscle function during mastication in *Macaca fascicularis*, Am. J. Phys. Anthropol., 88 (1992) 365–387.

Ito, T., Gibbs, C.H., Marguelles Bonnet, R, Lupkiewica, S.M., Young, H.M., Lundeen, H.C. and Mahon, P.E., Loading on the temporomandibular joints with five occlusal conditions, J. Prosthet. Dent., 56 (1986) 478–484.

Iwasaki, L.R., The Effect of Dentofacial Form on Chewing Efficiency in Humans, Ph.D. thesis, The University of Manitoba, 1992.

Jimenez, I.D., Dental stability and maximal masticatory muscle activity, J. Oral Rehabil., 14 (1987) 591–598.

Kawai, T., A new element in discrete analysis of plane strain problems, Seisan Kenkyu, 29 (1977) 204–207.

Kikuchi, M., Korioth, T.W.P. and Hannam, A.G., Bite force distribution during tooth clenching in man, J. Dent. Res., 73 (1994) 446 (abstr. 2755).

Kinzel, G.L., Van Sickle, D.C., Hillberry, B.M. and Hall, A.S., Jr., A preliminary study of the in vivo motion in the canine shoulder, Am. J. Vet. Res., 37 (1976) 1505–1510.

Koolstra, J.H., Van Eijden, T.M.G.J., Weijs, W.A. and Naeije, M., A three dimensional mathematical model of the human masticatory system predicting maximum possible bite forces, J. Biomech., 21 (1988) 563–576.

Kopp, S., Topographical distribution of sulphated glycosaminoglycans in human temporomandibular joint disks, J. Oral Path., 5 (1976) 265–276.

Kopp, S., Topographical distribution of sulphated glycosaminoglycans in the surface layers of the human temporomandibular joint, J. Oral Path., 7 (1978) 283–294.

Korioth, T.W.O. and Hannam, A.G., Effect of bilateral asymmetric tooth clenching on load distribution at the mandibular condyles, J. Prosthet. Dent., 64 (1990) 62–73.

Korioth, T., Romilly, D.P. and Hannam, A.G., Three-dimensional finite element stress analysis of the dentate human mandible, Am. J. Phy. Anthropol., 88 (1992) 69–96.

Kornecki, S., Mechanism of muscular stabilization process in joints, J. Biomech., 25 (1992) 235–245.

Mack, P.J., A functional explanation for the morphology of the temporomandibular joint of man, J. Dent., 12 (1984) 225–230.

McMillan, A.S. and Hannam, A.G., Motor-unit territory in the human masseter muscle, Archs. Oral Biol., 36 (1991) 435–441.

McMillan, A.S. and Hannam, A.G., Task-related behaviour of motor units in different regions of the human masseter muscle, Arch. Oral Biol., 37 (1992) 849–857.

Milam, S.B., Klebe, R.J., Triplett, R.G. and Herbert, D., Characterization of the extracellular matrix of the primate temporomandibular joint, J. Oral Maxillofac. Surg., 49 (1991) 381–391.

Minagi, S., Watanabe, H., Sato, T. and Tsuru, H., The relationship between balancing-side occlusal contact patterns and temporomandibular joint sounds in humans: proposition of the concept of balancing-side protection, J. Craniomandib. Disord. Facial Oral Pain, 4 (1990) 251–256.

Mohl, N.D., Functional anatomy of the temporomandibular joint. In: D. Laskin et al. (Eds), The President's Conference on the Examination, Diagnosis and Management of Temporomandibular Disorders, American Dental Association, Chicago, 1982, pp. 3–12.

Mohl, N.D., The temporomandibular joint. In: N.D. Mohl et al (Eds.), A Textbook of Occlusion, Quintesssence, Chicago, 1988, pp. 81–96.

Mongini, F., Preti, G., Calderale, P.M. and Barberi, G., Experimental strain analysis on the mandibular condyle under various conditions, Med. Biol. Eng. Comput., 19 (1981) 521–523.

Moss, M.L., Functional anatomy of the temporomandibular joint. In: L.Schwartz (Ed.), Disorders of the Temporomandibular Joint, W.B. Saunders, Philadelphia, 1959, pp 73–88.

Nelson, W.L., Physical principles for economies of skilled movements, Biol. Cybern., 46 (1983) 135–147.

Ng, F., Lagenbach, G., Beddoes, M. and Hannam, A., Dynamic modeling of musculoskeletal mechanics in the human jaw, J. Dent. Res., 73 (1994) 114 (abstr. 102).

Osborn, J.W., The disc of the human temporomandibular joint design, function and failure, J. Oral Rehabil., 12 (1985) 279–293.

Osborn, J.W. and Baragar, F.A., Predicted pattern of human muscle activity during clenching derived from a computer assisted model: symmetric vertical bite forces, J. Biomech., 18 (1985) 599–612.

Pruim, G.J., Ten Bosch, J.J. and De Jongh, H.J., Jaw muscle EMG-activity and static loading of the mandible, J. Biomech, 11 (1978) 389–395.

Pruim, G.J., Jongh, H.J. and Ten Bosch, J.J., Forces acting on the mandible during bilateral static bite at different bite force levels, J. Biomech., 13 (1980) 755–763.

Roth, T.E., Boldberg, J.S. and Behrents, R.G., Synovial fluid pressure determinants in the temporomandibular joint, OSOMOP, 57 (1984) 583–588.

Saizar, P., Centric relation and condylar movement: anatomic mechanism, J. Prosthet. Dent., 26 (1971) 581–591.

Sasaki, K., Hannam, A.G. and Wood, W.W., Relationships between the size, position and angulation of human jaw muscles and unilateral first molar bite force, J. Dent. Res., 68 (1989) 499–503.

Scherrer, P.K., Hillberry, B.M. and Van Sickle, D.C., Determining the in-vivo areas of contact in the canine shoulder, J. Biomech. Eng., 101 (1979) 271–278.

Smith, D.M., McLachlan, K.R. and McCall, W.D., A numerical model of temporomandibular joint loading, J. Dent. Res., 65 (1986) 1046–1052.

Soslowsky, L.J., Flatow, E.L., Biglioni, L.V., Powluk, R.J., Ateshian, G.A. and Mow, V.C., Quantitation of in situ contact areas at the glenohumeral joint: a biomedical study, J. Orthop. Res., 10 (1992) 524–534.

Standlee, J.P., Caputo, A.A. and Ralph, J.P., The condyle as a stress-disturbing component of the temporomandibular joint, J. Oral Rehab., 8 (1981) 391–400.

Taguchi, N., Nakata, S. and Oka, T., Three-dimensional observation of the temporomandibular joint disk in the rhesus monkey, J. Oral Surg., 38 (1980) 11–16.

Takanashi, K., Studies on the functional characteristics of the temporomandibular joint under biting force, Shikwa Gakuho, 79 (1979) 763–794.

Tanne, K., Miyasaka, J., Yamagata, Y., Sachdeva, R., Tsutsumi, S. and Sakuda, M., Three-dimensional model of the human craniofacial skeleton: method and preliminary results using finite element analysis, J. Biomed. Eng., 10 (1988) 246–252.

Throckmorton, G.S., Sensitivity of temporomandibular joint force calculations to errors in muscle force measurements, J. Biomech., 22 (1989) 455–468.

Throckmorton, G.S. and Throckmorton, L.S., Quantitative calculations of temporomandibular joint reaction forces, I. The importance of the magnitude of the jaw muscle forces. J. Biomech., 18 (1985) 445–452.

Triolo, R.J. and Moskowitz, G.D., The theoretical development of a multichannel time-series myoprocessor for simultaneous limb function detection and muscle force estimation, IEEE Trans. Biomed. Eng., 36 (1989) 1004–1017.

Van Eijden, T.M.G.J., Klok, E.M., Weijs, W.A. and Koolstra, J.H., Mechanical capabilities of the human jaw muscles studied with a mathematical model, Arch. Oral Biol., 33 (1988) 819–826.

Walker, P.S. and Hajek, J.V., The load-bearing area in the knee joint, J. Biomech., 5 (1972) 581–589.

272   *A. STOREY*

Wilkes, C.H., Arthropgraphy of the temporomandibular joint, Minn. Med., (1978), pp. 645–652.
Zajac, F.E. and Gordon, M.E., Determing muscle's force and action in multi-articular movement.
In: K. Pandolf (Ed.), Exercise and Sport Sciences Reviews (Baltimore), 17 (1989) 187–230.

Correspondence to: Arthur Storey, DDS, PhD, Department of Orthodontics, School of Dentistry, University of Texas Health Science Center, 7703 Floyd Curl Dr., San Antonio, TX 78204, USA. Tel: 210-567-3500; Fax: 210-567-2614.

Temporomandibular Disorders and Related Pain Conditions, Progress in Pain Research and Management, Vol. 4, edited by B.J. Sessle, P.S. Bryant, and R.A. Dionne, IASP Press, Seattle, © 1995.

15

Neuroendocrine and Immune Responses to Injury, Degeneration, and Repair

Kenneth M. Hargreaves,[a,b] Mark T. Roszkowski,[a] Douglass L. Jackson,[a] Walter Bowles,[a] Jennelle Durnett Richardson,[b] and James Q. Swift[c]

[a]*Division of Endodontics,* [b]*Department of Pharmacology, and* [c]*Division of Oral and Maxillofacial Surgery, University of Minnesota Schools of Dentistry and Medicine, Minneapolis, Minnesota, USA*

Chronic orofacial pain may be due to several factors, including biochemical and functional changes in peripheral tissues and the central nervous system (CNS), along with dysfunctional psychosocial interpretations of peripheral stimuli. Recent research has led to a greater understanding of peripheral pain mechanisms and their involvement in the development of pain. This knowledge base may contribute to a better understanding of chronic orofacial pain mechanisms, and provide new diagnosis and management strategies for affected patients.

Numerous physiologic systems are activated in response to tissue injury, degeneration, and repair. These responses include changes in the central, peripheral, and autonomic nervous systems, as well as activation of neuroendocrine, endocrine, and paracrine systems. However, not all responses can be considered adaptive. Indeed, many forms of chronic inflammation/injury are characterized by a substantial immunological component directed against host tissue (Birkedal-Hansen 1993). The collective action of these pathophysiological responses modulates the progression of the syndrome and the clinical response of the patient to treatment.

In reviewing research in this area, it is critical to evaluate the underlying experimental model. Due to the complexity and heterogeneity of clinical orofacial pain patients, and to ethical concerns restricting the level of experimental inquiry, it is likely that both clinical and animal studies will be required to determine the physiologic mechanisms of tissue injury, degeneration,

Table I
Factors modifying physiologic responses to
injury, degeneration, and repair

| Cellular composition of tissue (phenotypic defined responses) |
| Vascularity of tissue |
| Immunological status of tissue |
| Innervation density and fiber composition |
| Systemic factors (concurrent disease, stress, etc.) |
| Descending CNS influences |
| Local biomechanical factors |
| Species |

and repair. In addition to species-related issues, several additional factors may restrict the ability to generalize results from one model system to another (Table I). Clearly, the temporomandibular joint (TMJ) and oral tissues are not completely unique in their physiology. Instead of rejecting research from other model systems, the pertinent question is to determine the extent to which it is possible to generalize from various experimental models to clinical pain syndromes of interest. This issue is not trivial, because the major proportion of our database on pain and inflammation is derived from animal studies using nonorofacial model systems. This chapter reviews these studies, with the caveat that continuing research must determine the generalizability of these findings to temporomandibular disorders (TMDs), myalgia, and other orofacial pain conditions.

NEURAL RESPONSES TO INJURY AND INFLAMMATION

In contrast to a transient pain-producing stimulus (e.g., electric pulp test, venipuncture), pain associated with inflammation is associated with prolonged hyperalgesia, which can be characterized as spontaneous pain, a decrease in pain threshold, and an increase in responsiveness to suprathreshold stimuli (Willis 1985). Hyperalgesia is a common response to tissue injury, and appears to be due to combined peripheral and central mechanisms (Table II). In the periphery, activation and sensitization of certain primary afferent neurons is thought to contribute to hyperalgesia at the site of injury (Dubner and Bennett 1983; Willis 1985). This sustained peripheral response may also induce plasticity changes within the CNS (Table II).

In the CNS, several changes occur in response to tissue inflammation. A potentially important implication of central hyperalgesia is the proposal that

Table II
Factors that may contribute to hyperalgesia

Factor	Reference
Peripheral factors	
Sensitization of primary afferent neurons	Kumazawa et al. 1977; Schaible et al. 1986; Martin et al. 1987
Sympathetic-primary afferent interactions	Jänig and Kollman 1984; Levine et al. 1985; Roberts and Elardo 1985; Perl 1992
CNS factors	
Increased vesicular release from presynaptic terminals	Garry et al. 1992
Changes in postsynaptic receptors	Galeazza et al. 1992
Changes in second messenger systems	Meller and Gebhart 1993; Garry et al. 1994a,b
Changes in protooncogenes	Draisci and Iadarola 1989
Changes in endogenous opioids	Draisci and Iadarola 1989
Central sensitization	Woolf 1983; Wall and Woolf 1984; Cook et al. 1987; Hylden et al. 1989; Hu et al. 1992
Dark neurons	Sugimoto et al. 1990

relatively long-lasting changes may occur in the CNS in response to the afferent barrage that occurs during injury. It has been proposed that a persistent CNS component of hyperalgesia may contribute to some forms of chronic pain, and that this CNS component may persist even in the absence of continued peripheral nociceptor input (Coderre and Melzack 1992; Dubner and Ruda 1992). According to this hypothesis, chronic pain due to CNS hyperalgesia may prove refractory to therapeutic approaches designed to solely reduce peripheral afferent input (Table II). An additional implication is the rationale for preemptive analgesia, in which drugs administered prior to a procedure (e.g., surgery) may have increased analgesic effectiveness as compared to the same drug administered after surgery.

CLASSIFICATION AND ELECTROPHYSIOLOGIC RESPONSES OF NOCICEPTORS TO INFLAMMATION

Two major classes of nociceptive afferent nerve fibers, the A-delta-fibers and C-fibers, detect chemical mediators and physical forces associated with tissue injury. The classification and response properties of these neurons has been reviewed extensively (Dubner and Bennett 1983; Willis 1985; Sessle 1987; Hargreaves et al. 1995), so this chapter focuses on peripheral neuronal responses to inflammation.

The A-delta-fibers located in joints are distributed throughout ligaments and periosteum. These joint fibers can be classified according to their responsiveness to passive movement and to noxious stimulation (Schaible and Schmidt 1986). Under normal conditions, 30% of A-delta-fibers located in the cat knee joint respond only to noxious stimuli. These fibers are activated by chemicals such as prostaglandins as well as noxious joint movements. The A-delta-fibers in muscle are thought to be distributed throughout myofibrils, connective tissue, tendons, and endothelial walls (Stacey 1969). These fibers are activated by muscle contraction, but also respond to hypertonic saline, bradykinin, and potassium (Mense 1977). Current evidence suggests that A-delta-fibers are probably important for perceptions of joint pain but may only have a secondary role in mediating muscle pain (Willis 1985; Schaible and Schmidt 1986).

The second group of nociceptive fibers are unmyelinated, slowly conducting nerve fibers. Joints and muscle are innervated by similar unmyelinated C nociceptors (also known as group IV fibers), which have polymodal response properties (Kumazawa and Mizumura 1977). In normal cat knee joints, 34% of C-fibers are activated by noxious stimuli (Schaible and Schmidt 1986). Similar to the A-delta-fibers located in joints, C-fibers are activated by chemicals such as prostaglandins as well as noxious joint movements (Schaible and Schmidt 1986). The sensation of pain arising from muscle is thought to be mediated primarily by C polymodal nociceptors (Light 1992). In muscle, C-fiber afferents show little response to contraction, but respond vigorously to ischemia, potassium, bradykinin, and prostaglandins (Mense 1977; Dubner and Bennett 1983; Willis 1985; Sessle 1987; Light 1992). Activation of muscle C-fibers results in a prolonged alteration in spinal cord activity (i.e., increase in receptive field size of dorsal horn neurons) and flexion reflexes (Cook et al. 1987; Wall and Woolf 1984). This prolonged increase in spinal cord activity differs from the relatively brief responses that occur following stimulation of cutaneous C-fibers. Accordingly, injury to muscle may produce more extensive CNS changes than an equivalent amount of cutaneous injury.

In general, inflammatory mediators have two main effects on the peripheral nociceptive nerve ending. Mediators activate and/or sensitize certain peripheral nerve terminals and, as described below, also evoke peripheral release of neuropeptides such as substance P or calcitonin gene-related peptide (CGRP) (Dubner and Bennett 1983; Willis 1985; Martin et al. 1987; Sessle 1987; Jackson et al. 1992, 1993; Light 1992). While both C polymodal and A-delta-fibers can be sensitized to biochemical mediators, their susceptibility, at least to thermal stimuli, appears to differ. Studies from human and monkey skin indicate that C-fibers become sensitized at less intense noxious temperatures, while A-delta-fibers become sensitized at higher temperatures (Meyer and Campbell 1981). The sensory fibers that innervate joints can also become sensitized. During inflammation in joints, the spontaneous electrical activity of C- and A-delta-fibers more than doubles and their responses to non-noxious joint movements increase two to seven-fold (Schaible and Schmidt 1986, 1993).

The actual biochemical substances that mediate hyperalgesia are unknown, but probably vary depending on the tissue examined, the intervention employed, and the dependent measure evaluated. Numerous studies have evaluated the effects of inflammatory mediators on various dependent measures related to nociception. For example, prostaglandins, leukotrienes, bradykinin, histamine, serotonin, acetylcholine, potassium, interleukin-1, and hydrogen ions (e.g., low pH) all activate or sensitize primary afferent fibers located in skin, muscle, or joints (Mense 1977; Schaible and Schmidt 1986; Martin et al. 1987; O'Byrne et al. 1990; Steen et al. 1992; Schaible and Grubb 1993). In studies measuring a behavioral endpoint (e.g., flexion reflex or pain report), the administration of prostaglandins, leukotrienes, bradykinin, potassium, interleukin 1ß (IL-1ß) and dihydroxyicosotetraenoic acids (diHETES) into peripheral tissue produces behavior associated with nociception (Tyers and Haywood 1979; Rackham and Ford-Hutchinson 1983; Levine et al. 1984; Katori et al. 1986; Whalley et al. 1987; Ferreira et al. 1988). Collectively, these results suggest that these various biochemical mediators are capable of producing hyperalgesia with differential efficacy and time courses.

TISSUE DISTRIBUTION AND RESPONSES OF PERIPHERAL NEUROPEPTIDES TO INFLAMMATION

The cell body of the primary afferent nerve fiber synthesizes the neuropeptides substance P and CGRP (as well as other substances), which are transported both to the CNS and to the periphery. Recent studies have demonstrated that the dorsal root ganglion preferentially transports (nearly 80%) neuropeptides such as substance P and CGRP to *peripheral* endings of nerve terminals (Brimijoin 1980). These neuropeptides are highly concentrated in peripheral tissue such as joints and dental pulp, and electrical or chemical stimulation of peripheral nerves releases immunoreactive substance P and CGRP (Olgart et al. 1977; Yaksh 1988; Hargreaves et al. 1992; Jackson et al. 1992).

Several studies have evaluated the distribution of neuropeptides in peripheral tissues. Importantly, not all peripheral tissues contain the same proportion of neuropeptides. Rather, the target tissue appears to influence the chemical composition of the primary afferent fibers that innervate it (O'Brien et al. 1989). For example, as compared to unmyelinated fibers innervating skin, more unmyelinated fibers innervating joints contain immunoreactive CGRP (78% vs. 50%) and immunoreactive substance P (66% vs. 37%) (O'Brien et al. 1989). Thus, various tissues may differ in the relative contribution of

neuropeptides implicated in the modulation of tissue inflammation and repair.
Immunoreactive substance P is located in synovial tissue of several joints including the TMJ (Ichikawa et al. 1990; Kido et al. 1993) and knee (Grönblad et al. 1985). In the TMJ, both substance P and CGRP immunoreactivity tend to be more heavily concentrated in the anterior portion of the joint capsule (Kido et al. 1993). In addition, substance P binding sites (i.e., NK1) have also been identified in normal and inflamed synovium (Walsh et al. 1993).

Synovial fluid levels of immunoreactive substance P and CGRP are elevated in some (Appelgren et al. 1991; Larsson et al. 1991) but not all clinical studies of patients with inflamed joints (Larsson et al. 1989). Other neuropeptides such as neuropeptide Y, neurokinin A, and vasoactive intestinal peptide (VIP) also are elevated, or at least detectable, in synovial fluid (Larsson et al. 1989, 1991; Holmlund et al. 1991). Comparison of synovial neuropeptide levels between clinical studies has proven problematic due to differences in etiology, concurrent medications, and joint tissue, e.g., the TMJ may have higher levels than the knee joint (Holmlund et al. 1991).

Neuropeptides that are released during activation of certain afferent fibers (e.g., nociceptors) are thought to engage physiologic targets associated with the development of neurogenic inflammation. For example, administration of substance P and CGRP induces plasma extravasation in skin and exacerbates the effects of ongoing joint inflammation, or the effects of local infusion of bradykinin or histamine (Lembeck and Holzer 1979; Brain and Williams 1985; Levine et al. 1985, Cruwys et al. 1992; Scott et al. 1992). In addition, these peptides exhibit synergistic actions when co-administered (Brain and Williams 1985), and act to block their degradation (LeGreves 1985). Evidence indicates that electrical stimulation of peripheral nerves (including those that innervate joints) produces plasma extravasation due, at least in part, to release of these neuropeptides (Ferrell and Russell 1986; Holzer 1988). Extravasation permits the passage of blood-borne proteins (e.g., albumin, kininogen) and fluid into the injured tissue, contributing to the further release of plasma-derived inflammatory mediators (e.g., bradykinin) and to the development of edema. Moreover, passive immunization with anti-CGRP antisera or administration of a CGRP antagonist ($CGRP_{8-37}$) can inhibit the development of inflammation (Louis et al. 1989; Brain et al. 1991). Additional studies indicate that these neuropeptides alter blood flow in peripheral tissues including knee joint (Lam and Ferrell 1993b) and dental pulp (Gazelius et al. 1987; Kim et al. 1988).

Peripheral neuropeptides can also modulate inflammation by altering the release, metabolism, or actions of inflammatory mediators. Neuropeptides, such as substance P, act with other inflammatory mediators to stimulate histamine release from mast cells (Lembeck and Holzer 1979; Levine et al. 1985). Administration of substance P or the fragment SP_{7-11} to synoviocytes obtained from human joints stimulates these cells to secrete prostaglandin E_2 and collagenase and to proliferate in culture (Lotz et al. 1987; Halliday et al. 1993). In addition, substance P stimulates monocytes to release substances such as interleukin-1, interleukin-6, and tumor necrosis factor (Lotz et al. 1988).

Additional studies indicate that these neuropeptides, and possibly additional factors of primary afferent origin, are critical for the resolution of inflammation and the initiation of healing (Kjartannson and Dalsgaard 1987; Heden et al. 1989; Byers and Taylor 1993). For example, transection of peripheral nerves inhibits tissue healing and is associated with increased tissue necrosis; in contrast, local infusion of CGRP enhances tissue healing (Kjartannson and Dalsgaard 1987; Heden et al. 1989; Byers and Taylor 1993). Collectively, these studies indicate that certain primary afferent fibers not only detect and signal the occurrence of tissue damage, but they also modulate the development of tissue inflammation and healing. Accordingly, it is possible that delayed healing may be due, in part, to dysfunctional neuropeptide responses to inflammation.

Peripheral tissue content of immunoreactive substance P and CGRP is substantially altered during inflammation (Khayat and Byers 1988; Kimberly and Byers 1988; Byers et al. 1990; Buma et al. 1992; Grutzner et al. 1992; Buck et al. 1994), consistent with the hypothesis that these neuropeptides modulate the inflammatory and healing process. In general, injury of a mild-to-moderate intensity evokes an increase in peripheral content of these neuropeptides. Increases in peripheral neuropeptide levels are of neuronal origin, because transection of the afferent nerve abolishes the neuropeptide response to injury (Buck et al. 1994). In contrast, moderate to severe injury is associated with a decrease in tissue content of neuropeptides. For example, inflammation of the knee joint may lead to substantial reductions in immunoreactive levels of CGRP and substance P (Buma et al. 1992).

SYMPATHETIC NEUROMODULATORS

In addition to the A-delta and C-fiber nociceptors, evidence suggests that the sympathetic nervous system may also contribute to pain sensations by any of several proposed mechanisms. First, visceral afferents appear to travel with sympathetic efferents and to encode for visceral pain (Jänig and Kollman 1984). Second, sympathetic efferents may alter the responses of various primary afferent fibers thought to be involved with chronic pain conditions such as causalgia (Roberts 1985, 1988; Campbell et al. 1992; Engelstad et al. 1992; Perl 1992). And third, stimulations of sympathetic nerve fibers may alter the responses of certain nociceptors that have terminal endings in inflamed or injured tissue (Perl 1992). These findings suggest that the sympathetic nervous system may augment or modify activation of peripheral A-delta and C-fiber afferent nociceptors. In addition, several studies by Levine and colleagues have substantiated the hypothesis that sympathetic terminals may modulate the development of inflammatory responses to injury (Levine et al. 1985; Green et al. 1993a,b). Others have demonstrated reduced sympathetic-induced vasoconstriction during inflammation of the knee joint (Lam and Ferrell 1993a).

ENDOCRINE RESPONSES TO STRESS AND INFLAMMATION

In addition to neuronal responses to injury, several endocrine systems are activated during stress, inflammation, or injury (Table III). These circulating factors are important in initiating and coordinating numerous physiologic responses to inflammation. Although space limitations preclude a further discussion of these systems, several detailed reviews are available on this topic (Rose 1984; Garcia-Leme 1989; Ader 1990; Hargreaves 1990).

PARACRINE RESPONSES TO INFLAMMATION

A substantial amount of research in the last 20 years has focused on local (e.g., paracrine) mediators that act to alter tissue responses to injury, inflam-

Table III
Peripheral neuroendocrine responses to stress, inflammation, and tissue injury

Response	Increase over Baseline
Endocrine	
Pituitary-adrenal axis (ß-End, ACTH, cortisol)	2–5 fold
Prolactin	8–20 fold
Growth hormone	2–10 fold
Pituitary-thyroid axis	0?
Pituitary-gonadal axis	0?
Glucagon	0.5–1 fold
Insulin	0?
Renin-angiotensin	2–3 fold
Aldosterone	2–3 fold
Neuroendocrine	
Sympathoneural (NE, NPY)	0–32 fold
Adrenomedullary (Epi, DA)	0–300 fold

Source: Modified from Hargreaves 1990.
Note: ß-End = beta-endorphin; ACTH = adrenocorticotropic hormone; NE = norepinephrine; NPY = neuropeptide Y; Epi = epinephrine; DA = dopamine.

mation, and repair. Table IV provides a partial list of major classes of paracrine mediators. It is beyond the scope of this review to provide extensive detail on this burgeoning field; indeed, numerous symposia have been held on only one class of these paracrine factors (e.g., the cytokines). A greater understanding of the paracrine response and its regulation is important in elucidating tissue response to injury, degeneration, and repair.

Considerable research has focused on determining the actions and identifying tissue levels of arachidonic acid metabolites in joint inflammation. Levels of immunoreactive prostoglandin E_2 (iPGE$_2$) and leukotriene B_4 (iLTB$_4$) are elevated or correlated with symptoms in synovial fluid collected from TMJ and other joints (Trang et al. 1977; Atik 1990; Quinn and Bazan 1990). Cells isolated from synovium, or macro-phages collected from patients with inflamed joints, have increased ability to synthesize prostanoids such as PGE$_2$ (Seitz and Hunstein 1985; Moilanen 1989; Wittenberg et al. 1993). In contrast, cells isolated from cartilage, cortical bone, or cancellous bone from arthritic joints do not show elevated synthesis of eicosanoids (Wittenberg et al. 1993). The up-regulation of cyclooxygenase has been suggested to be T-cell dependent because it is not sustained in the inflamed joints of athymic rats (Sano et al. 1992). These biochemical studies, together with studies demonstrating the anti-inflammatory efficacy of nonsteroidal anti-inflammatory drugs (NSAIDs), are consistent with the hypothesis that certain eicosanoids may contribute to sustained joint inflammation.

Several studies have found elevated levels of histamine and related mast cell products (e.g., heparin, tryptase, chymase) in inflamed joints (Frewin et al

Table IV
Paracrine responses to inflammation and tissue injury

Cell-derived mediators
    Arachidonic acid metabolites (e.g., prostanoids, leukotrienes, thromboxane)
    Vasoactive amines
    Oxidants/free radicals
    Ions (e.g., potassium, hydrogen)
    Cytokines
    Immunoglobulins
    Amino acids
    Enzymes/proteases
Plasma-derived mediators
    Hageman factor
    Plasmin
    Kinins
    Complement

1986; Malone et al. 1986; Gruber 1989; Mican and Metcalfe 1990). In addition, H_2 receptors have been localized on articular fibroblasts and chondrocytes, suggesting that localized histamine levels may contribute to morphological alterations of joint degeneration (Taylor et al. 1985; Nakata et al. 1992).

Research into the immunological mediation of inflammation, degeneration, and repair represents one of the major research fronts over the last 20 years. This area has been reviewed extensively and is summarized in a number of recent reviews and symposium reports (Fantone 1990; Leadbetter et al. 1990; Birkedal-Hansen 1993). It is now recognized that the cellular and molecular host-immune response modulates many forms of chronic tissue injury, ranging from periodontal disease to chronic joint inflammation (Friedlander et al. 1990; Birkedal-Hansen 1993).

Several studies have implicated immune modulation of joint disease. Several animal models of joint inflammation indicate that both T- and B-cell responses can modulate the development of inflammation (Van Eden et al. 1985; Holmdahl et al. 1986; Brauer et al. 1988; Buchan et al. 1988; Haynes et al. 1988). Moreover, a T-cell clone that responds to a microbial antigen has been isolated; it cross-reacts with host collagen, leading to an autoimmune-mediated form of chronic joint injury (Van Eden et al. 1985). Indeed, adjuvant-induced arthritis can be considered infectious because transfer of T-cells from one animal to another can evoke joint degeneration (Whitehouse et al. 1969). Additional studies have pointed to the possible roles that macrophages or neutrophils may play in the development of joint inflammation (Alwan et al. 1989; Haas et al. 1992).

Several clinical studies have demonstrated elevated levels of cytokines in synovial tissues or fluid collected from inflamed joints. For example, IL-1, IL-6, and leukemia inhibitory factor are elevated during joint inflammation (Feldman et al 1990; Rosenbaum et al 1992; Waring et al. 1993). Many of these cytokines have pro-inflammatory actions when injected in vivo (Pettipher et al. 1986; Andrews et al. 1989; Baker et al. 1989; O'Byrne et al. 1990; Rosenbaum et al. 1992; Angel et al. 1993). However, not all inflammatory mediators are elevated during inflammation; levels of platelet activating factor (PAF) and tissue necrosis factor (TNF) are either not or barely detectable in synovial fluid of patients with inflamed joints (Neale et al. 1989; Quinn and Bazan 1990).

MICRODIALYSIS AS A METHOD TO EVALUATE PARACRINE RESPONSES TO INFLAMMATION

Despite considerable research, comparatively little is known regarding the tissue concentrations of these inflammatory mediators during inflammation and pain, their pharmacological modulation, and to what extent they are involved in mediating pain caused by different types of orofacial conditions. To address these issues, our research team has developed a microdialysis method that permits collection of inflammatory mediators in awake dental pain patients, who can provide verbal pain reports simultaneously (Hargreaves and Costello 1990; Roszkowski et al. 1992a,b, 1993; Swift et al. 1993).

Previous attempts to measure tissue levels of mediators generally have used methods such as needle aspirations or the insertion of a "push-pull" catheter in which saline is pumped into the tissue and then collected. These approaches are limited, however, in their utility and reliability due to: (1) concurrent collection of peptidases (e.g., kininases, kallikrein), which can alter mediator concentrations during the collection process and lead to inaccurate determination of mediator levels; (2) collection of precursors (e.g., kininogen), which can interfere with measurement assays; (3) inaccurate calculation of mediator levels as a result of dilution of mediator concentrations by an unknown factor (e.g., by introduction of saline into the inflamed tissue compartment); and (4) alteration of the inflammatory process by pumping exogenous fluid into the tissue.

Implanting microdialysis probes into inflamed tissue avoids the above limitations. By implanting a probe having a semipermeable membrane (molecular weight cutoff of 3000–20,000 daltons), it is possible to collect a dialysate that contains inflammatory mediators (most of which have a molecular weight less than 2000 daltons). Advantages of the microdialysis method include: (1) exclusion of peptidases and precursors at the tissue level; (2) quantitative recoveries of inflammatory mediators; and (3) minimal disruption of the inflamed tissue (i.e., saline is not being pumped into the tissue). The recent introduction of ultrafiltration probes eliminates the molecular weight cutoff limits observed with older microdialysis probes. In addition, new advances in measurement technology (e.g., immuno-polymerase chain reaction) greatly increase the ability to measure small levels of inflammatory mediators.

Our clinical studies have used microdialysis probes to collect tissue levels of immunoreactive bradykinin (iBK), $iPGE_2$, $iLTB_4$, substance P (iSP), and other mediators released into inflamed peripheral tissue. These inflammatory mediators were selected for their known pro-inflammatory actions. Most of our initial studies have used the oral surgery model, a well-recognized clinical model of acute pain and inflammation that easily permits the temporary implantation of microdialysis probes into awake patients who can simultaneously provide pain reports. Information obtained from this clinical model of acute orofacial pain not only provides greater knowledge of peripheral pain mechanisms in humans, but it also should provide a basis for comparison with results obtained by microdialysis studies conducted in patients with chronic orofacial pain.

The time-course studies indicate that iPGE$_2$, iBK, iLTB$_4$, and iSP are all detectable in tissue dialysates collected from the extraction site of awake patients after surgical removal of impacted third molars (Hargreaves and Costello 1990; Roszkowski et al. 1992a, 1993; Swift et al. 1993). The data in Table V illustrate typical values for peak concentrations of these mediators. Importantly, the peak concentrations of all four of these mediators are greater than the Kd values for binding of the mediators to their respective receptors (the Kd value is the concentration of the mediator that binds to 50% of its receptors). This comparison suggests that all of these mediators are present at physiologically relevant concentrations, and that they may contribute to the development of acute orofacial pain and inflammation.

Our ongoing studies are extending this method to additional models of inflammation. For example, periodontal patients represent a unique clinical model in which a standardized surgical procedure is performed on chronically inflamed tissue. Accordingly, microdialysis studies conducted in this patient population permit evaluation of how chronic inflammatory cells influence the molecular responses to a defined surgical intervention. The results of our preliminary studies suggest that the inflammatory response to a surgical intervention is substantially altered in the presence of chronic inflammatory cells. For example, peak tissue levels of iPGE$_2$ are more than 1000-fold greater after periodontal surgery as compared to tissue levels achieved after oral surgery (Table V).

Table V

Peak tissue levels of selected inflammatory mediators as measured by microdialysis probes implanted into models of orofacial inflammation

	Clinical Studies		Animal Studies	
Mediator	Oral Surgery	Perio. Surgery	Control TMJ	Inflamed TMJ
iPGE$_2$	5–7 nmol/l	261 µmol/l	0.2 nmol/l	1–2 nmol/l
iBradykinin	12–17 nmol/l	NM	0.04 nmol/l	0.2 nmol/l
iSubstance P	1 nmol/l	NM	NM	NM
iLTB$_4$	2–4 nmol/l	0.6 nmol/l	NM	NM

Source: Data from Hargreaves and Costello 1990; Roszkowski et al. 1992a,b, 1993; Swift et al. 1993; and O'Brien et al. 1994.

Note: Immunoreactive levels of these mediators were determined by RIA or ELISA. Tissue dialysates were collected using microdialysis probes implanted into awake postsurgical oral surgery patients (n = 15–50), periodontal surgery patients (n = 9), and anesthetized rabbits with inflamed TMJs (n = 21). The TMJ in the anesthetized rabbits was inflamed with local injection of carrageenan.

NM = not measured.

We have also conducted preliminary studies using a rabbit model of inflamed TMJ. Microdialysis probes are implanted in the TMJs of anesthetized rabbits. The joints are then inflamed by local administration of carrageenan, or saline is administered as a control. Synovial levels of iPGE$_2$ are elevated about five to six-fold, and levels of iBK are elevated about five-fold after inflammation of the TMJ (Table V). Both mediators are reduced by local or systemic administration of either an NSAID (ketoprofen) or a glucocorticoid (dexamethasone) (Roszkowski et al. 1992b).

Collectively, these microdialysis studies provide a biochemically based approach for: (1) identifying inflammatory mediators released in peripheral tissue of orofacial pain subjects; (2) determining their pharmacological regulation; and (3) evaluating their interactions and contributions to the development of pain and inflammation

CLINICAL RELEVANCE

The heterogeneous population of conditions that comprise chronic orofacial pain has rendered accurate diagnosis and effective symptom management problematic issues. Recent research on peripheral pain mechanisms offers new information on possible etiologies for activation of peripheral nociceptors that may contribute to chronic pain. Together with the newly developed microdialysis method, it is now possible to conduct biochemically based clinical and animal studies to evaluate the role of potential peripheral pain mechanisms that may contribute to various chronic orofacial pain conditions.

This approach is clinically significant because it offers the possibility of developing biochemically based diagnostic tests for including (or excluding) various peripheral etiologies contributing to a specific patient's chronic orofacial pain. This diagnostic information may allow the clinician to systematically elucidate the possible factors contributing to the pain state and provide some insight into the specific peripheral biochemical mechanisms contributing to the chronic pain condition. An additional opportunity afforded by this method is the development of improved therapeutic approaches for the management of the pain. Knowledge of basal levels of inflammatory mediators may permit a more rational selection of pharmacological and nonpharmacological treatments. Knowledge of post-treatment levels of inflammatory mediators may be equally important for evaluating treatment efficacy and optimizing patient care. Moreover, this approach may ultimately provide prognostic information for developing a unified approach for management of chronic orofacial pain.

ACKNOWLEDGMENT

Supported in part by National Institute of Dental Research grants DE09860, DE10096, DE07014, K16DE0027, and P30DE09737, and by a grant from the Oral and Maxillofacial Surgeons Foundation. JDR is supported by a pre-doctoral fellowship of the Howard Hughes Medical Institute.

REFERENCES

Ader, R., Felten, D. and Cohen, N., Interactions between the brain and the immune system, Ann. Rev. Pharmacol. Toxicol., 30 (1990) 561–602.

Alwan, W.H., Dieppe, P.A., Elson, C.J. and Bradfield, J.W., Hydroxapatite and urate crystal induced cytokine release by macrophages, Ann. Rheum. Dis., 48 (1989) 476–482.

Andrews, H.J., Bunning, R.A.D., Dinarello, C.A. and Russell, R.G.G., Modulation of human chondrocyte metabolism by recombinant human interferon ganna: in-vitro effects on basal and IL-1-stimulated proteinase production, cartilage degredation and DNA synthesis, Biochim. Biophys. Acta., 1012 (1989) 128–134.

Appelgren, A., Appelgren, B., Eriksson, S., Kopp, S., Lundeberg, T., Nylander, M. and Theodorsson, E., Neuropeptides in temporomandibular joints with rheumatoid arthritis: a clinical study, Scand. J. Dent. Res., 99 (1991) 519–521.

Atik, O.S., Leukotriene B_4 and prostaglandin E_2-like activity in synovial fluid in osteoarthritis, Prostaglandins Leukot. Essent. Fatty Acids, 39 (1990) 253–254.

Baker, D.G., Krakauer, K.A., Tate, G., Laposata, M. and Zurier, R.B., Suppression of human synovial cell proliferation by dihomo-y-liolenic acid, Arthritis Rheum., 32 (1989) 1273–1280.

Birkedahl-Hansen, H., Role of cytokines and inflammatory mediators in tissue destruction, J. Periodontal Res., 28 (1993) 500–510.

Brain, S. and Williams, T., Inflammatory oedema induced by synergism between calcitonin gene-related peptide (CGRP) and mediators of increased vascular permeability, Br. J. Pharmacol., 68 (1985) 855–848.

Brain, S. and Williams, T., Substance P regulates the vasodilatory actvity of calcitonin gene-related peptide, Nature, 335 (1988) 73–75.

Brain, S.D., Cambridge, H., Hughes, S.R. and Wilsoncroft, P., Evidence that calcitonin gene-related peptide contributes to inflammation in the skin and joint, Ann. N.Y. Acad. Sci., 657 (1992) 412–419.

Bräuer, R., Thoss, K., Henzgen, S. and Walldmann, G., Significance of cell-mediated and humoral immunity in the acute and chronic phase of antigen-induced arthritis in rabbits, Exp. Pathol., 34 (1988) 197–206.

Brimijoin, S, Lundberg, J, Brodin, E, Hokfelt T. and Nilsson G. Axonal transport of substance P in the vagus and sciatic nerves of the guinea pig, Brain Res., 191 (1980) 443–457.

Buchan, G., Barrett, T., Fujita, T., Taniguchi, T., Maini, R. and Feldmann, M., Detection of actvated T cell products in the rheumatoid joint using cDNA probes to Interleukin-2 (IL-2) IL-2 receptor and IFN-y, Clin. Exp. Immunol., 71 (1988) 295–301.

Buck, S., Reese, K., Kane, P. and Hargreaves, K.M., Pulpal exposure induces changes in levels of peripheral neuropeptides (abstract), J. Dent. Res., 73 (1994) 314.

Buma, P., Verschuren, D, Versleyen, D., Van der Kraan, P. and Oestreicher, P., Calcitonin gene-related peptide, substance P and GAP-43/B50 immunoreactivity in the normal and arthrotic knee joint of the mouse, Histochemistry, 98 (1992) 327–339.

Byers, M.R. and Taylor, P.E., Effect of sensory denervation on the response of rat molar pulp to exposure injury, J. Dent. Res., 72 (1993) 613–618.

Byers, M., Taylor, P., Khayat, B. and Kimberly, C., Effects of injury and inflammation on pulpal and periapical nerves, J. Endodontics, 16 (1990) 78–84.

Campbell, J., Meyer, R., Davis, K., and Srinivasa, R., Sympathetically maintained pain: a unifying hypothesis. In: W. Willis (Ed.), Hyperalgesia and Allodynia, Raven Press, New York, 1992, pp. 141–150.

Coderre, T. and Melzack, R., The contribution of excitatory amino acids to central senstization and persistent nociception after formalin-induced tissue-injury., J. Neurosci., 12 (1992) 3665–3670.

Cook, A., Woolf, C., Wall, P. and McMahon, S., Dynamic receptive field plasticity in rat spinal cord dorsal horn following C-primary afferent input, Nature, 33 (1987) 293–307.

Cruwys, S.C., Kidd, B.L., Mapp, P.I., Walsh, D.A. and Blake, D.R., The effects of calcitonin gene-related peptide on formation of intra-articular oedema by inflammatory mediators, Br. J. Pharm. 107 (1992) 116–119.

Draisci, G. and Iadarola, M., Temporal analysis of increases in c-fos, preprodynorphin and preproenkephalin mRNAs in rat spinal cord, Brain Res. Mol. Brain Res., 6 (1989) 31–37.

Dubner, R. and Bennett, G., Spinal and trigeminal mechanisms of nociception, Ann. Rev. Neurosci., 6 (1983) 381–418.

Dubner, R. and Ruda, M.A., Activity-dependent neuronal plasticity following tissue injury and inflammation, Trends Neurosci., 15 (1992) 96–102.

Engelstad, M., Garry, M., Jackson, D., Geier, H. and Hargreaves, K., Adrenergic inhibition of iCGRP release from capsaicin-sensitive fibers in dental pulp, Abstracts Society for Neuroscience, 18 (1992) 690.

Fantone, J.C., Basic concepts in inflammation. In: W.B. Leadbetter, J.A. Buckwalter, S.L. Gordon (Eds.), Sports-Induced Inflammation, American Academy of Orthopedic Surgeons, Park Ridge, Ill., 1990, p. 25.

Feldmann, M., Brennan, F.M., Chantry, D., Haworth, C., Turner, M., Abney, E., Buchan, G., Barrett, K., Barkley, D., Chu, A., Field, M. and Maini, R.N., Cytokine production in the rheumatoid joint: implications for treatment, Ann. Rheum. Dis., 49 (1990) 480–486.

Ferreira, S., Lorenzetti, B., Bristow, A. and Poole, S., Interleukin-1β as a potent hyperalgesic agent antagonized by a tripeptide analogue, Nature, 334 (1988) 698–670.

Ferrell, W.R. and Russell, J.W., Extravasation in the knee induced by antidromic stimulation of articular C fibre afferents of the anaesthetized cat, J. Physiol., 379 (1986) 407–416.

Frewin, D.B., Cleland, L.G., Jonsson, J.R. and Robertson, P.W., Histamine levels in human synovial fluid, J. Rheumatol., 13 (1986) 13–14.

Friedlander, G.E., Jokl, P. and Horowitz, M.C., The autoimmune nature of sports-induced injury: a hypothesis. In: W.B. Leadbetter, J.A. Buckwalter, S.L. Gordon (Eds.), Sports-Induced Inflammation, Am. Acad. Ortho. Surg., Ill., 1990, p. 619.

Galeazza, M., Stucky, C. and Seybold, V.S., Changes in [125I]h–CGRP binding in rat spinal cord in an experimental model of acute, peripheral inflammation, Brain Res., 591 (1992) 198–208

Garcia-Leme, J., Hormones and Inflammation, CRC Press, Boca Raton, Fla., 1989.

Garry, M.G. and Hargreaves, K.M., Enhanced Release of Immunoreactive CGRP and substance P from spinal dorsal horn slices occurs during carrageenan inflammation, Brain Res., 582 (1992) 139–142.

Garry, M.G., Durnett-Richardson, J., and Hargreaves, K.M., Carrageenan-induced inflammation alters levels of i-cGMP and i-cAMP in the dorsal horn of the spinal cord, Brain Res. 646 (1994a) 135–139.

Garry, M.G., Durnett Richardson, J. and Hargreaves, K.M., Sodium nitroprusside evokes the release of immunoreactive calcitonin gene-related peptide and substance P from dorsal horn slices via nitric oxide–dependent and nitric oxide–independent mechanisms. J. Neurosci., 14 (1994b) 4329–4337.

Gazelius, B., Edwall, B., Olgart, L., Lundberg, J., Hokfelt, T. and Fischer, J., Vasodilatory effects and coexistence of CGRP and substance P in sensory nerves of cat dental pulp, Acta Physiol. Scand., 130 (1987) 33–40.

Green, P.G., Luo, J., Heller, P.H. and Levine, J., Further substantiation of a significant role for the sympathetic nervous system in inflammation, Neuroscience, 55 (1993a) 1037–1043.

Green, P.G., Luo, J., Heller, P.H. and Levine, J.D., Neurogenic and non-neurogenic mechanisms of plasma extravasation in the rat, Neuroscience, 52 (1993b) 735–743.

Grönblad, G., Korkala, O., Liesi, P. and Karaharju, E., Innervation of synovial membrane and meniscus, Acta. Orthop. Scand., 56 (1985) 484–486.

Gruber, B., Activation of rheumatoid synovial mast cells: role of IgE–associated antiglobulins, Monogr. Allergy, 26 (1989) 120–134.

Grutzner, E., Garry, M. and Hargreaves, K.M., Effect of injury on pulpal levels of immunoreactive substance P and CGRP, J. Endodontics, 18 (1992) 553–557.

Haas, D.A., Nakanishi, O., MacMillan, R.E., Jordan, R.C. and Hu, J.W., Development of an orofacial model of acute inflammation in the rat, Arch. Oral Biol., 37 (1992) 417–422.

Halliday, D.A., McNeil, J.D., Betts, W.H. and Scicchitano, R., The substance P fragment SP-(7-11) increases prostaglandin E_2, intracellular Ca^{2+}, and collagenase production in bovine articular chondrocytes, Biochem. J., 292 (1993) 57–62.

Hargreaves, K.M., Neuroendocrine markers of stress, Anesthesia Prog., 37 (1990) 99–105.

Hargreaves, K.M. and Costello, A., Glucocorticoids suppress release of immunoreactive bradykinin from inflamed tissue as evaluated by microdialysis probes, Clin. Pharmacol. Ther., 48 (1990) 168–178.

Hargreaves, KM., Troullos, E. and Dionne, R., Pharmacologic rationale for the treatment of acute pain, Dent. Clin. North Am., 31 (1987) 675–694.

Hargreaves, K.M., Bowles, W.R. and Garry, M.G., An in vitro method to evaluate regulation of neuropeptide release fom dental pulp, J. Endodontics, 18 (1992) 597–600.

Hargreaves, K.M., Roszkowski, M., Jackson, DL. and Swift, J.Q., Peripheral pain mechanisms. In: J. Fricton and R. Dubner (Eds.), Orofacial Pain and Temporomandibular Disorders, Raven Press, New York, 1995, pp. 33–42.

Haynes, B.F., Grover, B.J., Whichard, L.P., Hale, L.P., Nunley, J.A., McCollum, D.E. and Singer, K.H., Synovial microenvironment–T cell interactions, Arthritis Rheum., 31 (1988) 947–953.

Heden, P., Jernbeck, J., Kjartansson, J. and Samuelson, U., Increased skin flap survival and arterial dilation by calcitonin gene-related peptide, Scand. J. Plast. Reconstr. Surg. Hand Surg., 23 (1989) 11–16.

Holmdahl, R., Klareskog, L., Rubin, K., Bjork, J., Smedegårde, G. and Jonsson, R., Role of T lymphocytes in murine collagen induced arthritis, Agents Actions, 19 (1986) 295–303.

Holmlund, A., Ekblom, A., Hansson, P., Lind, J., Lundeberg, T. and Theodorsson, E., Concentrations of neuropeptides substance P, neurokinin A, calcitonin gene-related peptide, neuropeptide Y and vasoactive intestinal polypeptide in synovial fluid of the human temporomandibular joint, Int. J. Oral Maxillofac. Surg., 20 (1991) 228–231.

Holzer, P., Local effector function of capsaicin-sensitive sensory nerve endings: involvement of tachykinins, calcitonin gene-related peptide and other neuropeptides, Neuroscience, 24 (1988) 739–768.

Hu, J, Sessle, B., Raboosoon, P., Dallel, R. and Woda, A., Stimulation of craniofacial muscle afferents induces prolonged facilitatory effects in trigeminal nociceptive brainstem neurones, Pain, 48 (1992) 53–60.

Hylden, J., Nahin, R., Traub, R. and Dubner, R., Expansion of receptor fields of spinal lamina I projection neurons in rats with unilateral adjuvant-induced inflamamtion, Pain, 37 (1989) 229–243.

IASP Subcommittee on Taxonomy, Pain terms: a list with definitions and notes on usage, Pain, 6 (1979) 249–252.

Ichikawa, H., Matsuo, S., Wakisaka, S. and Akai, M., Fine structure of calcitonin gene-related peptide-immunoreactive nerve fibres in the rat temporomandibular joint, Oral Biol., 35 (1990) 727–730.

Jackson, D., Aanonsen, L. Richardson, J.D., Wiski, B., Groves, N. and Hargreaves, K.M., Binding sites and actions of excitatory amino acids in bovine dental pulp (abstract), J. Dent. Res., 73 (1990) 190.

Jackson, D., Garry, M., Engelstad, M., Geier, H. and Hargreaves, K., Evaluation of iCGRP secretion from dental pulp in response to inflammatory mediators, Abs. Soc. Neurosci., 18 (1992) 689.

Jänig, W. and Kollman, W., The involvement of the sympathetic nervous system in pain, Arzneim Forsch. Drug Res., 34 (1984) 1066–1073.

Katori, M., Hon, Y., Uchida, K. and Harada, Y., Different modes of interaction of bradykinin with prostaglandins in pain and acute inflammation, Adv. Exp. Med. Biol., 198B (1986) 393–398.

Khayat, B. and Byers, M., Responses of nerve fibers to pulpal inflammation and periapical lesions in rat molars demonstrated by cacitonin gene-related peptide immunocytochemistry, J. Endodontics, 14 (1988)

Kido, M.A., Kiyoshima, R., Kondo, T., Ayasaka, N., Moroi, R., Terada, Y. and Tanaka, T., Distribution of substance P and calcitonin gene-related peptide-like immunoreactive nerve fibers in the rat temporomandibular joint, J. Dent. Res., 72 (1993) 592–598.

Kim, S., Dorscher-Kim, J., Liu, M.T. and Trowbridge, H.O., Biphasic pulp blood flow response to substance P in the dog as measured with radiolabelled microsphere injection method, Arch. Oral Biol., 33 (1988) 305–309.

Kimberly, C. and Byers, M., Inflammation of rat molar pulp and periodontium causes increased calcitonin gene-related peptide and axonal sprouting, Anat. Rec., 222 (1988) 289–300.

Kjartannson, J. and Dalsgaard, C., Calcitonin gene-related peptide increases survival of a musculocutaneous critical flap in the rat, Eur. J. Pharmacol., 42 (1987) 355–358.

Kumazawa, T. and Mizumura, K, Thin-fiber receptors responding to mechanical, chemical and thermal sdmulation in the skeletal muscle of the dog, J. Physiol., 273 (1977) 179–194.

Lam, F.Y. and Ferrell, W.R., Acute inflammation in the rat knee joint attenuates sympathetic vasoconstriction but enhances neuropeptide-mediated vasodilatation assesed by laser doppler perfusion imaging, Neuroscience, 52 (1993a) 443–449.

Lam, F.Y. and Farrell, W.R., Effects of interactions of naturally-occurring neuropeptides on blood flow in the rat knee joint, Br. J. Pharm., 108 (1993b) 694–698.

Larsson, J., Ekblom, A., Henriksson, K., Lundeberg, T. and Theodorsson, E., Immunoreactive tachykinins, calcitonin gene-related peptide and neuropeptide Y in human synovial fluid from inflamed knee joints, Neurosci. Lett., 100 (1989) 326–330.

Larsson, J., Ekblom, A., Henriksson, K., Lundeberg, T. and Theodorsson, E., Concentration of substance P, neurokinin A, calcitonin gene-related peptide, neuropeptide Y and vasoactive intestinal polypeptide in synovial fluid from knee joints in patients suffering from rheumatoid arthritis, Scand. J. Rheumatol., 20 (1991) 326–335.

Leadbetter, W.B., Buckwalter, J.A. and Gordon, S.L., Sports-Induced Inflammation: Clinical and Basic Concepts, Am. Acad. Ortho. Surg., Ill, 1990.

LeGreves P., Nyberg F., Terenius L. and Hokfelt T., CGRP is a potent inhibitor of substance P degradation. Eur. J. Pharmacol. 115 (1985) 309–311.

Lembeck, F.and Holzer, P., Substance P as a neurogenic mediator of antidromic vasodiation and neurogenic plasma extravasation, Arch. Pharmacol., 310 (1979) 175–183.

Levine, J., Lau, W., Kwiat, G. and Goetzl, E., Leukotriene B4 produces hyperalgesia that is dependent on ploymorphonuclear leukocytes, Science, 225 (1984) 743–745.

Levine, J., Moskowitz, M. and Basbaum, A., The contribution of neurogenic inflammation in experimental arthritis, J. Immunol., 135 (1985) 843s–847s.

Levine, J., Lam, D., Taiwo, Y., Donatoni, P. and Goetzl, E., Hyperalgesic properties of 15-liopoxygenase products of arachidonic acid, Proc. Nat. Acad. Sci. USA, 83 (1986) 5331–5334.

Light, A.R., The Initial Processing of Pain and Its Descending Control: Spinal and Trigeminal Systems, Karger, Basel, 1992.

Lotz, M., Carson, D. and Vaughan, J., Substance P activation of rheumatoid synoviocytes: neural pathway in pathogenesis of arthritis, Science, 235 (1987) 893–895.

Lotz, M., Vaughan, J. and Carson, D., Effect of neuropeptides on production of inflammatory cytokines by human monocytes, Science, 241 (1988) 1218–1221.

Louis, S., Johnstone, D., Russell, N., Jamieson, A. and Dockray, G., Antibodies to calcitonin-gene related peptide reduce inflammation induced by topical mustard oil but not that due to carrageenin in the rat, Neurosci Lett., 102 (1989) 257–260.

Malone, D.G., Irani, A.M., Schwartz, L.B., Barrett, K.E. and Metcalfe, D.D., Mast cell numbers and histamine levels in synovial fluids from patients with diverse arthritides, Arthritis Rheum., 29 (1986) 956–963.

Martin, H., Basbaum, A., Kwiat, G., Goetzl, E. and Levine, J., Leukotriene and prostaglandin sensitization of cutaneous high-threshold C- and A-delta mechanoreceptors in the hairy skin of rat hindlimbs, Neuroscience, 22 (1987) 651–659.

Meller, S. and Gebhart, G., Nitric oxide (NO) and nociceptive processing in the spinal cord, Pain, 52 (1993) 127–136.

Mense, S., Nervous outflow from skeletal muscle following chemical noxious stimulation., J. Neurophysiol., 267 (1977) 75–88.

Meyer, R. and Campbell, J., Myelinated nocicepdve afferents account for the hyperalgesia that follows a burn to the hand, Science, 213 (1981) 1527–1529.

Mican, J.M. and Metcalfe, D.D., Arthritis and mast cell activation, J. Allergy Clin. Immunol., 86 (1990) 677–683.

Moilanen, E., Effects of diclofenac, indomethacin, toldenamic acid and hydrocortisone on prostanoid production in healthy and rheumatic synovial cells, Agents Actions, 26 (1989) 342–347.

Morton, C. and Chahl, L., Pharmacology of the neurogenic oedema response to electrical stimulation of the saphenous nerve in the rat, Arch. Pharmacol., 314 (1980) 271–276.

Nakata, Y., Matsumura, F., Motoyoshi, H., Tamasaki, H., Fukuda, K. and Tanaka, S., Secretion of hyaluronic acid from synovial fibroblasts is enhanced by histamine: a newly observed metabolic effect of histamine, J. Lab. Clin. Med., 120 (1992) 707–712.

Neale, M.L., Williams, B.D. and Matthews, N., Tumour necrosis factor activity in joint fluids from rheumatoid arthiritis patients, Br. J. Rheumatol., 28 (1989) 104–108.

O'Brien, C., Woolf, C.J., Fitzgerald, M., Lindsay, R.M. and Molander, C., Differences in the chemical expression of rat primary afferent neurons which innervate skin, muscle or joint, Neuroscience, 32 (1989) 493–502.

O'Brien, T., Wolff, L., Roszkowski, M., and Hargreaves, K.M., Tissue levels of PGE2, LTB4 and pain after periodontal surgery (abstract), J. Dent. Res., 73 (1994) 379.

O'Byrne, E., Blancuzzi, V., Wilson, D., Wong, M. and Jeng, A., Elevated substance P and accelerated cartilage degradation in rabbit knees injected with interleukin-1 and tumor necrosis factor, Arthritis Rheum., 33 (1990) 1023–1027.

Ochoa, J. and Mair, W., The normal sural nerve in man. I. Ultrastructure and numbers of fibers and cells, Acta Neuropath. (Berlin), 13 (1969) 127–216.

Olgart, L., Gazelius, B., Brodin, E. and Nilsson, G., Release of substance P-like immunoreactivity from the dental pulp, Acta. Physiol. Scand., 101 (1977) 510–512.

Perl, E., Alterations in the responsiveness of cutaneous nociceptors: sensitization by noxious stimuli and the induction of adrenergic responsiveness by nerve injury. In: W. Willis (Ed.), Hyperalgesia and Allodynia, Raven Press, New York, 1992, pp 59–80.

Pettipher, E.R., Higgs, G.A. and Henderson, B., Interleukin 1 induces leukocyte infiltration and cartilage proteoglycan degradation in the synovial joint, Proc. Nat. Acad. Sci. USA, 83 (1986) 8749–8753.

Quinn, J H. and Bazan, N.G., Identification of prostaglandin E2 and leukotriene B4 in the synovial fluid of painful, dysfunctional temporomandibular joints, J. Oral Maxillofac. Surg., 48 (1990) 968–971.

Rackham, A. and Ford-Hutchinson, A., Inflammation and pain sensitivity: effects of leukotrienes D4, B4, and prostaglandin E1 in the rat paw, Prostaglandins, 25 (1983) 193–203.

Roberts, W. and Elardo, S., Sympathetic activation of A-delta nociceptors, Somatosens. Res. 3 (1985) 33–44.

Roberts, W. and Foglesong, M., II., Identification of afferents contributing to sympathetically evoked activity in wide-dynamic-range neurons, Pain, 34 (1988) 305–314.

Rose, R., Overview of endocrinology of stress. In: G. M. Brown (Ed.), Neuroendocrinology and Psychiatric Disorder, Raven Press, New York, 1984, pp 95–122.

Rosenbaum, J.T., Cugnini, R., Tara, D.C., Hefeneider, S. and Ansel, J.C., Production and modulation of interleukin 6 synthesis by synoviocytes derived from patients with arthritic disease, Ann. Rheum. Dis., 51 (1992) 198–202.

Roszkowski, M.T., Swift, J.Q. and Hargreaves, K.M., Prostaglandin E2 tissue levels increase following third molar extraction, J. Dent. Res., 71 (1992a) 178.

Roszkowski, M.T., Swift, J.Q., Alton, T. and Hargreaves, K.M., Prostaglandin E2 immunoreactivity is released during inflammation of the rabbit TMJ, Abs. Soc. Neurosci., 8 (1992b) 690.

Roszkowski, M.T., Swift, J.Q. and Hargreaves, K.M., Corticosteroids attenuate the local release of immunoreactive substance P following third molar surgery, J. Dent. Res., 72 (1993) 186.

Ruda, M.A. and Dubner, R., Molecular and biochemical events mediate neuronal plasticity following inflammation and hyperalgesia. In: W. Willis (Ed.), Hyperalgesia and Allodynia, New York, Raven Press, 1992, pp 311–327.

Sano, H., Hia, T., Maier, J.A., Crofford, L.J., Case, J.P., Maciag, T. and Wilder, R.L., In vivo cyclooxygenase expression in synovial tissues of patients with rheumatoid arthritis and osteoarthritis and rats with adjuvant and streptococcal cell wall arthritis, J. Clin. Invest., 89 (1992) 97–108.

Schaible, H. and Grubb, D., Afferent and spinal mechanisms of joint pain, Pain, 55 (1993) 5–54.

Schaible, H. and Schmidt, R., Discharge characteristics of receptors with fine afferents from normal and inflamed joints: influence of analgesics and prostaglandins, Agents Actions, 19 (suppl.) (1986) 99–117.

Scott, D.T., Lam, F.Y. and Ferrell, W.R., Acute inflammation enhances substance P-induced plasma protein extravasation in the rat knee joint, Regul. Pept., 39 (1992) 227–235.

Seitz, M. and Hunstein, W., Enhanced prostanoid release from monocytes of patients with rhematoid arthiritis and active systemic lupus erythematosus, Ann. Rheum. Dis. 44 (1985) 438–445.

Sessle, B., Neurophysiology of orofacial pain, Dent. Clin. N. Am., 31 (1987) 595–614.

Stacey, M., Free nerve endings in skeletal muscle of the cat, J. Anat., 105 (1969) 231–254.

Steen, K.H., Reeh, P.W., Anton, F. and Handwerker, H.O., Protons selectively induce lasting excitation and sensitization to mechanical stimulation of nociceptors in rat skin in vitro, J. Neurosci., 21 (1992) 86–95.

Sugimoto, T., Bennett, G. and Kajander, K., Transsynaptic degeneration in the superficial dorsal horn after sciatic nerve injury: effects of a chronic constriction injury, transection and strychnine, Pain, 42 (1990) 205–213.

Swift, J.Q., Garry, M.G., Roszkowski, M. and Hargreaves, K.M., Effect of flurbiprofen on tissue levels of immunoreactive bradykinin and acute post-operative pain, J. Oral Maxillofac. Surg., 51 (1993) 112–116.

Taylor, D.J., Yoffe, J.R., Brown, D.M. and Woolley, D.E., Histamine H_2 receptors on chondrocytes derived from human, canine and bovine articular cartilage, Biochem. J., 225 (1985) 315–319.

Trang, L.E., Granström L, and Lövgren, L., Levels of prostaglandins F_2 and E_2 and thromboxane B_2 in joint fluid in rheumatoid arthritis, Scand. J. Rheumatol., 6 (1977) 151–154.

Tyers, M. and Haywood, H;, Effects of prostaglandins on peripheral nociceptors in acute inflammation. In: K. Rainsford and A. Ford-Hutchinson (Eds.), Prostaglandins and Inflammation, Birkhauser, Basel, 1979, pp. 65–78.

Van Eden, W., Holoshitz, J., Nevo, Z., Frenkel, A., Klajman A. and Cohen, I., Arthritis induced by a T-lymphocyte clone that responds to mycobacterium tuberculosis and to cartilage proteoglycans, Proc. Nat. Acad. Sci. USA, 82 (1985) 5117–5120.

Wall, P. and Woolf, C., Muscle but not cutaneous C-afferent input produces prolonged increases in the excitability of the flexion reflex in the rat, J. Physiol., 356 (1984) 443–458.

Walsh, D., Salmon, M., Mapp, P., Wharton, J., Garrett, N., Blake, D. and Polak, J., Microvascular substance P binding to normal and inflamed rat and human synovium, J. Pharmacol. Exp. Ther., 267 (1993) 951–960.

Waring, P.M., Carroll, G.J., Kandiah, D.A., Buirski, G. and Metcalf, D., Increased levels of leukemia inhibitory factor in synovial fluid from patients with rheumatoid arthritis and other inflammatory arthritides, Arthritis Rheum., 36 (1993) 911–915.

Whalley, E., Clegg, S., Stewart, J. and Vavrek, R., The effect of kinin agonists and antagonists on the pain response of the human blister base, Arch. Pharmacol., 336 (1987) 652–655.

Whitehouse, D., Whitehouse, M. and Pearson, C., Passive transfer of adjuvant-induced arthritis and allergic encephalomyelitis in rats using thoracic duct lymphocytes, Nature, 224 (1969) 1322–1323.

Willis, W., The Pain System, Karger, Basel, 1985.

Wittenberg, R.H., Willburger, R.E., Kleemeyer, K.S. and Peskar, B.A., In vitro release of prostaglandins and leukotrienes from synovial tissue, cartilage, and bone in degenerative joint diseases, Arthiritis Rheum., 36 (1993) 1444–1450.

Woolf, C., Evidence for a central component of post-injury pain hypersensitivity, Nature, 306 (1983) 686–688.

Yaksh, T., Substance P release from knee joint afferent terminals: modulation by opioids, Brain Res., 458 (1988) 319–324.

Correspondence to: Kenneth M. Hargreaves, DDS, PhD, 8-166 Moos Tower, University of Minnesota School of Dentistry, Minneapolis, MN 55455, USA. Tel: 612-624-7682; Fax: 612-626-2655; E-mail: hargreav@lenti.med.umn.edu

Temporomandibular Disorders and Related Pain Conditions, Progress in Pain Research and Management, Vol. 4, edited by B.J. Sessle, P.S. Bryant, and R.A. Dionne, IASP Press, Seattle, © 1995.

16

Biomaterials and Biomechanics of Synthetic Materials for Tissue Replacement Prostheses

Jack E. Lemons

Departments of Surgery and Biomaterials, Division of Orthopaedic Surgery, Schools of Medicine and Dentistry, University of Alabama at Birmingham, Birmingham, Alabama, USA

The most recent period of active development in the biomaterial and biomechanical disciplines began during the late 1960s when clinicians, engineers, and basic scientists collaborated on mutual research interests (for example, during a symposium held at Clemson University in Clemson, South Carolina, in January 1969). The focus was on clearly delineated problems where surgical reconstructions had not fully satisfied the anticipated long-term clinical results. Individuals from physical and biological science-oriented backgrounds interacted across the surgical disciplines where cardiovascular, general, orthopedic, and dental groups converged (Hulbert et al. 1971; Homsy and Armadiades 1972). An advantage to this information transfer was that ideas on limitations and solutions to recognized problems were regularly exchanged. Over time and with growth and specialization, these collaborations have become more limited and subgroups now meet independently within the clinical and basic science-oriented professional societies (Cranin 1993; Society for Artificial Organs 1993; Orthopaedic Research Society 1994). A strongly held opinion is that multidisciplinary research represents a strength, and much could be gained through a re-emphasis on coordinations among the groups associated with surgical device applications, especially in the area of temporomandibular joint (TMJ) devices.

OVERALL CLASSIFICATIONS OF DEVICES INCLUDING
MECHANICAL AND PERCUTANEOUS FUNCTIONS

Surgical implant devices can be classified using: (1) areas of clinical applications within surgical disciplines; (2) the elements of synthetic materials and properties that define biomaterials; (3) force transfers and the mechanics of tissues and devices that provide the basis for biomechanics; and (4) physical and biological properties specific to the characteristics of synthetic implant biocompatibilities (Williams and Roaf 1973; Rubin 1983; von Recum 1986). The general aspects of device locations within various tissues are shown schematically in Fig. 1.

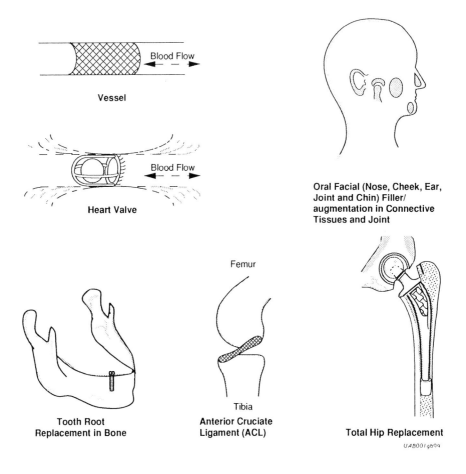

Fig. 1. Schematic representations of devices for cardiovascular, general, orthopedic, and dental surgical applications.

CLINICAL APPLICATIONS OF DEVICES

Most cardiovascular devices constructed from synthetic materials exist in direct contact with blood and therefore must include unique biomaterial surface and bulk properties (ASTM 1992). For example, vascular segmental replacements for blood vessels include openings within the device that permit initial blood penetration, followed by clotting and eventual tissue ingrowth to enhance mechanical stabilization. The mechanical properties of these porous tubelike devices have been selected so that biomechanical resiliencies are similar to the soft viscoelastic tissues replaced. A predominant cyclic motion during function is diametral expansion and contraction with pulsatile blood flow. Additionally, the device must provide a stable interconnection (anastomosis) along the proximal and distal ends of the synthetic vessel replacement. The chemistry of the biomaterial, especially the purity, uniformity, and topography of the device along blood-contacting surfaces is critical to minimize clotting and flow occlusion during the early stages after implantation. In this regard, very inert and compliant polymeric systems best satisfy both the mechanical and chemical conditions imposed by the cardiovascular system.

In contrast to vessel replacement, a heart valve must be constructed to include more rigid and wear-resistant biomaterials. These biomaterials also must be capable of remaining clean (deposit free) over time while in continuous contact with blood. Metals, carbons, and rigid (high-modulus) polymers have been selected because of combinations of desirable properties. In the cardiovascular system, any debris from a device or device-to-blood interactions cannot be tolerated by the host. Therefore, secondary debris from any source must be kept to an absolute minimum. Thus, cardiovascular applications of devices include special requirements that are site and function specific. Another aspect of this situation is that the devices must be capable of in vivo mechanical loading (deformation or valve cycle) at rates slightly greater than one per second to totals of about 40 million cycles per year. Synthetic biomaterials are incapable of repair in vivo, so the devices must be capable of providing long-term stability to achieve decades of in vivo service. This criterion is both chemically and mechanically demanding.

Devices for applications as replacements or augmentations within the general soft connective tissues, as with the cardiovascular devices, function at reduced mechanical loads as compared to orthopedic and dental total joint arthroplasties (TJA) and tooth root replacements (Fung et al. 1972). Also, the mechanical compliance factors of soft tissues tend to support the use of polymeric biomaterials, again because of similarities between tissue and synthetic material/mechanical properties. In contrast to the surfaces that continuously contact flowing blood, the general soft connective tissue implants usually interface with fibrous scar tissue. In addition, less than a million cycles of loading per year would be a normal functional situation. The surface purities and bulk mechanical properties thus become much less stringent, in that the clotting of blood does not represent a mode of failure. Also, decades of in vivo service results in much lower numbers of mechanical loading cycles.

If a device passes across cutaneous tissues, the requirements for simultaneous internal (tissue) and external environments must be considered for the same device construct. Percutaneous transitions across dry skin or wet mucosal surfaces introduce significantly different conditions, and device biomaterials and designs must be specific to the application. For example, biomaterial selections for a gastrointestinal access for bowel excretions differ significantly from a urethral tube replacement, and both differ from a blood or soft tissue access for dialysis, sampling, or pharmaceutical delivery. Each situation requires a special combination of biomaterial and design characteristics to meet the overall needs imposed by exposure to the internal and external environments.

Applications for dental and orthopedic load-bearing devices within the musculoskeletal system also impose special requirements for the prostheses (Lemons and Phillips 1991; McKinney 1991; Petty 1991). The interfacial conditions for interactions with bone under normal functional conditions have resulted in the selection of metals, alloys, ceramics, and some high-strength polymers, in part because of the higher magnitude loads associated with function. Joint replacement devices also require motions along articulating surfaces with loading cycles extending to millions per year (less than heart valves but greater than general soft tissue applications). Articulation and motion introduces a need for arthroplasty biomaterials with low friction and low wear rate. The properties of biomaterials correlated with attachment to bone are somewhat different from those that could simultaneously result in minimized wear during high-force transfer articulations. Thus, TJAs impose a new set of requirements.

The intraoral dental implant that is anchored into bone (endosteal) and supports the attachment of artificial teeth is an example of a device that crosses a mucosal (gingival) tissue region. Because these devices are anchored into bone and chewing forces are relatively high in magnitude (similar to orthopedic joint forces), some aspects of the prosthetic material and design selections must be different from prostheses for soft tissue applications. Therefore, dental implant devices often combine features of high-strength orthopedic arthroplasties and soft tissue percutaneous devices (Morrey 1991).

ELEMENTS AND BIOMATERIAL PROPERTIES

Synthetic biomaterials can be classified by interactions with the biological host. The following descriptions are specific to the chemical (and biochemical) properties of the synthetic biomaterials (Williams 1982). Inert substances should exhibit very limited biodegradation, and an anticipated result would be a minimal host response to small quantities of foreign elements. In contrast, the active substances should interact with the tissues at the beginning of implantation and the biomaterial-to-host response would be partially controlled (optimized) by this "bioactivity." However, in both situations, the terms *inert* and *active* are used to describe biomaterials used for long-term implants (i.e., the bulk of the implant would be retained). The concept of relative interactions along biomaterial surfaces and the host tissue involvement is shown schematically in Fig. 2.

As opposed to the inert and active biomaterials, the degradable synthetic substances dissolve or are resorbed by the host environment. The site, after healing and maturation, should return to normal site-specific tissues. In most cases, biodegradable implants are fabricated from substances that are metabolized following known physiological pathways (e.g., calcium phosphates, hydrogels, lactic and glycolic acids).

As an overall subclassification, the synthetic biomaterials can be listed using their atomic and structural characteristics, e.g., metals and alloys, ceramics or carbons, polymers, or these biomaterials in combination (mechanical mixtures) or composite (chemically bonded) structures. These groups provide a wide range of material, mechanical, and biological properties, plus a significant record of multidisciplinary investigations related to biocompatibility.

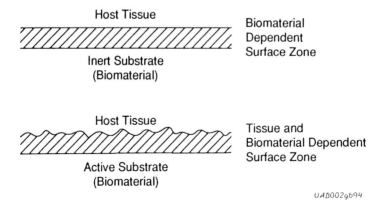

Fig. 2. Schematic representation of biomaterial-to-tissue interaction zones for inert and active synthetic substances.

National and international material standards exist for these classifications of synthetic biomaterials (ASTM 1992).

FORCE TRANSFER AND BIOMECHANICAL PROPERTIES

When devices are placed within tissues, various directions and magnitudes of mechanical forces will be transferred across the biomaterial-to-tissue interfaces and these are specific to the device, biomaterial, and application. In the case of the cardiovascular vessel replacement, the major force vectors introduced by the internal pressurization of the tubular conduits cause transverse and tangential (hoop) type mechanical stresses (mechanical stress is force-per-unit-area of transfer surface). In contrast, an anterior cruciate ligament (ACL) of the knee functions under tension and bending loading modes, while the bones directly adjacent to the hip and tooth root device are primarily loaded in compression. These modes of force transfer (tension, compression, and shear) are shown schematically in Fig. 3. Most importantly, for the biomaterial-to-tissue interface to remain stable over time, the types and magnitudes of these forces and stresses must be known, and the device design and biomaterial must be capable of withstanding and adequately transferring the associated mechanical stresses and strains (strain is deformation-per-unit-length of substance deformed) (McLean 1962).

Knowledge of the biomechanical properties of tissues specific to the intended implant device site and function is one requirement for prosthesis design and material selection. Obviously, the host conditions for blood, soft tissue, or bone tissue contact are key considerations. An overall intent within the research and development community has been to select materials and designs to maximize the in vivo longevities. As understanding of biomaterial-to-tissue interface interactions has increased through longer-term device applications and multidisciplinary communications, it has become possible to isolate and separate biomaterial conditions for attachment to bone or soft

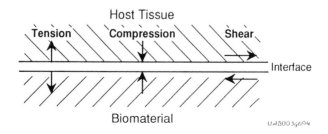

Fig. 3. Schematic drawing showing force vectors and conditions of tension, compression, and shear loading across a biomaterial-to-tissue interface.

tissues, as opposed to force transfer characteristics and conditions for articulation (valve and joint replacements). In this regard, knowledge of the host-tissues properties and the changes with disease and age must be included in the overall criteria for device selection. One key development has been the introduction of modular systems where different biomaterials can be combined and/or replaced within a single prosthesis (Morrey 1993). Also, new classes of substances or surface modifications have been introduced to accommodate the conditions for both attachment (porosities or coatings) to tissue and minimization of wear debris generation (harder materials, ion implantations, or coatings) during functional articulation.

BIOCOMPATIBILITY PROFILES FOR DEVICES AND ROLE(S) OF STANDARDIZED TESTING

Tissue responses to biomaterials have been compared in reference to known biological responses. Test methodologies and national standards exist for evaluating toxicity, hypersensitivity (allergy), and carcinogenicity to synthetic biomaterials (ASTM 1992). Because all substances of nonbiological origin are classified as foreign materials, these broad classifications for short- and long-term tissue responses and biocompatibility profiles can be used to develop independent protocols for different types of biomaterials, devices, and applications. Most initial evaluations for surgical devices emphasize toxicity profiles of the component materials based upon the long-term experience with bulk forms of metallic, ceramic, and polymeric biomaterials used within existing implant devices. It is important to emphasize that different toxicities (tissue interactions) are anticipated for bulk substances (biomaterials) versus finely divided particulates (debris) or ionic compounds and mers (unit structure of a polymer) from metallic, ceramic, or polymeric biomaterials. In most cases for standardized testing, all possible combinations are evaluated within laboratory environments, and tissue responses are tested over years of simulated applications (ASTM 1992).

Consensus standards for materials and devices have been established and accepted worldwide. Standards for medical and dental devices are published by the American Society for Testing and Materials (ASTM), Committee F-4, the American Dental Association (ADA), and other professional organizations. Additionally, all devices sold in interstate commerce must be reviewed and approved by the U.S. Food and Drug Administration (FDA). The available standards and reference documents provide protocols and detailed methods for the overall evaluations of synthetic materials for surgical implants and, importantly, these standards represent a significant resource for basic property data for intracomparisons among proposed applications.

BIOMATERIAL AND BIOMECHANICAL CONSIDERATIONS OF IMPLANT DEVICES

To provide more specific comparisons among the biomaterials and the applications of surgical implant devices, this section presents separate discussions on: (1) biomaterial elements and tissue interactions; (2) force transfer, mechanical properties, tissue attachment, and prosthesis articulations; and (3) biocompatibility considerations for synthetic biomaterials and devices.

BIOMATERIALS

Comparisons between synthetic biomaterials and host tissues can be evaluated by the elements and substances that are transferred across contacting interfaces and the adjacent surface zones. For the synthetic biomaterials, the surface and bulk properties must be independently considered. The basic considerations for elemental transfers along the tissue interfaces are depicted in Fig. 4. Exchanges from the outer surface where foreign substances are not a part of the biomaterial (surface impurities) represents one concept specific to tissue responses (Lemons 1975). The presence of surface impurities influences both short- and long-term biocompatibility profiles and represents an unanticipated result of tissue responses to foreign substances that were not intended as a part of the device (Lemons 1991). Fortunately, these types of impurity-based tissue interactions no longer exist for most applications due to controlled manufacturing, packaging, sterilizing, delivering, and implanting of devices.

Exchanges from within the surface zone include a region from the biomaterial plus the initial protein deposit associated with implantation (Davies 1991). An example would be titanium oxide on the surface of titanium and titanium alloy and the directly associated protein layer that forms at the time of implantation. Over the longer term, very thin (< 1 μm), directly adjacent soft and hard tissue could be considered as a part of this interaction region.

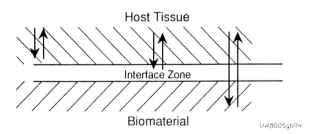

Fig. 4. Schematic representations of possible sources of elemental transfers across biomaterial-to-tissue interfaces.

The third consideration is transfer from the bulk (central) regions of the biomaterial (Buchanan et al. 1981). Examples would include corrosion of stainless steel where ions and compounds pass through the surface zones into the tissues or tissue fluid, tissue substance transport (e.g., liquids, water, salts) into polymers, or conversely selected leaching of products due to hydrolytic enzymatic reactions within the bulk structural regions of some biomaterials.

An extension of this same concept is shown in Fig. 5, which depicts a total hip replacement construct and the regional tissues (Morrey 1991). The listing of regions and component parts of the device and tissues demonstrate the complexity of the various interactions that include direct contacts with soft tissue, synovial and marrow fluids, and bone. In some situations, more than one type of biomaterial (e.g., metallic, ceramic, and polymeric) are in simultaneous contact and interaction with adjacent tissues and fluids. Also, at one location, the biomaterial(s) provide(s) a site for tissue attachment, while at another, a bearing-like surface for articulation and three-dimensional motion. Critical concerns develop when shear-oriented micromotions exist at sites intended for tissue attachment, or if wear debris (particulates) are generated during the interfacial sliding contact of articulation (McKellop et al. 1981; McKellop 1994). The considerations for biocompatibility are uniquely different for particulates generated from bulk-form synthetic biomaterials, in part

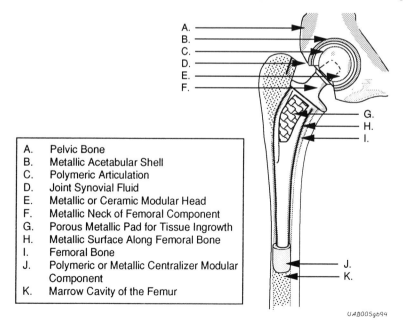

A. Pelvic Bone
B. Metallic Acetabular Shell
C. Polymeric Articulation
D. Joint Synovial Fluid
E. Metallic or Ceramic Modular Head
F. Metallic Neck of Femoral Component
G. Porous Metallic Pad for Tissue Ingrowth
H. Metallic Surface Along Femoral Bone
I. Femoral Bone
J. Polymeric or Metallic Centralizer Modular Component
K. Marrow Cavity of the Femur

Fig. 5. Total hip replacement construct.

because of particulate shape change, increased surface area, altered surface zones, and possibilities for local and systemic transport with accumulation(s) at sites where particulates may cause significantly adverse tissue responses (Goldring et al. 1993).

TISSUE INTERACTIONS

When a biomaterial such as titanium (Ti) is implanted into bone as a load-bearing orthopedic or dental prosthesis, and direct Ti-to-bone contact is the intended outcome, and the relative micromotions along the oxide-to-bone interface must be kept to a minimum during bone healing. If significant shear-type micromotions (> 150 μm) exist, the bone could become separated from the biomaterial surface by a zone of fibrous tissue (Pilliar et al. 1986). If motions continue between the Ti oxide and the fibrous soft tissue, particulate oxide debris could be transferred to the tissue environment (a black stain). An example of this phenomenon was the black colored regions noted in soft tissues adjacent to Ti bone plates used for bone fixation in orthopedics (Ferguson et al. 1962). This observation subsequently led to surface treatments of Ti and alloy surfaces by anodizing, nitriding, ion implanting, and other methods to minimize these types of transfers. In contrast, if the micromotions are controlled (small) after implantation, mineralized components of bone can be located directly adjacent to the biomaterial surface (osteointegration) and this condition minimizes particulate debris transfers (Lemons 1991). For example, device retrieval studies of dental root-form endosteal and orthopedic TJA devices have shown minimal debris within bone areas adjacent to osteointegrated Ti and Ti alloy implants (Lemons 1988; Davies 1991). Thus, for the same biomaterial, the interfacial conditions during healing and function significantly influence debris generation and, thereby, some aspects of biocompatibility profiles.

The articulating region of the TJA shown in Fig. 5 demonstrates the site of a femoral head (metallic or ceramic) and acetabular cup (ultra-high molecular weight polyethylene, UHMW-PE) contact and motion. Under anticipated articulating conditions, the surface interactions would be sliding motion without wear. If wear exists, the first level of damage is characterized as an adhesive type, where the polymeric surface zone is locally deformed and only small quantities of particulates are generated over time (McKellop et al. 1981), as depicted schematically in panel A of Fig. 6. If particulate debris of any type enters the bearing surface region, the mode of wear can be changed to abrasive (Fig. 6B), and the magnitude of (UHMW-PE) particulate generation is significantly increased. Some reports have given total hip arthtoplasty acetabular component linear wear rates of 0.1–0.5 mm per year over 10- to 20-year clinical evaluation periods (Charnley et al. 1969; Charnley and Halley

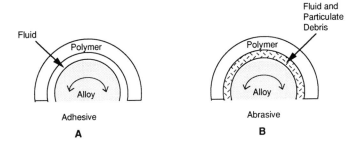

Fig. 6. Schematic representation of adhesive (**A**) and abrasive (**B**) wear conditions.

1975). This amount of polymer on a volume basis, if altered to particulates of micrometer dimensions during motion and wear, would represent a trillion or more particles distributed into the tissues of the host (McKellop 1994). This result, often called "Willert's phenomena" from early studies of Willert and co-workers, has significant biological implications (Willert and Buchhorn 1990). One of the concerns associated with the applications of recent modular designs using biological ingrowth for tissue fixation is that UHMW-PE particulates percolate along the device interfaces and can invade the bone tissues at localized regions in quantities capable of eliciting osteolytic reactions (Goldring et al. 1993). When severe, regional bone lysis has resulted in aseptic loosening and the loss of TJA constructs. In this context, most primary TJAs perform as intended (90–93% are never replaced), and conditions that result in a septic loosening and a need for revision over the long term occur in a low percentage (0–30%, depending upon the report) of the surviving device applications.

This same type of tissue interaction with particulate debris has been reported for other types of TJA, such as TMJ arthroplasty (AAOMS 1986) and for polymeric synthetic ligament replacements (Johnson et al. 1984). Reports associated with anterior cruciate ligament (ACL) devices introduced to orthopedic surgery showed that polymeric particulate debris could be generated during function through attachment site and condylar bone surface contacts with the ACL prosthesis. This debris was implicated in adverse soft and hard tissue reactions. One interesting correlation was the of polytetrafluoroethylene (PTFE) polymer in some THA, TMJ, and ACL devices. Debris from PTFE polymer devices has been recognized as an adverse particulate debris product for selected THA, TJA, and ACL devices (Charnley and Halley 1975; Johnson et al. 1984; AAOMS 1986). However, the results of a recent conference proceedings indicated that biological responses to particulate debris are more specific to the size and quantity of the debris than to the type of biomaterial (Macon et al. 1992).

Critical to the information described above is the need for more extensive and detailed analyses of devices and tissues retrieved from human applications. Another consideration is the need for a complete analysis of the numbers of devices that are lost due to specific phenomena, such as debris-originated tissue changes, as compared to those in place and functioning as anticipated. A combination of these interrelated data could then be used in benefit and risk assessments (Society for Biomaterials 1994).

From a research viewpoint, it would be beneficial to have separate information about the bulk and surface properties of biomaterials as components of devices versus information about reduced forms as particulates, ions, compounds, mers, and so forth. Also, more extensive standardized testing methods for evaluating biocompatibility profiles of synthetic biomaterials in different physical forms would be an advantage when associated with functional devices where biomechanical function is a simultaneously imposed test condition.

BIOMECHANICS

The mechanical and chemical property characteristics of implant biomaterials and designs directly influence device longevity (Williams 1982; von Recum 1986; Davies 1991; Morrey 1991; Petty 1991; ASTM 1992). Selected properties important to longevity include elastic modulus, ultimate tensile strength, elongation to fracture, and biomaterial surface chemistry (ASTM 1992).

Microstrain types and magnitudes along device-to-tissue interfaces can be determined, in part, by mechanical property similarities between the synthetic biomaterial and the adjacent tissue. For example, large differences in elastic moduli between the biomaterial and the adjacent tissue can result in microstrains that act as shear stress components along interfaces. In general, the biomaterial and design selections are made to minimize these types of strains. Microstrain distributions are controlled by providing design-based features (areas) along the implant surfaces that interdigitate with the tissues and thereby provide regions for force transfer where loading conditions are mostly compressive. Examples of biomaterial selections to minimize elastic modulus differences include low modulus polymers for soft tissue applications and higher modulus alloys and ceramics for applications with bone.

Biomaterial strength and elongation properties give measures of limits for force transfer, so that designs can be optimized to prevent the biomaterial structures from being broken down by functionally imposed mechanical stresses. To reemphasize a point made previously, the surface chemistry of the biomaterial and the attachment (or not) to the tissues are critical to the tissue interface conditions for biomechanical force transfer and stability. Therefore, to isolate biomaterial and biomechanical properties is not feasible, in that the in vivo function of devices includes a synergistic interaction among material and mechanical conditions.

BIOCOMPATIBILITY

The physical, mechanical, and chemical properties of surgical implant biomaterials are fundamental to initial tissue attachment after implantation and for stability over time. Because tissues change with function and aging, most devices are overdesigned to satisfy the extreme limits. In general, the strongest, most ductile, and most chemically inert biomaterials have been selected for device applications.

Another aspect of biocompatibility is the biomechanical responses of soft and hard tissue to mechanical loading. Studies have shown a direct relationship between microstrain magnitudes and tissue stabilities; for example, Fig. 7 presents mechanically induced microstrain magnitudes and bone stability relationships. As an extension of the microstrain data, when applied to surgical implant interfaces with bone, the data provide guidelines for prosthetic material and design selections. If stresses generated due to mechanical stress transfer result in microstrains of less than 1500, the bone would be expected to resorb over time due to "disuse" or low magnitude loading conditions (Roberts and Huiskies 1987; Cowin 1989). In contrast, if microstrains exceeded 2500 or greater, the local trauma could also result in bone resorption. Therefore, the designs of devices are selected in an attempt to achieve interfacial transfer conditions in the middle microstrain distribution range, so that the bone will be stabilized over time.

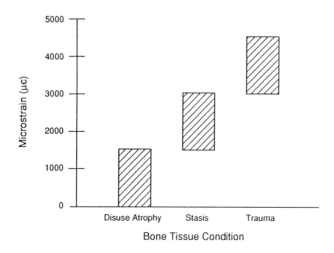

Fig. 7. Microstrain magnitudes and bone responses.

One of the more interesting and difficult questions to answer within the biomaterials and biomechanical research communities is the cause-effect relationship specific to why fibrous tissues exist adjacent to some inert biomaterial interfaces. For example, if evaluation of a device retrieved after some years of in vivo function demonstrates a fibrous tissue layer separating the biomaterial from the bone, why did the fibrous tissue zone evolve, given that device was originally placed in direct contact with bone?

Laboratory animal investigations have shown that selected biodegradation products (relatively reactive compounds) and larger concentrations of more inert substances (ions, mers, compounds, particulates, etc.) can cause bone to change into soft tissues. The reactive soft tissues that form could subsequently evolve to a passive fibrous tissue zone directly adjacent to prosthetic devices. Also, shear-oriented microstrains imposed during bone healing or improper (low or high) magnitude microstrains could also cause bone to evolve to soft tissue. Unfortunately, histological evaluations alone do not provide specific answers about the origin or dimensions of the fibrous tissue. In some situations, this type of soft tissue might be the more desirable functional condition (Branemark et al. 1985; Weiss 1986). Once again, a synergism exists between explanations based on either biomaterial (chemical) or biomechanical (mechanical) properties. This topic remains an active area for research.

In the area of biomechanical properties and the quantitative description of force transfer and its influence on tissue-to-biomaterial interfaces, finite element computer models and analyses are playing a significant role through enhancing the capabilities for expanded studies. The larger computer models using the capacities of supercomputer hard and software systems are leading to key insights into functional biomechanical properties for implant devices (Roberts and Huiskies 1987), another important area for expanded basic and applied research.

SUMMARY AND RECOMMENDATIONS

The various disciplines associated with the research, development, and applications of surgical implants have evolved significantly over the past three decades. Clearly, the ability to investigate biomaterial-to-tissue interfaces for all types of devices has advanced to a point where dimensions and concentrations can be measured at nanometer and nanogram levels. Models using supercomputers allow calculations of larger numbers of sample points (millions and above) from within three-dimensional models. Because of these capabilities, mechanisms of interactions between synthetic biomaterials and tissues are being evaluated more extensively and quantitatively. However, one limitation of this ever-increasing detail of study and specialization is a decrease in the multidisciplinary interactions among the professional disciplines. This chapter has attempted to demonstrate that important similarities exist among key issues related to prosthetic device attachments to tissue, functional motions, and wear-related phenomena, and that these issues span several surgical disciplines. Therefore, this firm recommendation is a strong proposal for increased levels of sponsored multidisciplinary interactions among the various surgical implant-related disciplines.

REFERENCES

AAOMS (American Association of Oral and Maxillofacial Surgeons), Review of Proplast® TMJ interpositional implants, Session at the annual meeting of the American Association of Oral and Maxillofacial Surgeons, New Orleans, La., September 1986.

ASTM (American Society for Testing and Materials), Annual Book of ASTM Standards, 13.01, Medical Implants, ASTM, Philadelphia, 1992.

Branemark, P.I., Zarb, G. and Albrektsson, T., Tissue Integrated Prostheses, Quintessence Publishing, Chicago, 1985.

Buchanan, R.A., Lemons, J.E., Griffin, C.D., Thompson, N.G. and Lucas, L.C., Effects of carbon coupling on the in vitro corrosion of cast surgical cobalt-base alloy, J. Biomed. Mater. Res., 15 (1981) 611–614.

Charnley, J. and Halley, D., Rate of wear in total hip replacement, Clin. Orthop., 112 (1975) 170.

Charnley, J., Kamangar, A. and Longfield, M., The optimum size of prosthetic heads in relation to the wear of plastic sockets in total replacement of the hip, Med. Biolog. Eng. Comput., 7 (1969) 31–67.

Cowin, S.C., Bone Biomechanics, CRC Press, Boca Raton, 1989.

Cranin, A. (Ed.), Entire issue of J. Oral Impl., 19 (1993).

Davies, J.E. (Ed.), The Bone-Biomaterial Interface, University of Toronto Press, Toronto, 1991.

Ferguson, A.B., Jr., Akahoshi, Y., Laing, P.G. and Hodge, E.S., Characteristics of trace ions released from embedded metal implants in the rabbit, J. Bone Joint Surg. (Am), 44A (1962) 323–336.

Fung, Y., Perrone, N. and Anliker, M., Biomechanics: Its Foundation and Objectives, Prentice-Hall, Englewood Cliffs, N.J., 1972.

Goldring, S., Clark, C. and Wright, T., The problem in total joint arthroplasty: aseptic loosening, J. Bone Joint Surg., 75A (1993) 799–802.

Homsy, C. and Armediades, C., Biomaterials for skeletal and cardiovascular applications, Biomedical Materials Symposium [special issue], J. Biomed. Mater. Res., 3 (1972).

Hulbert, S.F., Klawitter J.J., Lemons, J.E. and Wilson, C.N., Fabrication and evaluation of ceramic implant materials for replacement of teeth and bone: mechanical strength testing of highly porous calcium aluminate ceramics, Final Report: Contract no. NIH-70-2122, National Institutes of Health, Bethesda, Md., 1971.

Johnson, R., Eriksson, E., Haggmark, T. and Pope, M., Five to ten year follow-up evaluation after reconstruction of ACL, Clin. Orthop., 183 (1984) 122–140.

Lemons, J.E., Biomaterial considerations for dental implants, Part I: Metals and alloys, Alabama Academy of General Dentistry Sponsored Symposium on Dental Implants, J. Oral Impl., 4 (1975) 503–515.

Lemons, J.E., Dental implant retrieval analyses, J. Dent. Educ., 52 (1988) 748–756.

Lemons, J.E., Metals and alloys for devices in musculoskeletal surgery. In: B.F. Morrey (Ed.), Joint Replacement Arthroplasty, Churchill Livingstone, Edinburgh, 1991, pp. 13–21.

Lemons, J.E. and Phillips, R.W., Biomaterials for dental implants, In: C.E. Misch (Ed.), Contemporary Implant Dentistry, C.V. Mosby, St. Louis, 1991, pp. 259–278.

Macon, N.D., Lemons, J.E. and Niemann, K.M.W., Polymer particles in vivo: distribution in the knee, migration to lymph nodes and associated cellular response following ACL replacement. In: K. St. John (Ed.), ASTM Symposium on Particulate Debris from Medical Implants, ASTM STP 1144, ASTM, Philadelphia, 1992, p. 189.

McKellop, H., Presentation at the annual meeting of the Hip Society, American Academy of Orthopedic Surgeons, New Orleans, La., Feb. 1994.

McKellop, H., Clarke, I., Markolf, K. and Amstutz, H., Friction and wear properties of polymer, metal and ceramic prosthetic joint materials evaluated on a multichannel screening device, J. Biomed. Mater. Res., 15 (1981) 619–653.

McKinney, R.V., Jr. (Ed.), Endosteal Dental Implants, Mosby Year Book, St. Louis, 1991.

McLean, D., Mechanical Properties of Metals, Wiley, New York, 1962.

Morrey, B.F. (Ed.), Total Joint Arthroplasty, Churchill Livingstone, Edinburgh, 1991.

Morrey, B.F. (Ed.), Biological, Material, and Mechanical Considerations of Joint Replacement, Bristol-Myers Squibb/Zimmer Orthopaedic Symposium Series, Raven Press., New York, 1993.

Orthopaedic Research Society, Transactions of the 40th Annual Meeting of the Orthopaedic Research Society, New Orleans, La., 1994, Transactions of the Orthopaedic Research Society, Vol. 119, Secs. 1 and 2, 1994.

Petty, W. (Ed.), Total Joint Replacement, W. B. Saunders, Philadelphia, 1991.

Pilliar, R., Lee, J. and Maniatopoulos, C., Observations on the effect of movement on bone ingrowth into porous surfaced implants, Clin. Orthop., 208 (1986) 108–113.

Roberts, V.L. and Huiskies, R., Special issue on bone biomechanics, J. Biomech., 20 (1987).

Rubin, L.R. (Ed.), Biomaterials in Reconstructive Surgery, C. V. Mosby, St. Louis, 1983.

Society for Artificial Organs, Annual meeting, New Orleans, La., 1993.

Society for Biomaterials, Management requirements for a national implant data system, Paper presented at the planning conference of the Society for Biomaterials, Cape Cod, Mass., 1994.

von Recum, A. (Ed.), Handbook of Biomaterials Evaluation, Macmillan, New York, 1986.

Weiss, C.M., Tissue integration of dental endosseous implants: description and comparative analysis of fibro-osseous and osseous integration systems, J. Oral Impl., 12 (1986) 169–215.

Willert, H-G. and Buchhorn, G., Osteolysis in arthroplasty of the hip, Clin. Orthop., 258 (1990) 95–107.

Williams D.F., Biocompatibility of Orthopaedic Implants, Vol. I., CRC Press, Boca Raton, Fla., 1982.

Williams, D.F. and Roaf, R., Implants in Surgery, W.B. Saunders, Philadelphia, 1973.

Correspondence to: Jack E. Lemons, PhD, Professor and Director of Laboratory Research, Departments of Surgery and Biomaterials, 616 School of Dentistry Building, 1919 Seventh Avenue South, SDB Box 49, The University of Alabama at Birmingham, Birmingham, AL 35294-0007, USA. Tel: 205-934-9206; Fax: 205-975-6108.

Temporomandibular Disorders and Related Pain Conditions, Progress in Pain Research and Management, Vol. 4, edited by B.J. Sessle, P.S. Bryant, and R.A. Dionne, IASP Press, Seattle, © 1995.

17

Temporomandibular Joint Devices: Past, Present, and Future

Mark G. Fontenot

Department of Biomedical Engineering, Tulane University, New Orleans, Louisiana, USA

The use of temporomandibular joint (TMJ) devices in the United States escalated from a few in the mid-1960s, when Dow Corning (Midland, MI) labeled Silastic® brand sheeting for surgical correction of trismus, to thousands by 1986, when Vitek, Inc. (Houston, TX) developed and sold various TMJ devices such as the Proplast® TMJ Interpositional Implant (PTIPI) and the VK® (Vitek-Kent) Total TMJ Replacement System. In the late 1980s, TMJ Implants, Inc. (Golden, CO) and Techmedica, Inc. (Camarillo, CA) introduced production and custom TMJ devices, respectively.

However, in the early 1990s, patients, clinicians, and industry witnessed and endured widespread TMJ device failures. The most reported failures were associated with devices having an articular surface fabricated from Teflon® fluorinated ethylene propylene (FEP) (E.I. Dupont de Nemours and Co., Wilmington, DE) such as the VK I Teflon FEP fossa prosthesis (Vitek) and the PTIPI. In 1990, Vitek filed for voluntary bankruptcy, and the Food and Drug Administration (FDA) issued a safety alert and device recall directly affecting approximately 25,000 Proplast TMJ interpositional implants and indirectly affecting approximately 2000 VK prostheses. In January 1993, Dow Corning voluntarily suspended the sale of Silastic products for TMJ reconstruction. Also in 1993, OsteoMed (Dallas, TX) and Techmedica halted the sale of their custom TMJ devices. Presently, TMJ Implants, Inc., and ICSI (International Craniomandibular Surgical, Inc., La Crescenta, CA) are the only manufacturers offering production, noncustom devices for TMJ reconstruction.

Unfortunately, published engineering and clinical information is either sparse or lacking regarding TMJ biomechanics, the biomechanics of TMJ devices, prospective clinical outcomes surrounding various devices and associated treatment modalities, and the postoperative management of patients with and without artificial TMJ devices. At the same time, the population with TMJ devices is large and growing, challenging the dental and medical community and demanding outcomes data for devices and surgical modalities.

In an attempt to summarize events and issues surrounding TMJ devices, both past and present, this chapter relates the history of the development of TMJ devices. Because the literature is replete with articles discussing the performance of TMJ devices manufactured by Vitek, Inc., the chapter reviews the development of the VK TMJ System and the PTIPI. Finally, it presents a protocol for TMJ device development based on engineering design principles.

THE PAST: LESSONS FROM HISTORY

The challenge of surgically restoring mobility to osteoarthritic joints has captured the imagination of many surgeons throughout this century. Between 1940 and 1950, the brothers Judet in Paris, France, received acclaim for their acrylic femoral head prosthesis. The Judets based their choice of material on reported biocompatibility of acrylics in soft tissue and on rather limited mechanical testing (Eftekhar 1986). Continued problems with device failure, excessive wear, and loosening compelled the Judet brothers to abandon the prosthesis in the mid-1950s.

The Judet hip arthroplasty technique illustrated the short-term benefits of alloplastic hip arthroplasty. Intrigued by the Judet experience, Sir John Charnley began to concentrate his efforts on the biomechanics of materials and devices for alloplastic hip arthroplasty (Eftekhar 1986; Older 1986). In 1954, Charnley encountered a patient with a Judet acrylic femoral head replacement. Upon examination, he heard squeaking emanating from the alloplastic hip, indicating motion, contact, and friction. Inspired by his interest in joint physiology, Charnley performed experiments measuring physical quantities related to hip arthroplasty such as the coefficients of friction of articular cartilage against various materials with and without synovial fluid. Given the paucity of materials known and tried for alloplastic reconstruction at this time, Charnley concluded there was no hope of designing an artificial hip using synovial fluid as a lubricant (Eftekhar 1986). From these considerations, he decided in 1958 that the only viable option for alloplastic hip replacement was to consider materials that were intrinsically slippery between contacting surfaces, i.e., materials having low coefficients of friction.

Fluorocarbons such as Fluon® PTFE (polytetrafluoroethylene) type G-1 and G-2 (ICI, Ltd., London, UK) and Teflon TFE (tetrafluoroethylene) and Teflon FEP were, and are known, to have low coefficients of friction (Homsy 1982). Fluon PTFE and Teflon became commercially available in the late

1940s, and by the 1950s these fluorocarbons were used as implantable devices for cardiovascular prostheses (Girvin et al. 1956; Harrison 1957). In the late 1940s, animal studies were beginning to appear in the literature documenting tissue reactions to fluorocarbon polymers (Leveen and Barbario 1949). One report observed the formation of fibrosarcomata in rodents after implantation of Teflon films (Oppenheimer et al. 1952).

In a letter to Leidholt (Leidholt and Gorman 1965), Scurderi reported on limited clinical trials of a Teflon TFE acetabular prosthesis in 1958. He originally used a Teflon acetabular cup shaped like a Smith-Petersen mold to separate the steel femoral head from acetabular bone, but found that the Teflon deformed and showed wear. Scurderi also reported a foreign body reaction to Teflon particulate wear debris (Leidholt and Gorman 1965).

Charnley first attempted to resurface the acetabulum with a thin Fluon PTFE shell and encased the femoral condyle in a metal hollow ball (Eftekhar 1986). The early results were positive, but the in situ performance rapidly declined after 9 to 12 months. In a modified procedure, Charnley used a large diameter metal femoral head prosthesis against an acetabulum lined with a thin shell of PTFE. Again, the early results were positive, but in situ performance dramatically declined within 12 months, the first evidence that Fluon PTFE did not perform well in situ as a bearing material (Eftekhar 1986; Older 1986).

Critical in the development of an alloplastic hip was information surrounding the in situ service and environmental conditions of the hip such as load and contact geometry. Because this information was not available at the time, Charnley found it necessary to evaluate new device designs by clinical experimentation. In 1958, Charnley altered his technique and device design and implanted an alloplastic hip replacement employing stainless steel as the alloplastic stem and femoral head, which articulated against an acetabular cup fabricated from Fluon PTFE. As before, Charnley continued to fabricate acetabular cups fabricated from Fluon PTFE because of its commercial reputation as a material with a low coefficient of friction and chemical inertness (Charnley and Kamangar 1969).

After 300 total hip procedures, significant clinical problems compelled Charnley to abandon the Fluon PTFE acetabular cup and remove and revise the hip prosthesis (Charnley and Kamangar 1969; Eftekhar 1986; Older 1986). In 1969, Charnley reported on the wear rates of 100 stainless steel/Fluon PTFE total hip prostheses that had been removed from patients (Charnley and Kamangar 1969). Revision surgeries were necessary because failed or failing Fluon PTFE acetabular cups generated massive amounts of wear debris that caused "teflonomas," an undesirable tissue reaction producing pain and limited range of motion. In many of the cases the Fluon PTFE acetabular components had worn through.

Some of the mechanical and material properties of alloplastic-bearing materials considered in the design of the soft side in joint replacement are creep (or cold flow) and tensile strength. Soft side components fabricated from materials with low resistance to cold flow coupled with low tensile and yield strengths are not candidate materials for use in alloplastic joint devices. Materials possessing these characteristics have a high propensity to deform, wear, break down into particles, and fragment, which was vividly underscored by the clinical performance of fluorocarbon acetabular cups. The catastrophic performance of Fluon PTFE acetabular cups was attributed to its low resistance to cold flow and low yield strength, which deterred Charnley from further implantation due to the deleterious consequences of massive amounts of Fluon PTFE wear debris (Wright 1982).

However, Charnley and Kamangar (1969) did not feel that cold flow was a significant problem with Fluon PTFE. They described an experiment in which a 22-mm steel ball had been loaded into a socket machined into a block of PTFE. Under a static load of 76.3 kgf (kilograms force), no detectable deformity had manifested after more than seven years. Under this level of loading the mean contact pressure in the bearing was slightly below the static load carrying capacity of the PTFE, which is 2 MPa (Wright 1982). Therefore, excessive cold flow would not theoretically have been expected under these conditions. The static-load carrying capacity of PTFE was probably exceeded in many of the cases examined by Charnley and Kamangar (1969), and that cold flow may have contributed a significant portion to the apparent wear (Wright 1982).

At the 1963 Meeting of the American Academy of Orthopaedic Surgeons, Charnley stated that he no longer used Teflon (Leidholt and Gorman 1965). Charnley and the orthopedic community abandoned the use of PTFE fluorocarbon polymers in alloplastic joint arthroplasty in the 1960s because of better wear performance of ultra-high molecular weight polyethylene (UPE). Mechanical and material failure of PTFE generated large volumes of wear debris leading to premature clinical failures of these stainless steel/PTFE hips. Charnley reported that wear particles of PTFE gave rise to caseating granulomatous reaction seen histologically as amorphous, granular, slightly eosinophilic areas with large populations of foreign body giant cells (Homsy 1981). He postulated that the caseous material was the result of dead phagocytic giant cells that could not keep pace with the massive production of PTFE wear debris.

Charnley continued to report on the catastrophic failure of Fluon PTFE to the biomedical community. In 1976, he found the average clinical penetrative wear rate of PTFE to be 2.26 mm per year using a 22-mm diameter femoral head, whereas that for RCH 1000 UPE was observed to be 0.15 mm per year, a 15-fold difference (Wright 1982). His notion of selecting Fluon PTFE as the soft side bearing material in the alloplastic hip because of its low coefficient of friction and its reputation for chemical inertness proved to be calamitous. His experiences with fluorocarbon polymers have taught orthopedic surgeons a great lesson in selecting materials for the soft side components in joint prostheses.

In the late 1960s, Homsy, a professional chemical engineer, acquired a wealth of knowledge as an employee of E.I. Dupont de Nemours concerning Teflon fluorocarbon polymers such as Teflon PTFE and Teflon FEP. In the early 1970s, Homsy introduced Proplast, a porous composite material that was designed to stabilize devices by allowing fixations through the in-growth of tissue into its porous structure (Homsy et al. 1973). Proplast initially consisted of Teflon PTFE and vitreous carbon, and the resultant structure was both fibrous and porous with pore volume between 70 and 90 volume percent, with pore sizes between 50 and 400 microns and interpore connections greater than 80 microns. Eventually, Proplast was succeeded by Proplast II (Teflon PTFE – aluminum oxide) and Proplast HA (Teflon PTFE – hydroxylapatite).

In the 1970s, Homsy designed and fabricated devices for mandibular condyle resurfacing and TMJ disk replacement. These devices were manufactured using Teflon FEP film (10–15 mils) laminated to Proplast. In the early 1980s, he developed the VK I bilaminate polymer glenoid fossa prosthesis for partial and total TMJ reconstruction. The prosthesis consisted of a superior layer of Proplast II porous material laminated to a Nomex® (polyalamide fabric, Dupont) reinforced Teflon FEP bearing surface. Teflon FEP polymer thickness was 2 mm at the depth of the fossa prosthesis.

Criteria for selecting Teflon FEP as an alloplastic bearing surface was outlined by Homsy in 1986 when Kent and his co-workers (Kent et al. 1986) published their initial clinical experiences with the VK I Teflon FEP fossa prosthesis. Homsy selected Teflon FEP polymer in part on the basis of wear data he accumulated while investigating the rheological properties of sodium carboxymethylcellulose (SCMC) (Homsy et al. 1973; Kent et al. 1986). In 1973, Homsy used an apparatus designed by Lewis (1963) for measuring surface wear and friction of candidate prosthetic joint materials. The design was modified to measure rheological properties of SCMC-based pseudosynovial fluids (PSF) by using a thrust washer principle wherein an annulus of experimental material was rotated against a disk of mating material made from cobalt-chromium-molybdenum (Co-Cr-Mo) submerged in a reservoir of PSF. The pattern of cyclic loading attempted to mimic normal walking by imposing a square-wave oscillating load history at five times body weight, at a frequency of 36 cycles per minute, with a relative of speed of 5 cm/second between test and mating materials. Homsy et al. (1973) reported the drag profiles of PSF lubricants when Co-Cr-Mo was mated against high molecular weight polyethylene at a test stress of 6.67 kg/cm^2 (0.65 MPa) (Homsy et al. 1973). Wear rates were not given for polyethylene or any other materials.

In 1986, Homsy cited wear data of materials using the 1973 apparatus described above (Kent et al. 1986). Although, only rheological properties of PSF were published in 1973, wear rates were disclosed in 1986 for Teflon FEP, polyoxymethylene, acrylic, and Co-Cr-Mo. Results indicate that Teflon FEP polymer (0.018 mm/100,000 cycles) and polyoxymethylene (0.022 mm/100,000 cycles) had similar penetrative wear rates, acrylic (0.111 mm/100,000 cycles) had a less desirable rate, and Co-Cr-Mo showed galling and catastrophic wear (Kent et al. 1986).

Homsy in 1986 provided the qualification of test load and apparatus used to evaluate Teflon FEP polymer (Kent et al. 1986). Homsy indicated that the 1973 testing stress of 12 kg/cm^2 corresponded to a 12-kg total load across the TMJ, assuming that the effective articular interface between the condyle and fossa was on the order of 1 cm^2 (Kent et al. 1986). He cited from the dental literature and formulated the following biomechanical scenario. Normal bite force in the adult was reported to be 21 kgf (Hylander 1975), resulting in a single condylar reaction force of 75–80% of the biting force (Smith 1978). Subsequently, Homsy concluded that the maximum force through a single condyle corresponding to a normal bite force was 12.6 kg, thus correlating well with the test load he used in evaluating Teflon FEP polymer some 13 years earlier.

Although separated by 20 years, Charnley and Homsy selected the fluorocarbon polymers Fluon PTFE and Teflon FEP, respectively, primarily because of their low coefficients of friction. In both cases, these polymers incurred loading histories that exceeded the elastic limits of these materials, resulting in mechanical failure and explantation. Presumably, like Charnley, Homsy felt that cold flow was not a problem. Ironically, just as Charnley implanted PTFE acetabular components in 1958 only to have UPE ensue in 1962, the Teflon FEP fossa prosthesis was introduced by Vitek in 1982, only to be replaced in 1986 by UPE.

THE PRESENT: WHERE ARE WE NOW?

Techniques for TMJ alloplastic reconstruction can be categorized as interpositional arthroplasty, hemiarthroplasty or partial reconstruction, and total TMJ arthroplasty or total TMJ replacement.

TMJ devices intended for interpositional arthroplasty are placed either permanently or temporarily after surgical removal of the TMJ disk. Silastic medical grade sheeting, Silastic HP sheeting, Silastic TMJ implant HP (Wilkes Design), and the PTIPI were labeled and intended for use as devices in interpositional arthroplasty. These devices were positioned between the condyle and fossa and secured to the zygomatic arch with either sutures, wires, or screws. Presently, devices intended for interpositional arthroplasty are not commercially available.

TMJ devices intended for partial reconstruction of the TMJ are used to resurface either the mandibular condyle or glenoid fossa. The TMJ Fossa-Eminence™ Prosthesis System (TMJ Implants, Inc.) and the Articular Eminence Prosthesis (ICSI) are commercially available devices intended to resurface the fossa. These devices are secured to the zygomatic arch with screws.

TMJ devices intended for total TMJ replacement are placed to simultaneously resurface and replace the mandibular condyle and glenoid fossa. TMJ Implants, Inc., and ICSI market the only production devices for total TMJ replacement. The design and utilization of materials for these devices are the same. In particular, the alloplastic fossa prosthesis is fabricated from Co-Cr-Mo. The fossa prosthesis provides a trough for articulation with an alloplastic condyle formed of heat-cured polymethylmethacrylate (PMMA) onto a cast Co-Cr-Mo shank. Both, the condylar and fossa prostheses are secured to the mandible and zygomatic arch with screws.

OsteoMed and Techmedica offered custom devices for total TMJ replacement. OsteoMed's devices consist of a UPE fossa fastened to the zygomatic arch with screws and cemented with PMMA cement. The corresponding condylar prosthesis is fabricated from titanium alloy and Co-Cr-Mo and attached to the mandible with screws. Techmedica has offered custom TMJ devices since 1989. Techmedica's devices consist of a fossa prosthesis fabricated from titanium and UPE, with a condylar prosthesis fabricated from titanium and Co-Cr-Mo. The fossa and condylar prosthesis are secured to the bones in the joint with screws. Custom devices offered by OsteoMed and Techmedica are no longer available .

THE FUTURE: PROTOCOL FOR TMJ DEVICE DEVELOPMENT AND COMMERCIALIZATION

Designing for TMJ device safety and establishing effectiveness is a delicate interaction between engineering considerations and principles, surgical techniques and requirements, functional demand, anatomical boundary limitations, and material biocompatibility. Fig. 1 presents a protocol for TMJ device

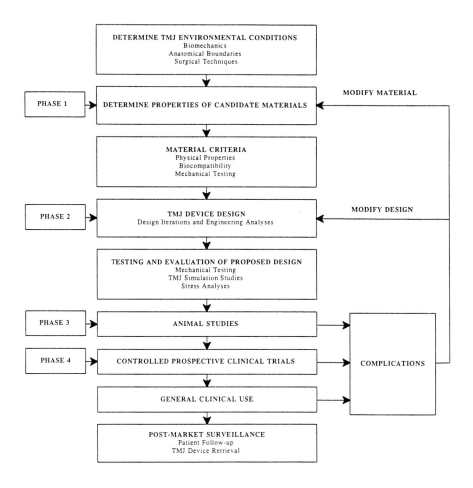

Fig. 1. Flow chart of a TMJ device development program.

development incorporating engineering design principles and clinical science.

In determining the service conditions for any TMJ device, the design team should have an understanding of the biomechanics of the TMJ, anatomical conditions, and the surgical techniques used to place the device. Once the design team has researched and assembled the services conditions in the joint and theoretical parameters for design, then design variations are contemplated and subjected to testing in the following manner.

PHASE 1: CRITERIA AND SCREENING OF MATERIALS

Phase 1 is a materials screening process to test and evaluate potential candidate materials. Those that satisfy minimum performance standards, such as mechanical strength and physical properties important in production of the device, become qualified for fabrication in end-use TMJ devices. Effects of sterilization on the properties of materials for consideration also should be addressed and possibly measured. The physical properties of candidate materials used in TMJ device fabrication can be measured by employing a variety of simple standard laboratory and mechanical testing procedures. Data concerning bulk physical properties such as static and fatigue strengths are often available from the raw materials supplier; however, additional information may be needed depending on standards that have been set by the TMJ device manufacturer regarding minimum values for bulk properties. Simple wear-screening devices, such as those reported in International Standards Organization 6474 (Ring-on-Disk) and American Society of Testing and Materials F 732-82 (Pin-on-Flat), may present an adequate method to assess resistance to wear and fatigue. In particular, accelerated laboratory wear testing of materials can offer efficient, low-cost techniques for evaluating many different materials while varying parameters such as geometry of mating surfaces and loading histories. Mechanisms of wear may also be identified and wear debris collected and examined or placed in laboratory animals to assess biocompatibility. If the proper physical properties are known or accessible through materials suppliers or testing laboratories, then the design process may proceed to Phase 2.

PHASE 2: IN VITRO EVALUATION OF THE PROPOSED TMJ DEVICE DESIGNS

Phase 2 is a TMJ device screening process to evaluate various designs under conditions that attempt to mimic the in vivo biomechanical environment. TMJ simulators can be constructed to screen device designs and material usages at this level of development. Evaluation of end-use TMJ device designs is costly because testing becomes significantly more complete with the introduction of simulation methods that require mechanization and machining of components that closely approximate the in vivo situation, as well as fabrication of iterative designs of potential end-use TMJ devices. Other information and important measurements can be collected from simulation such as wear debris, material creep, fatigue, and design integrity. However, we must be fully aware of the limitations of in vitro testing, because the in vivo situation is difficult and complicated to reproduce.

In Phase 2 evaluation of a TMJ device design, the most important mechanical properties of polymers used in TMJ reconstruction are the yield stress, creep resistance, and wear. The yield or flow stress controls whether instantaneous plastic deformation will occur under set prescribed loading conditions. Plastic deformation is critical because it can significantly increase wear and distort the implant. Under the influence of sustained loading forces, either compressive or tensile, polymers exhibit varying degrees of viscoelastic behavior and their deformation under loading increases with time, a characteristic known as cold flow. The static-load carrying capacity of a metal/polymer bearing assembly, such as a TMJ device, is governed by the magnitude of the compressive load to be supported. The bearing capacity is the mean surface pressure and is determined by dividing the applied compressive load by the projected support area of the bearing. For UPE the permissible mean surface pressure is 10 N/mm^2 (10 MPa), whereas for fluorocarbons such as PTFE and FEP it is on the order of 2 N/mm^2 (2 MPa). The limiting factor in a metal/polymer bearing in which the sliding partners move slowly or operate under full-fluid film lubrication, such as prosthetic joints, is the static-load carrying capacity of the bearing.

In 1988, Fontenot et al. reported on the laboratory wear performance of the PTIPI, VK I Teflon FEP, VK II UPE, and Silastic HP Sheeting. All devices were tested until failure; Table I gives the failure criteria based on accelerated in vitro wear testing. Penetrative wear rates per 100,000 cycles, at a 20-pound load, were calculated by dividing the average service life cycles of the implant by the thickness of the articular surface then presenting this value as a ratio per 100,000 cycles. Results from wear testing are given in Table II.

Wear testing created a wear trough coinciding with the path of oscillation of the VK condyle in all TMJ devices tested. In the PTIPI and VK I Teflon FEP fossa prosthesis, formation of the wear trough occurred simultaneous to structural deformation of the PTIPI and the VK I, which resulted from varying degrees of axial consolidation of the Proplast II and creep of the Teflon FEP surface. Microscopic inspection of the PTIPI revealed failure of the Teflon

Table I
Criteria to determine TMJ device failure using a TMJ simulator

TMJ Device	Criteria for Failure
PTIPI	Wear through the Teflon FEP surface
VK I and VK II	Wear through the Teflon FEP or UPE surface and into the Nomex fabric
Silastic HP Sheeting	Wear through the Silastic HP elastomer and into the Dacron fabric

Table II
Results from wear testing devices using a TMJ simulator

TMJ Device	Penetrative Wear Rate* (mm/100,000 cycles)
PTIPI	2.29
VK I FEP Fossa	1.18
VK II UPE Fossa	0.01
Silastic HP Sheeting	8.67

Source: Fontenot 1992a,b.
*20-lb load using a VK II condyle. TMJ devices were tested until failure defined in Table I.

FEP surfaces by a combination of wear-through coupled with fracture and fragmentation. Closer inspection at higher magnification reveals fracturing of the Teflon FEP surface, particulate wear debris, and areas of delamination of the Teflon FEP from Proplast II. Failure of the Teflon FEP surface resulted from material fatigue and thinning of the Teflon FEP film in the axial direction from wear, and thinning of the FEP film from material creep.

The in vitro implant service life and service cycles at a 20-pound load for the 1.3-mm PTIPI tested was 11.35 ($\pm$ 1.14) hours and 21,786 ($\pm$ 2188) cycles, respectively. The thickness of the Teflon FEP film of the PTIPI surface ranges from 10 mils (0.5 mm) to 15 mils (0.75 mm). Therefore, the range of values for the penetrative wear rate per 100,000 cycles was calculated to be 2.29 mm/100,000 cycles and 3.44 mm/100,000 cycles for Teflon thicknesses of 10 mils and 15 mils, respectively. The thickness Teflon FEP articular surface from a VK Teflon FEP fossa prosthesis is on the order of 2 mm. Dividing the average in vivo service life cycles of the VK Teflon FEP fossa by the Teflon FEP thickness of the articular surface gives an average linear wear rate of 1.184 mm/100,000 cycles at a load of 20 pounds.

PHASE 3: ANIMAL STUDIES

Animal experiments are commonly used for biofunctional device evaluation and biocompatibility testing. Some advantages of using animal models include biocompatibility assessment of material components, biologic response to wear debris, and biomechanical performance of the device. Some shortcomings of animal studies are unknown device loading and load history, miniaturization and modification of TMJ devices to accommodate anatomy, and compromised surgical placement due to lack of instrumentation or size of the animal's TMJ. Nevertheless, animal studies can provide significant insight into the performance of devices used in TMJ reconstruction. Although, qualification of a particular animal model as well as the corresponding miniature device can be difficult and costly, animal studies remain an important factor in the development of TMJ devices.

PHASE 4: CLINICAL TRIALS AND GENERAL USE EVALUATION

The most critical phase in the development of a device is encountered when the TMJ device is introduced into controlled clinical trials. At this phase, the clinical utility of a particular device is measured as well as the risks and benefits. If controlled clinical trials prove that the device is safe and effective, then the device may be released for general use under the statutes and guidelines set forth in the Medical Device Amendments of the Food, Drug, and Cosmetic Act of 1976 and the Safe Medical Device Act of 1990.

Biomechanical evaluation and clinical performance of devices can be assessed using a variety of methods and techniques. TMJ device retrieval and analysis provides essential information for TMJ device design protocols (Fig. 1). For example, we can correlate the effects of function to device integrity. In addition, examination of a removed implant also yields information concerning the in vivo performance of the implant, enhances conventional clinical data, and allows engineers to validate and qualify designs.

DISCUSSION

More than 500,000, and perhaps as many as 1,000,000 new patients seek some form of conservative management for their TMJ disorders each year from approximately 140,000 dental professionals (Fontenot 1992b). In other words, up to 0.4% of the U.S. population may seek some form of professional attention for a TMJ problem this year. Patients suffering from TMJ pathology and dysfunction commonly have facial pain and limited range of mandibular motion that can affect chewing, swallowing, and speech. Conservative management of these patients includes splint therapy, physical therapy, orthodontic therapy, adjustment of the teeth and occlusion, biofeedback, and pharmacologic therapy. If conservative management has been exhausted with limited results, such as failing to alleviate pain and/or limited range of motion, then surgical intervention with or without TMJ devices may be considered.

The art and armamentarium involved in TMJ surgery has experienced a dramatic increase since the mid-1980s. In 1988, as many as 42,000 TMJ arthroscopies and 35,000 open joint TMJ surgeries were performed in the United States. By 1991, those totals had risen to approximately 100,000 arthroscopies and 45,000 open joint procedures (Fontenot 1992b). Since 1965, at least 600,000 patients in the United States have had at least one TMJ surgery. Of these patients, 60,000 to 80,000 have received TMJ devices such as VK devices and other technologies developed and sold by Dow Corning and TMJ Implants, Inc. (Fontenot 1992b).

Currently, an estimated 4,000 TMJs annually undergo total TMJ reconstruction with either TMJ devices or autogenous rib grafts. Approximately 80% of these reconstructions are performed with rib grafts and the remaining 20% with TMJ devices. The performance and survivorship of rib grafts and TMJ devices used in total TMJ replacement is unknown. The estimated average age of the patients undergoing alloplastic TMJ replacement is approximately 35, with revision alloplastic TMJ replacement rates on the order of every three to seven years, which results in a substantial recurring patient population. It is estimated that the average patient who has undergone alloplastic TMJ arthroplasty may have as many as five revision arthroplasties over the lifetime. Consequently, the oral and maxillofacial surgical community desires an appropriate technology to service a large and growing population of patients requiring TMJ reconstruction.

In summary, TMJ device design and qualification is a delicate interaction between engineering considerations and principles, surgical technique and requirements, functional demand, anatomical boundary conditions, and biocompatibility. Clearly, the mechanobiological consequences of TMJ devices need to be evaluated. Poor TMJ device design and material selection has led to poor clinical outcome, premature revision surgery, and device failure. Biomechanical expectations from TMJ devices that have been prudently tested and evaluated should offer the surgical community and patient population predictable and reliable device.

REFERENCES

Charnley, J. and Kamangar, A., The optimum size of prosthetic heads in relation to wear of plastic sockets in total replacement of the hip, Med. Biol. Eng., 7 (1969) 31.
Eftekhar, N.S., The life and work of John Charnley, Clin. Ortho., 211 (1986) 10.
Fontenot, M.G., Biomechanical and clinical performance of TMJ devices, AAOMS scientific sessions, J. Oral Maxillofac. Surg., 51 (suppl.) 51 (1992a) 76.
Fontenot, M.G., Performance of TMJ devices. In: U.S. House Committee on Government Operations, Are FDA and NIH Ignoring the Dangers of TMJ-Jaw Implants?: Hearings before the House Committee on Government Operations, 102nd Cong., 4 June, 1992b.
Fontenot, M.G. and Kent, J.N., In vitro wear performance of Proplast TMJ disc implants, J. Oral Maxillofac. Surg., 50 (1992) 133.
Girvin, G.W., Wilhelm, M.C. and Merendino, K.A., The use of Teflon fabric as arterial grafts: an experimental study in dogs, Am. J. Surg., 92 (1956) 240.
Harrison, J.H., The use of Teflon as a blood vessel replacement in experimental animals, Surg. Gynecol. Obstet., 104 (1957) 81.
Homsy, C.A., Biocompatibility of perfluorinated polymers and composites of these polymers. In: D.F. Williams (Ed.), Biocompatibility of Clinical Implant Materials, Vol. II, CRC Series in

Compatibility, CRC Press, Boca Raton, Fla., 1982, pp. 60–73.

Homsy, C.A., Stanley, R.F. and King, J.W., Pseudosynovial fluids based on sodium carboxymeth-ylcellulose. In: Gabelnick and Litt (Eds.), Rheology of Biological Systems, C.C. Thomas, Springfield, Ill., 1973, pp. 278–298.

Hylander, W.L., The human mandible: lever or link? Am. J. Phys. Anthropol. 43 (1975) 227.

Kent, J.N., Block, M.S., Homsy, C.A., Prewitt, J.M. and Reid, R., Experience with a polymer glenoid fossa prothesis for partial or total TMJ reconstruction, J. Oral Maxillofac. Surg., 44 (1986) 520.

Leveen, H.H. and Barbario, J.R., Tissue reaction to plastics used in surgery with special reference to Teflon, Ann. Surg., 124 (1974) 49.

Leidholt, J.D. and Gorman, H.A., Teflon hip prosthesis in dogs, J. Bone Joint Surg. Am., 47 (1965) 1414.

Lewis, R.B., Wear of plastics: evaluation for engineering application, ASME Publication 83-WA-325, ASME, New York, 1963.

Older, J., A tribute to Sir John Charnley, Clin. Orthop., 211 (1986) 23.

Oppenheimer, B.S., Oppenheimer, E.T. and Hodge, E., Sarcomas induced in rats by embedding various plastic films, Proc. Soc. Exp. Biol. Med., 79 (1952) 336.

Smith, R.J., Mandibular biomechanics and temporomandibular joint function in primates, Am. J. Phys. Anthropol., 49 (1978) 341.

Wright, K.W.J., Friction and wear of materials and joint replacement prosthesis. In: D.F. Williams (Ed.), Biocompatibility of Orthopedic Implants, Vol. 2, CRC Series in Biocompatibility, CRC Press, Boca Raton, Fla., 1982, pp. 141–196.

Correspondence to: Mark G. Fontenot, DDS, MEng, 229 Marilyn Dr., Lafayette, LA 70503, USA. Tel: 318-988-3805; Fax: 318-988-3831.

Temporomandibular Disorders and Related Pain Conditions, Progress in Pain Research and Management, Vol. 4, edited by B.J. Sessle, P.S. Bryant, and R.A. Dionne, IASP Press, Seattle, © 1995.

18

Animal Models of Temporomandibular Disorders: How to Choose

Susan W. Herring

Department of Orthodontics, University of Washington, Seattle, Washington, USA

The characteristics of human temporomandibular* joints (TMJs) may not be adequately mimicked by common laboratory animals, calling into question the relevance of animal research. The choice of a model should depend on the question being asked. For normal TMJ function, the questions asked typically require that the animal model have comparable anatomy, occlusion, jaw movements, and biomechanics to those of humans. Some of these criteria are violated even by nonhuman primates, and all are violated by the commonly used rodents (rats, mice, guinea pigs) and carnivorans† (cats and dogs).

FORM AND FUNCTION OF THE TMJ

The morphological and functional variation in the TMJ is astonishing. Even the presence of a disk is variable. In monotremes and many marsupials, particularly carnivorous species, the disk is absent (Sprinz 1965). Even among placental mammals the disk can be lost as a simple developmental consequence of fetal paralysis (Herring and Lakars 1981).

The shapes of all TMJ components vary, and this variation is clearly correlated with the movements occurring at the joint. For example, in carnivorans the TMJ permits little if any protrusion, the movements being

---

* The term *temporomandibular* will be used throughout this chapter even though most of the animals discussed do not, strictly speaking, have a temporal bone. Instead, the petrosal and squamosal bones remain independent, so the jaw joint is actually "squamomandibular."

† This term refers to animals in the order Carnivora; it is not synonymous with "carnivores." For example, the giant panda is a carnivoran but is not a carnivore, and many people are carnivores but none are carnivorans.

rotation around a horizontal axis and to a lesser degree lateral translation (Scapino 1965). Correspondingly, the articulating surfaces are congruent and hingelike, and the disk is thin and uniform in thickness (Ström et al. 1988). In both function and morphology, the carnivoran TMJ is clearly an unsuitable model for humans.

Other mammals do exhibit protrusive movements of the condyles. Rodent TMJs are typically very long compared to their width, which is usually ascribed to the protrusion required for incision and considered an asset, because humans also protrude for incision. However, relative to body size, rodent protrusion is far more extensive than is ever seen in humans (Weijs 1975). Moreover, not only incision but also mastication in rodents relies on a long protrusive stroke of the working-side condyle, a mechanism that differs radically from the human power stroke, in which the working-side condyle rotates rather than translates.

It might be thought that animals with pronounced lateral grinding movements, such as rabbits and ungulates, would have TMJs similar to the human. Indeed, rabbits have emerged as the preferred model for TMDs (Macher et al. 1992; Ali et al. 1993). But rabbits actually resemble rodents in having small condyles in troughlike fossae and disks that are peaked in transverse section (Sprinz 1965; Weijs and Dantuma 1981). Sheep and goats contrast with humans in a different way. Their condyles are concave rather than convex, and their disks have elastic fibers in the center and venous sinuses in the front rather than the rear (Gillbe 1973). Furthermore, mastication in rabbits and ungulates such as sheep differs fundamentally from human chewing. In these animals the molar teeth form inclined planes that control the direction of the power stroke. In primates the low cusps of the teeth are much less important, the direction of the power stroke being determined instead by precise control of the musculature (Herring 1993a). The only domestic animal with a comparable dentition is the pig.

On grounds of morphology and masticatory movements, the closest resemblance to the human condition is found in other higher primates (monkeys and apes). Surprisingly, pigs are nearly as similar, perhaps even more so in details of disk anatomy (Ström et al. 1986; Bermejo et al. 1993). Both higher primates and pigs have bunodont dentitions, TMJ components like those of humans, and a short, muscle-controlled transverse power stroke. However, neither monkeys nor pigs are ideal models, differing from humans in occlusion, muscle orientation, TMJ configuration, and masticatory movements (Herring 1976; Byrd et al. 1978).

Whatever the anatomy of the joint in a species, functional manipulation can cause modification (Tuominen et al. 1993). The disk as well can be transformed by a change in function (Ferrari and Herring, unpublished observations). Adaptive remodeling reminds us that function determines form in a proximate sense as well as an evolutionary one. The sizes and shapes of TMJ components vary, both among and within species. Size correlates well with the magnitude of loading (Smith et al. 1983). The mechanism that matches joint size and loading is also probably growth rather than natural selection (Herring 1993b).

MUSCLE FORCES AND JOINT LOADING

Joint biomechanics has been repeatedly emphasized as the key to TMJ structure, function, malfunction, and repair. Loading is also a crucial element in regulating growth. Unfortunately, the theoretical predictions are complex and need to be validated by experimental measurements. Moreover, the loading of the human TMJ is a hotly debated topic, so it is not clear exactly what we should be modeling. In fact, the argument has become somewhat circular in that the only in vivo data available are from monkeys (Hylander and Bays 1979; Boyd et al. 1990), and these are usually simply assumed to hold true for humans as well.

Direction and magnitude of TMJ loading are byproducts of contracting jaw muscles. A simple static analysis of muscle vectors demonstrates that some laboratory animals differ strikingly from humans (Fig. 1). Most obvious as bad models are the rodents, frequently chosen for growth studies. Rodents have anteriorly positioned jaw muscles, with vectors typically passing through the bite point. Therefore, the mandible does not function as a lever and the TMJ is unloaded during mastication (Weijs and Dantuma 1975), quite different from the human condition. The extrapolation of rat data to humans, for example on the effect of functional appliances on condylar growth, is clearly not justified.

In other mammals, including humans, the jaw muscles are located more posteriorly and the resultant vector seldom if ever passes through the bite point; thus the mandible functions as a third-class lever and the TMJ is loaded in compression. However, there are still many variations (Fig. 1). The closer the resultant muscle force is to the bite point, the lower the reaction force on the joint. Thus, the highly protrusive orientation of the muscle resultant in rabbits (Weijs and Dantuma 1981) suggests lower TMJ loading than in higher primates and pigs. This light loading probably accounts for the small TMJs in rabbits.

The orientation of the load is also an important source of variation. The dominance of the temporalis muscle in carnivorans leads to a posteriorly inclined resultant (Fig. 1). Such a load along the axis of the condylar neck is

Fig. 1. Position of the jaw muscle resultant in representative mammals (not to scale). **a:** Rat. The resultant passes through the bite point, so the bite force equals the muscle force and the TMJ is not loaded. **b:** Rabbit. **c:** Pig. **d:** Human. **e:** Dog. Because the resultant is posterior to the bite point in b–e, muscle force exceeds bite force, and the TMJ is loaded. The load will generally be higher when the resultant is more distant from the bite point. Note that the resultant is retrusive in the dog, protrusive in the other species. Panel a is based on Weijs and Dantuma 1975, b on Weijs and Dantuma 1981, and d on Hylander 1985; c and e are from dissections.

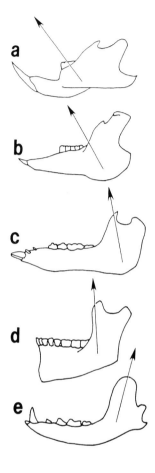

very different from the anteriorly directed loads in rabbits, ungulates, and primates.

The real value of animal studies of TMJ mechanics is the opportunity to make in vivo measurements. The dynamic nature of oral function defies computational methods because of the many variables involved. Storey (this volume) has reviewed evidence from monkeys that the TMJ is compressively loaded during mastication. Electromyographic observations on dogs (Dessem 1989) and rabbits (Weijs and Dantuma 1981) further indicate that differential muscle activation is used to minimize tensile (dislocating) loads on the condyle. Nevertheless, limited tensile loading occurs, at least in monkeys (Hylander and Bays 1979). Such dynamic reversals of strain direction are by no means unique to the monkey TMJ. We have recorded similar reversals in the zygomatic bone and suture of pigs (Herring and Mucci 1991), the critical factor being unilateral activity of the masseter muscle.

RECOMMENDATIONS

Differences in joint mechanics and jaw movements should eliminate rodents and carnivorans from any research seeking to illuminate TMJ function in humans. Rabbits are more suitable, and their small size and easy availability are assets for work requiring large samples. However, rabbit TMJ loading is probably relatively lighter than in humans, and mastication is differently controlled. Further, their small size makes surgical procedures and functional observations difficult. Ungulates such as sheep obviate the size problem but, like rabbits, differ from humans in masticatory control and disk anatomy. Higher primates and the pig are anatomically and functionally the closest to humans. Practical considerations of cost, size, and cooperation recommend the pig.

REFERENCES

Ali, A.M., Sharawy, M., O'Dell, N.L. and al-Beherey, G., Morphological alterations in the elastic fibers of the rabbit craniomandibular joint following experimentally induced anterior disk displacement, Acta Anat., 147 (1993) 159–167.

Bermejo, A., González, O. and González, J.M., The pig as an animal model for experimentation on the temporomandibular articular complex, Oral Surg., Oral Med., Oral Pathol., 75 (1993) 18–23.

Boyd, R.L., Gibbs, C.H., Mahan, P.E., Richmond, A.F. and Laskin, J.L., Temporomandibular joint forces measured at the condyle of *Macaca arctoides*, Amer. J. Orthod. Dentofacial Orthop., 97 (1990) 472–479.

Byrd, K.E., Milberg, D.J. and Luschei, E.S., Human and macaque mastication: a quantitative study, J. Dent. Res., 57 (1978) 834–843.

Dessem, D., Interactions between jaw-muscle recruitment and jaw-joint forces in *Canis familiaris*, J. Anat., 164 (1989) 101–121.

Gillbe, G.V., A comparison of the disc in the craniomandibular joint of three mammals, Acta Anat., 86 (1973) 394–409.

Herring, S.W., The dynamics of mastication in pigs, Arch. Oral Biol., 21 (1976) 473–480.

Herring, S.W., Functional morphology of mammalian mastication, Amer. Zool., 33 (1993a) 289–299.

Herring, S.W., Formation of the vertebrate face: epigenetic and functional influences, Amer. Zool., 33 (1993b) 472–483.

Herring, S.W. and Lakars, T.C., Craniofacial development in the absence of muscle contraction, J. Craniofac. Genet. Dev. Biol., 1 (1981) 341–357.

Herring, S.W. and Mucci, R.J., In vivo strain in cranial sutures: the zygomatic arch, J. Morphol., 207 (1991) 225–239.

Hylander, W.L., Mandibular function and temporomandibular joint loading. In: D.S. Carlson, J.A. McNamara and K.A. Ribbens (Eds.), Developmental Aspects of Temporomandibular Joint Disorders, Craniofacial Growth Series, Monograph 16, Center for Human Growth and Devolopment, University of Michigan, Ann Arbor, 1985, pp. 19–35.

Hylander, W.L. and Bays, R., An in vivo strain-gauge analysis of the squamosal-dentary joint reaction force during mastication and incisal biting in *Macaca mulatta* and *Macaca fascicularis*, Arch. Oral Biol., 24 (1979) 689–697.

Kantomaa, T. and Hall, B.K., Mechanism of adaptation in the mandibular condyle of the mouse, Acta Anat., 132 (1988) 114–119.

Macher, D.J., Westesson, P.L., Brooks, S.L., Hicks, D.G. and Tallents, R.H., Temporomandibular joint: surgically created disk displacement causes arthrosis in the rabbit, Oral Surg., Oral Med., Oral Pathol., 73 (1992) 645–649.

Scapino, R.P., The third joint of the canine jaw, J. Morphol., 116 (1965) 23–50.

Smith, R.J., Petersen, C.E. and Gipe, D.P., Size and shape of the mandibular condyle in primates, J. Morphol., 177 (1983) 59–68.

Sprinz, R., A note on the mandibular intra-articular disc in the joints of Marsupialia and Monotremata, Proc. Zool. Soc. Lond., 144 (1965) 327–338.

Ström, D., Holm, S., Clemensson, E., Haraldson, T. and Carlsson, G.E., Gross anatomy of the mandibular joint and masticatory muscles in the domestic pig (*Sus scrofa*), Arch. Oral Biol., 31 (1986) 763–768.

Ström, D., Holm, S., Clemensson, E., Haraldson, T. and Carlsson, G.E., Gross anatomy of the craniomandibular joint and masticatory muscles of the dog, Arch. Oral Biol., 33 (1988) 597–604.

Tuominen, M., Kantomaa, T. and Pirttiniemi, P., Effect of food consistency on the shape of the articular eminence and the mandible, Acta Odontol. Scand., 51 (1993) 65–72.

Weijs, W.A., Mandibular movements of the albino rat during feeding, J. Morphol., 145 (1975) 107–124.

Weijs, W.A. and Dantuma, R., Electromyography and mechanics of mastication in the albino rat, J. Morphol., 146 (1975) 1–34.

Weijs, W.A. and Dantuma, R., Functional anatomy of the masticatory apparatus in the rabbit (*Oryctolagus cuniculus* L.), Neth. J. Zool., 31 (1981) 99–147.

Correspondence to: Susan W. Herring, PhD, Department of Orthodontics, SM-46, University of Washington, Seattle, WA 98195, USA. Tel: 206-543-3203; Fax: 206-685-8163; E-mail: herring@u.washington.edu

Temporomandibular Disorders and Related Pain Conditions, Progress in Pain Research and Management, Vol. 4, edited by B.J. Sessle, P.S. Bryant, and R.A. Dionne, IASP Press, Seattle, © 1995.

Reaction Paper to Chapters 14–18

Alan G. Hannam

Department of Oral Biology, University of British Columbia, Vancouver, British Columbia, Canada

It is easy to see why modeling of human articular function has emerged as a useful way to study articular mechanics. Most methods needed to record physical events in and around the functioning articulation are too invasive to be used in living subjects. While animal models are valuable, as Herring and Fontenot (this volume) point out, the peculiarities of hominid musculoskeletal and dental morphology affect local biomechanics in ways that cannot be extrapolated readily from experiments on other species, primate or otherwise.

There are several advantages in creating working models. If it includes much of what is already known or assumed about the system, a model is a working hypothesis. Though theoretical, it permits a specific morphological reconstruction to perform real-life actions over time, while incorporating known physical laws and experimental data. Whether or not the model works plausibly, a working hypothesis is tested, and is available for criticism and modification. Designed properly, a good model can be easily altered to accommodate new, and often better, information. Simulation constantly questions the sources and quality of any biological data, and the reasonableness of assumptions when these data are unavailable. It also defines which data need to be gathered. Novel events may be predicted when the model is manipulated by the curious biologist or clinician, and it may be possible to verify them in subsequent experiments that otherwise may never have been performed. Finally, there is the prospect that models can be used to develop new devices. These may include research transducers, or devices with a therapeutic intent such as those outlined by Fontenot.

Clearly it would be naive to attempt to understand the mechanics of any articulation without a working knowledge of the forces responsible for the translation, rotation, compression, traction, shear and deformation that are believed to occur in the functioning joint. These forces are tensile, and generated by muscles. In the human jaw, they are spread widely across attachment sites that have complex patterns of motion, and are produced mostly by multipennate muscles that can contract differentially. Storey's chapter (this volume) reminds us that these muscles (or their components) have mostly been modeled as sets of static force vectors, tuned differentially according to assumptions of the muscles' cross-sectional sizes, their line of action, and their known or predicted levels of activation.

Lemons' chapter (this volume) argues convincingly for developing a formal rather than inferential understanding of biomechanical constraints in the regions affected by muscle forces. He would like to determine the physical properties of the tissues involved, and to use this information to define the changes that occur as a result of motion and loading. He suggests that this step is essential for designing devices that are tissue-compatible with respect to motion and force transfer.

The technical environment for advanced modeling by computer currently includes UNIX-based workstations (or supercomputers) that can be linked for both data transfer and interactive collaboration. This arrangement supports conjoint studies spanning large geographic distances. While there is software available for filtering and otherwise modifying data files from computerized tomography, magnetic resonance, or confocal-microscope images, for constructing wireframe meshes representing biological tissues and biomaterials, for analyzing induced stress, strain, and deformation by the finite element (FE) method, and for analyzing static and dynamic motion, these software packages are usually expensive, and often require site licenses. Almost all have a learning curve of many months, and are designed for use by engineers. It is highly desirable to have a continuous input from biological scientists when these packages are used; Storey refers to recent studies with such collaborations. Most software is not oriented toward the complex shapes and material properties found in biology, nor are the engineers who use them especially comfortable with the data biologists provide, which often include many generalizations, approximations, and assumptions.

Lemons' and Fontenot's pleas for cooperative efforts between specialists is pertinent because there are quite serious deficiencies in understanding the capabilities offered by different disciplines. For example, there is not a great deal of interaction between scientists involved in biomedical imaging, tissue reconstruction, musculoskeletal function, bioengineering, biomaterials, and tissue responses to changes in the physical environment. Many biological and clinical researchers do not seem to be fully aware of the tools available for biomechanical and bioengineering studies, nor realize how they may be adapted for use in biological systems.

Can some of Storey's, Fontenot's, and Lemons' needs and suggestions be met realistically with contemporary approaches? It is already possible to construct and validate FE models of the entire human mandible and its articulation. These models, of course, are imperfect, and require better representation of the trabecular structure of cancellous bone, the periodontium, and (as Storey suggests) the temporomandibular articulation. The occlusal surfaces of the teeth, which today can be modeled with very acceptable detail, have not been considered as collections of inclined planes with multiple zones of contact. Current models need a more sophisticated representation of distributed muscle tensions than has been the case, and as Storey indicates, none have yet correlated stress or strain analysis of articular structures (including ligaments) with jaw motion. This step is critical in explaining and understanding the biomechanical principles that govern the TMJ's function.

It is important to treat the craniomandibular system as a whole when modeling its biomechanics. For example, muscle contraction causes jaw motion, which affects the pattern of force distribution at both articular and dental sites. The motion is guided by these same morphological constraints. Jaw motion determines the way muscle attachments move. This differs regionally, and alters the contraction properties of the jaw muscles. Thus, even if CNS drive to the jaw muscle is smooth, mirroring patterns of amplitude and timing seen in EMG studies, the tensions that follow will differ, because they depend upon the physical state of each muscle, which changes dynamically in time and space. Storey and Herring allude to the recent development of a dynamic, muscle-driven jaw model, and it should now be clear why this was developed. Storey's concerns that neural feedback, and its effect on shaping muscle activation, have not been given enough attention are also valid. However, such factors are relatively easy to add as part of a muscle pattern-shaping algorithm once peripheral physical events (many of which are time and motion-dependent) are modeled satisfactorily. Local forces and motions (and their derivatives) at designated sites are the stimuli for the afferent neural signals that Storey would like to see shaping motor drive.

Theoretically, some of Lemons' needs could be met by whole-mandible models driven by muscle action, but he requires fine detail in his FE models, and reliable specifications of physical properties when he simulates relationships between biomaterials and biological tissues. One way of coping with this problem may be to use different models, i.e., to use relatively coarse, whole-system models to estimate expected forces and motions at key sites (e.g., the condylar neck), then to construct more detailed models of the specific area of interest. The latter would be driven by condylar-neck forces or motions only.

A good conceptual framework for explaining articular mechanics, and a formal means for predicting intra-articular physical events and relating these to regional morphology during static and dynamic function, would substantially benefit investigators wishing to understand how articular tissues respond to mechanically induced events, as well as assist investigators such as Herring and Hargreaves to select the appropriate animal model of TMJ function or injury in humans. Hargreaves and his colleagues (this volume) emphasize the important roles of injury and pain in association with the cascade of regional biochemical changes that accompany inflammation. Would it be useful to correlate injury and pain with physical events? While there are many ways of causing injury and pain, it might be worth using known physical insults in some future experiments rather than concentrating solely upon injections of known algesic chemicals to evoke neuroendocrine and immune responses. Obviously, the emphasis depends upon what is being studied, but if regional mechanical factors in muscle and joint are indeed believed to initiate or maintain any local injury or pain, it would seem sensible to manipulate them experimentally, and to do so within the framework of a multidisciplinary project.

Correspondence to: Alan G. Hannam, BDS, PhD, FDSRCS, Department of Oral Biology, University of British Columbia, Vancouver, BC, Canada V6T 1W5. Tel: 604-822-3750.

Part VII

Therapeutic Approaches to Temporomandibular Disorders

Temporomandibular Disorders and Related Pain Conditions, Progress in Pain Research and Management, Vol. 4, edited by B.J. Sessle, P.S. Bryant, and R.A. Dionne, IASP Press, Seattle, © 1995.

19

Prevention and Risk-Benefit of Early Treatment for Temporomandibular Disorders

James R. Fricton

Department of Diagnostic and Surgical Sciences, University of Minnesota School of Dentistry, Minneapolis, Minnesota, USA

A recent important advance in understanding orofacial pain and temporo-mandibular disorders (TMDs) is the conceptualization of these conditions as potential chronic pain syndromes distinctly different and more complex than acute pain (Check 1988; McNeil et al. 1990; Fricton 1991). Patients with chronic orofacial pain, like patients with chronic pain in other parts of the body, can have multiple drug dependencies, high stress levels, conflicts in relationships, disrupted lifestyles, impaired ability to perform vocational, so-cial, or recreational functions, and high health care use including multiple surgeries. In addition to being personally devastating, chronic pain is one of the most costly burdens on our health care system. Yet, chronic pain is benign and may, ultimately, be preventable.

However, there is considerable controversy in clinical practice and the scientific literature regarding what factors contribute to the development of orofacial pain and if it can be prevented. For example, it is unclear why some patients with acute orofacial injuries heal with little residual symptoms while others experience continuing pain and significant interference with their life-style, and need an exorbitant amount of health care. In addition, there is little research on the effectiveness of methods used to prevent acute injuries to the orofacial structures. It is also unclear what is the most effective method to treat early cases of acute orofacial pain to prevent the development of a chronic pain syndrome and what is the risk-benefit relationship of early treat-ment. This chapter discusses these clinical and scientific issues for orofacial pain disorders, particularly TMDs, their prevention, and risk/benefit issues of treatment.

ADVANCES IN OROFACIAL PAIN ASSESSMENT

The measurement of risk factors and criteria for orofacial pain diagnoses is a prerequisite for providing a scientific basis for clinical studies attempting to understand risk factors and the prevention of orofacial pain. Many authors have proposed that the multifactorial nature of pain disorders requires that they be conceptualized from a broad biopsychosocial model rather than the biomedical model traditionally used for acute problems (Bandura 1977; Engel 1977; Fricton 1985; Turk et al. 1987). This paradigm shift suggests that patients should be assessed from a multidimensional perspective determining both the physical diagnosis and the physical, behavioral, and psychosocial contributing factors. However, assessment of orofacial pain by the use of this model is complicated by the number of these diverse problems and the lack of traditional conceptual models to organize them and define the interrelationships between the various domains.

Advances have been made in defining both the physical and the psychosocial domains involved in chronic orofacial pain and providing instruments to measure them. In previous research on the physical parameters of TMDs, the Craniomandibular Index (CMI) and the Helkimo Index were developed to provide reliable and valid measures of the degree of jaw dysfunction and tenderness in TMDs and have been used as an epidemiological tool and an outcome measure (Fricton and Schiffman 1986, 1987; Dahlstrom et al. 1994). A more recent effort to develop standardized examination procedures and diagnostic criteria for TMDs resulted in the development of the research diagnostic criteria (RDC; Dworkin et al. 1992).

In defining psychosocial domains, the RDC for TMDs include an axis II to define common psychosocial dimensions of TMDs including depression, chronic pain grade, a symptom checklist, and jaw impact. In other research, both the McGill pain questionnaire (Melzack 1975) and Gracely's verbal descriptors (Gracely et al. 1979) provide tested methods to assess both affective and sensory dimensions of pain. The Chronic Illness Problem Inventory (Kames et al. 1984) and the West Haven–Yale Multidimensional Pain Inventory (Kerns et al. 1985) have been developed to assess the lifestyle and psychosocial characteristics of chronic pain patients. The Graded Chronic Pain Scale as defined by Von Korff and colleagues (1992) has been used to determine severity and impact of chronic pain. In the area of orofacial pain, IMPATH (Fricton et al. 1987b) and the TMJ Scale (Lundeen et al. 1988) have been developed to assess multidimensional contributing factors associated with TMDs and orofacial pain.

RISK FACTORS AND PREVENTION OF EARLY OROFACIAL PAIN

These and other methods of assessment have been used to examine different characteristics of chronic orofacial pain and provide some evidence of the progression and risk factors in the development of chronicity from an acute orofacial injury. Fig. 1 presents a model illustrating the onset and progression of orofacial pain to normal healing or to chronic injury. Table I lists potential predisposing or onset factors associated with the TMDs, the most common orofacial pain disorders. Evidence suggests that the onset of TMD pain can begin with an injury to the orofacial structures through macrotrauma from an event such as excessive or prolonged mouth opening during dental treatment, a motor vehicle accident, or a direct blow to the face or jaw. Although there has not been an in-depth study of these factors, one study of onset events for masticatory myofascial pain found trauma from these three events was related to the onset of pain in about 50% of cases of myofascial pain of masticatory system (Fricton et al. 1985). In most of the remaining cases, no specific event

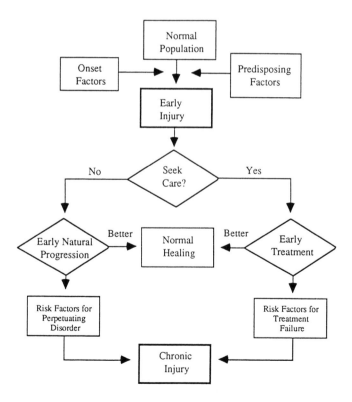

Fig. 1. Flow chart describing the early stages of progression of chronic orofacial pain from asymptomatic normal subjects to the onset of chronicity.

Table I
List of potential onset, predisposing, or perpetuating factors
in temporomandibular disorders

I. Onset factors
  A. Specific onset event: related to macrotrauma.
    1. Opening too wide.
    2. Opening mouth for too long a period.
    3. Blow to jaw or face.
    4. Motor vehicle accident.
    5. Biting on hard object.
  B. No specific onset event: related to cumulative microtrauma.
    1. Bruxism and other oral parafunctional habits.
    2. Overuse of jaw.
    3. Jaw tension from stressful situation, hurrying, and poor pacing.
    4. Musical instruments that use the jaw or mouth.
    5. Sustained poor jaw and head posture.
II. Predisposing or perpetuating risk factors
  A. Behavioral factors that cause microtrauma.
    1. Bruxism and other oral parafunctional habits.
    2. Overuse of jaw.
    3. Jaw tension from stressful situation, hurrying, and poor pacing.
    4. Musical instruments that use the jaw and mouth.
    5. Sustained poor jaw and head posture.
  B. Physical factors
    1. Systemic illness such as hypermobility and connective tissue disease.
    2. Malocclusion and skeletal abnormalities.
    3. Previous trauma or problems in the area.
    4. Presence of muscle tenderness or jaw dysfunction.
  C. Psychosocial factors
    1. Depression.
    2. Anxiety.
    3. Stressful life events.
    4. Social modeling.
    5. Chemical dependency.
    6. Sleep disorders.

or a stressful situation was noted, suggesting that other more indirect predisposing factors such as bruxism, clenching, postural abnormalities, reduced tolerance for pain, or other factors may be involved. In these cases, it was theorized that cumulative strain to the masticatory system from microtrauma may also lead to injury and onset of pain.

The literature examining methods to prevent TMDs is primarily anecdotal and based on theories of TMD onset or etiology. Because macrotraumatic events such as direct trauma or strain to the masticatory system play an important role in the onset of TMDs, some preventive efforts have been made through the use of mouth guards, particularly during sporting activity in children and adults. A study of the use of mouth pieces for children playing sports clearly documented the success of preventing injury to the orofacial structures and teeth (Scott et al. 1994). The mechanism of this protection may involve the cushioning effect of the splint when the mandible is abruptly forced against the maxilla. Rocobado (1984) has theorized that children and young adults develop TMDs because of imbalanced postural patterns in the orofacial, head, and neck structures. Thus, he advocates prevention efforts directed at improving proper tongue position on the palate, developing proper breathing patterns, and avoiding forward head posture and rounded shoulders. The possible role of occlusal factors in the prevention or development of TMDs is discussed more fully by McNamara (this volume).

PROGRESSION AND RISK FACTORS IN THE DEVELOPMENT OF CHRONIC OROFACIAL PAIN

Once an acute injury has occurred to the masticatory muscles or temporomandibular joints (TMJs), a large percentage of patients heal normally with few residual symptoms. However, in a small percentage of patients, the healing and recovery is delayed and a normal response to initial care is not achieved. Fig. 2 illustrates the progression and risk factors that may play a role in this process. The reasons for this delayed recovery are unclear, but factors ranging from psychosocial to physical have been implicated. Some authors have suggested that behavioral and psychosocial factors such as oral parafunctional habits, sleep disorders, stress, and depression play a significant role in perpetuation of orofacial pain disorders (Rugh and Solberg 1976; Kudrow and Stutrus 1979; Donaldson and Kroening 1980; Kroening 1980; Green et al. 1982; Moody et al. 1982; Rudy et al. 1989). These factors may have been present before the onset of the pain and predispose the patient to continued pain, treatment failure, and progressive impact of the pain on the lifestyle. Other issues such as secondary gain from pain behavior, litigation, and operant learning have been identified as significant contributing factors that reduce the prognosis for successful management (Fordyce and Steger 1979; Roberts and Reinhardt 1980; Wedel and Carlsson 1987). They may perpetuate the disorder by providing an environment that reinforces care-seeking behavior and conflicts with normal recovery from injury. However, only a few studies have examined which risk factors are involved in delayed recovery from an orofacial pain condition.

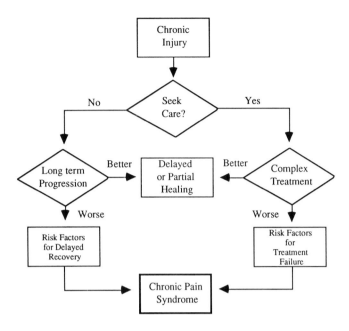

Fig. 2. Later stages of progression of a chronic orofacial pain disorder including risk factors for failed treatment, delayed recovery, and development of a chronic pain syndrome.

One such study (Olson 1987) identified illness, behavioral, and psychosocial variables prior to treatment and determined their ability to predict treatment success in two samples of chronic orofacial pain patients. The first sample of subjects included 94 patients diagnosed as having a chronic TMD with pain greater than six months. Prior to entering a conservative, interdisciplinary treatment program, each subject completed the IMPATH questionnaire of orofacial pain risk factors and was evaluated by a dentist using the CMI (a standardized measure of the physical impairment of the TMJ and surrounding musculature) and a symptom severity index (SSI). Treatment outcome (success or failure) was based on clinically significant decreases of at least one standard deviation in both the CMI and the SSI from pre- to post-treatment. The IMPATH questionnaire items were regressed on treatment outcome for a random sample of half the subjects (N = 47) to isolate the psychosocial and demographic items most predictive of treatment response. Discriminate analysis was then employed to test the predictive utility of the identified items for these subjects as part of the criterion group and then followed by cross-validation of the items on the remaining 47 subjects as the cross-validation group.

The most useful predictors of treatment outcome for the criterion group included patient self-report of low self-esteem, feeling worried, low energy, and poor sleep activity. Each appears to be a correlate of depression. The discriminate analysis employing these four items accounted for 49% of the variance in treatment response, was statistically significant ($P < .0001$), and correctly predicted treatment outcome for 41 of 47 subjects (87%) in the criterion group. The predictive utility of the identified items remained statistically significant when applied to the cross-validation group ($P < .01$), as the discriminate function employing the items correctly predicted treatment outcome for 37 of 47 subjects (79%) and explained for 28% of the variance in treatment response. Findings of this study suggest that pretreatment psychosocial information is useful in predicting treatment outcome for chronic TMDs, and the possibility that depression is a major factor that mediates treatment response for chronic pain patients.

In the second independent study Alter (1991) studied 51 female patients diagnosed with chronic orofacial pain of at least six months duration who were enrolled in a multidisciplinary outpatient orofacial pain treatment program. The SSI and the CMI were again used as the outcome measures with the same definition of success. In addition, the medical records of all patients were reviewed to determine the number of visits made to a health care provider and number of prescriptions written for the patients during the 12 months following termination of treatment. The resulting number was used as an index of utilization of health care (UHC) and served as the third measure of outcome. Risk factors were chosen among the items in the IMPATH instrument.

The IMPATH instrument was used as a pretest. Pretest and post-test scores were also gathered for all patients on the SSI, CMI, and UHC measures. Factor analysis was used to reduce the set of 108 potential predictor variables in IMPATH to a minimum. Four factors that represented the presence of depression, the presence of anxiety, social stressors (poor relationships, etc.), and an adverse history (e.g., presence in the home of a physically ill person who could provide a social modeling influence, long duration of illness, a history of sexual abuse) were identified as the most important predictors of outcome. Together, these four factors accounted for approximately one-third of the variance within the set of predictors. The four extracted factors were entered into multiple regression analyses after controlling for chronicity of pain, number of previous treatments received, length of time in treatment, number of treatment sessions, and pretreatment score on the relevant outcome measure. The combination of covariates and psychosocial predictors accounted for up to 71% of the variance in outcome.

McCreary and colleagues studied psychosocial factors in predicting outcome and found somatization or an overconcern regarding bodily function as the significant factor in predicting success of outcome (McCreary 1992). They used measures of pain intensity, jaw functioning difficulties, and satisfaction with treatment to determine success and the Minnesota Multiphasic Personality Inventory (MMPI), the Beck Depression Inventory, and the State-Trait Anxiety Inventory as psychosocial measures at pretreatment. The results showed that somatization was a major risk factor for treatment failure.

Despite these findings, other authors suggest that these psychosocial factors are only a consequence of chronic pain and instead cite physical factors such as severity of muscle dysfunction, the degree of joint pathology, or occlusal problems as a cause of perpetuation (Rasmussen 1981; Reeves et al. 1986; Wilkes 1989). For example, muscle pain and dysfunction is correlated with poor regular postural habits, muscle tension-producing habits, and sleep disturbance (Fricton et al. 1985; Blaustein and Scapino 1986). A common theory among dentists is that a malrelationship between the maxilla and mandible and the resulting malocclusion can cause static and functional postural strain to the muscle and joints, which in turn will cause continuation of pain and dysfunction, particularly if the masticatory system is also overloaded by oral habits, overchewing, and sustained muscle tension). The degree of joint pathology such as degeneration and disk displacement also may be a significant factor in causing continued inflammation in the TMJ and further pain and dysfunction (Wilkes 1978; Blaustein and Scapino 1986). Many clinicians, particularly surgeons, believe that correcting this structural pathology is the best method of encouraging healing in the joint and preventing progression to a chronic pain condition.

Each of these divergent theories attempts to explain the evolution of a chronic orofacial pain condition, but none have conclusive supporting evidence. Each factor may play some role in different patients, and the key to assessment is to evaluate all factors as possible contributors. However, we need more definitive research on the contribution of each factor in the progression of specific orofacial pain conditions, whether these factors can be changed, and if so, whether this will help prevent chronicity.

PREVENTION OF CHRONIC OROFACIAL PAIN WITH EARLY TREATMENT

Little research has been specifically directed at preventing the development of chronic orofacial pain after an acute injury. Standard treatment strategies typically encourage healing of the physical disorder, but little effort has been made to prevent reinjury by reducing risk factors. Traditionally, most treatments of chronic orofacial pain vary according to the clinician's favorite theory of etiology, as discussed earlier. Success of treatment is often compromised by approaches that only address part of the problem and do not consider all risk factors that delay healing or contribute to progression of the problem.

Given its proposed multifactorial nature, management of the TMDs may be most effective if conceived from a broader biopsychosocial model rather than the biomedical model traditionally used for acute problems (Engel 1977). This may be particularly true for patients with acute orofacial injuries who have several identified risk factors for delayed healing. This paradigm shift suggests that patients should be assessed from a multidimensional perspective determining both the physical diagnosis and the physical, behavioral, and psychosocial contributing factors. It has also been proposed that approaches to management follow these concepts by advocating long-term rehabilitation that addresses both the physical disorder and risk factors on an equal and integrated basis (Check 1988; McNeil 1993). This conceptual shift has provided significant impetus to the development of interdisciplinary teams for managing both acute orofacial injuries and chronic orofacial pain syndromes (Ng 1980; Fricton et al. 1987a). However, team concepts of management have yet to be studied in randomized clinical trials for either acute or chronic orofacial pain conditions.

Most investigations have been follow-up studies and clinical trials of multidisciplinary conservative care for TMDs; the best study to date was conducted by Mejersjo et al. (1983) and included splints, physical therapy, and psychological counseling. It indicated that TMD patients can improve both pain and dysfunction following long-term nonsurgical rehabilitation. Several other studies indicated that the addition of a psychologist to a team appears to improve treatment results. Rudy et al. (1989) studied the efficacy of intraoral appliances (IA) and/or biofeedback with stress management (BF/SM) in a six-week trial of TMD treatment. They conducted two experiments: the first compared IA to BF/SM, while the second examined both treatments in combination. The authors suggested that the combined treatment approach was more effective than either of the single treatments alone, particularly in pain reduction, at the six-month follow-up. Although patients were randomly assigned to the combined treatment group, treatment was brief (only six weeks' duration) and the study did not include a no-treatment control group. In a study of singular interventions of biofeedback and splint therapy, Dahlstrom and Carlsson (1984) demonstrated that both were effective treatment modalities with no significant differences in efficacy. Crockett et al. (1986) randomly assigned 21 women to one of three treatment conditions: splint and physiotherapy; relaxation, biofeedback, and stress management; or minimal treatment involving transcutaneous electrical nerve stimulation (TENS). Improvement was assessed through a dental examination, self-monitoring of pain, and an assessment of electromyographic (EMG) activity during resting and task conditions. All treatment programs produced similar changes.

Fricton and colleagues investigated the effect of an interdisciplinary team program on patients completed the program (completers), began but did not complete the program (noncompleters), and no treatment controls (Fricton et al. 1987a; Fricton and Dall'Arancio 1994). A prospective case-control group research design was used to evaluate efficacy in chronic orofacial pain patients. Primary diagnoses included all TMD diagnoses for myofascial/muscular pain, TMJ internal derangement, or TMJ degenerative joint disease. Of the 102 patients who were evaluated and began the program, 73 completed the program and were included in the treatment group. Eighteen were evaluated, but failed to continue the program and 11 were used as a no-treatment control group. Self-report questionnaires were completed by all patients at the initial evaluation and approximately one year later. The program included evaluation by a dentist, psychologist, and physical therapist, a group meeting with patient and team, and six months of individualized outpatient management designed to treat the diagnosis and reduce contributing factors. Treatment included a splint, exercises, and cognitive-behavioral therapy for identified contributing factors. Although a randomized study design was not used, the results showed that completers improved in symptom severity, use of health care, daily behaviors, and attitudes as compared to noncompleters and no-treatment controls.

RISK-BENEFIT DECISIONS IN TMD TREATMENT

The literature has included much discussion on the risk-benefit decisions associated with specific types of early TMD treatment, particularly those that are irreversible. The identification of structural joint problems associated with disk displacements in the TMJ has prompted the use of methods to correct this displacement. The most common of these corrective methods included surgical repair of the disk with or without implants and mandibular anterior positioning splints with and without occlusal treatment such as orthodontics and prosthodontics. Each of these treatments has significant associated risk and cost, and evidence suggests that long-term results of some cases are poor. Most recent publications support the concept that the TMDs are benign disorders that in most cases are mild in severity and fluctuate considerably over time; thus the use of irreversible and costly treatments has been criticized for having too high a risk and cost to warrant the questionable long-term benefits (McNeil et al. 1993).

Surgery has often been used to correct the structural problems in the TMJ, including arthroscopic surgery, meniscectomy, and disk repair procedures. With diskectomy, alloplastic implants were often used to provide interpositional support between the condyle and fossa. Recent studies show that these alloplastic implants are not able to withstand the biomechanical forces placed on them in the TMJ and in some patients break down, resulting in granulomatous immune reactions, degenerative changes, and continued pain and dysfunction (Valentine et al. 1989; Wagner and Mosby 1990). In some cases, these patients have developed severe dysfunction and deformity requiring many surgeries in an attempt to correct the problem, and also have developed a severe chronic pain syndrome. Currently, the extent of problems associated with TMD alloplastic implants and the characteristics of patients who have had them fail are not known. However, the FDA has prohibited most TMJ implants until further studies have been completed to determine their safety and efficacy. Other surgical techniques without the use of implants have had, in general, better long-term success in reducing pain and dysfunction but have never been compared to lower risk nonsurgical rehabilitative techniques, particularly for early-stage cases. For these reasons, most treatment guidelines for TMDs require unsuccessful treatment with nonsurgical care prior to considering surgery as an option (Table II).

Anterior positioning splints have also been used to treat TMJ disk displacements by permanently positioning the mandible in an anterior position to "recapture" the disk with the condyle (Molony and Howard 1986; Okeson 1988). Short-term results with this approach initially appeared promising in reducing both the joint noise and symptoms. However, because the splint holds the mandible in an anterior position, a malocclusion results with anterior prematurities and a posterior open bite. Many clinicians attempt to maintain this anterior position long term by changing the occlusion through orthodontic or prosthodontic treatment. Recent studies have found that in many

Table II
Criteria for performing TMJ surgery

1. Documented structural changes in the TMJ that may be surgically corrected.

2. Evidence that suggests symptoms and objective findings are a result of disk displacement or arthrosis.

3. Pain and/or dysfunction of such magnitude as to constitute a disability to the patient.

4. Prior unsuccessful treatment with a nonsurgical approach that includes a stabilization splint, physical therapy, and behavioral therapy for control of contributing factors.

5. Prior management of bruxism, oral parafunctional habits, and other medical and dental conditions (myofascial pain, etc.), or contributing factors that will affect outcome of surgery.

6. Patient consent after a discussion of potential complications, goals, success rate, timing, postoperative management, and alternative approaches, including no treatment.

Source: McNeil 1990.

cases, the long-term results are poor with return of clicking and pain despite permanent change in the occlusion. These findings, coupled with the higher risk and cost of treatment, have raised questions about continued use of permanent repositioning splints. In addition, studies of lower risk reversible treatments such as stabilization splints, physical therapy, and behavioral therapy show they offer successful alternatives.

As knowledge of the longitudinal progression of TMDs improves, it may become possible to determine if treatment actually alleviates pain and dysfunction more quickly than allowing the disorders to take their natural course. If so, clinical trials of specific interventions must be conducted to determine the relative efficacy and safety of treatments for the prevention of TMDs. Decisions regarding the appropriateness of treatments may then be made using both efficacy and safety data. Treatments of relatively similar efficacies for a specific TMD subtype can then be chosen for risk and cost. Treatment success for an individual patient often depends on addressing risk factors regardless of the treatment provided. Thus, the use of rehabilitation teams should be considered to improve long-term efficacy given that the benefits outweigh the consequent increase in costs.

SUMMARY

There is distinct gap in our knowledge of the longitudinal progression of chronic orofacial pain, and thus we have little understanding of issues of prevention and risk-benefit. We do not know what conditions or patient types most commonly become chronic, why they become chronic, if this progression can be prevented, and the best interventions. The recent methodological advances in studying TMDs allow us to begin investigations of these issues to improve our understanding of chronic orofacial pain. Future studies should focus on the following issues:

1. What physical, behavioral, and psychosocial factors play the most significant role in developing chronic orofacial pain after acute injury to the orofacial structures? For example, how does the primary diagnosis of muscle versus joint disorders in TMD patients influence progression? Does occlusal instability or a maxillomandibular malrelationship cause failure of early treatment of TMJ injuries, leading to chronicity? Are anxiety and depression consequential or antecedent factors in developing chronicity? Do bruxism or other oral habits in patient with an early injury continue to reinjure muscles and joints, resulting in further pain and chronicity?

2. What is the best strategy for treating early orofacial injuries to prevent the negative effects of chronic orofacial pain? Is a properly designed home care program sufficient or should individual risk factors for chronicity be identified and addressed in a rehabilitation program? Can these factors be effectively reduced in a rehabilitation treatment program as compared to usual somatic or home care treatment?

3. Can addressing risk factors in a team treatment program successfully improve patients and prevent the development of chronic orofacial pain as compared to usual somatic treatment or self-care? What are the risk-benefit issues of using more than home care for early injuries? Is surgery or other irreversible treatments warranted at an earlier point in injury of the TMJ? Does failed inadequate and inappropriate treatment lead to behavioral and psychosocial risk factors that will intensify lifestyle consequences of orofacial pain?

With future research to address these issues, we will be able to determine what is the best treatment or combination of treatments for patients with orofacial pain conditions. In addition, this knowledge will help us to prevent orofacial pain disorders.

REFERENCES

Alter, D., Discriminant Analysis of Psychosocial Factors in TMD Treatment, Ph.D. thesis, Chicago University, 1991.

Bandura, A., Self-efficacy: toward a unifying theory of behavior change, Psychol. Rev., 84 (1977) 191–215.

Blaustein, D.I. and Scapino, R.P., Remodeling of the temporomandibular joint disk and posterior attachment in disk, Plast. Reconstr. Surg., 78 (1986) 756–764.

Check, R., et al. Report of the Ad Hoc Committee on Craniomandibular and Temporomandibular Joint Disorders: Current Concepts of Diagnosis and Treatment, Minnesota Dental Association, Minneapolis, 1988.

Crockett, D.J., Foremann, M.E., Alden, L. and Blasberg, B., A comparison of treatment modes in the management of myofascial pain dysfunction syndrome, Biofeedback. Self Regul., 11 (1986) 279–291.

Dahlstrom, L. and Carlsson, S.G., Treatment of mandibular dysfunction: the clinical uselfulness of biofeedback in relation to splint therapy, J. Oral Rehabil., 11 (1984) 277–284

Dahlstrom,L., Keeling, S., Fricton, J., Hilsenbeck, S.,Clark, G. and Rugh, J., Evaluation of a training program intended to calibrate raters of temporomandibular disorders, Acta Odontol. Scand. (in press).

Donaldson, D. and Kroening, R., Recognition and treatment of chronic pain patients in dentistry, J.Am. Dent. Assoc., 99 (1980) 961–966.

Dworkin, S., LeReshce, L., Fricton, J., Huggins, K., Mohl, N., Orhbach, R., Sommers, E., Truelove, E. and Von Korff, M., Research diagnostic criteria: Axis I and Axis II and examination and history data, J. Orofacial Pain, 6 (1992) 327–345.

Engel, G.L., The need for a new medical model: a challenge for biomedicine, Science, 196 (1977) 129–135.

Fordyce, W.E. and Steger, J.C., Chronic pain. In: O.F. Pomerleau and J.P. Brady (Eds.), Behavioral Medicine: Theory and Practice, Williams & Wilkins, Baltimore, 1979, pp. 125–154.

Fricton, J., Behavioral and psychosocial factors in chronic craniofacial pain, Anesthesia Progress, 32 (1) (1985) 7–12.

Fricton, J., Recent advances in temporomandibular disorders and orofacial pain, J. Am. Dent. Assoc., 122 (1991) 25–32.

Fricton, J. and Dall'Arancio, D., Myofascial pain of the head and neck: longitudinal changes associated with an interdisciplinary treatment program, J. Musculoskeletal Pain, 2 (1994) 81–99.

Fricton, J. and Schiffman, E., Reliability of craniomandibular index, J. Dent. Res., 65 (1986) 1–6.

Fricton, J. and Schiffman, E., The craniomandibular index: validity, J. Prosth. Dent., 58 (1987) 221–228.

Fricton, J., Kroening, R., Haley, D. and Siegert, R., Myofascial pain and dysfunction of the head and neck: a review of clinical characteristics of 164 patients, Oral Surg. Oral Med. Oral Pathol., 57 (1985) 615–627.

Fricton, J.R., Hathaway, K.M. and Bromaghim, C., Interdisciplinary management of patients with TMJ and craniofacial pain: characteristics and outcome, J. Craniomandib. Disord. Facial Oral Pain, 1 (1987a) 115–122.

Fricton, J.R., Nelson, A. and Monsein, M., Impath: microcomputer assessment of behavioral and psychological factors in craniomandibular disorders, Journal of Craniomandibular Practice, 5 (1987b) 372–378.

Gracely, R.H., Dubner, R. and McGrath, P., Narcotic analgesia: fentanyl reduces intensity but not the unpleasantness of painful tooth pulp sensations, Science, 203 (1979) 1261–1263.

Green, C.D., Olson, R.E. and Laskin, D.M., Psychosocial factors in etiology progression and treatment of MPD syndrome, J. Am. Dent. Assoc., 105 (1982) 443–448.

Kames, L.D., Naliboff, B.D., Heinrich, R.L. and Schag, C.C., The chronic illness problem inventory: problem oriented psychosocial assessment of patients with chronic illness, Int. J. Psychiatric. Med., 14 (1984) 65–75.

Kerns, R.D., Turk, D.C., and Rudy, T.E., The West Haven–Yale multidimensional pain inventory (WHYMPI), Pain, 23 (1985) 345–386.

Kirveskari, P., Scientific evidence of occlusion and craniomandibular disorders, J. Orofacial Pain, 7 (1993) 235–240.

Kudrow, L. and Stutrus, B.J., MMPI pattern specificity in primary headache disorders, Headache, 19 (1979) 18–24.

Lundeen, T.F., Levitt, S.R.T. and McKinney, M.W., Clinical applications of the TMJ Scale, J. Cranio. Prac., 6 (1988) 339.

McCreary, C.P., Clark, G.T., Oakley, M.D. and Flack, V., Predicting response to treatment for temporomandibular disorders, J. Craniomandib. Disord. Facial and Oral Pain, 6 (3) (1992) 161–170.

McNeil, C. (Ed.), Temporomandibular Disorders: Guidelines for Evaluation, Diagnosis, and Management (American Academy of Orofacial Pain), Quintessence, Chicago, 1990.

McNeil, C. (Ed.), Temporomandibular Disorders: Guidelines for Evaluation, Diagnosis, and Management (American Academy of Orofacial Pain), Quintessence, Chicago, 1993.

Mejersjo, C. and Carlsson, G.E., Long-term results of treatment for temporomandibular joint pain-dysfunction, J. Prosthet. Dent., 49 (1983) 809–815.

Melzack, R., The McGill pain questionnaire: major properties and scoring methods, Pain, 1 (1975) 277–299.

Moloney, F. and Howard, J.A., Internal derangements of the temporomandibular joint III: anterior repositioning splint therapy, Aust. Dent. J. (1986) 30–39.

Moody, P.M., Kemper, J.T.,, Okeson, J.P., Calhoun, T.C. and Packe, M.V., Recent life changes and myofascial pain syndrome. J. Prosthet.Dent. 48 (1982) 328–30.

Ng, L.K. (Ed.), New Approaches to Treatment of Chronic Pain: A Review of Multidisciplinary Pain Clinics and Pain Centers. NIDA Research Monograph Series 36, U.S.Government Printing Office, Washington, D.C., 1980.

Okeson, J.P., Long-term treatment of disk-interference disorders of the temporomandibular joint with anterior repositioning occlusal splints, J. Prosthetic Dent., 60 (1988) 611–661.

Olson, T., Predictors of Outcome for Treatment of Temporomandibular Disorders, Ph.D. thesis, University of Minnesota, 1987.

Rasmussen, O.C., Description of population and progress of symptoms in a longitudinal study of temporomandibular arthropathy, Scand. J. Dent. Res., 89 (1981) 196–203.

Reeves, J.L., Jaeger, B. and Graff-Radford, S.B., Reliability of the pressure algometer as a measure of myofascial trigger point sensitivity, Pain, 24 (1986) 313–321.

Roberts, A.H. and Reinhardt, L., The behavioral management of chronic pain: long-term followup with comparison groups, Pain, 8 (1980) 151–162.

Rocabado, M., Diagnosis and treatment of abnormal craniocervial and craniomandibular mechanics. In: W.K. Solberg and G.T. Clark (Eds), Abnormal Jaw Mechanics: Diagnosis and Treatment, Quintessence, Chicago, 1984, pp. 141–159.

Rudy, T.E., Turk, D.C., Zaki, H.S. and Curtin, H.D., An empirical taxonmetric alternative to traditional classification of temporomandibular disorders, Pain, 36 (1989) 311–320.

Rugh, J. and Solberg, W.K., Psychological implications in temporomandibular pain and dysfunction, Oral Sciences Review, 7 (1976) 3–30.

Scott, J., Burke, F.J. and Watts, D.C., A review of dental injuries and the use of mouthgards in contact team sports, Br. Dent. J., 176 (1994) 310–314.

Turk, D. C. and Ruby, T.E.,. Towards a comprehensive assessment of chronic pain patients, Behav. Res. Ther., 25 (1987) 237–249.

Von Korff, M. , Ormel, J., Keefe, F. J. and Dworkin, S. F., Grading the severity of chronic pain, Pain, 50 (1992) 133–149.

Valentine, J.D., Jr., Reiman, B.E., Beuttenmuller, E.A and Donovan, M.G., Light and electron microscopic evaluation of Proplast II TMJ disc implants, J. Oral. Maxillofac. Surg., 47 (1989) 689–696.

Wagner, J.D. and, Mosby, E.L., Assessment of proplast-teflon disc replacements, J. Oral Maxillofacial Surgery, 48 (1990) 1140–1144.

Wedel, A. and Carlsson, G.E., Sick-leave in patients with functional disturbances of the masticatory system, Swed. Dent. J., 11 (1987) 53–59.

Wilkes,C.H., Arthrography of the temporomandibular joint in patient with the TMJ pain-dysfunction syndrome, Minn. Med., 61 (1978) 645–652.

Wilkes, C.H., Internal derangements of the temporomandibular joint: pathological variations, Otolaryngol. Head Neck Surg., 115 (1989) 469–477.

Correspondence to: James R. Fricton, DDS, MS, Associate Professor, Department of Diagnostic and Surgical Sciences, University of Minnesota School of Dentistry, Minneapolis, MN 55455, USA. Fax: 612-626-2653.

Temporomandibular Disorders and Related Pain Conditions, Progress in Pain Research and Management, Vol. 4, edited by B.J. Sessle, P.S. Bryant, and R.A. Dionne, IASP Press, Seattle, © 1995.

20

Integrating Behavioral and Dental Treatments: Utility of Customizing Protocols

Thomas E. Rudy[a] and Dennis C. Turk[b]

[a]Department of Anesthesiology and Critical Care Medicine, [b]Department of Psychiatry, and [a,b]Pain Evaluation and Treatment Institute, University of Pittsburgh Medical Center, Pittsburgh, Pennsylvania, USA

Temporomandibular disorders (TMDs) have interested clinicians since the 1930s. Most of the available classification systems for TMD focus on the presence or absence of a set of somatic symptoms (e.g., pain, joint noises) and physical signs (e.g., joint sounds, limitations of jaw opening, tenderness of muscles to palpation, radiographic findings). The diversity of signs, symptoms, and diagnoses associated with TMDs, however, has resulted in a proliferation of competing models upon which to make differential diagnoses and to explain the etiology, exacerbation, and maintenance of the signs and symptoms.

Several problems are inherent with existing systems that rely on oral dysfunctions/structural abnormalities (OD/SA). Some focus primarily on subjective reports of patients, whereas others use unstandardized examination and diagnostic procedures that place a heavy emphasis on clinical interpretation. Patients' self-reports of symptoms are known to be influenced by a wide range of factors in addition to objective physical pathology. Clinician assessment also may be affected by factors that are not associated directly with structural abnormalities. For example, Dworkin et al. (1988) noted the failure of many investigators to report on the reliability of OD/SA indices used to derive diagnostic classification systems, and their findings suggest that many of these indices have reliability coefficients that are inadequate for clinical and research purposes. Moreover, the predictive validity and clinical utility of many of these dental assessment and classification systems have not been addressed.

THE ROLE OF PSYCHOLOGICAL FACTORS IN TMDs

Several perplexing features of persistent symptomatic complaints in TMD patients has led numerous investigators to challenge physically based models of TMDs as inadequate and overly simplistic. For example, (a) patients with objectively determined equivalent degrees and types of tissue pathology vary widely in their reports of pain severity; (b) asymptomatic persons often reveal objective radiographic evidence of structural abnormalities; (c) conversely, patients with minimal objective physical pathology often complain of intense pain and other symptoms; (d) surgical procedures designed to inhibit pain sensations may fail to alleviate symptoms; and (e) OD/SA findings frequently are found to be uncorrelated with patients' responses to treatment, including widely disparate outcomes in patients with the same tissue pathology and treated with the same intervention.

These and many other apparent paradoxes suggest that broader conceptualizations of TMDs are needed to more adequately diagnose and treat this patient population. As with other chronic pain conditions, psychological factors have been hypothesized to explain why some TMD patients seem to be more distressed by symptoms and why only a small percentage of patients with symptoms actually seek treatment. Moreover, psychological variables such as emotional distress and secondary gain have been implicated to help explain why some patients do not respond to conventional therapy, or relapse after initial success following somatic treatments.

Similar to the OD/SA literature, research evaluating the role of psychological characteristics in TMDs has been both controversial and contradictory (Greene et al. 1982). The available research designed to identify specific psychological variables among TMD patients has proven equivocal (Rugh and Solberg 1976; Moss et al. 1982). For example, Oakley et al. (1989) reported that 28% (of 107) patients with TMDs showed signs of depression and 24% "high anxiety." In a retrospective study, Gallagher et al. (1991) reported that 41% of female TMD patients suffered from major depression. Keefe and Dolan (1986) compared groups of TMD and back pain patients and reported that both groups had high means scores for anxiety, depression, obsessive-compulsiveness, and somatization, and that there were no statistically significant differences between these two groups on these measures despite the fact that back pain patients were more disabled by their condition.

Others investigators, however, have found few differences in the degree of psychological distress between TMD patients and other medical patients with identified organic pathology. Rugh and Solberg (1976) reviewed 15 studies that investigated the personality characteristics of TMD patients; Speculand and Goss (1985) reviewed 10 additional studies examining psychological factors in TMD. Both reviews concluded that there was no clear TMD "personality profile"; although elevated levels of anxiety and depression were common, they have not been found consistently. Based on the diversity of findings and the lack of consistent results, Speculand and Goss concluded that there was little evidence to indicate that TMDs are correlated with any specific personality traits.

Similar inconsistencies have been found when TMD patients are compared with asymptomatic control subjects. Beaton et al. (1991) reported that on the average, TMD patients report more psychological symptoms than did healthy controls; whereas, Schnurr et al. (1990) reported that orofacial pain patients do not differ from healthy controls with regard to personality, coping skills, or attitudes toward health.

SUBGROUPS OF TMD PATIENTS BASED ON PSYCHOLOGICAL FACTORS

Several investigators have suggested that, similar to the heterogenous findings on somatic factors, TMD patients can be expected to display a diversity of psychological characteristics (Rudy et al. 1989; McCreary et al. 1991). From this perspective, TMD patients should not be considered as a psychologically homogeneous group. Thus, statistical analyses designed to test whether a set of psychological characteristics are related to all TMD patients' responses to treatment can be expected to lead to unreliable and contradictory findings similar to the dental classifications reviewed above.

This reconceptualization of the role of psychological factors has led to studies that are designed to identify subgroups of TMD patients who display similar patterns of response to psychological inventories. Instruments such as the Minnesota Multiphasic Personality Inventory (MMPI), Symptom Checklist-90 revised (SCL-90R), and Multidimensional Health Locus of Control (MHLC) have been used to identify patient subgroups (Butterworth and Deardorff 1987; Buckelew et al. 1990; McCreary et al. 1991). Turk (1990a,b) has suggested that in addition to measures of psychopathology (e.g., MMPI, SCL-90R), a range of psychosocial and behavioral factors (e.g., spouse support, feelings of control, activity levels) play an important role in chronic pain and should be evaluated and included in classification of these patients.

Turk and Rudy (1988) have demonstrated the reliability and preliminary validity of a classification of heterogeneous samples of pain patients based on the integration of both psychosocial and behavioral data. The primary hypothesis of this approach is that certain modal patterns among psychological factors recur in chronic pain patients and that these patterns represent homogeneous subgroups of patients that, at least to some extent, are independent of physical signs and symptoms. Using empirically-based classification methods, Rudy, Turk, and colleagues (Rudy et al. 1989; Turk and Rudy 1990) have demonstrated that the majority of TMD patients could be reliably classified into one of three subgroups based on psychosocial and behavioral factors. One group of patients (46%) labeled "dysfunctional," was characterized by higher levels of pain, symptoms that interfere with life activities, affective distress, and lower levels of activity and feelings of life control. A second group (22%), labeled "interpersonally distressed," was somewhat similar to the dysfunctional group; however, they differed in that they reported they experienced little support from significant persons in their environment and they received many negative responses and few solicitous responses or assistance related to their pain problem by significant others. The final group (32%), labeled "adaptive copers," was described as remaining active despite pain, feeling little psychological distress or life interference, and continuing to feel in control of their lives despite the presence of symptoms of TMDs.

Interestingly, Rudy et al. (1989) reported that the three subgroups of TMD patients described above did not differ in dental examination or radiographic findings. Thus, even though these groups appeared to manifest different psychological profiles, they did not differ in the common physical findings associated with TMDs. These results call into question the appropriateness of relying primarily upon physical factors for establishing TMD diagnoses and challenge the validity of basing treatment decisions exclusively on physical findings.

Turk and Rudy (1990) also compared TMD patients with chronic back pain (BP) and headache (HA) patients and found that regardless of diagnosis, the majority of patients could be classified reliably into one of these three groups. All three syndrome groups, however, were represented in each of the subgroups identified. Thus, it is possible that TMD, HA, and BP patients who are classified within the same psychosocial-behavioral subgroup may be more similar to each other than patients with the same physical diagnosis but who are classified within different psychosocial-behavioral subgroups. These findings also suggest that regardless of the physically based treatments provided, patients with different psychological characteristics may require additional treatments that target their unique characteristics. For example, the patients who were classified as dysfunctional demonstrate higher levels of psychological distress even when the physical findings are relatively minor. These patients are not likely to benefit from a treatment that does not address their psychological distress along with the physical basis of the symptoms.

PRELIMINARY EVIDENCE FOR THE CLINICAL UTILITY OF PSYCHOLOGICAL CLASSIFICATIONS

An important criticism of TMD classification strategies based on various psychological measures is that, to date, no research has demonstrated the clinical utility of these groupings (Palla 1992). That is, although subgroups have been reliably identified, no studies have demonstrated that this knowledge had any impact on response to treatment and, therefore, may be important in prescribing treatment.

UNDERSTANDING DIFFERENTIAL TREATMENT RESPONSE PATTERNS

One way to validate the clinical usefulness of any classification system is to demonstrate that patients with distinct pretreatment characteristics or profiles respond differentially on diverse outcome measures. Although it would be desirable for all patients to demonstrate major clinical improvement on each outcome measure, this is unlikely to occur in chronic pain samples due to patient heterogeneity as well as differential treatment response patterns that result because a specific treatment protocol may not be equally appropriate for all patients (Turk and Rudy 1992). Thus, for an empirically based classification system to have clinical utility, patients with specific characteristics would be expected to demonstrate greater improvement on measures that are most salient to their unique characteristics.

We examined the differential treatment response patterns of 122 TMD patients to a six-week treatment protocol comprised of a flat-plane occlusal splint and biofeedback/stress management treatment. Based on our previous findings (Turk et al. 1993), we hypothesized that all patients would derive some benefit from this combined dental and psychological treatment. However, we predicted that patients classified into distinct profile types would respond differently to selected outcome measures that are related directly to each subgroup's specific set of characteristics and problems.

We hypothesized that adaptive copers would demonstrate comparable levels of improvement on physical measures when compared with the dysfunctional and interpersonally distressed patient groups, but lower levels of improvement on psychological measures, because these patients have lower levels of psychological distress. By contrast, dysfunctional patients, characterized by higher levels of emotional problems, would show significant improvement on measures of psychological distress as well as physical measures. Also, because both the dysfunctional and interpersonally distressed groups were characterized by higher levels of pain intensity and life interference due to their pain, we hypothesized that they would report greater improvements in these areas than would the adaptive copers.

Nine dependent measures designed to tap physical, psychosocial, and behavioral outcome domains were collected prior to treatment initiation, at the posttreatment assessment, and at a six-month follow-up. Reliable change (RC) indices were computed for each patient on each of these nine outcome measures from pretreatment and six-month follow-up assessment scores. These nine indices for each subject were then analyzed with MANOVA, with cluster profile classification as the independent variable.

RC indices (Jacobson et al. 1984; Hageman and Arrindell 1993) were particularly useful in the present context because this methodology adjusted the differences between pretreatment and six-month follow-up scores for each of the nine outcome measures by its own specific standard error of measurement as well as its own reliability coefficient. The result of this approach is that these measures then are directly comparable to each other, despite unit or scaling differences in the original outcome measures. Additionally, RC indices can be referenced to the cumulative normal distribution, and values that exceed 1.96 are unlikely to occur ($P < 0.05$) unless an actual change in scores occurs between pretreatment and follow-up testing. An additional important aspect of RC indices is that they can be used to provide an individualized evaluation of clinical outcome data. Thus, each patient's progress can be determined, in addition to group effects.

The mean RC indices by patient profile for the nine treatment outcome measures are presented in Table I. A MANOVA for these indices, with patient profile as the independent variable, was statistically significant [$F(18,224)$ = 4.32, $P < 0.0001$]. Follow-up univariate ANOVAs indicated five of the nine indices were significantly different (all $Ps < 0.01$) across patient profiles (Table I). Tukey HSD post-hoc tests indicated: (1) as predicted, the dysfunctional group displayed larger reductions in depression (Beck Depression Inventory, BDI; Beck et al. 1961), catastrophizing (Coping Strategies Questionnaire, CSQ; Rosenstiel and Keefe 1983), and life interference from pain (Multidimensional Pain Inventory, MPI; Kerns et al. 1985) when compared with the RC scores of the interpersonally distressed and the active copers; (2) adaptive copers had smaller reductions in pain severity (McGill Pain Questionnaire, MPQ; Melzack 1987) than did dysfunctional and interpersonally distressed patients; and (3) patients classified as interpersonally distressed showed significantly smaller changes in maximum unassisted opening compared with patients classified as dysfunctional or adaptive copers (Table I).

The results of this study confirmed our hypotheses regarding differential responses on outcome criteria that are most relevant to primary patient characteristics. Specifically, although the majority of patients demonstrated and

Table I
Pretreatment to follow-up mean reliable change indices by patient profile

Change Index Scale	Patient Profile[1]			F value[2]
	DYS	ID	AC	
Physical				
Muscle palpation pain	3.85	3.86	3.73	0.02
	(3.52)[3]	(2.89)	(3.75)	
TMJ palpation pain	1.92	1.61	1.81	0.25
	(2.29)	(1.67)	(1.77)	
Unassisted mandibular opening, no pain	1.57	1.72	2.13	0.73
	(2.45)	(2.11)	(2.03)	
Maximum unassisted mandibular opening	1.16[a4]	0.47[b]	2.08[a]	4.59*
	(2.04)	(2.30)	(2.49)	
Psychosocial				
MPQ short form, total score	3.69[a]	3.54[a]	1.96[b]	6.91**
	(2.66)	(2.17)	(2.06)	
BDI, total score	2.39[a]	0.91[b]	0.60[b]	6.06*
	(3.23)	(2.52)	(1.63)	
CSQ, catastrophizing	2.75[a]	1.08[b]	1.09[b]	13.90**
	(1.63)	(1.75)	(1.80)	
MPI, life interference from pain	3.11[a]	1.61[b]	0.72[b]	24.30**
	(2.03)	(1.71)	(0.89)	
Behavioral				
Oral-parafunctional habits scale	3.86	3.35	3.25	0.73
	(3.08)	(1.97)	(2.24)	
Sample size	50	32	40	—

[1] DYS = dysfunctional, ID = interpersonally distressed, AC = adaptive coper.

[2] *df*s for F tests are 2,119.

[3] Numbers in parentheses are standard deviations.

[4] Means with the same superscript letters for significant F tests are not significantly different at the $P < 0.05$ level, based on Tukey HSD post-hoc tests.

  * $P < 0.01$

 ** $P < 0.001$

maintained improvements in response to a standard treatment protocol, the dysfunctional patients displayed significantly greater improvements on measures of pain, catastrophizing, depression, and disability, when contrasted with the interpersonally distressed and adaptive coper patient subgroups. Using the methods developed by Hageman and Arrindell (1993) to compute RC indices, we found these results exceeded effects that may simply be due to the regression to the mean problem, that is, changes in scores with repeated testing when the measures used are less than perfectly reliable. These findings also have important methodological implications for clinical investigators in that they demonstrate the advantages and increased accuracy of not combining psychologically heterogeneous samples when interpreting the results of treatment outcome studies.

CUSTOMIZING TREATMENTS BASED ON PSYCHOLOGICAL CHARACTERISTICS

Typically, treatment outcome studies of TMDs provide the same treatment, either physically or psychologically based, to all patients. The result of this practice has produced equivocal results because not all patients are receiving a treatment that specifically addresses their problems. Moreover, relapse would be expected to be high given that significant contributions to the patients' problems are not addressed directly.

Previous research has demonstrated that the use of intraoral appliances can produce rapid improvement in pain for TMD patients (Turk et al. 1993). Moreover, biofeedback also has been effective in several studies (Funch and Gale 1984; Turk et al. 1993). As we noted, the combination of intraoral appliances and biofeedback is more effective in the long-term maintenance of beneficial effects than is either of the treatments alone (Turk et al. 1993); however, many patients, while significantly improved, still had residual problems. Based on the suggestions regarding individualizing treatments (Turk 1990b), it would be expected that other treatment components might augment the positive effects promoted by more common treatment protocols.

Recently, we completed a study (Rudy et al. 1994) designed to determine the efficacy of customizing a treatment to a specific subset of TMD patients, those classified as dysfunctional. This group of patients is characterized by higher levels of pain and emotional distress compared to other groups of TMD patients. We predicted that a treatment matched to these patients' psychological features would demonstrate greater improvement in pain severity and depressed mood, compared to dysfunctional TMD patients who receive a more generic treatment protocol that has been shown generally to be beneficial (the combined treatment described above, Turk et al. 1993). Thus, we hypothesized an incremental rather than an absolute effect.

Forty-eight TMD patients empirically classified as dysfunctional were enrolled in the study. Each subject had an extensive oral/dental and psychological evaluation before and after treatment, and at six months following treatment. All patients received a standardized six-week treatment program that combined a flat, full-arch interocclusal appliance with biofeedback and stress management training (IA/BF condition). The psychological treatment consisted of six one-hour sessions of both biofeedback-assisted relaxation and stress management training. This treatment has been proven effective for TMD patients (Turk et al. 1993). Twenty-four randomly assigned patients received the IA/BF treatment described above plus a standardized cognitive therapy (CT) for depression protocol, based on the work of Beck et al. (1979).

As described in the previous study, reliable change (RC) indices, derived from pretreatment and six-month follow-up evaluations, were computed for each subject for nine scales from the dental and psychological evaluations. MANOVA, followed by ANOVAs, were used to test for significant differences between the IA/BF and IA/BF+CT treatment conditions on the treatment outcome change indices.

ANOVA analyses indicated that the mean changes from pretreatment to six months were statistically significant for both treatment conditions (generic and customized) on all nine outcome measures. The means and standard deviations for the nine RC indices by treatment condition are displayed in Table II. A MANOVA indicated significant differences existed between the two treatment groups $[F(9,31) = 2.53, P < 0.001]$. Follow-up ANOVA analyses indicated four of the nine RC indices were significantly different (Table II). These differences included: (1) muscle palpation pain; (2) unassisted mandibular opening, no pain; (3) total pain score on the short form of the MPQ; and (4) Beck Depression score.

These findings suggest that a treatment that addressed both physical and psychological features, namely an intraoral appliance and biofeedback/stress management, produced significant improvement on physical examination measures, self-reported measures of pain and depressed mood, and on self-reported parafunctional oral habits. The addition of a treatment component tailored to the emotional distress of patients classified as dysfunctional added significantly to the treatment outcome. Specifically, the addition of psychological therapy for depression led to greater improvement in depressed mood than did the more generic treatment protocol. Moreover, the addition of the psychological therapy led to significant improvements both on self-reported and muscle palpation pain. Thus, although the generic treatment proved to be effective, there was an incremental effect of adding a treatment component that directly addressed patients' emotional distress.

We are now evaluating whether patients in the other psychosocial-behavioral subgroups identified, namely "adaptive copers" and "interpersonally distressed," also display incremental benefits from an individualized treatment directed to their specific characteristics.

Table II
Pretreatment to follow-up mean reliable change indices by treatment condition

| Change Index Scale | Treatment Condition[a] | | F value[b] |
	IA/BF	IA/BF+CT	
Physical			
Muscle palpation pain	2.47	4.91	10.88**
	(2.37)[c]	(2.35)	
TMJ palpation pain	2.09	1.99	0.02
	(2.17)	(2.68)	
Unassisted mandibular opening, no pain	1.14	2.17	4.30*
	(1.71)	(1.47)	
Maximum unassisted mandibular opening	0.98	1.52	0.69
	(2.38)	(1.80)	
Psychosocial			
MPQ short form, total score	3.25	4.76	4.49*
	(2.57)	(1.97)	
BDI, total score	3.41	5.58	14.15***
	(1.96)	(1.74)	
CSQ, catastrophizing	2.34	2.01	0.27
	(1.85)	(2.30)	
MPI, life interference from pain	2.46	1.86	0.78
	(2.33)	(1.97)	
Behavioral			
Oral-parafunctional habits scale	3.98	3.98	0.01
	(3.41)	(2.83)	
Sample size	20	21	—

[a] IA = interocclusal appliance, BF = biofeedback and stress management training, CT = cognitive therapy.

[b] dfs for F tests are 1,39.

[c] Numbers in parentheses are standard deviations.

  * $P < 0.05$
 ** $P < 0.01$
*** $P < 0.001$

TREATMENT IMPLICATIONS OF A DUAL-DIAGNOSTIC APPROACH

The results of the studies reviewed in the previous section suggest that a dual-diagnostic approach may be most appropriate for TMD patients, as recommended in the recent Research Diagnostic Criteria for TMDs (Dworkin and LeResche 1992). From this perspective, patients with TMD signs and symptoms would be given two diagnoses based upon two axes, one based on oral-dental/structural abnormalities and a second based on specific psychosocial and behavioral characteristics.

A dual-diagnostic approach and subsequent treatment planning should make use of these two classification axes *simultaneously*. For example, it might be suggested that the physical treatment should be directed toward the disease classification and other treatments would supplement this by focusing on a classification based on relevant psychological characteristics. Adopting such an approach would serve the valuable function of encouraging diagnosticians to think concurrently in terms of the two relevant areas for TMDs. Finally, a dual-diagnostic system hopefully would encourage clinicians to creatively combine physical and psychological treatment modalities that are tailored to the presenting characteristics of the patient, rather than viewing these treatment approaches as mutually exclusive. However, carefully designed and controlled clinical trials are needed to evaluate the incremental advantages of integrated treatment protocols, particularly their long-term efficacy and cost effectiveness, before recommending them for widespread adoption.

ACKNOWLEDGMENT

Preparation of this chapter was supported by USPHS Research Grant R01 DE07514 from the National Institute of Dental Research, National Institutes of Health, Bethesda, Maryland, USA.

REFERENCES

Beaton, R.D., Egan, K.J., Nakagawa-Kogan, H. and Morrison, K.N., Self-reported symptoms of stress with temporomandibular disorders: comparisons to healthy men and women, J. Prosthet. Dent., 65 (1991) 289–293.

Beck, A.T., Ward, C.H., Mendelson, M., Mock, J. and Erbaugh, J., An inventory for measuring depression, Arch. Gen. Psychiatry, 4 (1961) 461–471.

Beck, A.T., Rush, A.J., Shaw, B.F. and Emery, G., Cognitive Therapy for Depression, Guilford Press, New York, 1979.

Buckelew, S.P., Shutty, M.S., Hewett, J., Landon, J., Morrow, K. and Frank, R.G., Health locus of control, gender differences and adjustment to persistent pain, Pain, 42 (1990) 287–294.

Butterworth, J.C. and Deardorff, W.W., Psychometric profiles of craniomandibular pain patients: identifying specific subgroups, J. Craniomandib. Pract., 5 (1987) 225–232.

Dworkin, S.F. and LeResche, L. (Eds.), Research diagnostic criteria for temporomandibular disorders, J. Craniomandib. Disord. Facial Oral Pain, 6 (1992) 301–355.

Dworkin, S.F., LeResche, L. and Derouen, T., Reliability of clinical measurement in temporomandibular disorders, Clin. J. Pain, 4 (1988) 89–99.

Funch, D.P. and Gale, E.N., Biofeedback and relaxation therapy for chronic temporomandibular joint pain: predicting successful outcomes, J. Consult. Clin. Psychol., 52 (1984) 928–935.

Gallagher, R.M., Marbach, J.J., Raphael, K.G., Dohrenwend, B.P. and Cloitre, M., Is major depression comorbid with temporomandibular pain and dysfunction syndrome? A pilot study, Clin. J. Pain, 7 (1991) 219–225.

Greene, C.S., Olson, R.E. and Laskin, D.M., Psychological factors in the etiology, progression, and treatment of MPD syndrome, J. Am. Dent. Assoc., 105 (1982) 443–448.

Hageman, W.J.M. and Arrindell, W.A., A further refinement of the reliable change (RC) index by improving the pre-post difference score: introducing RC-ID, Behav. Res. Ther., 31 (1993) 693–700.

Jacobson, N.S., Follette, W.C. and Revenstorf, D., Psychotherapy outcome research: methods for reporting variability and evaluating clinical significance, Behavior Therapy, 15 (1984) 336–352.

Keefe, F.J. and Dolan, E., Pain behavior and pain coping strategies in low back pain and myofascial pain dysfunction syndrome patients, Pain, 24 (1986) 49–56.

Kerns, R.D., Turk, D.C. and Rudy, T.E., The West Haven-Yale Multidimensional Pain Inventory (WHYMPI), Pain, 23 (1985) 345–356.

McCreary, C.P., Clark, G.T., Merril, V. and Oakley, M.A., Psychological distress and diagnostic subgroups of temporomandibular patients, Pain, 44 (1991) 29–34.

Melzack, R., The short-form McGill Pain Questionnaire, Pain, 30 (1987) 191–197.

Moss, R.A., Garrett, J. and Chiodo, J.F., Temporomandibular joint dysfunction and myofascial pain dysfunction: parameters, etiology and treatment, Psychol. Bull., 92 (1982) 331–346.

Oakley, M.E., Clark, G.T., McCreary, C.P., Solberg, W.K., Flack, V.F. and Pullinger, A.G., Dentists' ability to detect psychological problems in patients with temporomandibular disorders and chronic pain, J. Am. Dent. Assoc., 118 (1989) 727–730.

Palla, S., Review and commentary, clinical sciences: research diagnostic criteria for temporomandibular disorders, J. Craniomandib. Disord. Facial Oral Pain, 6 (1992) 350–355.

Rosenstiel, A.K. and Keefe, F.J., The use of coping strategies in chronic low back pain patients: relationship to patient characteristics and current adjustment, Pain, 17 (1983) 33–44.

Rugh, J.D. and Solberg, W.K., Psychological implications in temporomandibular pain and dysfunction, Oral Sci. Rev., 1 (1976) 3–15.

Rudy, T.E., Turk, D.C., Zaki, H.S. and Curtin, H.D., An empirical taxometric alternative to traditional classification of temporomandibular disorders, Pain, 36 (1989) 311–320.

Rudy, T.E., Turk, D.C., Kubinski, J.A. and Zaki, H.S., Differential treatment responses of TMD patients as a function of psychological characteristics, Pain (1994) in press.

Schnurr, R.F., Brooke, R.I. and Rollman, G.B., Psychosocial correlates of temporomandibular joint pain and dysfunction, Pain, 42 (1990) 153–165.

Speculand, B. and Goss, A.M., A review of psychological factors in temporomandibular joint dysfunction pain, Int. J. Oral Surg., 14 (1985) 131–137

Turk, D.C., Psychological assessment of patients with persistent pain. I. Traditional views, Pain Management, 3 (1990a) 165–172.

Turk, D.C., Psychological assessment of patients with persistent pain. II. Alternative views, Pain Management, 3 (1990b) 227–237.

Turk, D.C. and Rudy, T.E., Toward an empirically-derived taxonomy of chronic pain patients: integration of psychological assessment data, J. Consult. Clin. Psychol., 56 (1988) 233–238.

Turk, D.C. and Rudy, T.E., The robustness of an empirically derived taxonomy of chronic pain patients, Pain, 42 (1990) 27–35.

Turk, D.C. and Rudy, T.E., Multiaxial assessment and taxometric classification. In: D.C. Turk and R. Melzack (Eds.), Handbook of Pain Assessment, Guilford Press, New York, 1992, pp. 409–428.

Turk, D.C., Zaki, D.S. and Rudy, T.E., Effects of intraoral appliance and biofeedback/stress management alone and in combination in treating pain and depression in patients with temporomandibular disorders, J. Prosthet. Dent., 70 (1993) 158–164.

Correspondence to: Thomas E. Rudy, PhD, Pain Evaluation and Treatment Institute, University of Pittsburgh Medical Center, 4601 Baum Blvd., Pittsburgh, PA 15213, USA. Tel: 412-518-3100; Fax: 412-682-6214.

Temporomandibular Disorders and Related Pain Conditions, Progress in Pain Research and Management, Vol. 4, edited by B.J. Sessle, P.S. Bryant, and R.A. Dionne, IASP Press, Seattle, © 1995.

21

Pharmacologic Treatments for Temporomandibular Disorders

Raymond A. Dionne

Neurobiology and Anesthesiology Branch, National Institute of Dental Research, National Institutes of Health, Bethesda, Maryland, USA

Pharmacologic intervention in the management of chronic orofacial pain is usually considered adjunctive on the assumption that more definitive treatments will eventually correct the underlying pathophysiologic process. As described elsewhere in this volume, many putative therapies for chronic orofacial pain have not withstood the scientific scrutiny of well-controlled clinical trials. Additionally, the possible adverse effects of long-term use of drugs for benign pain may not be as harmful to patients as the iatrogenic effects of failed dental or surgical procedures or the immunologic response to the placement of foreign objects into the temporomandibular joint (TMJ). The use of drugs often can be the primary approach to treating depression associated with chronic pain or to inhibiting inflammatory processes that may contribute to temporomandibular disorders (TMDs). This chapter reviews the scientific basis for the use of drugs in the management of TMDs as adjunctive to other therapeutic modalities and as the primary treatment.

Despite the large body of literature on therapeutic modalities for chronic orofacial pain, few studies have evaluated pharmacologic treatments in a well-controlled fashion. The population of patients with TMDs is heterogeneous; patients with myogenous pain are often not distinguished in clinical drug trials from those who have TMJ disorders such as degenerative arthritis or displacement of the meniscus (Fassbender 1975; Goss et al. 1985). Observations by clinicians and case series often fail to use standardized methods for measurement of pain and dysfunction. The main evidence of a positive treatment outcome too often is the clinician's impression of improvement or the patient's failure to seek further treatment (Greene 1976; Okeson et al. 1983). Another major weakness in previous studies has been the lack of an adequate control group receiving either a placebo or a drug with known efficacy as a positive control, or a no-treatment group. These deficiencies in study design are particularly significant given the high rate of success reported for manipulations such as placebo splints, placebo drug, sham occlusal equilibration, positive doctor-patient relationship, and enthusiastically presented treatment (Greene and Laskin 1972; Laskin and Greene 1972; Goodman et al. 1976).

Another factor that may affect the evaluation of drug therapies is the fluctuating nature of orofacial pain, which may undergo remissions and exacerbations independent of treatment (Magnuson et al. 1986). Concurrent psychological problems, which occur frequently in this population, also may influence the onset of symptoms, reporting of pain levels, and response to treatment (Moody et al. 1982; Greene et al. 1983; Speculand et al. 1983). Many patients eventually improve even if they fail an initial course of therapy (Greene and Laskin 1974) or receive no treatment at all (Magnusson et al. 1986), suggesting that the natural history of this condition may be one of exacerbations and remissions. Such responses may explain the high rate of success reported in loosely controlled studies of many therapeutic modalities used for TMDs.

A wide variety of drug classes have been described for chronic orofacial pain, ranging from short-term treatment with nonsteroidal anti-inflammatory drugs (NSAIDs) and muscle relaxants for pain of muscular origin to chronic administration of antidepressants for less well characterized pain (MacDonald and Phero 1991). In general, enthusiastic claims of efficacy based on clinical observations are superseded by equivocal findings of efficacy and belated recognition of adverse effects or toxicity associated with long-term administration (e.g., elevated incidence of renal failure with chronic NSAID use). The use of a drug for chronic orofacial pain should be based on documented therapeutic efficacy in one or more well-controlled clinical trials, an acceptable side effect liability, and minimal potential for systemic toxicity with chronic administration. Clinical use of a drug that does not meet these criteria can be considered a nonvalidated clinical practice and requires further evaluation in controlled clinical trials, full disclosure to the patient of the unproven nature of the drug for the indication, and consideration of the medicolegal ramifications of off-label use of a drug approved for another indication.

ANTIDEPRESSANTS

Antidepressant drugs have been used for more than 30 years (Magni 1991) for the management of pain from a wide variety of conditions, including chronic orofacial pain (McNeill 1993). Based on a relatively large number of published studies, a consensus is emerging on whether drugs of this class have analgesic properties or act through alleviation of depression, the appropriate dose range for analgesia, and whether drugs with specificity for one neurotransmitter have a better therapeutic ratio than drugs with multiple effects in the central nervous system (e.g., amitriptyline; Onghena and Van Houdenhove 1992). Three independent reviews of controlled studies of the use of antidepressants for pain management indicate that their analgesic effects are largely independent of antidepressant activity (Egbunike and Chaffee 1990; Magni 1991; Onghena and Van Houdenhove 1992). The analgesic effects can be differentiated from placebo, are seen at doses lower than those usually effective in depression, and can occur in patients who are not depressed.

Studies in nondental chronic pain, primarily diabetic and postherpetic neuropathy, indicate that drugs which inhibit reuptake of both serotonin and norepinephrine, such as amitriptyline, are more efficacious than drugs which are selective for either neurotransmitter. Max and colleagues (1987, 1992) demonstrated that amitriptyline relieved the symptoms of painful diabetic neuropathy, while fluoxetine, a serotonin reuptake blocker, was ineffective. Similarly, single doses of two 5-HT$_1$ agonists, buspirone and m-chlorophenyl-piperazine, were ineffective in neuropathic pain patients (Kishore-Kumar et al. 1989).

Clonidine, an alpha-2-adrenergic agonist, also is efficacious in some, but not all, neuropathic pain patients (Zeigler et al. 1992). Conversely, desipramine, which is a relatively selective blocker of norepinephrine reuptake, was equally efficacious with amitriptyline for painful diabetic neuropathy (Max et al. 1992). If these observations can be extrapolated to orofacial pain, blockade of norepinephrine reuptake is critical to the use of antidepressants for chronic pain.

Indirect evidence that antidepressants produce analgesia independent of the alleviation of depression comes from studies with low doses of amitriptyline in chronic pain patients. Sharav et al. (1987) demonstrated that a low dose (mean 23.6 mg) of amitriptyline was as effective for chronic orofacial pain as a higher dose (mean 129 mg), the usual daily antidepressant dose being 75–150 mg (Baldessarini 1985). A daily dose of 25 mg amitriptyline for three weeks was also demonstrated to be superior to placebo in a variety of patients with chronic nonmalignant pain (McQuay et al. 1992). A dose-response comparison of 25, 50, and 75 mg amitriptyline demonstrated increased analgesia with increasing dose and improved sleep with the 75-mg dose, but significantly higher incidence of adverse effects at the 75-mg dose (McQuay et al. 1993). Zitman and colleagues (1990) also reported analgesia with 75 mg amitriptyline and improved sleep over six weeks but considered the magnitude of the effect modest. If antidepressants produced therapeutic effects through alleviation of depression, the doses needed would be similar to those needed for depression.

THERAPEUTIC IMPLICATIONS

The clinical use of antidepressants for chronic nonmalignant pain in the orofacial region should be considered when other treatments have failed or if depression accompanies the pain. Tricyclic antidepressants with both serotonergic and noradrenergic effects (e.g., amitriptyline or doxepin) should be employed (Onghena and Van Houdenhove 1992). Lower dosages should be used initially for nondepressive patients, with antidepressant doses reserved for depressed patients and given in collaboration with a clinician experienced in the diagnosis and treatment of psychiatric illness. The sedative effects of antidepressants may be useful when patients have sleeping problems and may help to reduce the use of hypnotics (Onghena and Van Houdenhove 1992). Dose will usually be limited by anticholinergic side effects (dry mouth, constipation, blurred vision, and urinary retention) and should be adjusted in response to individual variation in analgesic response and side effects. Cardiovascular effects ranging from postural hypotension to serious ventricular arrhythmias can occur, especially in patients with preexisting heart disease; medical consultation or parallel management should be considered in patients at risk.

Although approximately 40 placebo-controlled studies have been identified in the literature regarding the use of antidepressants for chronic pain, only three evaluated their use for orofacial pain, and one of those was published nearly 30 years ago (Lascelles 1966). The two most recent studies (Feinmann 1983; Sharav et al. 1987) evaluated amitriptyline in a total of only 121 patients. More clinical research is needed to determine prognostic factors in this patient population predictive of analgesic responsiveness to antidepressants and to determine which drugs have the most favorable balance of analgesia and side effect liability. While patients with depressive symptoms accompanying pain may best benefit from the use of antidepressants, dentists may not recognize depressive patients who may be suicidal. Psychiatric evaluation should be considered if depressive symptoms are marked or suicidal ideation present.

BENZODIAZEPINES

Drugs of the benzodiazepine class frequently are administered to chronic pain patients, often for prolonged periods, despite long-standing professional concern over their ability to produce dependence. A survey of 114 consecutive new patients at an academic pain center found that 38% were taking one or more benzodiazepines, with the majority being chronic users for one to two years (King and Strain 1990). The most common indication (86%) for the use of the benzodiazepine was to improve sleep, yet the authors concluded that these patients reported as many sleep problems as new patients not taking benzodiazepines. While the efficacy of benzodiazepines for chronic pain is not generally recognized, their long-term administration is controversial owing to adverse effects, potential for abuse and dependence, and the possibility of initiating or exacerbating depression. Conversely, several studies have demonstrated therapeutic effects of benzodiazepines for musculoskeletal pain (fibromyalgia, TMD-associated myofascial pain), suggesting that their use for chronic orofacial pain be reexamined.

Administration of clonazepam to patients with chronic TMD–associated myofascial pain was demonstrated to be superior to placebo in a double-blind 30-day trial (Harkins et al. 1991). Subjects reported a reduction in pain at all sites tested, with several sites reaching significance despite the small sample size (N = 10 per group). No instances of dependence or withdrawal symptoms were noted after discontinuation of the drug after 30 to 60 days, albeit the small sample size limits generalization. In a larger study (N = 78), patients with fibromyalgia meeting the published criteria for primary fibrositis/ fibromyalgia syndrome (Russell et al. 1986) received alprazolam, ibuprofen, or a combination of the two in comparison with placebo (Russell et al. 1991). Improvement in patient rating of disease severity and tenderness upon palpation was significant in the alprazolam plus ibuprofen group after six weeks. It was not clear whether alprazolam or ibuprofen was primarily responsible for the improvement seen. Four patients from the placebo group withdrew because of side effects, compared with only two withdrawals among all three active drug groups, suggesting that the doses of ibuprofen (2400 mg daily) and alprazolam (0.5–3.0 mg daily) were well tolerated. A total of 52 patients completed 24 weeks of open-label treatment with the combination; the authors report that many patients tapered their alprazolam dosage by one or more tablets (0.5 mg) per day below the level offered, contrary to a pattern of drug abuse.

A similar study in 39 patients with chronic orofacial pain of myogenic origin evaluated ibuprofen (mean dose 2400 mg/day), diazepam (mean dose 17 mg/day), and the combination of the two in comparison with placebo in a four-week double-blind trial (Singer et al. 1987). Pain, as measured by a visual analog scale, decreased significantly in the diazepam and diazepam plus ibuprofen groups but not in the ibuprofen or placebo groups. Analysis of variance showed a significant drug effect for diazepam but not for ibuprofen, indicating that the pain relief was attributable to diazepam. Depression showed a tendency toward improvement on both the depression adjective checklist and the Zung depression scale in the groups receiving diazepam; there was also a trend for less anxiety in the benzodiazepine groups. The small sample size (9–11 per group) in this study limits generalization of the findings, but the data are supportive of benzodiazepine-mediated relief of symptoms in chronic orofacial pain of myogenic origin.

A recent review addressed several commonly held beliefs regarding the long-term use of benzodiazepines for chronic pain (Dellemijn and Fields 1994). The authors concluded, based in part on the studies reviewed above, that chronic use of benzodiazepines is effective for some pains of presumed musculoskeletal origin. They suggest, however, that the antidepressant effects attributed to triazolo-benzodiazepines, such as alprazolam, may be artifactual because of overlaps in diagnostic criteria used for depression and anxiety disorders and the impact of the sedative effects on rating scales used to assess depression. These authors also conclude that benzodiazepines in high doses produce reversible side effects mistakenly interpreted as depression, rather than actually initiate endogenous depression. The literature reviewed indicates that a high proportion of chronic pain patients have some type of depressive syndrome, which may develop concomitantly with the chronic pain state rather than be drug induced.

THERAPEUTIC IMPLICATIONS

The scientific literature does not provide unequivocal support for either the use of benzodiazepines or their condemnation on the basis of lack of efficacy or potential toxicity. Like all drugs, they should be used only in patients whose symptoms suggest potential efficacy and should not be prescribed in large amounts permitting dose escalation without professional supervision or the development of dependence with long-term therapy. Patients whose pain appears to be of musculoskeletal origin may benefit from a two- to four-week course of a benzodiazepine, possibly in combination with an NSAID. Lack of efficacy or the onset of sedative side effects or depressive symptoms should be an indication to reduce the dose or discontinue the benzodiazepine. If difficulties in sleep onset or duration are the primary complaint, consideration should be given to the use of a benzodiazepine indicated for hypnosis to minimize drug effects during the day. Patients who appear to have depressive symptoms prior to therapy should be referred to a psychiatrist for consultation and possible antidepressant therapy rather than prescribed a benzodiazepine with putative antidepressant properties. In any event, therapy with a benzodiazepine should not be extended beyond a few weeks, as the natural course of myofascial pain combined with conservative therapy will likely result in a lowering of symptomology to acceptable levels that would not justify the risks of pharmacologic intervention. Patients who fail such a therapeutic course should be reevaluated rather than "managed" with long-term benzodiazepine treatment.

MUSCLE RELAXANTS

Drugs thought to reduce skeletal muscle tone are often administered to patients with chronic orofacial pain to help prevent or alleviate the increased muscle activity attributed to some forms of TMDs (McNeill 1993). While the use of benzodiazepines is sometimes rationalized on the basis of putative muscle-relaxing properties, drugs of this class decrease muscle tone only at doses that produce central nervous system depression. Muscle relaxants are thought to decrease muscle tone without impairment in motor function by acting centrally to depress polysynaptic reflexes. Other drugs with sedative properties, such as barbiturates, also depress polysynaptic reflexes, making it difficult to assess whether centrally acting skeletal muscle relaxants actually are muscle relaxants as opposed to nonspecific sedatives (Elenbaas 1980).

Carisoprodol is one of the oldest drugs of this class, having first been evaluated for chronic orofacial pain in a study published in 1960. A double-blind placebo-controlled clinical evaluation found carisoprodol to be equally efficacious (5 of 17 patients improved) with placebo (5 of 17 improved), with a similar incidence of side effects (Schwartz et al. 1960). Similarly, carisoprodol could not be differentiated from placebo in a double-blind comparison to placebo in 60 patients (Gallardo et al. 1975). A critical review of centrally acting skeletal muscle relaxants concluded that carisoprodol and related propanediols were better than placebo for acute musculoskeletal disorders but less effective for chronic conditions (Elenbaas 1980).

A possible exception is cyclobenzaprine (Flexeril), which is effective in some chronic musculoskeletal disorders (Elenbaas 1980). Cyclobenzaprine is superior to placebo for pain in the cervical and lumbar regions associated with skeletal muscle spasms (Bercel 1977; Brown and Womble 1978) and reduces electromyographic signs of muscle spasm (Basmajian 1978). While not directly assessed for TMDs, these findings suggest efficacy for muscle relaxation in the orofacial region.

THERAPEUTIC IMPLICATIONS

There appears to be a discrepancy between the common clinical use of skeletal muscle relaxants and the results of controlled clinical trials evaluating their efficacy in comparison with placebo. Further studies are needed to document whether they are specific for muscle relaxation or produce nonspecific depression, thereby reducing muscle tone. Little supporting evidence exists for their efficacy in chronic orofacial pain of myogenic origin, nor is it clear if they provide an additive effect with exercise or splint therapy aimed at muscle relaxation. Given this modest scientific support, clinicians should probably limit the use of skeletal muscle relaxants to a brief trial in conjunction with physical therapy regimens.

NONOPIOID ANALGESICS

Nonopioid analagesics comprise a heterogenous class of drugs including the salicylates (aspirin and diflunisal), para-aminophenol derivatives (primarily acetaminophen), and the NSAIDs (ibuprofen and many others). Despite their diverse structures, nonopioid analgesics have similarly therapeutic effects, oral efficacy, and side effect profiles. They are better tolerated than opioids by ambulatory patients, have fewer sedative effects, and are much less likely to produce tolerance or dependence. Conversely, the hazards of long-term administration of these drugs are belatedly being recognized as an increased incidence of serious toxicity to the gastrointestinal (GI) tract and kidneys. The use of nonopioid analgesics rests on the same principles that apply to all other drugs: demonstrated efficacy for the indication (chronic orofacial pain), an acceptable side effect liability, and safety over prolonged periods.

Review of the primary literature reveals few well-controlled studies suggesting that daily use of nonopioid analgesics offers benefit for chronic orofacial pain (Truelove 1994). Standard texts (Dworkin et al. 1990) and summaries of expert opinion (McNeill 1993) often provide recommendations for specific drugs and doses, but either do not provide support for these recommendations or extrapolate from chronic inflammatory conditions such as arthritis. Yet, the results of two placebo-controlled studies suggest that NSAIDs are ineffective for chronic orofacial pain. Administration of ibuprofen 2400 mg per day for four weeks could not be separated from placebo in a group of patients with chronic orofacial pain characterized as myogenic in origin (Singer et al. 1987). Comparison of piroxicam 20 mg daily to placebo for TMD pain (N = 28) also failed to demonstrate any therapeutic advantage for the NSAID (Gordon et al. 1990).

The lack of clinical studies to support the efficacy of NSAIDs for TMDs becomes more important when contrasted with the growing body of data on the serious toxic effects of NSAIDs when given chronically. Suppression of prostaglandins by aspirin and NSAIDs is not limited to the site of injury and also results in alteration of renal blood flow and of normal function in the GI mucosa. The resultant changes in the GI tract can manifest as localized irritation, ulceration, occult blood loss, or even frank hemorrhage. Retrospective studies have established an association between ingestion of aspirin or NSAIDs and increased risk of upper GI bleeding (Holvoet et al. 1991; Laporte et al.

1991; Kaufman et al. 1993). Meta-analysis of 16 controlled studies suggests that users of NSAIDs have a three-fold greater risk of developing serious adverse GI events than nonusers and that this risk is greater in persons over 60 years of age (Gabriel et al. 1991).

NSAIDs alter renal blood flow by interfering with the synthesis in the kidney of prostaglandins involved in the autoregulation of blood flow and glomerular filtration (Clive and Stoff 1984). Approximately 1% (500,000) of Americans exposed to NSAIDs yearly will develop detectable renal function abnormalities (Whelton and Hamilton 1991). The inhibitory effects of NSAIDs on renal prostaglandin production leads to acute, reversible renal failure in 0.5–1% of patients who take NSAIDs on a chronic basis (Whelton and Hamilton 1991). The most significant renal side effect of NSAIDs is hemo-dynamically mediated acute renal failure, which occurs in individuals with preexisting reduced renal blood perfusion. Retrospective analysis of patients with end-stage renal disease requiring hemodialysis demonstrated an association between chronic NSAID use (defined as more than 5000 pills over the lifetime) and a nine-fold increased risk of end-stage renal disease (Perneger et al. 1994). Aspirin was not associated with increased risk but heavy acetaminophen use (more than 5000 pills over the lifetime) was associated with an appropriately 2.5-fold increase in kidney failure requiring hemodialysis.

THERAPEUTIC IMPLICATIONS

The lack of clinical evidence of a therapeutic effect for nonopioid analgesics in the symptomatic treatment of chronic orofacial pain must by weighed against the potential for serious toxicity with chronic use. A short trial of an NSAID may be considered in patients with an apparent inflammatory component to the pain. A lack of therapeutic effect after a 7–10 day trial or the development of any GI symptoms should prompt discontinuation of the NSAID. Patients with risk factors for GI or renal disease should be managed cautiously with NSAIDs or acetaminophen and not for prolonged periods of time.

RESEARCH NEEDS FOR PHARMACOLOGIC MANAGEMENT OF TMDs

Review of the drug classes most commonly used for TMDs does not reveal a wealth of data upon which to base therapy. The wide variety of other drug modalities currently in clinical use for chronic orofacial pain have even less scientific support. Given the potential for serious toxicity that can accompany long-term administration of drugs that are safe enough to be mar-

keted without a prescription (i.e., the NSAIDs), a lack of demonstrated efficacy for drugs with even greater potential toxicity may indicate risk to the
patient without therapeutic benefit. A need exists for well-controlled studies
of drugs in the chronic orofacial pain patient population, for periods that
approximate their use clinically, with appropriate indices of therapeutic efficacy and toxicity, and in comparison with a group receiving placebo medication to control for cyclic fluctuation in symptomology. In the interim, clinicians who treat patients with TMDs should consider the use of many drug
classes to be nonvalidated clinical practice that carries the burden of proof of
efficacy and liability for adverse outcomes.

REFERENCES

Baldessarini, R.J., Drugs and the treatment of psychiatric disorders. In: A.G. Gilman, L.S.,
    Goodman, T.W. Rall and F. Murad (Eds.), The Pharmacological Basis of Therapeutics, 7th
    ed., Macmillan, 1985, p. 419.
Basmajian, J.V., Cyclobenzaprine hydrochloride effect on skeletal muscle spasm in lumbar region
    and neck: Two double-blind controlled clinical and laboratory studies, Arch. Phys. Med.
    Rehabil., 59 (1978) 58–63.
Bercel, N.A., Cyclobenzaprine in the treatment of skeletal muscle spasm in osteoarthritis of the
    cervical and lumbar spine, Curr. Ther. Res., 22 (1977) 462–468.
Brown, B.R. and Womble, J., Cyclobenzaprine in intractable pain syndromes with muscle spasm,
    JAMA, 240 (1978) 1151–1152.
Clive, D.M. and Stoff, J.S., Renal syndromes associated with nonsteroidal anti-inflammatory
    drugs, N. Engl. J. Med., 310 (1984) 563–572.
Dellemijn, P.L.I. and Fields, H.L., Do benzodiazepines have a role in chronic pain management?
    Pain 57 (1994) 137–152.
Dworkin, S.F., Truelove, E.L., Bonica, J.J. and Sola, A., Facial and head pain caused by myofacial
    and temporomandibular disorders. In: J.J. Bonica (Ed.), The Management of Pain, Lea &
    Febiger, Philadelphia, 1990, pp. 727–745.
Egbunike, I.G. and Chaffee, B.J., Antidepressants in the management of chronic pain syndromes,
    Pharmacotherapy, 10 (1990) 262–270.
Elenbaas, J.K., Centrally acting oral skeletal muscle relaxants, Am. J. Hosp. Pharm., 37 (1980)
    131–132.
Fassbender, H.G., Pathology of Rheumatic Diseases, Springer-Verlag, New York, 1975, pp.
    303–314.
Feinmann, C., Psychogenic facial pain: presentation and treatment, J. Psychosom. Res., 27 (1983)
    403–410.
Gabriel, S.E., Jaakkimainen, L. and Bombardier, C., Risk of serious gastrointestinal complications
    related to use of nonsteroidal anti-inflammatory drugs, Ann. Int. Med., 115 (1991) 787–796.
Gallardo, F., Molgo, J., Miyazaki, C. and Rossi, E., Carisoprodol in the treatment of myofascial
    pain-dysfunction syndrome, J. Oral Surg., 33 (1975) 655–658.
Goodman, P., Greene, C.S. and Laskin, D.M., Response of patients with myofascial pain-dysfunc-
    tion syndrome to mock equilibration, J. Am. Dent. Assoc., 92 (1976) 755–758.
Gordon, S.M., Montgomery, M.T. and Jones, L.D., Comparative efficacy of piroxicam versus
    placebo for temporomandibular pain (abstract), J. Dent. Res., 69 (1990) 218.
Goss, A.N., Speculand, D.B. and Hallet, E., Diagnosis of temporomandibular joint pain in patients
    seen at a pain clinic, J. Oral Maxillofac. Surg., 43 (1985) 110–114.

Greene, C.S., The fallacies of clinical success in dentistry, J. Oral Med., 31 (1976) 52–55.

Greene, C.S. and Laskin, D.M., Splint therapy for the myofascial pain-dysfunction (MPD) syndrome: a comparative study, J. Am. Dent. Assoc., 84 (1972) 624–628.

Greene, C.S. and Laskin, D.M., Long-term evaluation of conservative treatment for myofascial pain-dysfunction syndrome, J. Am. Dent. Assoc., 89 (1974) 1365–1368.

Greene, C.S., Oleson, R.E. and Laskin, D.M., Psychosocial factors in the etiology, progression, and treatment of MPD syndrome, J. Am. Dent. Assoc., 105 (1983) 443–448.

Harkins, S., Linford, J., Cohen, J., Kramer, T. and Cueva, L., Administration of clonazepam in the treatment of TMD and associated myofascial pain: a double-blind pilot study, J. Craniomandib. Disord., 5 (1991) 179–186.

Holvoet, J., Terriere, L., Van Hee, W., Verbist, L., Fierens, E. and Hautekeete, M.L., Relation of upper gastrointestinal bleeding to non-steroidal anti-inflammatory drugs and aspirin: a case-control study, Gut, 32 (1991) 730–734.

Kaufman, D.W., Kelly, J.P., Sheehan, J.E., Laszlo, A., Wilholm, B.-E., Alfredsson, L., Koff, R.S. and Shapiro, S., Non-steroidal anti-inflammatory drug use in relation to major upper gastrointestinal bleeding, Clin. Pharmacol. Therapy, 53 (1993) 485–494.

King, S.A. and Strain, J.J., Benzodiazepine use by chronic pain patients, Clin. J. Pain., 6 (1990) 143–147.

Kishore-Kumar, R., Schafer, S.C., Lawlor, B., Murphy, D.L. and Max, M.B., Single doses of serotonin agonists buspirone and m-chlorophenylpiperazine do not relieve neuropathic pain, Pain, 37 (1989) 223–227.

Laporte, J.-R., Carne, X., Vidal, X., Moreno, V. and Juan, J., Upper gastrointestinal bleeding in relation to previous use of analgesics and nonsteroidal and anti-inflammatory drugs, Lancet, 337 (1991) 85–89.

Lascelles, R.G., Atypical facial pain and depression, Br. J. Psychiatry, 112 (1966) 651–659.

Laskin, D.M. and Greene, C.S., Influence of the doctor-patient relationship on placebo therapy for patients with myofascial pain dysfunction (MPD) syndrome, J. Am. Dent. Assoc., 85 (1972) 892–894.

Magni, G., The use of antidepressants in the treatment of chronic pain, Drugs, 42 (1991) 730–748.

Magnusson, T., Egermark-Eriksson, I. and Carlsson, G.E., Five-year longitudinal study of signs and symptoms of mandibular dysfunction in adolescents, J. Craniomandib. Pract., 4 (1986) 338–343.

Max, M.B., Culnane, M., Schafer, S.C., Gracely, R.H., Walther, D.J., Smoller, B. and Dubner, R., Amitriptyline relieves diabetic neuropathy pain in patients with normal or depressed mood, Neurology, 37 (1987) 589–596.

Max, M.B., Lynch, S.A., Muir, J., Shoaf, S.E., Smoller, B. and Dubner, R., Effects of desipramine, amitriptyline, and fluoxetine on pain in diabetic neuropathy, N. Engl. J. Med., 326 (1992) 1250–1256.

McDonald, J.S. and Phero, J.C., Evaluation of chronic pain conditions of the head and neck: a multidisciplinary approach. In: R.A. Dionne and J.C. Phero (Eds.), Management of Pain and Anxiety in Dental Practice, Elsevier, Amsterdam, 1991, pp. 361–382.

McNeill, C., Temporomandibular Disorders, Quintessence, Chicago, 1993, p. 87.

McQuay, H.J., Carroll, D. and Glynn, C.J., Low dose amitriptyline in the treatment of chronic pain, Anaesthesia, 47 (1992) 646–652.

McQuay, H.J., Carroll, D. and Glynn, C.J., Dose-response for analgesic effect of amitriptyline in chronic pain, Anaesthesia, 48 (1993) 281–285.

Moody, P.M., Kemper, J.T., Okeson, J.P., Calhoun, T.C. and Parker, M.W., Recent life changes and myofascial pain syndromes, J. Prosthet. Dent., 48 (1982) 328–330.

Okeson, J.P., Moody, D.M., Kemper, J.T. and Haley, J.V., Evaluation of occlusal splint therapy and relaxation procedures in patients with temporomandibular disorders, J. Am. Dent. Assoc., 107 (1983) 420–424.

Onghena, P. and Van Houdenhove, B., Antidepressant-induced analgesia in chronic non-malignant pain: a meta-analysis of 39 placebo-controlled studies, Pain, 49 (1992) 205–219.

Perneger, T.V., Whelton, P.K. and Klag, M.J., Risk of kidney failure associated with the use of acetaminophen, aspirin, and non-steroidal anti-inflammatory drugs, N. Engl. J. Med., 331 (1994) 1675–1679.

Russell, I.J., Fletcher, E.M., Michalek, J.E., McBroom, P.C. and Hester, G.G., Treatment of primary fibrositis/fibromyalgia syndrome with ibuprofen and alprazolam, Arthritis Rheum., 34 (1991) 552–560.

Schwartz, L., Kutscher, A.H., Yavelow, I., Cobin, H.P. and Brod, M.S., Carisoprodol in the management of temporomandibular join pain and dysfunction: a preliminary investigation, Ann. N.Y. Acad. Sci., 86 (1960) 245–249.

Sharav, Y., Singer, E., Schmidt, E., Dionne, R.A. and Dubner, R., The analgesic effect of amitriptyline on chronic facial pain, Pain, 31 (1987) 199–209.

Singer, E.J., Sharav, Y., Dubner, R. and Dionne, R.A., The efficacy of diazepam and ibuprofen in the treatment of chronic myofascial orofacial pain, Pain (1987) S83.

Speculand, B., Goss, A.N., Hughes, A., Spence, N.D. and Pilowsky, I., Temporomandibular joint dysfunction: pain and illness behavior, Pain, 17 (1983) 139–150.

Truelove, E.L., The chemotherapeutic management of chronic and persistent orofacial pain, Dent. Clin. North Am., 38 (1994) 669–688.

Whelton, A. and Hamilton, C.W., Nonsteroidal anti-inflammatory drugs: effects on kidney function, J. Clin. Pharmacol., 31 (1991) 588–598.

Zeigler, D., Lynch, S.A., Muir, J., Benjamin, J. and Max, M.B., Transdermal clonidine versus placebo in painful diabetic neuropathy, Pain, 48 (1992) 403–408.

Zitman, F.G., Linssen, A.C.G., Edelbroek, P.M. and Stijnen, T., Low dose amitriptyline in chronic pain: the gain is modest, Pain, 42 (1990) 35–42.

Correspondence to: Raymond A. Dionne, DDS, PhD, 9000 Rockville Pike, Bldg. 10, Rm. 1N-103, Bethesda, MD 20892, USA. Tel: 301-496-0294; Fax: 301-496-1005.

Temporomandibular Disorders and Related Pain Conditions, Progress in Pain Research and Management, Vol. 4, edited by B.J. Sessle, P.S. Bryant, and R.A. Dionne, IASP Press, Seattle, © 1995.

22

The Efficacy of Physical Medicine Treatment, Including Occlusal Appliances, for a Population with Temporomandibular Disorders

Glenn T. Clark,[a] Jae-Kap Choi,[a] and Phyllis A. Browne[b]

[a]University of California Los Angeles School of Dentistry, Los Angeles, and [b]Division of Physical Therapy, Chapman University, Orange, California, USA

More than 30 years ago, Laszlo Schwartz reviewed the scope of physical medicine treatments available for temporomandibular disorders (TMDs) (Schwartz 1959), and Ulf Posselt described the various occlusal appliances used to treat TMDs (Posselt 1962). Since then, the use of physical medicine procedures, including occlusal appliances, has grown steadily. Yet, the question remains, "What is the efficacy of these physical medicine based treatments for a TMD population?"

Before answering this question, we must define the term TMDs. It is a global descriptor used to characterize several clinical problems affecting the muscles of mastication and the temporomandibular joint (TMJ). There are three major categories of TMDs. *Intracapsular dysfunctions of the TMJ* can be divided into the following subcategories: (1) clicking joints, (2) locked joints, (3) painful TMJ, and (4) polyarthritic diseases. *Myogenous pain and dysfunction* can be separated into three subcategories: (1) myalgia and myositis, (2) trismus or splinting, and (3) dyskinesia. *Mandibular mobility dysfunctions* include hyper- and hypomobility problems. Hypermobility is a true dislocation of the mandibular condyle during jaw opening or open locking. Open locking is the inability to close the mandible from a wide open (not dislocated) position. Hypomobility problems are due to joint derangements and abnormalities that interfere with full translation and sometimes rotation of the condyle (e.g., joint adhesions and/or ankylosis), or to muscle and fascial contractures that limit full muscle extension. Because of space limitations, this chapter will address only the first two major categories, which are far more prevalent than true mandibular mobility dysfunctions. Unfortunately, few of the studies on the efficacy of physical medicine procedures for TMD described in this chapter are well controlled or employ random-assignment and unbiased comparative research methods. Most are uncontrolled case studies and technique articles. Randomized, controlled trials are cited when available.

PHYSICAL MEDICINE PROCEDURES FOR INTRACAPSULAR DYSFUNCTION

CLICKING JOINTS

Structural abnormality of the TMJ has been blamed for producing the clinical phenomena called TMJ clicking, disk-condyle incoordination, or disk displacement with reduction (Ireland 1953). TMJ clicking, a symptom resistant to treatment, has been managed primarily with four approaches: (1) an exercise-avoidance regime, (2) a dental appliance that stops the click while worn (usually by repositioning the mandible), (3) open (diskoplasty) and closed surgical manipulation (arthroscopy) of the disk, and (4) infusion of a hyaluronate solution into the joint (Bertolami et al. 1993; Liu and Clark 1993).

The exercise-avoidance approach was first advocated by Schwartz (1959) to help reduce TMJ clicking. Patients may learn to avoid the clicking during normal function, even though it is still present on wide jaw opening movements. The efficacy of the approach is debatable. Avoidance of a persistent click was reportedly ineffective in eliminating the jaw-joint clicking phenomena (Messenger and Barghi 1987). In young patients with more recent onset TMJ click problems, some exercises reportedly helped eliminate the click (Au and Klineberg 1993), although the degree to which spontaneous remission would have occurred in this these patients was not examined. The avoidance approach seems logical empirically and may be a reasonable treatment alternative for a patient with a persistent TMJ click (Kirk and Calabrese 1989). Epidemiologic research suggests that most clicking patterns do not change and few develop into or lead to serious TMJ locking or degenerative joint disease (Greene et al. 1982; Lundh et al. 1987). There are no data on the efficacy of this therapeutic approach compared to a no treatment approach; the data that have been collected are not from a randomized controlled trial (RCT).

The use of stabilization and repositioning occlusal appliances for the treatment of TMJ clicking is discussed in a later section. The management of TMJ clicking with open surgical manipulation such as disk plication, diskoplasty, or closed surgical manipulation such as arthroscopic lavage and/

or arthroscopically assisted disk plication is beyond the scope of this chapter.

Joint surface lubrication using sodium hyaluronate (HA) is the most recent physical medicine technique to be considered for TMJ clicking. Data from other joints (knee) where HA infusion has been used suggest that a high molecular weight hyaluronate has the potential to be a conservative, safe, efficacious, and essentially hazard-free adjunctive "lubricating" agent to reduce joint friction and promote healing of intracapsular disorders (Rydell and Balazs 1971; Peyron and Balazs 1974; Namiki et al. 1982; Ruth and Swites 1985). In one study, a multisite RCT, injections of HA were moderately efficacious for the management of painful symptoms associated with TMJ clicking, but the clicking did not disappear (Bertolami et al. 1993). HA infusion is limited at present because it has not yet been approved by the FDA for intra-articular use in humans in the United States.

LOCKED JOINTS

Recurrent, momentary locking that prevents normal jaw opening is a common pattern in many patients; this condition has been described by some as "closed locking." A patient with frequent intermittent closed locking can progress to continuous closed locking. It is assumed that the reduced joint translation is due to a combination of adherence, deformation, and displacement of the disk. Closed locking (also described as acute onset hypomobility of the TMJ and diskal displacement without reduction) has been managed with three primary approaches: (1) manual reduction, typically performed by a dentist or physical therapist, in the very early stages of the problem, (2) arthroscopic surgical procedure, or (3) arthrocentesis procedure (involving saline infusion) to increase joint mobility.

Although the reported success of manual reduction varies widely, typically less than half of all attempted cases have a quick return of normal mobility. Segami and colleagues (1990) reported that manual manipulation was successful in 26 of 30 cases. Arthrographic imaging, however, showed a normal disk position following manipulation in only a few of their cases. These reports are all case series descriptions; no RCT has been performed in which manual reduction is compared with the other two treatments (arthroscopy or arthrocentesis). Many authors who report success also describe a post manipulation protocol involving the insertion of a mandibular repositioning appliance on the assumption that the clicking and locking would recur if no appliance were used (McCarty 1980; Friedman et al. 1982a; Friedman and Weisberg 1985). No RCT has addressed whether the appliance is necessary after manipulation. Actually, the frequent suggested use of such a protocol implies that the results of manual reduction are short term.

Arthroscopy of the TMJ for the patient with closed locking was introduced in 1986 (Sanders 1986) and soon replaced open surgical diskoplasty and disk plication operations. Indications for TMJ arthroscopy are continuous, painful, closed locking and a failure of the manual reduction or arthrocentesis procedures to resolve the problem. No RCTs have been conducted for TMJ open or closed surgery. It is thus impossible to distinguish the surgical effect from the postoperative physical therapy program or the steroid injections used in most cases.

The third and most current treatment method for an acute closed locking condition is arthrocentesis. Only three papers have described this procedure (Murakami et al. 1987; Ross 1989; Nitzan et al. 1991). All three reported success rates comparable to those given for arthroscopy (greater than 80%); none of these studies was an RCT comparing arthrocentesis to arthroscopy and/or manual manipulation. By comparison, even if no attempt is made to mobilize a locked joint, patients will eventually experience a near full restoration of jaw mobility and a substantial decrease in painful symptoms (Rasmussen 1981; Mejersjo and Carlsson 1983; Carlsson 1985; McNeill 1985). This improvement, however, is generally slower than might occur following an arthroscopic surgical or arthrocentesis procedure. Regardless of the therapeutic method, the amount of pain and lost mobility in these chronically locked joints is usually minimal after 6 to 12 months. Researchers have observed that the signs of crepitation and arthrotic remodeling are present in some of the untreated closed lock patients. It is not known if the occurrence of these signs is less likely following successful arthroscopy or arthrocentesis.

LOCALIZED TMJ PAIN

The two major expected causes of localized TMJ pain are macrotrauma (trauma due to an external force to the jaw) and microtrauma (trauma due to parafunctional loading) (Friedman et al. 1982b). Trauma produces articular tissue injury with subsequent inflammation and pain, and may result in localized bony arthrotic changes. Five approaches have been described for the management of a painful TMJ: (1) a jaw rest/soft diet/nonsteroidal anti-inflammatory drug (NSAID) regime, (2) topically applied anti-inflammatory modalities such as ice and/or transcutaneously applied anti-inflammatory medications such as aspirin or corticosteroid-based ointments, induced by phonophoresis or electrophoresis (Griffin et al. 1967; Wing 1982; Gangarosa 1983), (3) a dental occlusal appliance to alter jaw function and reduce articular surface loading, (4) open surgical arthrotomy or closed (arthroscopic) surgical lavage and lysis of the TMJ, and (5) injection or ingestion of a corticosteroid medication (Kopp et al. 1985, 1987; Wenneberg et al. 1991).

In general, the jaw rest/soft diet/NSAID approach is the first recommended therapy when joint pain is acute and due to identifiable macrotrauma. In addition, gentle mobilization techniques and active range of motion exercises may be recommended if joint motion is restricted due to pain (Wyke 1975; Maitland 1979; Carstensen 1986). Intuition dictates that such an approach is reasonable even though no RCT has been performed to test its validity or efficacy relative to other approaches. If joint pain appears to be caused by repeated parafunctional behavior (e.g., bruxism), an occlusal stabilization appliance may be added to the treatment regime. It has not been proven whether an occlusal appliance can alter loading in the TMJ, but clinically it does seem to alter parafunctional behaviors. (The clinical case-based data on the efficacy of occlusal appliances for joint pain are presented in a later section.) The rest/soft diet/NSAID method in combination with an occlusal appliance approach has not been compared to other available approaches using RCT testing.

No RCTs have evaluated the efficacy of topically applied anti-inflammatory modalities or transcutaneously induced anti-inflammatory medications for TM pain (Olson 1972; Toller 1973; Burgess et al. 1986). However, there are many generally positive case-based reports in the physical medicine literature in which these methods have been used. One study of chronic back and neck pain patients compared these modalities, among others, with a control condition of manual therapy only and reported no clear benefits of one approach versus the other (Koes et al. 1992). The efficacy of surgical arthrotomy, arthroscopy, and corticosteroid injection is not within the scope of this chapter.

POLYARTHRITIC DISEASE INVOLVING THE TMJ

Radiographic changes indicative of osteoarthritic joint disease involving the TMJ and other body joints are quite common (Solberg 1986; Pullinger and Seligman 1987). When crepitus or multiple clicking sounds occur, the likelihood of radiographic confirmation of an osseous joint disease is greater. The TMJ is less commonly the site of polyarthritic inflammatory joint diseases (e.g., rheumatoid arthritis, scleroderma).

Nonpharmacologic physical medicine procedures have not been reported to reverse or arrest any polyarthritic joint disease process. However, the same physical medicine procedures described for localized TMJ pain management are commonly prescribed to provide symptomatic treatment for TMJ pain of polyarthritic origin and its secondary myogenous symptoms. In addition, stretching and range of motion exercises are commonly prescribed to maintain or increase joint mobility when a hypermobility is being induced from the polyarthritic process (Yavelow et al. 1973; Bush 1984; Friedman and Weisberg

1984). The latter occurs because when intra-articular osseous changes exist, patients often avoid movement of the involved joint. Although movement avoidance is appropriate for acute joint pain, joint mobilization is generally considered important in the management of chronic joint pain (Kraus 1988; Okeson 1989). Unfortunately, no data from RCT are available in which the efficacy of these procedures was tested in the TMJ afflicted with polyarthritic disease.

PHYSICAL MEDICINE PROCEDURES FOR MYOGENOUS DYSFUNCTION

MYALGIA

Myalgia (muscle pain) and occasionally an associated myositis (swelling) may be present in the masticatory musculature. The pathologic changes are not fully known; pain and swelling are generally considered to be due to local tissue inflammation and/or a localized hypoxia of the muscle (Raft et al. 1968; Moller 1981). Chronic regional muscle pain is typically described as myofascial pain dysfunction. Pain occurring in at least three of the four body quadrants is called fibromyalgia. An association has been demonstrated between masticatory muscle parafunctions and the symptoms of masticatory myalgia (Rubin 1981; Yemm 1985). These parafunctions are variable and include sleep-associated tooth grinding behaviors, i.e., bruxism (Rugh and Solberg 1975), skeletal muscle activity while awake due to habitual oral behaviors (e.g., clenching or abnormal jaw posturing), and protective muscle activity (trismus) induced by regional pain. Less commonly, acute myalgia and myositis in the masticatory muscles may occur as a result of local trauma to the jaw muscle (Brooke and Stenn 1978). Numerous physical medicine procedures are used to treat chronic myalgia and myositis symptoms in the orofacial region (Table I) (Gold et al. 1983; Laskin and Block 1986; Clark 1987; Clark et al. 1990).

No RCTs have been performed to compare the effectiveness of the rest/ soft diet/NSAID treatment program with a no-treatment approach for acute onset myalgia and myositis in the masticatory muscles. Nevertheless, these methods are commonly prescribed to provide symptomatic treatment for acute muscle pain problems.

When a muscle disorder is recalcitrant to treatment and therefore considered chronic, other methods are traditionally prescribed such as topically applied pain relief and inflammation-reducing modalities (e.g., ultrasound and/or ice and heat pack applications to the injured site). The proposed mechanism by which these modalities provide pain relief and inflammation reduction is via an increase in regional arterial perfusion. Although no specific evidence

Table I
Physical medicine procedures for the management of myalgia and myositis

Rest/soft diet/NSAIDs

Topically applied pain-relief modalities

Postural awareness and range of motion exercises

Deep tissue massage and muscle stretching

Transcutaneous pain relief techniques (e.g., ultrasound, TENS, and/or muscle stimulation)

Acupuncture and/or trigger point injections

Occlusal appliances

Muscle relaxation techniques (e.g., biofeedback)

exists for the masticatory muscles, these methods have been proven clinically effective by physical therapists treating other body parts (Cordray and Krusen 1959; Fountain and Gersten 1960; Keene 1985). Few, if any, authors question the conservative use of cold for an acute traumatic injury and even for some of the more resistant subacute problems. Conversely, it is unclear whether thermal agents are appropriate and efficacious for chronic myalgia problems. A comparative study, published in abstract form only, of ultrasound versus electrical stimulation and jaw exercises for a TMD patient group with chronic muscle pain found that all treatments were partially helpful but no significant difference resulted among these methods (Eisen et al. 1984).

Postural awareness and range of motion exercises are typically used when, upon evaluation, the myalgia symptoms appear to be related to mandibular muscle parafunction. No RCT data have been reported demonstrating that these exercises are more effective than a no-treatment approach for myalgia and myositis in the masticatory muscles. These same statements apply for deep tissue massage and stretching techniques, which are used to relax chronically contracted muscles, stretch related tissue, alter motor patterns, and increase the patient's postural awareness.

The efficacy of transcutaneous electrical nerve stimulation (TENS) procedures has been challenged. Several controlled trials indicate they have no greater benefit than a placebo therapy program (Block and Laskin 1980; Graff-Radford et al. 1989; Deyo et al. 1990). Other transcutaneous therapies such as ultrasound, cold lasers, and slow-frequency electrical pulsing devices for muscle stimulation also generally lack any RCT data to prove their efficacy. Soft (cold) lasers have been investigated as a tool for wound healing and muscle pain relief. Usually pain free, the cold laser is aseptic, nonthermal, and noninjurious to tissues. The proposed empirical biostimulatory effects include accelerated collagen synthesis, increased vascularity of healing tissue, and decreased pain (Seitz and Kleinkort 1986). Most studies of cold laser therapy have focused on chronic musculoskeletal, rheumatologic, and neurologic pain conditions (Goldman et al. 1980; Walker 1983; Kleinkort and Foley 1984; Snyder-Mackler and Bork 1988; Strang et al. 1988; Zakariasen and Dederich 1988). The results have been mixed and the majority of the studies lacked proper research design. The use of laser irradiation of musculoskeletal trigger points as a substitute for direct local anesthetic injections is promising, but additional work is needed. A decrease in trigger point pain has been reported following irradiation in a sample of patients with neck and lower back pain (Snyder-Mackler and Bork 1988; Olavi et al. 1989; Snyder-Mackler et al. 1989). Two case studies have been published in which cold laser treatment was used on persistent TMJ pain (Hansson 1985; Palano et al. 1985) and resulted in decreased pain, decreased crepitation, and increased range of motion; however, the studies lacked controls, blinding, and adequate sample sizes.

Several recent studies have been published in which an RCT method was used to compare acupuncture to occlusal appliances for the treatment of TMD problems (Johansson et al. 1991; List et al. 1992). Both treatment methods have generally resulted in a substantial improvement in chronic muscle pain symptoms immediately after the treatment period and at the one year follow-up. These data are encouraging and hold promise for acupuncture as a therapeutic method of managing local myalgia and myositis in the masticatory system.

The efficacy of local anesthetic injections into tender areas or "trigger points" for regional myalgia and myositis has not been substantiated with RCT-based research. However, numerous case reports describe how anesthetic blocking of the tender areas in an involved muscle has helped a patient (Bonica 1957; Bell 1969; Toller 1976). Stress-management and muscle-relaxation techniques such as biofeedback therapy are also commonly used in patients who complain of stress-tension problems and/or have strong diurnal parafunctional habits (see Rudy and Turk, this volume, for an assessment of the efficacy of these behavioral methods).

TRISMUS AND SPLINTING

Trismus and splinting of the masticatory muscles results in a decreased range of voluntary jaw opening (Tveteras and Kristensen 1986). Limited mandibular movements may also occur for several nonmuscular reasons. For this discussion, however, decreased range of mandibular movement is assumed to be a protective reflex induced during opening in which jaw-opening muscles are inhibited and jaw-closing muscles are excited. A common physical medicine approach for patients with complaints of trismus is ice and/or vapocoolant spray application to the skin over the painful muscle followed by stretching of the involved muscles (Schultz 1947; Schwartz 1954; Burgess et al. 1986).

Except as a diagnostic test, this approach is not typically recommended for acute (less than five days) trismus caused by a recent injury or trauma. If the condition is caused by acute psychological distress, the patient must be referred to a psychologist (Salmon et al. 1972). In most cases, acute traumatic and hysterical trismus are self-limiting and resolve in 7–14 days as the injury heals or the emotional crisis passes. If prolonged trismus develops following this approach, re-evaluation of the original diagnosis is appropriate. In these cases, prolonged trismus may develop due to ongoing microtraumatic/jaw muscle parafunctions or an unusual healing process.

Advocates of vapocoolant spray and stretch procedures claim that stretching helps alleviate chronic myofascial pain and dysfunction by desensitizing the "trigger point" in the muscle (Travell 1976). Although the validity of this proposed mechanism is not proven, the clinical effectiveness of this procedure has been accepted. The application of spray and stretch procedures in cases without muscle shortening, however, is not logical. In fact, vigorous overstretching can produce muscle microtearing and is potentially damaging. Trismus is usually a symptom secondary to regional pain. Thus, treatment of trismus without appropriate management of the underlying pathology is not likely to be efficacious.

Other treatment approaches for trismus involve high-voltage galvanic stimulation as well as ultrasound of the involved muscles (Kahn 1980; Esposito et al. 1984). These treatments reduce pain and inflammation and, if followed by stretching procedures, alleviate the trismus response. Similar to other physical medicine procedures, these treatments must be repeated frequently to be effective in increasing mandibular range of motion. When posttreatment relief is transient, greater attention must be paid to etiologic factors. As with myalgia, RCT data are needed to identify the most efficacious physical medicine approach for the management of trismus.

DYSKINESIA

Clinically evident, mild abnormality in jaw movement is best described as muscle incoordination or a learned dyskinesia. It is rarely a significant clinical problem (Clark and Lynn 1986). It may, however, be an indicator of early muscle dysfunction. This form of dysfunction is thought to reflect poor proprioceptive control of the muscles due to disuse, pain avoidance, or incoordination. For this reason, patients may be given exercises to increase proprioceptive awareness of their jaws (Yavelow et al. 1973; Voss et al., 1985; Monteiro and Clark 1988).

The goal is to relieve the myalgic pain as the patient's motor control improves. Theoretically, this improvement results from increased awareness of the muscles. As this occurs, the patient is better able to recognize when the muscles are contracting and when they are relaxed (Monteiro and Clark 1988). The above motor control problem should not be confused with true involuntary orofacial dyskinesia (e.g., focal mandibular dystonia or facial tics). These latter conditions are neurologic disorders and should be evaluated and treated as such (Klawans et al. 1988).

OCCLUSAL APPLIANCES FOR INTRACAPSULAR DYSFUNCTION

The most commonly used appliances for treatment of TMDs are stabilization and repositioning devices. This chapter focuses on the empirical indications for using these two devices and, where research is available, presents the efficacy of each device. Unfortunately, as with the other physical medicine procedures, most evaluations of occlusal appliances for the treatment of TMDs are not controlled comparative studies but uncontrolled case studies and technique articles.

TMJ CLICKING

As mentioned, TMJ clicking is the symptom most resistant to treatment (Greene and Laskin 1972). Some studies have reported improvement of other symptoms (e.g., pain) with a stabilization appliance, but few of the subjects exhibited diminished clicking (Agerberg and Carlsson 1974; Goharian and Neff 1980; Mejersjo and Carlsson 1983). In a published study in which subjects with TMJ clicking were randomly assigned to one of two treatments (repositioning versus stabilization appliances), those using the stabilization appliance had no change in joint clicking (Lundh et al. 1985). Finally, Helkimo and Westling (1987) compared the outcome of 55 cases with a diagnosis of disk displacement (both with and without reduction) with 342 other cases with TMD and no disk displacement. All cases had conventional treatment (physical therapy and stabilization appliances). After one year, 69% of disk displacement subjects improved while 74% of other TMD patients improved.

Repositioning appliances have been used extensively to treat clicking since Farrar first described their use for TMJ disk displacement in 1971. Clark (1984) subsequently reported on 25 patients with TMJ clicking treated with a repositioning appliance and followed prospectively for one to two years. Ten of 20 patients (50%) available at follow-up still had clicking. Within the same group, 70% had improvement in pain symptoms measured with a categorical scale questionnaire. In a second study, Clark and colleagues (1988) again reported similar results for clicking reduction (39%) and improvement of other symptoms (39%) at 19 months follow-up. Le Bell and

Kirveskari (1985) and Okeson (1988) also had similar results when they described a substantially greater improvement in symptoms (e.g., pain) other than clicking at follow-up. Moloney and Howard (1986) reported that only 36% of 241 repositioning cases followed for three years maintained an absence of clicking. They suggested the repositioning device was less effective on late-opening than early-opening clicks.

In contrast, Anderson and colleagues (1985) compared 10 patients who received repositioning and 10 who received stabilization appliances. They claimed that after a 90-day treatment period, clicking was gone in 80% of the repositioned group and in none of the stabilization appliance group. In fact, two cases in the stabilization appliance group became locked during treatment. They further reported that pain symptoms improved in 60% of the repositioned group and in none of the stabilization appliance group. Lundh and colleagues (1985) also compared repositioning to other techniques. They randomly assigned 72 subjects to either a stabilization splint, a repositioning appliance, or a wait list condition. At one year clicking was present in all subjects in the stabilization appliance group and in 81% of the wait list group. The repositioning appliance stopped the clicking in 22 of 24 cases, but clicking returned in 18 cases after use of the repositioning appliance was stopped. One case became locked. They recommended permanent repositioning of the jaw for longlasting effect, and subsequently conducted such a study (Lundh et al. 1988). They reported that the permanently repositioned group had a continued cessation of clicking while the other two groups did not. Lundh and Westesson (1989) reported three-year results for 15 of these clicking cases after exchanging the removable repositioning appliance with cemented posterior tooth onlays. Thirteen were click-free after treatment, and 82% had normal disk position (two cases had anterior disk position).

JOINT PAIN

Two studies reported improvement of joint pain with the use of stabilization appliances (Agerberg and Carlsson 1974; Carraro and Caffesse 1978). Magnusson and Carlsson (1980), in contrast, reported no effect of appliances on joint pain at follow-up.

OCCLUSAL APPLIANCES FOR MYOGENOUS DYSFUNCTION

MYALGIA

Myalgia is generally considered to be a function of local tissue inflammation, vascular alterations in the muscle, and pain referred from other sources.

The pathophysiologic changes in the muscle tissue are not established. Occlusal splints have been used for many years to treat this condition under the assumption that masticatory muscle parafunction contributes to the pain production (Fuchs 1975; Carlsson et al. 1979; Kawazoe et al. 1980; Hamada et al. 1982; Rugh 1982).

Clark et al. (1979, 1981) evaluated the relationship between nocturnal muscle parafunction, myogenous pain symptoms, and stabilization appliances. Fifty-two percent (N = 25) of the myofascial pain dysfunction patients had significantly reduced nocturnal muscle activity levels and 80% experienced overall improvement in pain symptoms when full-arch stabilization splints were used. They reported that patients with more severe symptoms were less likely to be helped with occlusal appliances as a sole treatment modality. Others also have demonstrated a good correlation between occlusal appliance therapy and reduction of bruxism (Solberg et al. 1975) and relief of masticatory muscle pain (Greene and Laskin 1972; Agerberg and Carlsson 1974). Agerberg and Carlsson (1974) reported decreased myalgia symptoms in 71% of patients wearing stabilization appliances. Several other studies reported similar positive results with the stabilization device (Greene and Laskin 1972; Carraro and Caffesse 1978; Magnusson and Carlsson 1980).

Except for the studies where masseter electromyographic (EMG) activity was measured directly, most prior studies did not assess whether the muscle pain patients had parafunctional behaviors or were strictly exhibiting muscle pain that might be described as myofascial in character (i.e., spontaneous onset, daytime occurrence with a clear stress component to its fluctuation). This distinction might be important because occlusal appliances could work differently on these two patterns of muscle pain. Patients who have parafunction-aggravated myalgia might be more likely to respond to stabilization appliances. Pierce and Gale (1988) conducted an RCT on 100 subjects to evaluate the efficacy of stabilization appliances against biofeedback, exercises, no treatment, and auditory feedback at night (triggered by tooth clenching). The stabilizing appliance and the auditory feedback significantly interfered with bruxism. Unfortunately, they did not report or evaluate muscle pain levels in these subjects. In another RCT performed on the efficacy of stabilization appliances for the specific management of myofascial pain patients, Dao and colleagues (1994) found no remarkable efficacy for stabilization appliances compared to two placebo controls. These data suggest that the primary mechanism for the reported efficacy of the stabilization appliance (especially in myofascial patients without strong oral parafunction) is nonspecific and likely to be more behavioral in its treatment action. A stabilization appliance does appear to be a strong behavior-modifying device. In an RCT-based study, Turk et al. (1993) reported that the occlusal appliance approach was as effective as a biofeedback/stress management program for pain reduction in TMD patients, and that when combined, the two therapies (appliances and biofeedback) were more effective than either one alone.

It appears that at least for chronic myofascial pain of spontaneous onset, the mechanism of the stabilization appliance is not known and might best be considered a behavior-modifying device. Several studies have shown that the stabilization appliance is a moderately powerful treatment for modifying parafunctional activities in the jaw. Conversely, in the myalgia patient without a strong parafunctional origin to symptoms, these appliances are comparable to both acupuncture treatment and most other behavioral therapies. Further, when a credible pseudotherapy has been used in clinical trials on pain of musculoskeletal origin, stabilization appliances have not proven to be superior to other treatments. When either stabilization appliances or behavioral therapy for TMDs are compared to a no-treatment or wait-list program, patients almost always report these treatments to be strongly helpful, while the no-treatment program has a weak effect.

TRISMUS

Anecdotally, it is widely known that appliances are used with great effect to treat trismus, probably because they alter parafunctional behaviors. Unfortunately, there is no specific research on the effect of splints on trismus.

DYSKINESIA AND MUSCLE INCOORDINATION

Several investigators have studied the effect of appliances on motor coordination (McCall et al. 1976; Beard and Clayton 1980; Monterio and Clark 1988). These studies suggest that occlusal appliances improve motor skills in patients who exhibit reduced coordination, but are not helpful (except as protective devices) in any patient with a true involuntary motor abnormality.

FINAL RECOMMENDATIONS

Before summarizing the above information into a set of recommendations to help clinicians select logical treatment methods and to help researchers establish the future agenda of investigations needed to advance the discipline, we offer the following perspective for consideration. First, the typical problems seen in TMD patients are not usually disabling or extremely longlasting. Even when TMD symptoms are prolonged for more than six months, they are not disabling and, in most patients do not interfere substantially with the patient's work life or social life (except eating). For this reason, conservative reversible treatments with reasonable efficacy should be selected and advocated for a vast majority of TMD problems. Second, a conceptual framework for organizing and understanding the available treatments is helpful. In this regard, the most common method of treatment for TMD problems includes a combination of techniques derived from a physical medicine model (e.g., physical therapy and physical medicine procedures applied at home or in the office including dental occlusal appliances) and a behavioral medicine model (e.g., counseling, biofeedback, stress management, and relaxation training). These two models are generally considered reversible treatments with low morbidity and high efficacy.

Because some conditions afflicting the TMJ produce a clear and substantial interference in function, two additional minimally invasive models of care are commonly used: the pharmacologic model (e.g., NSAIDs, antidepressant medications, antispasmodic medications, and steroid injections), and the closed-joint surgical manipulation model (e.g., arthrocentesis and arthroscopy). Both these latter models carry greater potential risks than do the physical and behavioral medicine models. If selected for the right patient and used in the right situation, they should have low morbidity and good efficacy. Finally, in all areas of medicine, it is assumed that if a correct and specific diagnosis is made, appropriate and logical treatment will follow. Unfortunately, diagnosis is difficult and the choice of therapy is not simple. Treatments are selected based on numerous factors including cost, risk-benefit ratio, prior experience, degree of invasiveness, the patient's confidence in the care provider, and the care provider's judgment regarding which treatment would best help the patient. There is no substitute for prior experience in making the best treatment choice.

CLICKING

The sparse research and clinical observation data indicate that the clicking TMJ is not cured by the use of avoidance-exercise therapy. This approach may be viable for slowing the progression of a dysfunctional clicking joint, but there is no experimental verification. Neither the open diskoplasty, the arthroscopic lavage, or disk plication methods, which have been advocated for the painful TMJ click, have been reviewed for efficacy. Data suggest that the stabilization appliance has poor efficacy for management of TMJ clicking. For repositioning appliances, the short-term (one year or less) data suggest that these appliances can clearly modify, if not eliminate, some TMJ clicking problems. The long-term data, however, are less convincing, with approximately one-third or fewer of these patients experiencing a permanent change in their clicking pattern. The cost of reconstructing (surgically, orthodontically, or prosthetically) a permanently repositioned occlusion is also substantial. This approach does not seem warranted except in rare cases. The studies upon which conclusions regarding the efficacy of repositioning for TMJ clicking are based have several design problems. Few of the studies used random assignment and none were "double-blind" evaluation studies. There are no good objective methods of measuring clicking over a prolonged period in the natural environment. All prior data are based on patient self-report or a laboratory-based measurement of clicking. Laboratory-based assessments are useful, but the frequency of the problem in the day-to-day routine is more relevant than the loudness of a click in the laboratory. The development of portable, long-term TMJ noise measuring technology would be beneficial in future studies of TMJ clicking. Finally, the criteria for selecting cases that "require" permanent repositioning are not clear and need to be refined and tested.

Until well-designed research is performed that compares the above treatments for TMJ clicking against newer, minimally invasive methods such as hyaluronate infusion into the joint, no definitive prediction can be made regarding which treatment is the most efficacious, has the lowest morbidity, and the best longevity. Further, the entire phenomenon of clicking needs investigation to determine if early and still painless clicks are more likely to progress into painful dysfunctional clicks that induce a truly prolonged interference in jaw movement.

LOCKING

Since the mid-1970s, the patient with acute onset loss of TMJ motion has been managed with methods that directly invade or manipulate the joint. For a 10-year period (from approximately 1978 to 1988), open TMJ disk repositioning surgery was widely performed. This procedure was described as a method for treating closed lock problems (Wilkes 1978a,b). Since the advent of arthroscopic surgery , the closed locking problem has been managed with this less invasive method. Whether manual manipulation, arthrocentesis, or arthroscopic lavage or lysis is the best way to manage these cases has not been established. Until more research compares these treatment methods, no definitive prediction can be made regarding which treatment is the most efficacious and has the lowest morbidity and the best longevity. A clear problem with all prior research is that the method of measuring passive jaw opening is not standardized. Methodologic research is needed. Maximum passive opening is the interincisal distance achieved by stretching the patient's jaw open with the examiner's fingers. The resulting value is partially dependent on the level of force applied by the examiner. Further, additional information about the natural course of an untreated closed locking condition is needed because some cases of closed lock will resolve fully without invasive therapy and others will progress to a rapid degeneration of the articular surfaces. The anatomic and functional status of the disk itself or of the intracapsular fluid constituents might be important variables in prognosis. At present, decisions about treatment for individual cases should be based on both the patient's history and at least a two-week period of continued pain and disability from the closed locking condition even after appropriate, noninvasive pharmacologic and physical medicine therapy has been attempted. Clinical logic encourages initial use of the therapy with the lowest morbidity.

JOINT PAIN

Few well-designed clinical outcome research studies have been conducted to specifically evaluate the efficacy of individual physical medicine techniques to relieve TMJ pain beyond a brief therapeutic period. The exceptional studies include randomized comparison trials of corticosteroid and sodium hyaluronate infusions for TMJ pain management associated with TMJ arthritis. Clinical case reports and therapeutic logic generally support the claim that the rest/soft diet/NSAID approach is helpful for acute trauma-induced joint pain; however, its efficacy in chronic TMJ pain is not proven. Chronic TMJ pain appears to respond only weakly to the stabilization appliance. Better scientific research is needed to evaluate its efficacy for this condition. Clearly, comparative studies are needed to determine the relative effectiveness of treatment approaches (i.e., physical-medicine versus pharmacologic versus surgical therapy). TMJ pain rarely occurs as an isolated problem and secondary myogenous symptoms are usually present. Identifying the cause of the problem is essential, because treatment will provide only transient relief if the cause persists (e.g., a systemic arthritis disorder). More reliable and valid methods (e.g., joint fluid markers of inflammation) are needed to assess and quantify joint pain (versus adjacent muscle pain).

TMJ POLYARTHRITIS

The efficacy of physical medicine procedures for symptomatic management of the TMJ due to a polyarthritic disease process has not been well studied. Nevertheless, these procedures are widely used for other body joints. It is logical to assume that physical medicine procedures (especially the postural awareness and range of motion exercises) can reduce secondary arthritic symptoms. Education of the patient on how to reduce the strain on an arthritic joint may be the critical factor. Nowhere in the medical literature is there any scientific evidence that nonpharmacologic physical medicine, including occlusal appliances, can reverse or stop the bony erosive process of any substantial polyarthritic disease. Although intra-articular steroid injections have been widely accepted as the standard approach for an isolated inflamed joint, the relative efficacy of other pharmacologic agents for management of TMJ arthritis of a polyarthritic nature is beyond the scope of this chapter. Separate literature citations regarding the efficacy of occlusal appliances for managing polyarthritis pain symptoms do not exist. Stabilization appliances might actually have a greater value in the patient with substantial polyarthritic destruction of the TMJ than in the TMJ pain patient without arthritic change. The former often has a disturbed dental occlusion (e.g., open bite). In these cases, the stabilization appliance is theoretically serving to support the disturbed occlusion.

MYALGIA/MYOSITIS

Limited studies have tested commonly used modalities for muscle pain (i.e., exercise, stretching, and thermal agents) for their individual efficacy for myogenous jaw pain. The more invasive modalities such as trigger point injections, acupuncture, TENS, muscle stimulation, and cold lasers, have not been fully tested for efficacy. The most reasonable data on physical medicine modalities for treatment of chronic jaw muscle pain concerns acupuncture. However, if a credible pseudoacupuncture treatment were tested in an RCT, these findings might weaken. Additional testing of acupuncture versus a control condition and other myalgic management methods seems warranted. Comparative studies of various physical medicine methods of treating musculoskeletal pain in other anatomic areas have not consistently rated one method better than another. Further, testing of traditional physical medicine procedures against behavioral medicine methods (e.g., biofeedback or other stress management methods) showed a similar efficacy. Until the therapeutic effectiveness of one approach or modality can be well correlated with a specific clinical, etiologic-based diagnosis, the physical medicine modalities selected for the treatment of chronic myalgia will continue to be based solely on the clinician's best judgment and experience. Use of occlusal appliances for masticatory muscle pain is likely to be no more or less effective than any other approach. None of the physical medicine methods (including occlusal appliances) have been shown to be superior to a credible pseudotherapy control condition, which suggests that a strong behavioral component is present in most physical medicine methods.

TRISMUS/SPLINTING

The potential of physical medicine modalities to interrupt a significant masticatory muscle trismus response (of extracapsular origin) is well recognized by most clinicians. Unfortunately, there is no clear experimental evidence regarding the use of various physical medicine modalities, including occlusal appliances, for trismus.

DYSKINESIA/MUSCLE INCOORDINATION

The literature does not support the effectiveness of any physical medicine procedures in the management of involuntary motor disorders except as a purely palliative measure. Exercise methods involving movement feedback can help mild masticatory muscle incoordination problems if they are learned behaviors. Additional research is needed to compare the various treatment methods for masticatory muscle pain, trismus, and movement incoordination problems. Available data suggest that occlusal appliances have a strong and helpful effect on jaw muscle incoordination.

REFERENCES

Agerberg, G. and Carlsson, G.E., Late results of treatment of functional disorders of the masticatory system: a follow-up by questionnaire, J. Oral Rehabil., 1 (1974) 309–316.

Anderson, G.C., Schulte, J.K. and Goodkind, R.J., Comparative study of two treatment methods for internal derangement of the temporomandibular joint, J. Prosthet. Dent., 53 (1985) 392–397.

Au, A.R. and Klineberg, I.J., Isokinetic exercise management of temporomandibular joint clicking in young adults, J. Prosthet. Dent., 70 (1993) 33–39.

Beard, C.C. and Clayton, J.A., Effect of occlusal splint therapy on TMJ dysfunction, J. Prosthet. Dent., 44 (1980) 324–335.

Bell, W.H., Nonsurgical management of the pain-dysfunction syndrome, J. Am. Dent. Assoc., 79 (1969) 161–170.

Bertolami, C.N., Gay, T., Clark, G.T., Rendell, J., Shetty, V., Liu, C. and Swann, D.A., Use of sodium hyaluronate in treating temporomandibular disorders, J. Oral Maxillofac. Surg., 51 (1993) 232–242.

Block, S.L. and Laskin, D.M., The effectiveness of transcutaneous nerve stimulation (TNS) in the treatment of unilateral MPD syndrome (abstract), J. Dent. Res., 59 (spec. iss. A) (1980) 519.

Bonica, J.J., Management of myofascial pain syndrome in general practice, JAMA, 164 (1957) 732–738.

Brooke, R. and Stenn, P., Postinjury myofascial pain dysfunction syndrome: Its etiology and prognosis, Oral Surg. Oral Med. Oral Pathol., 45 (1978) 846–850.

Burgess, J., Sommess, E., Truelove, E. and Dworkin, F., Effects of ice, sketch, and reflex inhibition on TMD (abstract), J. Dent. Res., 65 (1986) 307.

Bush, F.M., Physical therapy for mandibular movement - jaw pain (abstract), J. Dent. Res., 63 (1984) 172.

Carlsson, G.E., Longterm effects of treatment of craniomandibular disorders, J. Craniomandib. Pract., 3 (1985) 337–342.

Carlsson, G.E., Ingervall, B. and Kocak, G., Effect of increasing vertical dimension on the masticatory system in subjects with natural teeth, J. Prosthet. Dent., 41 (1979) 284–289.

Carraro, J.J. and Caffesse, R.G., Effect of occlusal splints on TMJ symptomatology, J. Prosthet. Dent., 40 (1978) 563–566.

Carstensen, B., Indications and contraindications of manual therapy for temporomandibular joint dysfunction. In: G. Grieve (Ed.), Modern Manual Therapy, Churchill Livingstone, New York, 1986, pp. 700–705.

Clark, G.T., Treatment of jaw clicking with temporomandibular repositioning: an analysis of 25 cases, J. Craniomandib. Pract., 2 (1984) 263–270.

Clark, G.T., The diagnosis and treatment of painful temporomandibular disorders. In: F. Curro (Ed.), The Dental Clinics of North America, W.B. Saunders, Philadelphia, 1987, pp. 645–674.

Clark, G.T. and Lynn, P., Horizontal plane jaw movements in controls and temporomandibular joint clinic patients, J. Prosthet. Dent., 55 (1986) 730–735.

Clark, G.T., Beemsterboer, P.L., Solberg, W.K. and Rugh, J.D., Nocturnal electromyographic evaluation of myofascial pain dysfunction in patients undergoing splint therapy, J. Am. Dent. Assoc., 990 (1979) 607–611.

Clark, G.T., Beemsterboer, P.L. and Rugh, J.D., Nocturnal masseter muscle activity and the symptoms of masticatory dysfunction, J. Oral Rehabil., 8 (1981) 279–286.

Clark, G.T., Lanham, F. and Flack, V.F., Treatment outcome for consecutive TMJ clinic patients, J. Craniomandib. Disord., 2 (1988) 87–95.

Clark, G.T., Seligman, D., Solberg, W. and Pullinger, A., Guidelines for the treatment of temporomandibular disorders, J. Craniomandib. Disord. Facial Oral Pain, 4 (1990) 80–88.

Cordray, Y.M. and Krusen, E.M., Use of hydrocollator packs in the treatment of neck and shoulder pains, Arch. Phys. Med. Rehabil., 40 (1959) 105–108.

Dao, T.T.T., Lavigne, G.J., Charbonneau, A., Feiue, J.S. and Lund, J.P., The efficacy of oral splints in the treatment of myofascial pain of the jaw muscles: a controlled clinical trial, Pain, 56 (1994) 85–94.

Deyo, R.A., Walsh, N.E., Martin, D.C., Schoenfeld, L.S. and Ramamurthy, S., A controlled trial of transcutaneous electrical nerve stimulation (TENS) and exercise for chronic low back pain, N. Engl. J. Med., 322 (1990) 1627–1634.

Eisen, R., Kaufman, A. and Greene, C., Evaluation of physical therapy for MPD syndrome patients (abstract), J. Dent. Res., 63 (1984) 344.

Esposito, C.J., Veal, S.J. and Farman, A.G., Alleviation of myofascial pain with ultrasound therapy, J. Prosthet. Dent., 51 (1984) 106–108.

Farrar, W.B., Diagnosis and treatment of anterior dislocation of the articular disc, New York J. Dent., 41 (1971) 348–351.

Fountain, F.P. and Gersten, J.W., Decrease in muscle spasm produced by ultrasound, hot packs, and infrared radiation, Arch. Phys. Med. Rehabil., 41 (1960) 293–298.

Friedman, M.H. and Weisberg, J., Joint play movements of the temporomandibular joint: clinical considerations, Arch. Phys. Med. Rehabil., 65 (1984) 413–417.

Friedman, M.H. and Weisberg, J., Temporomandibular joint disorders: diagnosis and treatment, Quintessence, Chicago, 1985, pp. 75–159.

Friedman, M.H., Anstendig, H.S. and Weisberg, J., Treatment of disc dysfunction, J. Clin. Orthodont., 16 (1982a) 408–411.

Friedman, M.H., Weisberg, J. and Agus, B., Diagnosis and treatment of inflammation of the temporomandibular joint, Semin. Arthritis Rheum., 12 (1982b) 44–51.

Fuchs, P., The muscular activity of the chewing apparatus during night sleep, J. Oral Rehabil., 2 (1975) 35–48.

Gangarosa, L.P., Iontophoresis in dental practice, Quintessence, Chicago, 1983, pp. 59–66.

Goharian, R.K. and Neff, P.A., Effect of occlusal retainers on temporomandibular joint and facial pain, J. Prosthet. Dent., 44 (1980) 206–208.

Gold, N., Greene, C.S. and Laskin, D.M., TENS therapy for treatment of MPD syndrome (abstract), J. Dent. Res., 62 (1983) 244.

Goldman, J.A., Chiapella, J., Casey H., Bass, N., Graham, J., McClatchey, W., Dronavalli, R.V., Brown, R., Bennett, W.J., Miller, S.B., Wilson, C.H., Pearson, B., Haun, C., Persinski, L., Huey, H. and Muckerheide, M., Laser therapy of rheumatoid arthritis, Lasers Surg. Med., 1 (1980) 93–101.

Graff-Radford, S.B., Reeves, J.L., Baker, R.L. and Chiu, D., Effects of transcutaneous electrical nerve stimulation on myofascial pain and trigger point sensitivity, Pain, 37 (1989) 1–5.

Greene, C.S. and Laskin, D.M., Splint therapy for the myofascial pain-dysfunction (MPD) syndrome: a comparative study, J. Am. Dent. Assoc., 84 (1972) 624–628.

Greene, C.S., Turner, C. and Laskin, D.M., Long term outcome of TMJ clicking in 100 MPD patients (abstract), J. Dent. Res., 61 (1982) 218.

Griffin, J.E., Echternach, J.L., Price, R.E. and Touchstone, J.C., Patients treated with ultrasonic driven hydrocortisone and with ultrasound alone, Phys. Ther., 47 (1967) 594–601.

Hamada, T., Kotani, H., Kawazoe, Y. and Yameda, S., Effect of occlusal splints on the EMG activity of masseter and temporal muscles in bruxism with clinical symptoms, J. Oral Rehabil., 9 (1982) 119–123.

Hansson, T.L., Infrared laser in the treatment of craniomandibular arthrogenous pain, J. Prosthet. Dent., 61 (1985) 614–617.

Helkimo, E. and Westling, L., History, clinical findings, and outcome of treatment of patients with anterior disk displacement, Cranio, 5 (1987) 269–276.

Ireland, V.E., The problem of the clicking jaw, J. Prosthet. Dent., 3 (1953) 200–212.

Johansson, A., Wenneberg, B., Wagersten, C. and Haraldson, T., Acupuncture in treatment of facial mandibular pain, Acta Odontol. Scand., 49 (1991) 153–158.

Kahn, J., Iontophoresis and ultrasound for post surgical temporomandibular tissues and paresthesis, Phys. Ther., 60 (1980) 307–308.

Kawazoe, Y., Kotani, H., Hamada, T. and Yamada, S., Effect of occlusal splints on the electromyographic activities of masseter muscles during maximum clenching in patients with myofascial pain-dysfunction syndrome, J. Prosthet. Dent., 43 (1980) 578–580.

Keene, J., Ligament and muscle-tendon unit injuries. In: J. Gould and G. Davies (Eds.), Orthopedic and Sports Physical Therapy, Mosby, St. Louis, 1985, pp. 146–152.

Kirk, W. and Calabrese, D., Clinical evaluation of physical therapy management of internal derangement of temporomandibular joint, J. Oral Maxillofac. Surg., 47 (1989) 113–119.

Klawans, H., Tanner, C. and Goetz, C., Epidemiology and pathophysiolgy of tardive dyskinesias. In: J. Jankovich and E. Tolosa (Eds.), Facial Dyskinesias, Advances in Neurology, Vol. 49, Raven Press, New York, 1988, pp. 185–197.

Kleinkort, J.A. and Foley, R., Laser acupuncture: its use in physical therapy, Am. J. Acupunct., 12 (1984) 51–56.

Koes, B.W., Bouter, L.M., van Mameren, H., Essers, A.H.M., Verstegen, G.M.J.R., Hofhuizen, D.M., Houben, J.P. and Knipschild, P.G., A blinded randomized clinical trial of manual therapy and physiotherapy for chronic back and neck complaints: physical outcome measures, J. Manipulative Physiol. Ther., 15 (1992) 16–23.

Kopp, S., Wenneberg, B., Haraldson, T. and Carlsson, G.E., The short-term effect of intra-articular injections of sodium hyaluronate and corticosteroid on temporomandibular joint pain and dysfunction, J. Oral Maxillofac. Surg., 43 (1985) 429–435.

Kopp, S., Carlsson, G.E., Haraldson, T. and Wenneberg, B., Long-term effect of intra-articular injections of sodium hyaluronate and corticosteroid on temporomandibular joint arthritis, J. Oral Maxillofac. Surg., 45 (1987) 929–935.

Kraus, H., The use of surface anesthesia in the treatment of painful motion, JAMA, 16 (1941) 2582–2583.

Kraus, S., Physical therapy management of temporomandibular joint dysfunction. In: S. Kraus (Ed.), TMJ Disorders, Management of the Craniomandibular Complex, Churchill Livingstone, New York, 1988, pp. 150–158.

Laskin, D.M. and Block, S., Diagnosis and treatment of myofacial pain-dysfunction (MPD) syndrome, J. Prosthet. Dent., 56 (1986) 75–84.

Le Bell, Y. and Kirveskari, P., Treatment of reciprocal clicking of the temporomandibular joint using a mandibular repositioning splint and occlusal adjustment, Proc. Finn. Dent. Soc., 81 (1985) 251–255.

List, T., Helkimo, M., Anderson, S. and Carlsson, G.E., Acupuncture and occlusal splint therapy in the treatment of craniomandibular disorders. Part I: A comparative study, Swed. Dent. J., 12 (1992) 125–141.

Liu, C. and Clark, G.T., Sodium hyaluronate injections in synovial joints. In: G.T. Clark, B. Sanders and C.N. Beertolami (Eds.), Advances in Diagnostic and Surgical Arthroscopy of the Temporomandibular Joint, W.B. Saunders, Philadelphia, 1993, pp. 157–162.

Lundh, H. and Westesson, P., Long-term follow-up after occlusal treatment to correct abnormal temporomandibular joint disk position, Oral Surg. Oral Med. Oral Pathol., 67 (1989) 2–10.

Lundh, H., Westesson, P., Kopp, S. and Tillstrom, B., Anterior repositioning splint in the treatment of temporomandibular joints with reciprocal clicking: comparison with a flat occlusal splint and an untreated control group, Oral Surg. Oral Med. Oral Pathol., 60 (1985) 131–136.

Lundh, H., Westesson, P. and Kopp, S., A three-year follow-up of patients with reciprocal temporomandibular joint clicking, Oral Surg. Oral Med. Oral Pathol., 63 (1987) 530–533.

Lundh, H., Westesson, P., Jisander, S. and Eriksson, L., Disk-repositioning onlays in the treatment of temporomandibular joint with disk displacement: comparison with a flat occlusal splint and with no treatment, Oral Surg. Oral Med. Oral Pathol., 66 (1988) 155–162.

Magnusson, T. and Carlsson, G.E., Treatment of patients with functional disturbances in the masticatory system: a survey of 80 consecutive patients, Swed. Dent. J., 4 (1980) 145–153.

Maitland, J., Peripheral Manipulation, 2nd ed., Butterworths, London, 1979, pp. 318–329.

McCall, W.D., Bailey, J.O. and Ash, M.M., A quantitative measure of mandibular joint dysfunction: phase plane modelling of jaw movement in man, Arch. Oral Biol., 21 (1976) 685–689.

McCarty, W., Diagnosis and treatment of internal derangements of the articular disc and mandibular condyle. In: W.K. Solberg and G.T. Clark (Eds.), Temporomandibular Joint Problems, Quintessence, Chicago, 1980, pp. 145–168.

McNeill C., Nonsurgical management of internal derangements. In: C.A. Helms, R.W. Katzberg and M.F. Dolwick (Eds.), Radiology Research and Education Foundation, Quintessence, Chicago, 1985, pp. 193.

Mejersjo, C. and Carlsson, G.E., Long term results of treatment for temporomandibular joint pain-dysfunction, J. Prosthet. Dent., 49 (1983) 809–815.

Messenger, K. and Barghi, N., The effect of function and rest on the amplitude of the TMJ click, J. Oral Rehabil., 14 (1987) 261–266.

Messenger, K., Barghi, N., Burgar, C. and Rey, R., Effect of exercise and rest on amplitude of TMJ click (abstract), J. Dent. Res., 61 (1982) 350.

Moller, E., The myogenic factor in headache and facial pain. In: Y. Kawamura and R. Dubner (Eds.), Oral Facial Sensory and Motor Functions, Quintessence, Tokyo, 1981, pp. 225–239.

Moloney, F. and Howard, J.A., Internal derangements of the temporomandibular joint: anterior repositioning splint therapy, Aust. Dent. J., 31 (1986) 30–39.

Monteiro, A.A. and Clark, G.T., Mandibular movement feedback versus occlusal appliances in the treatment of masticatory muscle dysfunction, J. Craniomandib. Disord. Facial Oral Pain, 2 (1988) 41–47.

Murakami, K., Matsuki, M., Iizuka, T. and Ono, T., Recapturing of persistent anteriorly displaced disc by mandibular manipulation after pumping and hydraulic pressure to the upper joint cavity of the temporomandibular joint, J. Craniomandib. Pract., 5 (1987) 17–24.

Namiki, O., Toyoshima, M. and Morisaki, N., Therapeutic effect of intra-articular injection of high molecular weight hyaluronic acid on osteoarthritis of the knee, Int. J. Clin. Pharmacol. Ther. Toxicol., 20 (1982) 501–507.

Nitzan, D.W., Dolwick, M.F. and Martinez, G.A., Temporomandibular joint arthrocentesis: a simplified treatment for severe, limited mouth opening, J. Oral Maxillofac. Surg., 49 (1991) 1163–1167.

Okeson, J.P., Long-term treatment of disk-interference disorders of the temporomandibular joint with anterior repositioning occlusal splints, J. Prosthet. Dent., 60 (1988) 611–616.

Okeson, J.P., Management of Temporomandibular Joint Disorders and Occlusion, Mosby, St. Louis, 1989, pp. 371–384.

Okeson, J.P., Moody. P.M., Kemper, J.T. and Haley, J.V., Evaluation of occlusal splint therapy and relaxation procedures with temporomandibular disorders, J. Am. Dent. Assoc., 107

(1983) 420–424.

Olavi, A., Pekka, R., Pertti, K. and Pekka, P., Effects of the infrared laser therapy at treated and non-treated trigger points, Acupunct. Electrother. Res., 14 (1989) 9–14.

Olson, J., A review of cryotherapy, Phys. Ther., 52 (1972) 840–853.

Palano, D., Martelli, M., Avi, R., Gaurneril, L. and Palmeri, B., A clinic statistical investigation of laser effect in the treatment of pain and dysfunction of the temporomandibular joint (TMJ), Med. Laser Report No. 2, (1985) 21–29.

Peyron, J.G. and Balazs, E.A., Preliminary clinical assessment of Na-hyaluronate injection into human arthritic joints, Path. Biol., 22 (1974) 731–736.

Pierce, C.J. and Gale, E.N., A comparison of different treatments for nocturnal bruxism, J. Dent. Res., 67 (1988) 597–601.

Posselt, U., Physiology of Occlusion and Rehabilitation, F.A. Davis, Philadelphia, 1962, pp. 242–248.

Pullinger, A. and Seligman, D., Temporomandibular joint osteoarthrosis: a differentiation of diagnostic subgroups by symptom history and demographics, J. Craniomandib. Disord. Facial Oral Pain, 1 (1987) 251–256.

Raft, G.H., Johnson, E.W. and LaBan, M.M., The fibrositis syndrome, Arch. Phys. Med. Rehabil., 49 (1968) 155–162.

Rasmussen, O.C., Description of population and progress of symptoms in a longitudinal study of temporomandibular joint arthropathy, Scand. J. Dent. Res., 89 (1981) 196–213.

Ross, J.B., The intracapsular therapeutic modalities in conjunction with arthrography: case reports, J. Craniomandib. Disord. Facial Oral Pain, 3 (1989) 35–43.

Rubin, D., Myofascial trigger point syndromes: an approach to management, Arch. Phys. Med. Rehabil., 62 (1981) 107–110.

Rugh, J.D., Muscle activity studies of MPD in the natural environment (abstract), J. Dent. Res., 61 (1982) 175 (Abstract No. S-24).

Rugh, J.D. and Solberg, W.K., Electromyographic studies of bruxist behavior before and during treatment, J. Calif. Dent. Assoc., 3 (1975) 56–59.

Ruth, D.T. and Swites, B.J., Comparison of the effectiveness of intra-articular hyaluronic acid and conventional therapy for the treatment of naturally occurring arthritic conditions in horses, Equine Pract., 7 (1985) 25

Rydell, N. and Balazs, E.A., Effect of intra-articular injection of hyaluronic acid on the clinical symptoms of osteoarthritis and on granulation tissue formation, Clin. Orthop., 80 (1971) 25–32.

Salmon, T.N., Tracy, N.H. and Hiatt., N.R., Hysterical trismus (conversion reaction): report of a case, Oral Surg., 34 (1972) 187–191.

Sanders, B., Arthroscopic surgery of the temporomandibular joint: treatment of internal derangement with persistent closed lock, Oral Surg. Oral Med. Oral Pathol., 62 (1986) 361–372.

Schultz, L.W., A curative treatment for subluxation of the temporomandibular joint or of any joint, J. Am. Dent. Assoc., 24 (1937) 1947–1950.

Schultz, L.W., Report of ten years of treating hypermobility of the temporomandibular joint, J. Oral Surg., 5 (1947) 202–207.

Schwartz, L., Ethyl chloride treatment of limited painful mandibular movement, J. Am. Dent. Assoc., 48 (1954) 497–507.

Schwartz, L., Disorders of the Temporomandibular Joint, W.B. Saunders, Philadelphia, 1959, pp. 222–251.

Segami, N., Murakami, K. and Iizuka, T., Arthrographic evaluation of disk position following mandibular manipulation technique for internal derangement with closed lock of the temporomandibular joint, J. Craniomandib. Disord. Facial Oral Pain, 4 (1990) 99–108.

Seitz, L.M. and Kleinkort, J.A., Low-power laser: its applications in physical therapy. In: S.L. Michlovitz and S.L. Wolf (Eds.), Thermal Agents in Rehabilitation, F.A. Davis, Philadelphia, 1986, pp. 217–238.

Snyder-Mackler, L. and Bork, C.E., Effect helium-neon laser irradiation on peripheral sensory nerve latency, Phys. Ther., 68 (1988) 223–225.

Snyder-Mackler, L., Barry, A., Perkins, A. and Soucek, M., Effects of helium-neon laser irradiation on skin resistance and pain in patients with trigger points in the neck and back, Phys. Ther., 69 (1989) 336–341.

Solberg, W.K., Temporomandibular disorders: functional and radiological considerations, Br. Dent. J., 160 (1986) 195–200.

Solberg, W.K., Clark, G.T. and Rugh, J.D., Nocturnal electromyographic evaluation of bruxing patients undergoing short-term splint therapy, J. Oral Rehabil., 2 (1975) 215–223.

Strang, R., Moseley, H. and Carmichael, A., Soft lasers—have they a place in dentistry? Br. Dent. J., 165 (1988) 221–225.

Toller, P., Osteoarthrosis of the mandibular condyle, Br. Dent. J., 134 (1973) 223–231.

Toller, P., Non-surgical treatment of dysfunctions of the temporo-mandibular joint., Oral Sci. Rev., 7 (1976) 70–85.

Travell, J., Myofascial trigger points: clinical view. In: J.J. Bonica and D. Albe-Fessard (Eds.), Proceedings of the First World Congress on Pain, Advances in Pain Research and Therapy, Vol 1, Raven Press, New York, 1976, pp. 919–926.

Turk, D.C., Zaki, H.S. and Rudy, T.E., Effect of intraoral appliance and biofeedback/stress management alone and in combination in treating pain and depression in patients with temporomandibular disorders, J. Prosthet. Dent., 70 (1993) 158–164.

Tveteras, K. and Kristensen, S., The etiology and pathogenesis of trismus, Clin. Otolaryngol., 11 (1986) 383-387.

Voss, D., Ionta, M. and Meyers, B., Proprioceptive Neuromuscular Facilitation Patterns and Techniques, 3rd ed., Harper and Row, Philadelphia, 1985, pp. 302-308.

Walker, J., Relief from chronic pain from low-power laser irradiation, Neurosci. Lett., 43 (1983) 339–344.

Wenneberg, B., Kopp, S. and Grondahl, H-G., Long-term effect of intra-articular injections of a glucocorticoid into the TMJ: a clinical and radiographic 8-year follow-up, J. Craniomandib. Disord. Facial Oral Pain, 5 (1991) 11–18.

Wilkes, C.H., Arthrography of the temporomandibular joints in patients with the TMJ pain-dysfunction syndrome, Minn. Med., 61 (1978a) 645–652.

Wilkes, C.H., Structural and functional alterations of the temporomandibular joint, Northwest. Dent., 57 (1978b) 287–294.

Wing, M., Phonophoresis with hydrocortisone in the treatment of temporomandibular joint dysfunction, Phys. Ther., 62 (1982) 32–33.

Wyke, B., Articular neurology and manipulative therapy. In: Glasgow, Twomey, and Scull (Eds.), Aspects of Manipulative Therapy. 2nd ed., Churchill Livingstone, Edinburgh, 1975, pp. 1–4.

Yavelow, I., Forster, I. and Wininger, M., Mandibular relearning, Oral Surg., 36 (1973) 632–641.

Yemm, R., A neurophysiological approach to the pathology and aetiology of the temporomandibular joint dysfunction, J. Oral Rehabil., 12 (1985) 343–353.

Zakariasen, K. and Dederich, D., Lasers in dentistry. "Star Wars." Dreaming or a future reality? Can. Dent. Assoc. J., 54 (1988) 27–30.

Correspondence to: Glenn T. Clark, DDS, MS, UCLA School of Dentistry, 73-017 Center for the Health Sciences, 10833 Le Conte Ave., Los Angeles, CA 90024-1668, USA. Tel: 310-206-8045; Fax: 310-825-0921.

Temporomandibular Disorders and Related Pain Conditions, Progress in Pain Research and Management, Vol. 4, edited by B.J. Sessle, P.S. Bryant, and R.A. Dionne, IASP Press, Seattle, © 1995.

23

The Relationship of Occlusal Factors and Orthodontic Treatment to Temporomandibular Disorders

James A. McNamara, Jr.,[a] Donald A. Seligman,[b] and Jeffrey P. Okeson[c]

[a]Department of Orthodontics and Pediatric Dentistry and Center for Human Growth and Development, The University of Michigan, Ann Arbor, Michigan, USA, [b]Section of Orofacial Pain and Occlusion, School of Dentistry, University of California Los Angeles, Los Angeles, California, USA, and [c]Orofacial Pain Center, Department of Oral Health Practice, College of Dentistry, University of Kentucky, Lexington, Kentucky, USA

The diagnosis and treatment of temporomandibular disorders (TMDs) has been a focus of many in dentistry for much of this century, due in part to the presumed association of TMDs to occlusion of the teeth. Many occlusally related claims have been made and numerous therapies advocated, including occlusal appliance therapy, anterior repositioning appliances, occlusal adjustment, restorative procedures, and orthodontic/orthognathic treatment. Conversely, many types of dental interventions, including routine orthodontic treatment, have been alleged to cause TMDs.

HISTORICAL PERSPECTIVE

One of the first practitioners to call attention to the possible relationship of occlusion to temporomandibular joint (TMJ) problems was Costen (1934), an otolaryngologist who noted that many of his patients who had pain in the TMJ region seemed to benefit from therapeutic alteration of their occlusion, particularly in the vertical dimension. This apparently logical association of mandibular dysfunction to occlusion stimulated some interest within the dental community in the diagnosis and treatment of TMJ-related problems. Even though most of Costen's original concepts have been discredited, his suggestion of using bite opening appliances became the treatment protocol of choice for many clinicians (e.g., Bleiker 1938; Pippin 1940). During the next decade, however, others began to question the effectiveness of bite-raising appliances (e.g., Harvey 1940; Brussels 1949), and alternative treatments were sought.

In the 1950s and 1960s, interest increased in the treatment of TMD through permanent adjustments of the occlusion (e.g., Gerry 1947; Ramfjord 1961). At this time, emphasis shifted to masticatory pain disorders, with the etiology of these disorders often related to occlusal disharmony (e.g., Perry and Harris 1954; Jarabak 1956).

The diversity and multifactorial nature of the TMDs began to be recognized in the 1960s and 1970s, with the role of stress and other psychological states acknowledged as contributing factors (Moulton 1955; Laskin 1969; Solberg et al. 1972; Rugh and Solberg 1985). Later the role of intracapsular problems, specifically disk interference disorders, was described (Farrar 1971; McCarty 1980) and clarified further as improved diagnostic methodologies (e.g., CT scans, magnetic resonance imaging) became available.

It was only in the 1980s that the breadth of the multifactorial nature of the TMDs was appreciated. Attempts were made to bring together basic scientists and clinicians in interdisciplinary symposia (e.g., Laskin et al. 1983; Carlson et al. 1985; Stohler and Carlson 1994). The American Academy of Orofacial Pain issued and subsequently revised a so-called white paper entitled *Craniomandibular* (later *Temporomandibular) Disorders: Guidelines for Classification, Assessment, and Management* (McNeill 1990, 1993). Gradually categories of TMD became defined, with masticatory muscle pain, internal (disk) derangement, and degenerative joint disorders becoming recognized as distinct and sometimes coexisting conditions.

Thus, the emphasis on occlusal therapies (e.g., occlusal appliances, occlusal adjustment) as singular treatments for TMD gradually has given way to the recognition that TMDs are a cluster of related conditions of the TMJ and the masticatory musculature that have many overlapping symptoms and signs. TMDs may be classified as a subgroup of disorders (Bell 1982; Okeson 1993) of the general musculoskeletal system. Orofacial pain patients may suffer from a variety of conditions, including systemic-related problems as well as articular, neuromuscular, neurologic, neurovascular, and behavioral disorders (McNeill 1993).

OCCLUSAL FACTORS AND THE TMDs

Numerous clinical studies have investigated the relationship of occlusal factors and the signs and symptoms associated with the TMDs in relatively large patient and nonpatient populations. Some studies reported statistically significant associations, while others did not, and few common trends were apparent. For example, Nilner (1986) examined 749 juveniles and adolescents and reported that TMD signs and symptom were associated with centric slides and balancing-side contacts. Egermark-Eriksson and colleagues (1983), after examining a random sample of 402 children, reported that occlusal supracontacts as well as many characteristics of unusual occlusion (i.e., anterior crossbite, anterior open bite, Class II malocclusion, Class III malocclusion) were associated with signs and symptoms of TMDs. Similarly, Brandt (1985) in a study of 1342 children noted a positive correlation of overbite, overjet, and anterior open bite with TMDs.

In contrast, other investigators have reported no such associations, including DeBoever and Adriaens (1983) in 135 TMD patients, Gunn and co-workers in 151 migrant children, and Dworkin and colleagues (1990) upon examining 592 subjects in a health maintenance organization.

EVALUATION OF PREVIOUS STUDIES

As can be seen from the above-mentioned studies, there is no universal agreement as to the relationship of occlusal factors to the TMDs. These differences in findings can be explained in part by problems in study design. According to Seligman (1994), some of the problems are as follows:

Symptoms are not disease states. The most common type of study used in TMD research is an investigation of symptoms. This approach is problematic because isolated symptoms are not the same as disease. Any actual association of a symptom to a specific disease state may be obscured when only isolated symptoms are monitored. For example, the report of joint clicking would not differentiate disk displacement due to osteoarthrosis from simple soft tissue internal derangement. Similarly, latent muscle tenderness to palpation may reflect problems within a specific muscle group or may indicate global chronic fibromyalgia. If the differences among symptoms are subtle, overlapping symptoms can mask distinguishing morphological differences by including too many different pathological processes in the analysis.

Lack of differential diagnosis. Most investigations have grouped subjects into a single disease category without differentially diagnosing each patient. Thus, often it is unclear as to which disease process is being studied. Further, many patient studies are purely descriptive and do not compare patient populations with equivalent populations of healthy persons.

Unrepresentative samples. In some studies, the sample population does not represent the target population, particularly with regard to age and gender. For example, it is inappropriate to extrapolate to adults with osteoarthritis or fibromyalgia the findings from children, who rarely appear as patients with these conditions. The sample should match the target population as closely as possible, especially with regard to age and gender.

Lack of factor definition. The definitions of the factors being studied must be made clear in operational terms, with specific criteria established for each variable. For instance, when multiple occlusal factors are grouped together into an overall variable termed "malocclusion," it is difficult to determine exactly which factors are being investigated. A factor such as posterior crossbite in one patient must be shown to have the same impact on the analysis as does a deep overbite in another patient. And if the efficacy of poorly defined occlusal treatments is examined (e.g., occlusal equilibration) and the treatment is focused on the correction of a wide range of occlusal conditions rather than on the elimination of a single condition (e.g., slides between centric relation and centric occlusion), the interpretation of the results of the treatment will be difficult.

Multifactorial analysis not used. Combinations of factors must be studied together in a multifactorial analysis, rather than separately (Seligman 1994). Isolated pair-wise or sensitivity-specificity analyses attribute either major responsibility or no significant role to the occlusal factors that they examine. It is obvious that individual occlusal factors do not act in isolation from one another, and to suggest otherwise is inappropriate. With multiple factor analysis, an estimate can be made of the relative contribution of each factor in characterizing the patient.

Inappropriate groupings of data. Every attempt should be made to consider continuous variables over the entire range of their occurrence, otherwise an artificial or arbitrary skewing of the results may occur. Further, the transformation of real data to unvalidated severity scales should be avoided. If a transformation is to be performed, the individual measures in the severity scale must be shown to be roughly equivalent. For example, the number of muscles tender to palpation can be quantified. To deem this information useful, it must be shown that that a certain number of tender muscles is of greater concern than another number, and that there is no threshold of a minimum number of muscles before an effect is noted.

If several unrelated symptoms are included in a severity scale (e.g., clicking, crepitus, muscle tenderness), the investigator must prove that the weighted input ascribed to each variable is valid. In addition, if one sign or symptom is emphasized in a given scoring system (e.g., muscle tenderness over clicking), this preference for one type of factor also must be shown to be valid.

The observations of Seligman (1994) illustrate the necessity of examining previous studies not necessarily on the basis of the conclusions stated by the authors, but rather by the groups studied, the criteria used, and the methods of analysis employed.

CRITICAL REVIEWS OF THE LITERATURE

Two of the most comprehensive reviews that have considered the relationship of occlusion to the TMDs have been published by Seligman and Pullinger (1991a,b), one considering *morphological* occlusal relationships and the second *functional* occlusal relationships. These reviews were compiled in an attempt to determine consensus on the roles of various occlusal factors on the pathophysiology of TMDs. These investigators considered only original research articles and emphasized those that used appropriate methodology, in particular research that evaluated diagnostic groups or disease states rather than symptoms. The reader is referred to these articles for an in-depth literature review on each subject.

Morphological occlusal relationships

Seligman and Pullinger (1991a) considered five identifiable factors related to the static occlusion.

1. Overbite/open bite. The vertical overlap of the teeth should be considered as a continuous variable. Large overbite is common in nonpatient populations, so this variable cannot be used to define a patient population. Studies that do not consider overbite as a continuous variable report mixed results, with a majority reporting no or very selective associations. If overbite is considered as a continuous variable, there is consensus that minimal overbite in adults is associated with osteoarthrosis. A reduced overbite may be a result of osseous changes in the joint, rather than vice versa.

Skeletal anterior open bite is of particular significance. This condition is characterized as a negative vertical overlap of the anterior teeth that often is combined with occlusal contacts only in the molar region. Skeletal open bite is not common in asymptomatic nonpatients and usually is associated with disease states demonstrating intracapsular changes (e.g., osteoarthrosis). Larheim and co-workers (1983) among others have noted that these occlusal changes may be a result of, rather than the cause of, these osseous changes. Skeletal anterior open bite in adults should be distinguished from anterior open bite in children, which may arise from different causes (e.g., thumb sucking, abnormal tongue posture) and may be self-correcting.

2. Overjet. The horizontal overlap of the teeth does not seem to be associated with TMJ symptoms or disease. Seligman and Pullinger (1991a) note one exception, namely the higher prevalence of large overjet in patients with osteoarthropathies of the TMJ. Pullinger and Seligman (1991) found that although larger overjets were associated with osteoarthrosis patients who had a prior history of disk derangement, no such association was evident in derangement patients without osteoarthrosis. Despite the association with osteoarthrosis, large overjet is common in nonpatient populations as well, and thus this measure lacks specificity in defining patient groups.

3. Crossbite. Most previous studies of crossbite have considered younger patient populations (e.g., Egermark-Eriksson 1982; Lieberman et al. 1985; DeBoever and van den Berghe 1989). Although asymmetrical muscle activity has been reported in children with unilateral posterior crossbite (Troelstrup and Møller 1970; Ingervall and Thilander 1975), there is little evidence that this type of morphologic relationship leads to TMJ symptomatology (e.g., Pullinger et al. 1988; Runge et al. 1989). Most patient studies report no greater prevalence of crossbite in patients as compared to nonpatients (e.g., Helöe and Helöe 1975; Mohlin and Kopp 1978).

Crossbites persisting in adults typically are skeletal in origin and do not appear to provoke TMD symptoms or disease. Thus, the correction of crossbites in adults to prevent potential TMD problems does not seem warranted.

4. Posterior occlusal support. Loss of posterior tooth support has been associated with osteoarthrosis (Granados 1979; Whittaker et al. 1985), but this association becomes questionable when the evaluation is controlled for age effects (Whittaker et al. 1990). However, research on this topic in patient populations is scant.

One of the few research groups to consider the longitudinal relationship of the loss of posterior teeth to the health of the masticatory system has been conducted by Käyser and associates (Käyser 1981; Witter 1993). They have shown that the adaptive capacity of the masticatory system over years is great, and that most people with loss of molar support have acceptable masticatory function and no increased amount of TMD signs and symptoms. Thus, no conclusions can be drawn regarding the benefits of prosthetically replacing missing posterior teeth as a preventative measure for TMDs.

5. Asymmetrical contact in retruded cuspal position. If imbalances of tooth contacts exist in retruded cuspal position (RCP)/centric relation, they may be most obvious in younger patient populations (Egermark-Eriksson et al. 1983), and as with a loss of posterior dental support, may be associated with age. No associations of this type of disorder and TMDs have been reported in older populations. Prophylactic adjustment of the natural occlusion is not indicated based on published studies, but the establishment of bilateral contact in RCP may be a prudent restorative goal.

Functional occlusal relationships

Seligman and Pullinger (1991b) reviewed similar published research concerning the relationship of the functional movements of the mandible to the TMDs.

Balancing and working occlusal contacts. Most controlled surveys fail to demonstrate any association between occlusal supracontacts and TMD signs or symptoms in symptomatic nonpatients or in populations of TMD patients. Occlusal supracontacts are so common and variable (e.g., Argerberg and Sandstrom 1988) that they lack the sensitivity and specificity for defining a present or potential TMD population. Further, a precise and reproducible method for determining the presence of occlusal supracontacts does not exist.

Slides between centric relation and centric occlusion. According to Seligman and Pullinger (1991b), most past studies report little association between the length of the slide between RCP/centric relation and ICP (intercuspal position)/centric occlusion and signs or symptoms of disorders in asymptomatic persons. Studies of patients with radiographically determined osteoarthrosis report longer slides in arthrosis patients than in controls (Akerman et al. 1988; Seligman and Pullinger 1989), a finding that indicates that osseous remodeling or condylar lysis can be accompanied by an increased slide. In none of the studies is the amount of the slide handled as a continuous variable, thus adding bias to the interpretation of the data.

Occlusal guidance pattern. While there is evidence that occlusal guidance patterns can alter muscle activity levels (e.g., Shupe et al. 1984; Belser and Hannam 1985), there is little evidence to suggest that a given guidance pattern can provoke TMD symptomatology. Little is known concerning the role of specific guidance patterns in particular patient populations.

Parafunction. Bruxism and clenching often are cited as etiologic factors in the development of TMDs, but similar to occlusal interferences, these activities (especially bruxism) seem to be endemic in the general population (Seligman et al. 1988). Furthermore, comparisons of groups identified according to self-reports of parafunctional activities are suspect because of the universality of this activity and the lack of definition as to the quantification of severity measures. Seligman and Pullinger (1991b) stated that there is increasing evidence that parafunction is not associated with chronic occlusal factors, and thus reversible rather than nonreversible treatment should be provided in attempts to prevent or minimize possible harmful effects of this activity (Okeson 1993).

Dental attrition. There is no evidence from most nonpatient studies that dental attrition is associated with signs or symptoms of TMDs. Men show greater attrition severity than do women, yet they have fewer TMD symptoms. Once again, patients with osteoarthrosis have the most notable occlusal changes, often demonstrating advanced rates of attrition. These changes may be secondary to the occlusal changes resulting from the arthrosis.

MULTIPLE ANALYSIS OF OCCLUSAL FACTORS

The studies cited above considered the significance or nonsignificance of occlusal factors relative to the TMDs as isolated factors. Pullinger and colleagues (1993) used a blinded multifactorial analysis to determine the *weighted influence* of each factor acting in combination with the other factors. The interaction of 11 occlusal factors was considered in randomly collected but strictly defined diagnostic groups compared to asymptomatic controls.

The asymptomatic controls were considered the "gold standard," in that the subjects in this group lacked signs and symptoms and had no history of TMDs. The samples were demographically representative, and the occlusal factors studied were collected blindly and strictly defined. A multiple logistic regression model was used for simultaneous assessment of the relative odds of each potential occlusal factor. The outcome always was the disease classification versus the asymptomatic controls.

Findings in healthy subjects

Wide variation in occlusal features were noted in the asymptomatic control group, including overjet from −1 mm to 6 mm, overbite from −2 mm to 10 mm, midline discrepancies to 5 mm, anteroposterior molar relationships from −6 mm to 6 mm, molar asymmetries of from 0 to 6 mm, and RCP-ICP slides up to 2 mm in length. In addition, a wide variety of crossbites, asymmetrical slides, retruded posterior contacts, and severe attrition facets were observed. Skeletal anterior open bite relationships were not observed. Thus, variations in occlusal morphology are the norm in healthy persons, indicating the capacity of the human masticatory system to adapt to a wide variety of morphological and functional features.

Pullinger and co-workers (1993) proposed a new definition of "normal" within the context of TMDs, that being those occlusal features that exist without significant elevated risk of disease. Such "normal" features include RCP-ICP slides of 2 mm or less, deep overbite, minimal overjet, midline discrepancies, all Angle classifications of occlusion, unilateral RCP contacts, and less than five missing posterior teeth. These factors alone cannot define either TMD patients or asymptomatic normals.

Findings in patient populations

No single occlusal factor was able to differentiate patients from healthy subjects. Four occlusal features, however, occurred mainly in TMD patients and were rare in normals: the presence of a skeletal anterior open bite, RCP-ICP slides of greater than 2 mm, overjets of greater than 4 mm, and five or more missing and unreplaced posterior teeth. Unfortunately, these signs are rare not only in healthy persons, but also in patient populations, indicating limited diagnostic usefulness of these features.

Pullinger and co-workers (1993) concluded that many occlusal parameters that traditionally were believed to be influential contribute only minor amounts to the change in risk in the multiple factor analysis used in their study. They reported that although the relative odds for disease were elevated with several occlusal variables, clear definition of disease groups was evident only in selective extreme ranges and involved only a few subjects. Thus, they concluded that occlusion cannot be considered the most important factor in the definition of TMDs.

Pullinger and colleagues (1993) noted, however, that the results of their study indicated that occlusal factors do contribute to TMDs. Combinations of two to five of the occlusal parameters, involving eight of the eleven factors, contributed to risk for disease. These investigators stated that more commonly used statistical methods, such as robust pair-wise testing, would have ignored some of these variables. The minor elevation in odds ratio revealed by the multiple factor analysis indicates that specific occlusal factors are making some biological contribution and thus cannot be ignored. They state further that a biological system must adapt to its various morphological features until stability is achieved, and some occlusal features may place greater adaptive demands on the system. While most persons compensate without problems, adaptation in others may lead to a greater risk of dysfunction.

Some occlusal differences between diagnostic groups were reported (Pullinger et al. 1993). For a clinically perceptible influence to be significant, Pullinger and co-workers stated that an occlusal feature would need at least to double the risk of disease (at least a 2:1 mean odds ratio). Only five occlusal conditions reached this threshold:

1. Anterior open bite. The highest odds ratio was for anterior open bite, and this occlusal manifestation was seen predominantly in both the osteoarthrosis and the myalgia-only groups, an observation noted previously by Seligman and Pullinger (1991a) and Stegenga (1991). For anterior open bite to be shown as an etiologic factor in the development of osteoarthritis, some evidence of this occlusal factor should exist in other diagnostic groups thought to be conditions often preceding osteoarthrosis. However, anterior open bite was not common in disk displacement disorders, with or without reduction. Further, Pullinger and co-workers (1993) noted that most osteoarthrosis and myalgia patents did not have anterior open bite.

2. Overjets greater than 6–7 mm. Overjets of greater than 4 mm were associated with the likelihood of osteoarthrosis, the same disease groups as the anterior open bite populations. There was no contribution to the patients with TMJ derangement. Pullinger and co-workers (1993) stated that some large overjets in adults can be secondary to the condylar repositioning seen with advanced osteoarthrosis. An overjet of 6 mm or larger was needed for a subject to be assigned to one of these disease classifications with an odds ratio of at least 2:1. The occurrence of a progressively increasing overjet in adults should alert the clinician to evaluate a patient for other signs of TMD disease.

3. RCP-ICP occlusal slides. Small occlusal slides, mostly under 1 mm, were common in all patient groups and normals, but sagittal slides longer than 2 mm were found in the disease groups only. None of the asymptomatic subjects had occlusal slides greater than 2 mm, and only 6% had slides longer than 1 mm. Pullinger and co-workers (1993) found that larger slides occasionally were associated with degenerative changes within the TMJ. A slide of 5 mm or greater would be necessary to reach a 2:1 odds ratio threshold for notable risk, and this ratio never was observed in the patients. Thus, the effective clinical contribution of this factor was minimal.

Because an occlusal slide has not been shown to be a contributor to the etiology of TMDs, the prophylactic elimination of most slides through occlusal equilibration procedures is not indicated. Even in the presence of what may appear to be symptoms associated with an occlusal slide, the removal of a large discrepancy between centric relation and centric occlusion may not be advisable because the slide may be a consequence of an articular disorder (e.g., primary arthrosis) rather than a result of occlusal factors.

These three factors that have emerged from the multiple factor analysis have a primary association with osseous and ligamentous changes within the articular compartments of the TMJ. These occlusal factors may in fact be a result of, rather than a cause of, these joint changes.

4. Unilateral maxillary lingual crossbite. This occlusal feature, occurring in about 10% of the adult population, has a greater risk for assignment to the TMJ derangement groups. Nearly one-fourth of the nonreducing disk displacement patients had this feature, and the odds ratio that a person with this type of crossbite also would have TMJ disk displacement *with* reduction was over 3:1 (Pullinger et al. 1993). Similar odds ratios were seen for the disk displacement group *without* reduction (2.6:1) and also in the osteoarthrosis patients with a history of disk displacement (1.96:1).

Pullinger and co-workers (1993) noted that the persistence into adulthood of an odds ratio for disease association indicates that the adaptive response in a small percentage of subjects may be less than optimal and leads to the suggestion that functional adaptation to a unilateral posterior crossbite in childhood may be made at the expense of the articular disk through the development of internal derangement, including a few that eventually progress to arthrosis. These investigators believe that a case can be made for the treatment of children with unilateral crossbites to reduce the adaptive demands on the masticatory system. Conversely, the orthodontic correction of unilateral crossbite in adults to prevent TMJ derangement development probably is not warranted, because skeletal adaptation already has occurred.

5. Missing posterior teeth. In the samples studied by Pullinger and colleagues (1993), extensive posterior tooth loss was not common. Five or more posterior teeth needed to be missing before the odds ratio of assignment to disease groups assumed a minimal critical ratio of 2:1 for osteoarthrosis with disk displacement history and primary osteoarthrosis and also for disk displacement with reduction. Age is associated with both osteoarthrosis (Pullinger and Seligman 1987) and tooth loss (Agerberg and Bergenholz 1989), indicating that the increase in odds ratio in patients with osteoarthrosis with more than four missing teeth also may be a reflection of age.

Much of the increase in tooth loss in the patients characterized by disk displacement with reduction, a group of patients generally younger than those in the osteoarthrosis groups, was a result of premolar extraction as part of an orthodontic treatment. Pullinger and co-workers (1993) noted that the contribution of the extraction of two to four teeth per se, for example as part of an orthodontic treatment protocol, was negligible in most cases when other variables were controlled. As mentioned earlier, longitudinal studies of patients with multiple missing posterior teeth have shown acceptable masticatory function without increased signs and symptoms of TMDs (Käyser 1981; Witter 1993).

The multifactorial analysis of Pullinger and co-workers (1993) has shown that, except for a few defined occlusal conditions, there is a relatively low risk of occlusal factors associated with the TMDs. In a subsequent reanalysis of these data, Seligman (1994) has estimated that overall contribution of occlusal factors in defining TMD patients probably ranges from 10% to 20%, which leaves 80–90% of the characteristics of TMD patients unexplained by their occlusion.

None of these studies can identify a cause and effect relationship of occlusal factors to TMDs. However, the correlation coefficients usually are in the 0.3 range and explain less than 10% of the variation. In a specific disease state, the causative agent usually explains 80–90% of the variation.

ORTHODONTIC TREATMENT AND THE TMDs

Although TMDs have long been recognized by orthodontists as a clinical problem, little emphasis was placed on the diagnosis and treatment of TMDs within the specialty until about the mid-1980s. Traditionally, scant mention was made of TMD treatment in the curricula of graduate programs in orthodontics, and only cursory examinations of the TMJ region were conducted in routine orthodontic clinical examinations in private practice.

However, the interest of the orthodontic community was awakened abruptly in the late 1980s following litigation that alleged that orthodontic treatment was the proximal cause of TMDs in orthodontic patients, with substantial monetary judgments awarded to several plaintiffs (Pollack 1988). This litigious climate stimulated the American Association of Orthodontists not only to sponsor a series of risk management teleconferences and newsletters, but also to underwrite research concerning the relationship of orthodontic treatment to TMDs. This series of clinical studies, published in the January 1992 issue of the *American Journal of Orthodontics and Dentofacial Orthopedics*, found that orthodontic treatment generally is not a primary factor in TMDs. Yet, this controversy is not settled, as is indicated by the Thompson (1994) article that cites faulty intercuspation of the teeth and dental intrusions into the freeway space as two of the many etiologic factors that may lead to TMJ dysfunction and its sequelae.

REVIEW OF THE LITERATURE

Prior to ten years ago, surprisingly few methodologically sound clinical studies regarding the relationship between orthodontic treatment and the TMDs had been published. In a comprehensive review of the literature published between 1966 and 1988, Reynders (1990) divided 91 publications into three categories: viewpoint articles, case reports, and sample studies. The most numerous were *viewpoint articles* (N = 55), publications that usually were anecdotal in nature, stating the opinions of the author regarding the orthodontic-TMD relationship. Little (or more commonly no) data were presented to support the opinion. Further, Reynders (1990) notes that 23 of the 55 viewpoint articles were published in *The Functional Orthodontist*, with articles advancing the concepts that orthodontic treatment can either cause or cure TMDs.

The second most frequent type of article (N = 30) was the *case report*, which described the influence of certain orthodontic treatment modalities on the signs and symptoms of dysfunction in one or more patients. The least numerous (N = 6) were in the third category of *sample studies*, investigations that reported data from large sample groups. These studies varied in quality, often having the same methodological problems and limitations as discussed previously for studies of occlusal factors. Since 1988, a substantial number of clinical investigations have considered the association of orthodontics and TMDs (Table I).

Viewpoint articles, of course, are not suitable for critical evaluation of associations between two entities such as orthodontic treatment and TMDs; they are, however, useful in identifying questions that may be worthy of scientific investigation. Some of these questions are:

- What is the prevalence of signs and symptoms of TMDs in orthodontically untreated populations?

Table I
Major studies of the relationship between orthodontic treatment
and signs and symptoms of TMDs

Author	Sample	Appliance	Ext. vs Nonext.*	Relationship
Sadowsky and Begole 1980	75 treated 75 untreated	Fixed	Yes	No
Larsson and Rönnerman 1981	23 treated	Fixed	No	Improvement
Janson and Hasund 1981	60 treated 30 untreated	Fixed Functional	Yes	Improvement
Sadowsky and Polsen 1984	207 treated 214 untreated	Fixed	No	No
Pancherz 1985	22 treated	Functional	No	No
Dibbets and van der Weele 1987	135 treated	Fixed Functional	Yes	No
Dahl et al. 1988	51 treated 47 untreated	Fixed Functional	No	No
Smith and Freer 1989	87 treated 28 untreated	Fixed	No	No
Sadowsky et al. 1991	160 treated	Fixed	Yes	No
Dibbets and van der Weele 1992	92 treated	Fixed Functional	Yes	No
Luecke and Johnston 1992	42 patients	Fixed	Yes	No
Artun et al. 1992	63 treated	Fixed	Yes	No
Kremenak et al. 1992a	65 treated	Fixed	Yes	No
Kremenak et al. 1992b	109 treated	Fixed	No	No
Egermark and Thilander 1992	402 mixed	Fixed Functional	No	Improvement
Paquette et al. 1992	63 orthodontic patients	Fixed	Yes	No
Luppanapornlarp and Johnston 1993	62 orthodontic patients	Fixed	Yes	No
Beattie et al. 1994	63 orthodontic patients	Fixed	Yes	No

* "Yes" indicates that the study included both extraction and nonextraction patients.

- Does orthodontic treatment lead to a greater incidence of signs and symptoms of TMDs?

- Does the type of appliance (e.g., fixed vs. functional, orthodontic vs. orthopedic) make a difference?

- Does the removal of teeth as part of an orthodontic protocol lead to a greater incidence of TMDs?

- Can orthodontic treatment lead to a posterior displacement of the mandibular condyle?

- Should the occlusions of orthodontic patients be treated to specific gnathologic standards?

- Does orthodontic treatment prevent TMDs?

Although the literature on the relationship of orthodontics to TMDs is not as extensive as that on the occlusal/TMD relationship, the questions outlined above have been addressed in numerous recent studies. Many of the investigations considered more than one question. These reports are discussed in detail below.

Occurrence of signs and symptoms of TMDs in healthy persons

We previously have seen the importance of studying healthy asymptomatic populations in assessing the relationship of occlusal factors to TMDs. Such is the case when considering orthodontic populations.

Numerous epidemiological studies have examined the prevalence of signs and symptoms associated with TMDs in a wide variety of subject populations. In general, the prevalence is significant, with an average of 32% reporting at least one symptom of TMDs and an average of 55% demonstrating at least one clinical sign.

Cross-sectional epidemiological studies of specific adult nonpatient populations indicate that at any given time, between 40% and 75% have at least one sign, and about one-third report at least one symptom of TMDs (Rugh and Solberg 1985; Schiffman and Fricton 1988; De Kanter et al. 1993). According to Montegi and co-workers (1992), the point prevalence of symptoms in children and teenagers is lower, about 12–20%.

Because of the longitudinal nature of orthodontic treatment (e.g., 2–3 years for adolescents; 5–7 years for patients starting a two-phase treatment protocol in the early mixed dentition), an understanding of the changes in the signs and symptoms of TMDs in a healthy population is essential. Several investigators have noted that signs and symptoms of TMDs generally increase in frequency and severity, beginning in the second decade of life (Egermark-Eriksson et al., 1987; Agerberg and Bergenholz 1989; Salonen et al. 1990). Wänman and Agerberg (1990) have noted that the incidence of joint sounds in young adults in their late teens can be as high as 17.5% over a two-year period. Thus, the occurrence of joint sounds during orthodontic treatment must be considered within the context of longitudinal changes in a comparable untreated population studied during the same time interval.

Orthodontic treatment versus no treatment

Two of the first investigations sponsored by the National Institutes of Health to consider the relationship between orthodontics and TMDs were initiated about 15 years ago (Table I). These research efforts considered the prevalence of TMDs and the status of the "functional occlusion" (to be discussed later) in large groups of subjects who had undergone orthodontic treatment at least 10 years previously.

Sadowsky and Begole (1980) reported on the findings from a University of Illinois study of 75 adult subjects who as adolescents at least 10 years previously had been treated with full orthodontic appliances. The treated group was compared to a group of 75 adults with untreated malocclusions. In a subsequent article by Sadowsky and Polsen (1984), the sample from the Illinois study (increased to 96 treated and 103 controls) was compared to a treatment group of 111 subjects who had been treated at least 10 years previously at the Eastman Dental Center and a control group of 111 subjects with untreated malocclusions. In the two studies, 15–21% of the subjects had one or more signs of TMDs and 29–42% had at least one or more symptoms of TMDs, usually joint sounds. There were no statistically significant differences between the treated and untreated groups (Sadowsky 1992). The results of these two studies provide evidence to support the concept that orthodontic treatment performed during adolescence generally did not increase or decrease the risk of developing TMDs later in life.

Larsson and Rönnerman (1981) conducted another study of the long-term effects of orthodontic treatment. They evaluated 23 adolescent patients who had been treated orthodontically at least 10 years earlier. Eighteen of the patients were treated with fixed appliances, while five patients received activator treatment. Using the Helkimo index (Helkimo 1974) as an evaluative tool, they recorded mild dysfunction in eight patients, while one patient had severe dysfunction. Comparing their results to published epidemiological studies, Larsson and Rönnerman (1981) stated that comprehensive orthodontic treatment can be undertaken without fear of creating TMD problems.

Dahl and co-workers (1988) examined 51 subjects five years after the completion of orthodontic treatment. Signs and symptoms of TMDs were noted and compared to the findings from a similar group of 47 untreated persons. According to the authors, "nobody really had craniomandibular disorders" in either group. Severe symptoms (e.g., difficulties in wide opening, locking, pain on mandibular movement) typically were not observed; however, mild symptoms (e.g., joint sounds, muscle fatigue, stiffness of the lower jaw) were observed more frequently in the untreated group than in the treated group, a difference that was statistically significant. Dahl and co-workers (1988) noted that the number of subjects in both groups who had at least one mild symptom was relatively high (70% in the treated group, 90% in the untreated group), especially in comparison to the previously mentioned investigation of Larsson and Rönnerman (1981), which reported a 27% occurrence of mild dysfunction in their treated patients. They reported that differences between samples may be due as much to measuring differences (e.g., lack of factor definition, differences in the interpretation of the criteria of the Helkimo index) as to a true reflection of differences between groups.

Rendell and colleagues (1992) examined 462 patients receiving treatment in an orthodontic graduate clinic (90% adolescents, 10% adults), using a modification of the Helkimo (1974) index. Eleven of the patients had TMD signs/symptoms prior to treatment. During the 18-month study period, none of the patients who had been sign/symptom-free at the beginning of treatment developed signs or symptoms of TMDs. No clear or consistent changes in the levels of pain and dysfunction occurred during the treatment period in those patients with preexisting signs or symptoms. Rendell and co-workers (1992) concluded that a relationship could not be established in their patient population between orthodontic treatment and either the onset or the change in severity of TMD signs and symptoms.

One of the few clinical studies to report positive findings is the investigation of Smith and Freer (1989), who examined 87 patients treated with full orthodontic appliances in adolescence. About two-thirds of the sample had permanent teeth removed as part of the treatment protocol. The treated group was compared to an untreated control group of 28 subjects. Four years following the end of retention, symptoms were found in 21% of the treated group and 14% of the controls, a difference that was not significant statistically. However, the investigators noted a single sign that was statistically significant, the association between what they termed *soft clicks* and previous treatment. Soft clicks were found in 64% of the treatment group and 36% of the untreated group. However, they did not find any difference in joint sounds (i.e., crepitus as determined by stethoscopic examination) between the two groups. Interestingly, the authors concluded the article by stating: "The null hypothesis that there is a significant association between orthodontic treatment and occlusal or joint dysfunction has been rejected by nearly all previously reported studies and continues to be rejected by the present study."

Relatively few prospective studies have examined the relationship of orthodontics to TMDs. The two major investigations have been conducted at the University of Groningen in the Netherlands (to be discussed later) and at the University of Iowa (Kremenak et al. 1992a,b). In the latter ongoing study, 30 new orthodontic patients have been enrolled annually since 1983. The investigators are using the method of Helkimo (1974) to collect TMD data prior to orthodontic treatment and at yearly intervals following the completion of treatment. Patients were treated by comprehensive edgewise appliances with and without extractions. No longitudinal data on a comparable untreated population were obtained.

Kremenak and co-workers (1992b) have reported data from pretreatment and posttreatment examinations from 109 patients. Data on follow-up examinations from one to six years posttreatment were available on declining samples sizes of 92, 56, 33, 19, 11, and 7 subjects. No significant differences were noted between mean pretreatment and posttreatment Helkimo scores for any of the various groupings. Ninety percent of the patients had Helkimo scores that remained the same or improved, and 10% had scores that worsened (an increase of 2–5 Helkimo points). Kremenak and colleagues (1992a,b) concluded that the orthodontic treatment experienced by their sample was not an important etiologic factor for TMD.

Hirata and co-workers (1992) examined 102 patients before and after orthodontic treatment for signs of TMDs. Findings from this group were compared to findings from 41 untreated subjects matched for age. The incidence of TMD signs for the treatment and control groups was not significantly different.

Type of orthodontic mechanics used

In the other major longitudinal study of this subject, Dibbets and colleagues (Dibbets and van der Weele 1987, 1991, 1992) followed 171 patients, of whom 75 were treated with the Begg technique (most patients had extractions as part of their treatment protocol), 66 with activator therapy, and 30 with chin cups. The *pretreatment* documentation revealed a strong association between age and the prevalence of signs and symptoms: from 10% at age 10 years, signs increased to 30% at 15 years while symptoms increased to over 40%. They also noted that at the end of treatment, the fixed appliance group had a higher percentage of objective symptoms than did the functional group, but no differences existed at the 20-year follow-up (Dibbets and van der Weele 1992).

Janson and Hasund (1981) conducted a similar study of adolescent patients with Class II, division 1 malocclusion examined five years out of retention. Thirty patients underwent a two-phase treatment regimen (headgear/ activator therapy followed by fixed appliances) without the removal of teeth, while 30 patients were treated using fixed appliances following the removal of four premolars. An additional 30 untreated subjects served as controls. One or more symptoms were reported in about 42% of the subjects overall (treated and untreated), with similar findings for the clinical dysfunction index (Helkimo 1974).

One prospective study examined the effect of functional mandibular advancement in patients with Class II, division 1 malocclusion. Pancherz (1985) used the banded Herbst appliance only in 22 adolescent patients with Class II, division 1 malocclusion during a treatment period of six months. Following an initial incisal edge-to-edge bite registration, Pancherz reported that a number of patients complained of muscle tenderness during the first three months of treatment. However, 12 months following treatment the number of subjects with symptoms was the same as before treatment.

Extraction and TMDs

Viewpoint articles and texts have strongly associated the extraction of premolars with the occurrence of TMDs in orthodontic patients (e.g., Bowbeer 1985; Witzig and Yerkes 1985; Witzig and Spahl 1987), publications that are long on opinion and short on data.

The clinical studies that have dealt with this issue have not shown a relationship between premolar extraction and TMDs. For example, Sadowsky and co-workers (1991) reported findings on 160 patients, 54% of whom were treated with extraction treatment strategies. Joint sounds were monitored before and after treatment in 87 extraction patients and 68 nonextraction orthodontic patients. Before treatment, 25% of patients had joint sounds whereas 16.5% had sounds after treatment. Similarly, 14% of patients had reciprocal clicking; only 8% had clicking after treatment. The investigators concluded that their findings did not indicate a progression of signs and symptoms to more serious problems during treatment. They also reported no increase in the risk of developing joint sounds regardless of whether teeth were removed or not.

The long-term effect of extraction and nonextraction edgewise treatments were compared in 63 patients with Class II, division 1 malocclusions who were identified by discriminant analysis as being equally amenable to the two treatment strategies (Paquette et al. 1992; Beattie et al. 1994). This study found no difference between extraction and nonextraction samples for a menu of 62 signs and symptoms (e.g., muscle palpation, joint function) that commonly are thought to be characteristic of TMDs. A follow-up study by

Luppanapornlarp and Johnston (1993) that examined an additional 62 "clear-cut" patients (those in the tail of the distribution) also noted that both extraction and nonextraction samples demonstrated similar findings.

The longitudinal studies at Iowa also have addressed this question. Kremenak and colleagues (1992a) followed three groups of patients: 26 patients treated with nonextraction, 25 patients with four premolars extracted, and 14 patients with two upper premolars extracted. No significant intergroup differences between mean pretreatment or posttreatment Helkimo scores were noted. A small but statistically significant improvement in Helkimo scores was observed posttreatment in both the nonextraction group and the four premolar extraction group.

Dibbets and van der Weele (1991) followed 111 of the original 172 orthodontic patients in the Groningen study over a 15-year period. In this group, a nonextraction approach was used in 34% of the patients, four premolars were extracted in 29%, and other extraction patterns were used in the remaining 37%. Functional appliances were used in 39%, fixed appliances (Begg) were used in 44%, and chin cups in 17% of the patients. Symptoms increased from 20% to 62%; signs of clicking and crepitus increased from 23% to 36% after four years and then stabilized. In contrast to the finding from the first 10 years, during which the three treatment groups showed no difference with regard to clicking, after 15 years this symptom was seen more often in the premolar extraction group. The authors noted, however, that clicking was higher in the premolar extraction group before treatment was started and concluded that the original growth pattern, rather than the extraction protocol, was the most likely factor responsible for the TMD complaints seen many years posttreatment. These investigators also noted that for a substantial number of patients, symptoms of TMDs appeared and disappeared during the course of study. In the 20-year follow-up, the difference had disappeared completely (Dibbets and van der Weele 1992). They also noted that even though the overall incidence of symptoms increased with time, many previously symptomatic children became asymptomatic at the time of subsequent evaluations.

Finally, in the multiple factor analysis of occlusal factors described previously, Pullinger and co-workers (1993) noted that the contribution of the extraction of two to four teeth per se, for example as part of an orthodontic treatment protocol, was negligible in most cases when other variables were controlled.

Orthodontic treatment and posterior condylar displacement

Several viewpoint articles have asserted that a wide variety of traditional orthodontic procedures (e.g., premolar extraction, extraoral traction, retraction of upper anterior teeth) cause TMD signs and symptoms by producing a distal displacement of the condyle (e.g., Bowbeer 1986; Wyatt 1987). This allegation is opposite to that of the gnathologist's approach to condylar position, a topic that will be considered in the next section.

Gianelly and co-workers (1988) used corrected tomograms to evaluate condylar position before orthodontic treatment in 37 consecutive patients aged 10 to 18 years and compared them with tomograms from 30 consecutive patients treated with fixed appliances (edgewise or Begg) and the removal of four premolars. No differences in condylar position were noted between groups. The position of the condyle tended to be centered within the glenoid fossa, but wide variation in condylar position was noted in both groups.

Luecke and Johnston (1992) evaluated the pretreatment and posttreatment records of 42 patients treated with fixed appliances in conjunction with the removal of two upper premolars. The results of this study indicated that the majority of patients (about 70%) undergo a forward mandibular displacement and a slight opening rotation of the mandible. The remainder of the sample had distal movement of the condyle. Incisor changes were essentially unrelated to condylar displacement during treatment. Luecke and Johnston (1992) stated that a change in the spatial position of the mandible is a function of changes in the anteroposterior position of the occluding buccal segments, rather than the relatively nonoccluding incisors. These observations also are supported by the findings of Tallents and co-workers (1991).

The recall studies of Paquette and co-workers (1992) and Luppanaporn-larp and Johnston (1993) have reported no differences between groups with regard to TMD signs and symptoms. They also noted that both extraction and nonextraction treatments produced a mean mesial displacement of the mandible.

Artun and colleagues (1992) also investigated the relationship of orthodontic treatment to posterior condylar displacement. Sixty-three female patients were evaluated after routine fixed appliance treatment (29 with extraction and 34 without extraction). Condylar position was measured in percent anterior and posterior displacement from absolute concentricity on the basis of sagittally corrected tomograms. The investigators did note a mean difference in condylar position between the two treatment groups, but the difference was due mainly to the occurrence of *presumed* anteriorly displaced condyles in the nonextraction group (data on the pretreatment position of the condyle were not obtained). They noted that the condyles in patients with clicking were in a more posterior position, but condylar position varied widely in all samples, and this variation also extended to different tomographic sections within the same condyle. They concluded that any posterior condylar position was not due to orthodontic treatment.

Gnathologic principles and orthodontic treatment

Several viewpoint articles (e.g., Williamson 1976; Roth 1981) have maintained that TMDs may result from a failure to treat orthodontic patients to gnathologic standards that include the establishment of a "mutually protected occlusion" and proper seating of the mandibular condyle within the glenoid fossa (in contrast to the more anterior position of the condyle advocated by the so-called "functional orthodontists"). The gnathologists claim that nonfunctional occlusal contacts, when introduced through orthodontic treatment, can lead to signs and symptoms of TMDs.

The discussion of the relationship of occlusion and malocclusion to TMDs presented earlier in this paper illustrates the lack of association between most occlusal factors and TMDs. Pullinger and co-workers (1993) reported that small occlusal slides, mostly under 1 mm, are common in asymptomatic subjects as well as TMD patients. Only when a slide between RCP and ICP becomes extreme (5 mm or greater) does the odds ratio for disease become elevated. Thus, finishing orthodontic treatment with a modest slide typically is within the adaptive capabilities of most patients.

Sadowsky and Begole (1980) and Sadowsky and Polsen (1984) evaluated the prevalence of nonfunctional occlusal contacts in patients at least 10 years after orthodontic treatment. They noted a high incidence of such occlusal contacts in both orthodontic and control groups. Similar findings have been reported by Cohen (1965) and Rinchuse and Sassouni (1983).

It probably is prudent to establish morphological treatment goals that mimic what is observed in untreated occlusion judged normal or ideal, such as the "six keys of ideal occlusion" advocated by Andrews (1972, 1989), and to treat a patient orthodontically so that there is a minimal (< 2 mm) slide between RCP and ICP. The establishment of an occlusion that meets gnathologic ideals probably is unnecessary, particularly in adolescent patients, and sometimes the attainment of a gnathologic ideal may be impossible in certain adult patients.

Orthodontic treatment to prevent TMDs

This last concept is probably the most difficult to investigate, given the prevalence of signs and symptoms of TMDs in healthy persons and the many types of orthodontic treatment philosophies, goals, and techniques in existence today. The question of whether orthodontic treatment can prevent TMDs is complicated further by many of the unsubstantiated viewpoint articles that claim preventive capabilities of nonextraction treatment, functional appliances, and some of the more nontraditional orthodontic treatment protocols (e.g., second molar extraction and third molar replacement) that have been advocated vigorously (e.g., Wilson 1971; Mehta 1984; Stack 1985; Witzig and Spahl 1987).

As discussed above, most studies that have compared treated and untreated populations have found no differences between groups in the occurrence of TMD signs and symptoms. One of the few investigations that found improved TMD health in a treated group was the sample studied by Magnusson and co-workers (1986) and Egermark and Thilander (1992). These investigators reevaluated at five and 10 years, respectively, a group of 402 children and adolescents who originally had been evaluated cross-sectionally by Egermark-Eriksson (Egermark-Eriksson et al. 1981; Egermark-Eriksson 1982). The sample originally was divided into three groups according to age (7, 11, and 15 years). About one-third of the sample had received orthodontic treatment at the end of the final examination period. Bruxism awareness and subjective symptoms of TMDs increased in all age groups, with symptoms slightly more pronounced in untreated subjects. The investigators also noted that clicking recorded at the first examination may disappear at subsequent examinations and that clicking may appear at subsequent intervals regardless of whether the subject had orthodontic treatment. As in many previous studies, the Helkimo (1974) index was used to measure clinical signs of TMDs in the oldest age group (25 years). The clinical dysfunction index outcome was lower in those experiencing orthodontic treatment than in those who had not.

As mentioned earlier, a trend toward decreased prevalence of TMD signs and symptoms in treated patients also was noted by Sadowsky and Polsen (1984) and Dahl and co-workers (1988). The signs and symptoms of TMDs in the previously treated orthodontic patients seldom were so severe that it could be said that these patients suffered from TMDs (even if they had signs and symptoms).

SUMMARY

In this chapter, we have attempted to review the current literature regarding the interaction of morphologic and functional occlusal factors relative to the TMDs. We have cited the review articles of Seligman, Pullinger, and colleagues (Seligman and Pullinger, 1991a,b; Pullinger et al. 1993) as comprehensive reviews of the literature on this subject. Of particular importance is the methodological weakness of previously published studies, particularly with regard to the sample groups, the criteria used for evaluation, and the method of analysis employed.

The multiple factor analysis of Pullinger and co-workers (1993) has indicated a relatively low association of occlusal factors in characterizing TMDs.

This association, however, is not zero, and several occlusal features characterized the diagnostic groups:

1. Skeletal anterior open bite.
2. Overjets greater than 6–7 mm.
3. RCP/ICP slides greater than 4 mm.
4. Unilateral lingual crossbite.
5. Five or more missing posterior teeth.

The first three factors often are associated with TMJ arthropathies and may be the result of an osseous or ligamentous change within the temporomandibular articulation. Overall, Seligman (1994) estimates that the total contribution of occlusal factors to the multifactorial characterization of TMD patients is about 10–20%, with other factors, both pronounced and subtle, interacting and providing the remaining 80–90% of the differences between patients and healthy subjects.

The second part of this paper reviewed the current literature regarding the relationship of orthodontic treatment to the TMDs. Although this subject became a focus of conversation within the dental and legal communities in the late 1980s, little substantive research on this topic was available until recently.

The findings of current research on this subject can be summarized as follows:

1. Signs and symptoms of TMDs occur in healthy persons.
2. Signs and symptoms of TMD increase with age, particularly during adolescence. Thus, TMDs that originate during treatment may not be related to the treatment.
3. Orthodontic treatment performed during adolescence generally does not increase or decrease the odds of developing TMDs later in life.
4. The extraction of teeth as part of an orthodontic treatment plan does not increase the risk of TMDs.
5. There is no elevated risk for TMDs associated with any particular type of orthodontic mechanics.
6. Although a stable occlusion is a reasonable orthodontic treatment goal, not achieving a specific gnathologic ideal occlusion does not result in TMD signs and symptoms.
7. No method of TMD prevention has been demonstrated.

8. When more severe TMD signs and symptoms are present, simple treatments usually can alleviate them in most patients.

The results of this review agree in principle with the observations of Behrents and White (1992) regarding the orthodontic/TMD interface.

According to the existing literature, the relationship of the TMDs to occlusion and orthodontic treatment is minor. The important question that still remains in dentistry is how this minor contribution can be identified within the population of TMD patients. As mentioned above, future research should be directed toward developing a more complete understanding of these occlusal factors so that reliable criteria can be developed to assist the dental practitioner in deciding when dental therapy plays a role in the management of TMDs. Reliable criteria likely would spare many TMD patients significant dental therapies and related health costs. Until such criteria are developed, the dental profession should be encouraged to manage TMD symptoms with reversible therapies, only considering permanent alterations of the occlusion in patients with unique circumstances.

FUTURE DIRECTIONS

Because there is so little evidence of notable occlusal contribution to TMDs, future research should concentrate on discerning other contributors to TMD etiology. Orthodontic therapy, while also showing little evidence that it is a significant contributor to TMD disease development, has not yet been evaluated through a multifactorial analysis that can assess its relative contribution. Future research should attempt to correct this deficiency by collectively evaluating all potential orthodontic treatment contributors within a single analysis.

Finally, because occlusion has been shown to make a small percentage contribution to TMDs in some persons, it should be evaluated with other possible contributors in a further multifactorial analysis. If orthodontic therapy proves to be a significant contributor, even if the contribution is small as is suggested by past research, it also should be included. In the end, owing to the multiple potential contributory factors in TMD etiology, it is unlikely that any single factor will dominate, and the prediction of TMDs can be accomplished only through simultaneous consideration of many factors acting together. Unfortunately, the research to prove or deny this hypothesis still is lacking, and the ultimate aim of all future etiologic investigations should be to provide estimates of the relative and simultaneous contributions of all potential risk factors.

ACKNOWLEDGMENT

The authors thank Dr. Gary Carter and Ms. Kim Huner for their help in preparing the extensive bibliography for this chapter. We also thank Drs. Lysle E. Johnston, Jr., Christian S. Stohler, Gunnar E. Carlsson, and J.H.M. Dibbets for their critical reviews of the manuscript.

REFERENCES

Agerberg, G. and Bergenholz, A., Craniomandibular disorders in adult population of West Bothnia, Sweden, Acta Odontol. Scand., 47 (1989) 129–140.

Agerberg, G. and Sandstrom, R., Frequency of occlusal interferences: a clinical study in teenagers and young adults, J. Prosthet. Dent., 59 (1988) 212–217.

Akerman, S., Kopp, S., Nilner, M., Petersson, A. and Rohlin, M., Relationship between clinical and radiologic findings of the temporomandibular joint in rheumatoid arthritis, Oral Surg. Oral Med. Oral Pathol., 66 (1988) 639–643.

Andrews, L.F., Straightwire: The Concept and Appliance, L.A. Wells, San Diego, 1989.

Andrews, L.F., The six keys to normal occlusion, Am. J. Orthod., 62 (1972) 296–309.

Artun, J., Hollender, L.G. and Truelove, E.L., Relationship between orthodontic treatment, condylar position, and internal derangement in the temporomandibular joint, Am. J. Orthod. Dentofacial Orthop., 101 (1992) 48–53.

Beattie, J.R., Paquette, D.E. and Johnston, L.E., Jr., The functional impact of extraction and non-extraction treatments: a long-term comparison in "borderline," equally-susceptible Class II patients, Am. J. Orthod. Dentofacial Orthop., 105 (1994) 444–449.

Behrents, R.G. and White, R.A., TMJ research: responsibility and risk, Am. J. Orthod. Dentofacial Orthop., 101 (1992) 1–3.

Bell, W.E., Clinical Management of Temporomandibular Disorders, Year Book Medical Publishers, Chicago, 1982.

Belser, U.C. and Hannam, A.G., The influence of altered working side occlusal guidance on masticatory muscle and related jaw movement, J. Prosthet. Dent., 53 (1985) 406–413.

Bleiker, R.F., Ear disturbances of temporomandibular origin, J. Am. Dent. Assoc., 25 (1938) 1390–1399.

Bowbeer, G.R.N., Saving the face and the TMJ, Funct. Orthod., 2 (1985) 32–44.

Bowbeer, G.R.N., Saving the face and the TMJ—Part 2, Funct. Orthod., 3 (1986) 9–39.

Brandt, D., Temporomandibular disorders and their association with morphologic malocclusion in children. In: D.S. Carlson, J.A. McNamara, Jr. and K.A. Ribbens (Eds.), Developmental Aspects of Temporomandibular Joint Disorders, Monograph 16, Craniofacial Growth Series, Center for Human Growth and Development, University of Michigan, Ann Arbor, 1985.

Brussels, I.J., Temporomandibular joint disease: differential diagnosis and treatment, J. Am. Dent. Assoc., 39 (1949) 532–554.

Carlson, D.S., McNamara, J.A., Jr. and Ribbens, K.A. (Eds.), Developmental Aspects of Temporomandibular Joint Dysfunction, Craniofacial Growth Series monograph 16, Center for Human Growth and Development, The University of Michigan, Ann Arbor, 1985.

Cohen, W.E., A study of occlusal interferences in orthodontically treated occlusions and untreated normal occlusions, Am. J. Orthod., 51 (1965) 647–689.

Costen, J.B., A syndrome of ear and sinus symptoms dependent upon disturbed function of the temporomandibular joint, Ann. Otol., 43 (1934) 1–15.

Dahl, B.L., Krogstad, B.O., Øgaard, B. and Eckersberg, T., Signs and symptoms of craniomandibular disorders in two groups of 19-year-old individuals, one treated orthodontically and the other not, Acta Odontol. Scand., 46 (1988) 89–93.

DeBoever, J.A. and Adriaens, P.A., Occlusal relationship in patients with pain-dysfunction symptoms in the temporomandibular joint, J. Oral. Rehabil., 10 (1983) 1–7.

DeBoever, J.A. and van den Berghe, L., Longitudinal study of functional conditions in the masticatory system in Flemish children, Community Dent. Oral Epidemiol., 15 (1989) 100–103.

De Kanter, R.J.A.M., Truin, G.J., Burgersdijk, Van T. Hof., M.A., Battistuzzi, P.G.F.C.M., Kalsbeek, H. and Käyser, A.F., Prevalence in the Dutch adult population and a meta-analysis of signs and symptoms of temporomandibular disorders, J. Dent. Res., 72 (1993) 1509–1518.

Dibbets, J.H.M. and van der Weele, L.T., Orthodontic treatment in relation to symptoms attributed to dysfunction of the temporomandibular joint: a ten year report of dysfunction of the University of Groningen study, Am. J. Orthod., 91 (1987) 193–199.

Dibbets, J.H.M. and van der Weele, L.T., Extraction, orthodontic treatment and craniomandibular dysfunction, Am. J. Orthod. Dentofac. Orthop., 99 (1991) 210–219.

Dibbets, J.H.M. and van der Weele, L.T., Long-term effects of orthodontic treatment, including extractions, on signs and symptoms attributed to CMD, Eur. J. Orthod., 14 (1992) 16–20.

Dworkin, S.F., Huggins, K.H., LeResche, L., Von Korff, M., Howard, J., Truelove, E. and Sommers, E., Epidemiology of signs and symptoms in temporomandibular disorders: clinical signs in cases and controls, J. Am. Dent. Assoc., 120 (1990) 273–281.

Egermark, I. and Thilander, B., Craniomandibular disorders with special reference to orthodontic treatment: an evaluation from childhood to adulthood, Am. J. Orthod. Dentofacial Orthop., 101 (1992) 28–34.

Egermark-Eriksson, I., Mandibular dysfunction in children and in individuals with dual bite (thesis), Swed. Dent. J., Suppl. 10 (1982).

Egermark-Eriksson, I., Carlsson, G.E. and Ingervall, B., Prevalence of mandibular dysfunction and orofacial parafunction in 7, 11 and 15 year old Swedish children, Eur. J. Orthod., 3 (1981) 163–172.

Egermark-Eriksson, I., Ingervall, B. and Carlsson, G.E., The dependence of mandibular dysfunction in children on functional and morphologic malocclusion, Am. J. Orthod., 83 (1983) 187–194.

Egermark-Eriksson, I., Carlsson, G.E. and Magnusson, T., A long-term epidemiologic study of the relationship between occlusal factors and mandibular dysfunction in children and adolescents, J. Dent. Res., 67 (1987) 67–71.

Farrar, W.B., Diagnosis and treatment of anterior dislocation of the articular disc, New York J. Dent., 41 (1971) 348–351.

Gerry, R.G., The clinical problems of the temporomandibular articulation, J. Am. Dent. Assoc., 34 (1947) 26.

Gianelly, A.A., Hughes, H.M., Wolgemuth, P. and Glidea, G., Condylar position and extraction treatment, Am. J. Orthod. Dentofac. Orthop., 93 (1988) 201–205.

Granados, J., The influence of the loss of teeth and attrition on the articular eminence, J. Prosthet. Dent., 42 (1979) 78–85.

Gunn, S.M., Woolfolk, M.W. and Faja, B.W., Malocclusion and TMJ symptoms in migrant children, J. Craniomandib. Disord. Facial Oral Pain, 2 (1988) 196–200.

Harvey, W., Investigation and survey of malocclusion and ear symptoms, with particular reference to ototic barotrauma (pains in ears due to change in altitude), Br. Dent. J., 85 (1940) 219–255.

Helkimo, M., Studies on Function and Dysfunction of the Masticatory System, Elanders Boktryckeri AB, Kungsbacka, 1974.

Helöe, B. and Helöe, LA., Characteristics of a group of patients with temporomandibular joint disorders, Community Dent. Oral Epidemiol., 3 (1975) 72–79.

Hirata, R.H., Heft, M.W., Hernandez, B. and King, G.J., Longitudinal study of signs of temporomandibular disorders (TMD) in orthodontically treated and untreated groups, Am. J. Orthod. Dentofac. Orthop., 101 (1992) 35–40.

Ingervall, B. and Thilander, B., Activity of temporal and masseter muscles in children with a lateral forced bite, Angle Orthod., 45 (1975) 249–258.

Janson, M. and Hasund, A., Functional problems in orthodontic patients out of retention, Eur. J. Orthod., 3 (1981) 173–179.

Jarabak, J.R., An electromyographic analysis of muscular and temporomandibular joint disturbances due to imbalance in occlusion, Angle Orthod., 26 (1956) 170–190.

Käyser, A.F., Shortened dental arches and oral function, J. Oral Rehabil., 8 (1981) 457–462.

Kremenak, C.R., Kinser, D.D., Harman, H.A., Menard, C.C. and Jakobsen, J.R., Orthodontic risk
factors for temporomandibular disorders (TMD). I: Premolar extractions, Am. J. Orthod.
Dentofac. Orthop., 101 (1992a) 13–20.

Kremenak, C.R., Kinser, D.D., Melcher, T.J., Wright, G.R., Harrison, S.D., Ziaja, R.R., Harman,
H.A., Ordahl, J.N., Demro, J.G., Menard, C.C., Doleski, K.A. and Jakobsen, J.R., Orthodon-
tics as a risk factor for temporomandibular disorders (TMD) II, Am. J. Orthod. Dentofac.
Orthop., 101 (1992b) 21–27.

Larheim, T.A., Storhaug, K. and Tveito, L., Temporomandibular joint involvement and dental
occlusion in a group of adults with rheumatoid arthritis, Acta Odontol. Scand., 41 (1983)
301–309.

Larsson, E. and Rönnerman, A., Mandibular dysfunction symptoms in orthodontically treated
patients ten years after completion of treatment, Eur. J. Orthod., 3 (1981) 89–94.

Laskin, D.M., Etiology of pain-dysfunction syndrome, J. Am. Dent. Assoc., 79 (1969) 147–153.

Laskin, D., Greenfield, W., Gale, E., Rugh, J., Neff, P., Alling, C., and Ayer, W.A. (Eds.), The
President's Conference on the Examination, Diagnosis and Management of Temporomandibular Disorders, American Dental Association, Chicago, 1983.

Lieberman, M.A., Gazit, E., Fuchs, C. and Lilos, P., Mandibular dysfunction in 10–18 year old
schoolchildren as related to morphological malocclusion, J. Oral. Rehabil., 12 (1985) 209–214.

Luecke, P.E. and Johnston, L.E., Jr., The effect of maxillary first premolar extraction and incisor
retraction on mandibular position: testing the central dogma of "functional orthodontics," Am.
J. Orthod. Dentofac. Orthop., 101 (1992) 4–12.

Luppanapornlarp, S. and Johnston, L.E., Jr., The effects of premolar-extraction: a long-term
comparison of outcomes in "clear-cut" extraction and nonextraction Class II patients, Angle
Orthod., 63 (1993) 257–272.

Magnusson, T., Egermark-Eriksson, I. and Carlsson, G.E., Five-year longitudinal study of signs
and symptoms of mandibular dysfunction in adolescents, J. Craniomand. Pract., 4 (1986)
338–344.

McCarty, W., Diagnosis and treatment of internal derangements of the articular disc and mandibular condyle. In: W.K. Solberg and G.T. Clark (Eds.), Temporomandibular Joint Problems:
Biologic Diagnosis and Treatment, Quintessence, Chicago, 1980.

McNeill, C., Craniomandibular Disorders: Guidelines for Classification, Assessment, and Management. The American Academy of Craniomandibular Disorders. Quintessence, Chicago, 1990.

McNeill, C., Temporomandibular Disorders: Guidelines for Classification, Assessment, and Management. The American Academy of Orofacial Pain. Quintessence, Chicago, 1993.

Mehta, J., Incorporating functional appliances in a traditional fixed appliance practice, Funct.
Orthod., 1 (1984) 30–32.

Mohlin, B. and Kopp, S., A clinical study on the relationship between malocclusion, occlusal
interferences and mandibular pain and dysfunction, Swed. Dent. J., 2 (1978) 105–112.

Montegi, E., Miyasaki, H. and Oguka, I., An orthodontic study of temporomandibular joint
disorders. Part I: Epidemiologic research in Japanese 6–18 year olds, Angle Orthod., 62
(1992) 249–256.

Moulton, R.E., Psychiatric considerations in maxillofacial pain, J. Am. Dent. Assoc., 51 (1955)
408–414.

Nilner, M., Functional disturbances and diseases of the stomatognathic system: a cross-sectional
study, J. Peridodontol., 10 (1986) 211–238.

Okeson, J.P., Management of Temporomandibular Disorders, 3rd ed., Mosby Year Book, St.
Louis, 1993.

Pancherz, H., The Herbst appliance—its biological effect and clinical use, Am. J. Orthod., 87
(1985) 1–20.

Paquette, D.E., Beattie, J.R. and Johnston, L.E., Jr., A long-term comparison of non-extraction and bicuspid-extraction edgewise therapy in "borderline" Class II patients, Am. J. Orthod. Dentofac. Orthop., 102 (1992) 1–14.

Perry, H.T. and Harris, S.C., The role of the neuromuscular system in functional activity of the mandible, J. Am. Dent, Assoc., 48 (1954) 665–673.

Pippin, B.N., A method of repositioning the mandible in the treatment of lesions of the temporo-mandibular joint, Washington Univ. Dent. J., 6 (1940) 107–120.

Pollack, B., Cases of note: Michigan jury awards $850,000 in ortho case: a tempest in a teapot, Am. J. Orthod. Dentofac. Orthop., 94 (1988) 358–359.

Pullinger, A.G. and Seligman, D.A., TMJ osteoarthrosis: a differentiation of diagnostic subgroups by symptom history and demographics, J. Craniomand. Disord. Facial Oral Pain, 1 (1987) 251–256.

Pullinger, A.G. and Seligman, D.A., Overbite and overjet characteristics of refined diagnostic groups of temporomandibular disorder patients, Am. J. Orthod. Dentofac. Orthop., 100 (1991) 401–415.

Pullinger, A.G. and Seligman, D.A., The degree to which attrition characterizes differentiated patient groups of temporomandibular disorders, J. Orofacial. Pain, 7 (1993) 196–208.

Pullinger, A.G., Seligman, D.A. and Solberg, W.K., Temporomandibular disorders, Part II: Occlusal factors associated with temporomandibular joint tenderness and dysfunction, J. Prosthet. Dent., 59 (1988) 363–367.

Pullinger, A.G., Seligman, D.A. and Gornbein, J.A., A multiple regression analysis of the risk and relative odds of temporomandibular disorders as a function of common occlusal features, J. Dent. Res., 72 (1993) 968–979.

Ramfjord, S.P., Dysfunctional temporomandibular joint and muscle pain, J. Prosthet. Dent., 11 (1961) 353–374.

Rendell, J.K., Norton, L.A. and Gay, T., Orthodontic treatment and temporomandibular disorders, Am. J. Orthod. Dentofac. Orthop., 101 (1992) 84–87.

Reynders, R.M., Orthodontics and temporomandibular disorders: a review of the literature (1966–1988), Am. J. Orthod. Dentofac. Orthop., 97 (1990) 463–471.

Rinchuse, D.J. and Sassouni, V., An evaluation of functional occlusal interferences in orthodontically treated and untreated subjects, Angle Orthod., 53 (1983) 122–130.

Roth, R.H., Functional occlusion for the orthodontist, Part I, J. Clin. Orthod. 15 (1981) 32–41.

Rugh, J.D. and Solberg, W.K., Oral health status in the United States: temporomandibular disorders, J. Dent. Educ., 49 (1985) 398–404.

Runge, M.E., Sadowsky, C., Sakols, E.I. and BeGole, E.A., The relationship between temporo-mandibular joint sounds and malocclusion, Am. J. Orthod. Dentofac. Orthop., 96 (1989) 36–42.

Sadowsky, C., The risk of orthodontic treatment for producing temporomandibular disorders: a literature review, Am. J. Orthod. Dentofacial Orthop., 101 (1992) 79–83.

Sadowsky, C. and Begole, E.A., Long-term status of temporomandibular joint function and functional occlusion after orthodontic treatment, Am. J. Orthod., 78 (1980) 201–212.

Sadowsky, C. and Polsen, A.M., Temporomandibular disorders and functional occlusion after orthodontic treatment: results of two long-term studies, Am. J. Orthod., 86 (1984) 386–390.

Sadowsky, C., Theisen, T.A. and Sakols, E.I., Orthodontic treatment and temporomandibular joint sounds: a longitudinal study, Am. J. Orthod. Dentofac. Orthop., 99 (1991) 441–447.

Salonen, L., Hellden, L. and Carlsson, G.E., Prevalence of signs and symptoms of dysfunction in the masticatory system: an epidemiologic study in an adult Swedish population, J. Craniomand. Disord. Facial Oral Pain, 4 (1990) 241–250.

Schiffman, E. and Fricton, J.R., Epidemiology of TMJ and craniofacial pain. In: J.R. Fricton and K.M. Hathaway (Eds.), TMJ and Craniofacial Pain: Diagnosis and Management, IEA Publ., St. Louis, 1988.

Seligman, D.A., Occlusal risk factors in craniomandibular disorders: recommendations for diagnostic examination and treatment, Presentation and abstract at the European Academy Craniomandibular Disorders, Hamburg, 1994.

Seligman, D.A. and Pullinger, A.G., Association of occlusal variables among refined TM patient diagnostic groups, J. Craniomandib. Disord. Facial Oral Pain, 3 (1989) 227–236.

Seligman, D.A. and Pullinger, A.G., The role of intercuspal occlusal relationships in temporomandibular disorders: a review, J. Craniomandib. Disord. Facial Oral Pain, 5 (1991a) 96–106.

Seligman, D.A. and Pullinger, A.G., The role of functional occlusal relationships in temporomandibular disorders: a review, J. Craniomandib. Disord. Facial Oral Pain, 5 (1991b) 265–279.

Seligman, D.A., Pullinger, A.G. and Solberg, W.K., The prevalence of dental attrition and its association with factors of age, gender, occlusion and TMJ symptomatology, J. Dent. Res., 67 (1988) 1323–1333.

Shupe, R.J., Mohamed, S.E., Christensen, L.V., Finger, I.M. and Weinberg, R., Effects of occlusal guidance on jaw muscle activity, J. Prosthet. Dent. 51 (1984) 811–818.

Smith, A. and Freer, T.J., Post-orthodontic occlusal function, Austral. Dent. J., 34 (1989) 301–309.

Solberg, W.K., Flint, R.T. and Brantner, J.P., Temporomandibular joint pain and dysfunction: a clinical study of emotional and occlusal components, J. Prosthet. Dent., 28 (1972) 412–427.

Stack, B., Orthopedic/orthodontic case finishing techniques on TMJ patients, Funct. Orthod., 2 (1985) 28–44.

Stegenga, B., Temporomandibular joint osteoarthrosis and internal derangement: diagnostic and therapeutic outcome assessment, Drukkerij Van Denderen BV, Groningen, The Netherlands, 1991.

Stohler, C.S. and Carlson, D.S., Biological and Psychological Aspects of Orofacial Pain, Craniofacial Growth Series monograph 29, Center for Human Growth and Development, The University of Michigan, Ann Arbor, 1994.

Tallents, R.H., Catania, J. and Sommers, E., Temporomandibular joint findings in pediatric populations and young adults: a critical review, Angle Orthod., 61 (1991) 7–16.

Thompson, J.R., The individuality of the patient and the temporomandibular joints, Am. J. Orthod. Dentofacial Orthop., 105 (1994) 83–87.

Troelstrup, B. and Møller, E., Electromyography of the temporalis and masseter muscle in children with unilateral crossbite, Scand. J. Dent. Res., 78 (1970) 425–430.

Wänman, A. and Agerberg, G., Etiology of craniomandibular disorders: evaluation of some occlusal and psychosocial factors in 19-year-olds, J. Craniomandib. Disord. Facial Oral Pain, 5 (1991) 35–44.

Whittaker, D.K., Davies, G. and Brown, M., Tooth loss, attrition, and temporomandibular joint changes in a Romano-British population, J. Oral Rehabil., 12 (1985) 407–419.

Whittaker, D.K., Jones, J.W., Edwards, P.W. and Molleson, T., Studies on the temporomandibular joints of an 18th century London population (Spitalfields), J. Oral. Rehabil., 17 (1990) 89–97.

Williamson, E.H., Occlusion: understanding or misunderstanding, Angle Orthod., 46 (1976) 86–93.

Wilson, H.E., Extraction of second molars in orthodontics, Orthodontist, 3 (1971) 18–24.

Witter, D.J., A 6 year follow-up study of the oral function in shortened dental arches, Thesis, University of Nijmegen, The Netherlands, 1993.

Witzig, J.W. and Spahl, T.J., The Clinical Management of Basic Maxillofacial Orthopedic Appliances, Volume I: Mechanics, PSG Publishing, Littleton, Mass., 1987.

Witzig, J.W. and Yerkes, I.M., Functional jaw orthopedics: mastering more technique. In: H. Gelb (Ed.), Clinical Management of Head, Neck and TMJ Pain and Dysfunction, 2nd ed., W.B. Saunders. Philadelphia, 1985.

Wyatt, W.E., Preventing adverse effects on the temporomandibular joint through orthodontic treatment, Am. J. Orthod., 91 (1987) 493–499.

Correspondence to: James A. McNamara, DDS, PhD, Department of Orthodontics and Pediatric Dentistry, The University of Michigan, Ann Arbor, MI 48109-1078, USA. Tel: 313-763-1565; Fax: 313-747-4024

Temporomandibular Disorders and Related Pain Conditions, Progress in Pain Research and Management, Vol. 4, edited by B.J. Sessle, P.S. Bryant, and R.A. Dionne, IASP Press, Seattle, © 1995.

24

Surgical Management of Temporomandibular Joint Disorders

Louis G. Mercuri

Department of Surgery, Stritch School of Medicine, Loyola University of Chicago, and Division of Oral and Maxillofacial Surgery and Dental Medicine, Loyola University Medical Center, Maywood, Illinois, USA

Temporomandibular disorders (TMDs) have been defined as a collective term embracing a number of clinical problems that involve the musculature and/or the temporomandibular joint (TMJ) itself. The term TMDs refers to a group of conditions that are often called TMJ by the public. Unfortunately, this ambiguous term, TMJ, has also been used by physicians, dentists, and in the literature to describe all the myriad pain problems that patients experience in association with the head, neck, jaws, and muscles in this anatomical region of the body. This imprecision in the use of terms has led to a great deal of confusion. This chapter presents the following definitions:

There are two distinct categories of TMDs:

Masticatory and cervical muscle fatigue/spasm/pain and dysfunction. This category describes specific painful and debilitating *extra-articular* maladies of the head, neck, and jaws:

1. Myofascial pain

2. Myofibrosis

3. Myositis

4. Myofunctional disorders

Although the etiology of these conditions is poorly understood, these problems are usually considered to result from the abuse of the masticatory and cervical musculature secondary to abnormal parafunctional habits such as bruxism, clenching of the teeth, and compromising head posture in response to stress and/or myofascial pain. However, if not controlled or eliminated, these problems could, in some cases, cause intra-articular pathology due to muscle-induced joint overloading.

Intra-articular biomechanical dysfunction. This category describes the specific pathologic entities that occur to the *intra-articular* structures of the TMJ:

1. Developmental abnormalities
   a. Agenesis
   b. Hypoplasia
   c. Hyperplasia
2. Neoplasia
   a. Benign
   b. Malignant
   c. Metastatic
3. Traumatic
   a. Subluxation
   b. Dislocation
   c. Fracture
      i. Intracapsular
      ii. Extracapsular
   d. Internal derangement
4. Arthritis
   a. Infectious
   b. Traumatic
   c. Rheumatoid
   d. Osteoarthrosis
   e. Metabolic
5. Ankylosis
   a. Extra-articular
   b. Intra-articular

The important distinction between these two categories of TMDs is that they are based on pathophysiologic etiology and thus guide treatment appropriately. Masticatory and cervical muscle pain and dysfunction may not be primarily centered in the joint itself, so treatment should be directed to conditions outside of the joint. When abnormal anatomy and associated pathology of the joint cause biomechanical dysfunction of the TMJ, treatment directed to the joint is more appropriate.

The health consequences of TMDs can be devastating. Dependence on pain medications, decreased productivity, and disability are common. Most patients who have extra-articular TMDs can be successfully treated and rehabilitated with a combination of rest, medication, change in habits, and an orthotic appliance. Those patients whose TMD cause is intra-articular pathology, however, often cannot be treated successfully without surgical intervention. Misdiagnosis leading to surgical treatment of extra-articular problems creates a potentially even more devastating scenario and may be the reason there is much confusion on this subject in the literature. As with any disease process, proper initial diagnosis is paramount to the success of any form of therapy.

Biomechanical dysfunctions associated with other joints in the body generally require surgical intervention to correct the anatomical discrepancies and return the patient to function. It is beyond the scope of this chapter to discuss all of the surgical treatments of intra-articular dysfunction on the TMJ, as listed above. A discussion of the pathogenesis and treatment of these entities can be found in the literature (Mercuri 1991). This chapter will be restricted to a review of the surgical procedures used to manage one of the biomechanical dysfunctions affecting the TMJ—internal derangement. It reviews the most advanced techniques for surgical management of internal derangement and recommends further directions in research.

HISTORICAL BASIS FOR THE SURGICAL MANAGEMENT OF INTERNAL DERANGEMENT

Sir Astley Cooper first used the term *internal derangement* to describe dysfunction in the joints of the extremities in a treatise on bone and joint surgery published in 1822 (Morris 1930). In 1887, Annandale used this term to report a surgery he performed in a young female patient with a clicking painful joint (Annandale 1887). This was the first published use of the term *internal derangement* in association with the TMJ.

For the next 50 years, the concept of TMJ internal derangement was discussed in the medical literature as *the* cause of all TMJ pain and dysfunction (Lanz 1909; Pringle 1918; Wakeley 1929). The disk was deemed to be the whole problem because it was out of its appropriate anatomical position. It was assumed that the disk had to be either repositioned or removed surgically to treat patients with TMJ pain and dysfunction. Costen (1934) proposed that the lack of posterior teeth, rather than internal derangement, was the cause of TMJ problems, and thereby ceded the problem to dentistry, where it has since remained.

Therapy for the painful and dysfunctional TMJ, as well as facial pain in general, was thus placed into the hands of dentists. Interest in the orthopedic and surgical concept of internal derangement waned as dental concepts of condylar position, malocclusion, gnathology, and overstretched/understretched masticatory muscles were proposed in an attempt to explain the TMJ enigma.

Schwartz (1955, 1956, 1959) introduced the psychophysiologic theory of facial and TMJ pain in the late 1950s. This concept was redefined by Laskin (1969), who introduced the term *myofascial pain dysfunction syndrome* (MPD) into the literature. The concept that higher central nervous system processes could affect the anatomy was difficult for the occlusion-oriented therapists to accept.

During the mid to late 1950s and through the 1960s, a few surgeons still believed that TMJ surgery such as high condylectomy, condylotomy, or diskectomy were the procedures of choice (Dingman and Moorman 1951;

Ireland 1951; Kiehn 1952; Silver and Simon 1956; Henny 1957). But for the most part, the dental profession's therapeutic approach focused on teeth and plastic appliances (Dawson 1974; Shore 1976).

In the 1970s, it became obvious to the profession that the problem of TMJ and facial pain was much more complex than first realized. Enamel grinding, plastic appliances, and Valium were not solving the problem to their satisfaction, despite statements in the literature extolling the virtues of mechanically based treatment modalities. Dentistry often assumes a direct cause/effect relationship for problems: bacteria/caries, poor oral hygiene/periodontal disease, nonrestorable teeth/pain; and the solutions are always mechanical: caries/fillings, periodontal disease/gingival therapy such as scaling and gingivectomy, and nonrestorable teeth/extractions. Applying this paradigm to the problem posed by TMJ and facial pain creates the following expectation: the clinician sees the effect, finds the cause, treats it mechanically, and the problem goes away. This simplistic mechanical approach to problem solving led to a rediscovery of the concept of internal derangement as *the* mechanical cause of all TMJ and some facial pain problems, irrespective of the true pathology. This concept was even extended to chronic headache, athletic prowess, and sexual function and dysfunction.

Internal derangement, as a mechanistic concept, was perfect for this paradigm (Farrar 1972, 1978). The disk belongs on top of the condyle, because that is the way it is always represented in textbooks and journal articles. Arthrography was resurrected to render an opinion on the physiologic nature of the resultant radiograph despite its drawback of inducing a nonphysiologic situation during the procedure (Wilkes 1978; Katzberg 1979). Imaging techniques became even more sophisticated, further displaying the displaced disk. Computerized tomography (CT) scans were touted in the literature (Cohen et al. 1985; Hoffman et al. 1986) and at meetings, until it was realized that the image of the supposedly culprit disk was really an artifact or fatty tissue. Then came magnetic resonance imaging (MRI), a new noninvasive imaging tool, which led to further condemnation of the disk as the culprit (Katzberg et al. 1985).

Nonsurgeons began their quest to "recapture" this displaced piece of fibrocartilage, the disk, with plastic appliances (Gausch and Kulmer 1977; Weinberg 1979). Anterior repositioning mandibular splints (ARMS), and mandibular occlusal repositioning appliances (MORA) were two mainstays in nonsurgical therapy. Mandibles were repositioned forward with appliances, teeth were orthodontically repositioned or covered with gold or porcelain to accommodate this new jaw position, and the patients were pronounced cured in the subsequent anecdotal case reports. Whole new "institutes" were dedicated solely to deal with recapturing the elusive disk and restoring the occlusal discrepancies that resulted from "treatment."

Surgeons quickly embraced this concept. Often the plastic appliances were ineffective against the elusive disk, especially in the chronic headache patient with no functional TMJ problem. A surgical procedure was therefore deemed necessary to directly capture the disk with a suture and return it to its rightful and proper position atop the condyle.

The surgical literature of the late 1970s and early 1980s was filled with reports of various techniques to accomplish this mission (McCarty and Farrar 1979; Mercuri et al. 1982; Marciani and Ziegler 1983; Tiner and Dolwick 1983; Stith 1984; Weinberg 1984; Walker and Kalamchi 1987; Kerstens et al. 1989). A review of the articles related to open surgical correction of internal derangement during this period reveals that the reported success rate ranged from 77% to 100% (Zeitler and Porter 1993). There was, however, no standard for determining the actual therapeutic success among the various studies.

Newer techniques and materials were introduced for surgical treatment of the TMJ. A whole generation of patients had their disks removed and replaced with autogenous (Georgiade 1962; Ionnides and Freihofer 1988; Pogrel and Kaban 1990) and alloplastic (Christensen 1964; Gallagher and Wolford 1982; Kiersch 1984) materials, many of the latter resulting in significant iatrogenic injury (Rooney et al. 1988; Ryan 1989; Baraducci et al. 1990).

The introduction in the mid-1980s of the arthroscope, along with advances in imaging technology, opened new vistas on the internal structure and function of the TMJ (Murakami and Hoshino 1982; Sanders 1986; McCain 1988). Joint function could now be directly visualized without having to open the joint surgically. Many raised the same criticism of this modality that was raised against arthrography as a diagnostic tool—that it was nonphysiologic. But diagnostic and therapeutic arthroscopy of the TMJ has probably stimulated more scientific analysis of TMJ function and dysfunction than any tool in the past. The therapeutic success of surgical arthroscopy ranged from 70% to 96% (Zeitler and Porter 1993), but most of these studies were preliminary and often defined untested criteria for abnormality. Indeed, a review of the arthroscopy literature reveals a paucity of random assignment, controlled, and scientifically sound clinical trials.

This most sophisticated of instruments to date, along with advancements in MRI, proved to be two-edged swords. They revealed displaced disks not only in symptomatic patients, but also in asymptomatic volunteers, as well as in the asymptomatic contralateral joints of symptomatic patients. Arthroscopy and MRI also revealed that anterior repositioning splints and disk repositioning surgery did not always reposition disks, but in many cases actually caused further anterior displacement (Moore 1989; Montgomery et al. 1989, 1991; Moses 1989). Cadaver studies also questioned the concept of disk displacement as the cause of all TMJ, headache, and facial pain problems. These studies revealed disk displacement to be a relatively common finding, ranging from 33% to 56% of the specimens examined, a much higher percentage than would be expected given the prevalence of the problem (Solberg et al. 1984; Rohlin et al. 1985). Scientific evidence is still lacking regarding the clinical significance of disk displacement in the TMJ. Further, these studies suggest that disk repositioning may not be essential to achieve clinical success.

LAVAGE OF THE TMJ

One of the results of the intense interest in TMJ diagnostic and surgical arthroscopy was investigation into the chemical mediators of pain found in the fluid lavaged from affected joints (Quinn and Bazan 1990). It is now suggested that pain relief after arthroscopic lysis and lavage may be due to the removal of the inflammatory substances from the joint with the lavage, and the subsequent injection of steroids (Clark and Liu 1993). The role of postoperative physical therapy and the possibility of spontaneous remission must also be addressed.

The success with lysis and lavage arthroscopic surgery led to the development of TMJ arthrocentesis. In this less invasive technique, joint lavage can be accomplished using needle puncture, thus avoiding the introduction of the arthroscope (Nitzan et al. 1991). Murakami and his associates (1994) reported on a comparison of this technique to splint therapy and arthroscopic lysis and lavage in patients with TMJ locking. They found success in unlocking the affected TMJ in 70% of the cases by the use of arthrocentesis, 56% of the cases by a splint, and 91% of these cases by arthroscopic lysis and lavage. Once again, these studies were not randomized or controlled.

As Clark has stated, it is clear that additional series of well-designed comparative diagnostic methodology studies are still needed (Clark and Liu 1993). Those studies should define the specific conditions being evaluated and the stage of the condition at which the use of a particular diagnostic method is appropriate. The American Society of Temporomandibular Joint Surgeons (1992) has attempted in its *Guidelines* to provide such a staging for internal derangement (Table I). The American Association of Oral and Maxillofacial Surgery (1992) has published indications and outcome expectations for TMJ surgery, including internal derangements, but did not include a staging profile.

TMJ REPLACEMENT SURGERY

Total TMJ replacement surgery has become essential for two reasons: (1) Misdiagnosis or overdiagnosis leading to inappropriate intra-articular surgery

Table I
Staging of internal derangement of the TMJ

Stage	Signs and Symptoms	Imaging	Surgical
I Early	Painless clicking No restricted motion	Slightly forward disk Normal TMJ osseous contours	Normal disk form Slight anterior displacement Passive incoordination (clicking)
II Early/ intermediate	Occasional painful clicking Intermediate locking Headaches	Slightly forward disk Early disk deformity Normal bone	Anterior disk displacement Thickened disk
III Intermediate	Frequent pain Joint tenderness Headaches Locking Restricted motion Painful chewing	Anterior disk displacement Moderate to marked disk thickening Normal TMJ osseous contours	Anterior disk displacement Variable adhesions Normal bone
IV Intermediate/ late	Chronic pain Headache Restricted motion	Anterior disk displacement Marked disk thickening Abnormal bone contours	Degenerative re- modeling of bone Osteophytes Adhesions Disk deformity without perforation
V Late	Variable pain Joint crepitus Painful function	Anterior disk displacement with disk perforation and gross deformity Degenerative osseous changes	Gross degenerative changes of disk and bone Disk perforation Multiple adhesions

Source: American Society of Temporomandibular Joint Surgeons 1992.

in patients suffering from extra-articular TMDs. As would be expected, further operations in such cases result in multiple failed attempts to resolve pain. This scenario leads to mutilation and devascularization of the normal TMJ bony and soft tissue anatomy and associated mandibular dysfunction. (2) The use of inappropriate alloplastic materials as replacements for components of the TMJ which, when these materials fail, results in severe and destructive reactions leading once again to anatomic mutilation and jaw pain and dysfunction.

Both situations require either allogenic or alloplastic reconstruction. It is beyond the scope of this chapter to present the absolute indications for each, but it is generally accepted that allogenic reconstruction is preferred when sufficient vascularity remains in the host bed. Unfortunately, this is not the situation in most of the multiply operated failed cases, which require an alloplastic total TMJ replacement prosthesis.

A total prosthesis must be proven safe and effective in prospective, well-controlled, multicenter clinical trials, and must be constructed of materials proven safe and effective in other forms of joint replacements, such as knees and hips. The orthopedic literature contains a plethora of data on these materials and their performance in vivo and in vitro. Given the many patients who need an alloplastic TMJ replacement, any new TMJ prosthesis must be evaluated in a scientific manner before widespread clinical use. An example of a multicenter clinical trial of a new TMJ prosthesis was recently reported after four years of careful data collection (Mercuri et al. 1995).

CRITERIA FOR TMJ SURGERY

The current status of TMJ surgery in the international community of oral and maxillofacial surgeons in the early 1990s is reflected in a report of the Second International Consensus Meeting on TMJ Surgery (Goss 1993). The consensus definition from this meeting for the term internal derangement was "a localized mechanical fault of the joint which interferes with its smooth action." Osteoarthrosis was defined as "a noninflammatory disorder of a moveable joint characterized by deterioration and abrasion of articular connective tissues and also by formation of new bone at the articular surfaces" (Goss 1993). It was agreed that a range of imaging techniques could be used to determine the morphologic state of the joint, but it was recommended that surgery not be performed without the demonstration by imaging of a pathologic condition amenable to surgery.

De Bont and Stegenga (1993) reported that MRI showed disk displacement in asymptomatic patients. Disk displacement thus may represent extremes of normal variation. Further, osteoarthrosis could result in disk displacement, suggesting that internal derangement may be a sign of a range of conditions rather than a single entity. It is now recognized that there is not a direct relationship between the morphogenic condition of the joint (pathology) and the clinical symptoms. Although the morphologic condition may relate to the physical symptoms of clicking and locking, such mechanical explanations do not necessarily relate to pain.

The consensus of the meeting was that a candidate for TMJ surgery must meet all three of the following criteria:

1. Appropriate nonsurgical treatment should have been tried and have failed. A six-month period was considered appropriate.

2. The patient has requested treatment including, if necessary, surgery.

3. There are no medical or psychiatric contraindications to surgery.

Consensus could not be reached on the specific recommendations for surgical procedures because valid outcome evaluations between surgical methods were lacking (Goss 1993). Holmlund (1993) reported that TMJ surgery treatment outcome studies in the literature do not specify inclusion and exclusion criteria, methods of assignment, and definitions of outcome criteria. Further, in many studies, the treatment is not a single procedure but a combination of different procedures. The number of variables introduced into such studies confound the results. These factors, he states, lead to surgical follow-up studies of limited value.

The general consensus on surgical management of TMJ disorders was that surgery should be aimed at conserving existing tissue in the joint, consistent with the degree of the disorder. Arthroscopy should be considered in the early stages. Arthrotomy should be used to restore normal joint function and structure, if possible.

OUTCOME MEASURES FOR EVALUATING SUCCESS

There was also consensus on the need to develop clearly defined, scientific, long-term outcome criteria by which the results of clinical trials should be evaluated. It was noted, however, that generalized ideal criteria are inappropriate for individual patients, because treatment outcomes in patients with end-stage disease would be less likely to fulfill all of the ideal criteria for success.

The following criteria for success were discussed (Goss 1993):

1. Pain absent or so mild that it does not concern the patient. Absence of pain is ideal, but significant pain reduction in intensity and frequency would be satisfactory. Visual analogue scales were recommended for scoring pain and evaluating change.

2. Range of motion of 35 mm interincisal and 6 mm lateral and protrusive. The consensus was that these ranges correlated well with patients' subjective feelings of well-being postoperatively.

3. Absence of joint sounds.

4. Regular diet that, at worst, avoids tough or hard foods. The patient is minimally inconvenienced by the diet.

5. Return of normal imaging appearance. This is either dependent on the stage of disease at presentation or unobtainable, or both. Stabilization of degenerative change is a more appropriate goal.

6. Absence of significant complications.

7. Absence of symptoms for at least two years.

FUTURE RESEARCH FOR TMJ SURGERY

The Consensus Meeting highlighted the following areas that required further investigation (Goss 1993):

1. Basic research into the biomechanics of the TMJ and the role of inflammation, including chemical mediators and degenerative and morphologic changes in the causation of pain.

2. The etiology and pathogenesis of internal derangements and osteoarthrosis and their relationship.

3. The diagnosis and staging of internal derangements.

4. Prospective studies, which should be done in the following areas:
   a. The interrelationship between surgical and nonsurgical therapy.
   b. Arthrocentesis, arthroscopy, and arthrotomy.
   c. Total joint replacement.
   d. Comparative studies among
      i.   disk repositioning, lysis, and lavage
      ii. disk replacement and diskectomy alone
      iii. autogenous vs. alloplastic disk replacement.

Holmlund (1993) recommended that these studies include the following features: goals of treatment, prospective design, inclusion and exclusion criteria, proper assessment methods, defined outcome criteria, lengthy follow-up period, minimal dropout, and appropriate statistical analysis. It is generally recognized that randomized clinical trials are the best method of evaluating treatment in patients because random allocation makes it less likely that outcome differences relate to the treatment and not to the selection bias inherent in uncontrolled or nonrandomized studies (Korn and Baumrind 1991).

CONCLUSIONS

Surgery is indicated in the treatment of intra-articular biomechanical dysfunctional pathology of the TMJ (see list above) when there is demonstrable evidence of anatomical abnormality with appropriate imaging, as well as evidence that surgical correction of that anatomical abnormality will result in decreased symptomatology and improvement of function. It appears that arthrocentesis, arthroscopic surgery, and arthrotomy are appropriate procedures for dealing with the various stages of internal disk derangement (Table I). To determine scientifically which procedure is most appropriate for each stage of disease, the profession needs prospective, multicenter, well-controlled surgical studies based on the criteria outlined by Goss (1993) and Holmlund (1993).

REFERENCES

American Association of Oral and Maxillofacial Surgeons, Special Committee on Parameters of Care, Parameters of care for oral and maxillofacial surgery, J. Oral Maxillofac. Surg., 50 (1992) 121–144.

American Society of Temporomandibular Joint Surgeons, Guidelines for Diagnosis and Management of Disorders Involving the Temporomandibular Joint and Related Musculoskeletal Structures, American Society of Temporomandibular Joint Surgeons, Minneapolis, 1992.

Annandale, R., On displacement of the intra-articular cartilage of the lower jaw and its treatment by operation, Lancet, 1 (1887) 411.

Baraducci, J., Thompson, D. and Scheffer, R., Perforation into the middle cranial fossa as a sequel to the use of a Proplast-Teflon implant for TMJ reconstruction, J. Oral. Maxillofac. Surg., 48 (1990) 496–498.

Christensen, R., Mandibular joint arthrosis corrected by insertion of a cast vitallium glenoid fossa prosthesis, Oral Surg., 17 (1964) 712–722.

Clark, G.T. and Liu, G., Arthroscopic treatment of the human temporomandibular joint. In: G.T. Clark, B. Sanders, and C.N. Bertolami (Eds.), Advances in Diagnostic and Surgical Arthroscopy of the Temporomandibular Joint, W.B. Saunders, Philadelphia, 1993, pp. 85–91.

Cohen, H., Ross, S. and Gordon, R., Computerized tomography as a guide in the diagnosis of temporomandibular joint disease, J. Am. Dent. Assoc., 11 (1985) 57–60.

Costen, J.B., Syndrome of ear and sinus symptoms dependent upon disturbed function of the temporomandibular joint, Ann. Otol. Rhinol. and Laryngol., 43 (1934) 3–15.

Dawson, P.E., Evaluation, Diagnosis and Treatment of Occlusal Problems, C.V. Mosby, St. Louis 1974.

de Bont, L.M.E. and Stegenga, B., Pathology of temporomandibular joint internal derangement and osteoarthosis, Int. J. Oral Maxillofac. Surg., 22 (1993) 71–74.

Dingman, R.O. and Moorman, W.C., Meniscectomy in the treatment of lesions of the temporomandibular joint, J. Oral Surg., 9 (1951) 214–224.

Farrar, W.B., Differentiation of temporomandibular joint dysfunction to simplify treatment, J. Prosthet. Dent., 28 (1972) 629–636.

Farrar, W.B., Characteristics of condylar path in internal derangements of the TMJ, J. Prosthet. Dent., 39 (1978) 319–323.

Gallagher, D.M. and Wolford, L.M., Comparison of silastic and proplast in the temporomandibular joint after condylectomy, J. Oral Maxillofac. Surg., 40 (1982) 627–630.

Gausch, K. and Kulmer, S., The role of retrodisclusion in the treatment of the TMJ patient, J. Oral Rehab., 4 (1977) 29–32.

Georgiade, N., The surgical correction of temporomandibular joint dysfunction by means of autogenous dermal grafts, Plast. Reconstr. Surg., 30 (1962) 68–73.

Goss, A.N., Toward an international consensus on temporomandibular joint surgery, Int. J. Oral Maxillofac. Surg., 22 (1993) 78–81.

Henny, F.A. and Baldridge, O.L., Condylectomy for the persistently painful temporomandibular joint, J. Oral Surg., 15 (1957) 24–31.

Hoffman, D.C., Berliner, L., Manzione, J., Saccaro, R. and McGivern, B.E., Jr, Use of direct sagittal computed tomography in the diagnosis and treatment of internal derangements of the temporomandibular joint, J. Am. Dent. Assoc., 113 (1986) 407–411.

Holmlund, A.B., Surgery for TMJ internal derangement, Int. J. Oral Maxillofac. Surg., 22 (1993) 75–77.

Ionnides, G. and Freihofer, H., Replacement of the damaged intra-articular disc of the TMJ, J. Craniomaxillofac. Surg., 16 (1988) 273–278.

Ireland, V.E., The problem of the clicking jaw, Proc. R. Soc. Med., 44 (1951) 363–372.

Katzberg, R.W., Arthrotomography of the temporomandibular joint: a new technique and preliminary observations, Am. J. Radiol., 132 (1979) 949–953.

Katzberg, R.W., Schenck, J., Roberts, D., Tallents, R.H., Manzione, J., Hart, H.R., Foster, T.H., Wayne, W.S. and Bessette, R.W., Magnetic resonance imaging of the temporomandibular joint meniscus, Oral Surg., 59 (1985) 332–335.

Kerstens, H.C.J., Tuinzing, D.B. and VanDerKwast, W.A.M., Eminectomy and discoplasty for correction of the displaced temporomandibular joint disc, J. Oral Maxillofac. Surg., 47 (1989) 150–152.

Kiehn, C.L., Meniscectomy for internal derangement of the temporomandibular joint, Am. J. Surg., 83 (1952) 364–373.

Kiersch, T.A., The use of Teflon-Proplast implants for meniscectomy and disc repair in the temporomandibular joint. In: AAOMS Clinical Congress on Reconstruction and Biomaterials: Current Assessment and Temporomandibular Joint: Surgical Update, Program Outlines and Abstracts, New York, New York, 1984.

Korn, E.L. and Baumrind, S., Randomized clinical trials with clinician preferred treatment, Lancet, 337 (1991) 149–152.

Lanz, W., Discitis mandibularis, Zentralbl Chir, 36 (1909) 289.

Laskin, D.M., Etiology of the pain dysfunction syndrome, J. Am. Dent. Assoc., 79 (1969) 147–153.

Marciani, R. and Ziegler, R., Temporomandibular joint surgery: a review of fifty-one operations, J. Oral Surg., 56 (1983) 472–476.

McCain, J.P., Arthroscopy of the human temporomandibular joint, J. Oral Maxillofac. Surg., 46 (1988) 648–655.

McCarty, W.L. and Farrar, W.B., Surgery for internal derangements of the temporomandibular joints, J. Prosthet. Dent., 42 (1979) 191–196.

Mercuri, L.G., Temporomandibular joint surgery. In: P.H. Kwon and D.M. Laskin (Eds.), Clinicians Manual of Oral and Maxillofacial Surgery, Quintessence, Chicago, 1991, pp. 339–354.

Mercuri, L.G., Campbell, R.L. and Shamaskin, R.G., Intra-articular meniscus dysfunction surgery, Oral Surg., 54 (1982) 613–621.

Mercuri, L.G., Wolford, L.M., Sanders, B., White, R.D., Hurder, A. and Henderson, W., Custom CAD/CAM total TMJ reconstruction system: preliminary milticenter report of a 4-year clinical study, J. Oral Maxillofac. Surg., 53 (1995) 106–115.

Montgomery, M.T., VanSickels, J.E. and Harms, S.E., Arthroscopic TMJ surgery: effects on signs, symptoms, and disc position, J Oral Maxillofac Surg., 47 (1989) 1263–1271.

Montgomery, M.T., VanSickels, J.E. and Harms, S.E., Success of temporomandibular joint arthroscopy in disc displacement with and without reduction, Oral Surg., 71 (1991) 651–659.

Moore, J.B., Coronal and sagittal TMJ meniscus position in asymptomatic subjects by MRI. In:

Proceedings of the American Association of Oral and Maxillofacial Surgeons' Annual Meeting, American Association of Oral and Maxillofacial Surgeons, San Francisco, 1989.

Morris, J.H., Chronic recurring temporomandibular joint subluxation, Surg. Obstet. Gynecol., 50 (1930) 483–491.

Moses, J.J., The effect of arthroscopic surgical lysis and lavage of the superior joint space on TMJ disc position and mobility, J. Oral Maxillofac. Surg., 47 (1989) 674–678.

Murakami, K.I. and Hoshino, K., Regional anatomical nomenclature and arthroscopic terminology in human temporomandibular joints, Okajimas Folia Anat. Japan, 58 (1982) 745–760.

Murakami, K.I., Hosaka, H., Haraguchi, H., Segami, N. and Iizuka, T., Arthrocentesis vs other non-surgical and surgical treatment for TMJ locking. In: C.N. Bertolami (Ed.), Proceedings of the UCLA International Symposium on Controversies in Oral and Maxillofacial Surgery, UCLA School of Dentistry, Continuing Education, Los Angeles, 1994.

Nitzan, D.W., Dolwick, M.F. and Martinez, G.A., Temporomandibular joint arthrocentesis: a simplified treatment for severe, limited mouth opening, J. Oral Maxillofac. Surg., 49 (1991) 1163–1167.

Pogrel, M. and Kaban, L., The role of the temporalis fascia and muscle flap in temporomandibular joint surgery, J. Oral Maxillofac. Surg., 48 (1990) 14–19.

Pringle, J., Displacement of the mandibular meniscus and its treatment, Br. J. Surg., 6 (1918) 385–392.

Quinn, J.H. and Bazan, N.G., Identification of prostaglandin E2 and leukotriene B4 in the synovial fluid of painful, dysfunctional TMJ, J. Oral Maxillofac. Surg., 48 (1990) 968–971.

Rohlin, M., Westesson, P.L. and Eriksson, L., The correlation of joint sounds with joint morphology in fifty-five autopsy specimens, J. Oral Maxillofac. Surg., 43 (1985) 194–200.

Rooney, T., Haug, R., Toor, A. and Indresano, A.T., Rapid condylar degeneration after glenoid fossa prosthesis insertion, J. Oral Maxillofac. Surg., 46 (1988) 240–246.

Ryan, D., Alloplastic implants in the temporomandibular joint, Oral Maxillofac. Clin. N. Am., 1 (1989) 427–441.

Sanders, B., Arthroscopic surgery of the temporomandibular joint: treatment of internal derangement with persistent closed lock, Oral Surg., 62 (1986) 361–372.

Schwartz, L.L., Pain associated with the temporomandibular joint, J. Am. Dent. Assoc., 51 (1955) 393–397.

Schwartz, L.L., Temporomandibular joint pain-dysfunction syndrome, J. Chron. Dis., 3 (1956) 284–293.

Schwartz, L.L., Disorders of the Temporomandibular Joint, W.B. Saunders, Philadelphia, 1959.

Shore, N.A., Temporomandibular Joint Dysfunction and Occlusal Equilibration, 2nd ed., J.B. Lippincott, Philadelphia,1976.

Silver, C.M. and Simon, S.D., Meniscus injuries of the temporomandibular joint, J. Bone Surg., 38-A (1956) 541–552.

Solberg, W.K., Hanson, T. and Nordstrom, B., Morphologic evaluation of young adult TMJs at autopsy, J. Dent. Res., 63 (1984) 228 (abstr 518).

Stith, H.E., Surgical treatment of internal derangements of the temporomandibular joint: review of 198 joints. In: Proceedings of the American Association of Oral and Maxillofacial Surgeons' Annual Meeting, American Association of Oral and Maxillofacial Surgeons, New York, 1984.

Tiner, B.D. and Dolwick, M.F., Surgical correction of internal derangement of the TMJ: five year results. In: Proceedings of the American Association of Oral and Maxillofacial Surgeons' Annual Meeting, American Association of Oral and Maxillofacial Surgeons, Las Vegas, 1983.

Wakeley, C., The causation and treatment of displaced mandibular cartilage, Lancet, 2 (1929) 543–545.

Walker, R.V. and Kalamchi, S., A surgical technique for the management of internal derangement of the temporomandibular joint, J. Oral Maxillofac. Surg., 45 (1987) 299–305.

Weinberg, L.A., Role of condylar position in TMJ pain-dysfunction syndrome, J. Prosthet. Dent., 41 (1979) 636–643.

Weinberg, S., Eminectomy and meniscoplasty for internal derangements of the temporomandibu-

lar joint: rationale and operative technique, Oral Surg., 57 (1984) 241–249.
Wilkes, C.H., Arthrography of the temporomandibular joint, Minn. Med., 67 (1978) 645–652.
Zeitler, D.L. and Porter, B.T., A retrospective study comparing arthroscopic surgery with arthrotomy
    and disc repositioning. In: G.T. Clark, B. Sanders and C.N. Bertolami (Eds.), Advances in
    Diagnostic and Surgical Arthroscopy of the Temporomandibular Joint, W.B. Saunders, Phila-
    delphia, 1993, pp. 47–60.

Correspondence to: Louis G. Mercuri, DDS, MS, Division of Oral and Maxillofacial Surgery and Dental Medicine, Loyola University Medical Center, 2160
South First Ave., Maywood, IL 60153, USA. Tel: 708-216-6907; Fax: 708-216-
5560.

Temporomandibular Disorders and Related Pain Conditions, Progress in Pain Research and Management, Vol. 4, edited by B.J. Sessle, P.S. Bryant, and R.A. Dionne, IASP Press, Seattle, © 1995.

25

The Temporomandibular Joint Alloplastic Implant Problem

Larry M. Wolford,[a] Charles H. Henry,[b]
Afzal Nikaein,[c] Joseph T. Newman,[d] and
Thomas C. Namey[e]

[a]Department of Oral and Maxillofacial Surgery, Baylor College of Dentistry, and private practice at Baylor University Medical Center, Dallas, Texas, USA; [b]Former fellow in oral and maxillofacial surgery with Dr. L. Wolford, Baylor University Medical Center, Dallas, Texas, now in private practice, Keene, New Hampshire, USA; [c]Transplantation Immunology Laboratory, Baylor University Medical Center, Dallas, Texas, USA; [d]Department of Immunology, Baylor University Medical Center, Dallas, Texas, USA; [e]Departments of Medicine, Pediatrics, Nutrition, and Exercise Science, University of Tennessee Graduate School of Medicine, and Department of Medicine, University of Tennessee, Knoxville, Tennessee, USA

Alloplastic implants have been used extensively for temporomandibular joint (TMJ) reconstruction. The most commonly used implant materials were Proplast-Teflon (Vitek, Inc., Houston, TX) and Silastic (Dow-Corning, Midland, MO). Others have included polymethylmethacrylate (PMMA), polyethylene, and various metals. The Vitek TMJ implants and prostheses used Proplast-Teflon (PT) as a major component of their devices. PT and Silastic TMJ implants have resulted in numerous complications, including fragmentation, foreign body giant cell reaction, particle migration, pain, lymphadenopathy, severe osteoarthritis, bone resorption, and perforation into the middle cranial fossa, (Timmis et al. 1986; Heffez et al. 1987; Ryan 1989; Yih and Merrill 1989; Wagner and Mosley 1990).

The human body cannot degrade these polymers, and severe local and systemic reactions thus occur. We have conducted several studies to evaluate the local and systemic effects of these materials.

TREATMENT OUTCOMES FOR TMJ RECONSTRUCTION AFTER PROPLAST-TEFLON IMPLANT FAILURE

A retrospective study was conducted by Henry and Wolford (1993) on 107 patients with 163 joints previously treated with PT implants. The average length of patient follow-up was 84.6 months (range 59 to 126 months). Only 12% of the joints showed no significant osseous changes radiographically. Forty-five patients still had PT implants in place; 36% of those patients had significant pain requiring medication, 25% had developed an anterior open-bite and malocclusion, 9% had limited vertical opening, and only 40% were asymptomatic. It is predicted that all of these TMJ implants will eventually fail. TMJ reconstruction after PT implant failure was performed with five different autologous tissues or a total joint prosthesis. Autologous tissues used to reconstruct the TMJ and the rates of success with these were as follows: (1) temporalis fascia and muscle graft 13%, (2) temporalis fascia and muscle graft with sagittal split ramus osteotomy 31%, (3) dermis graft 8%, (4) conchal cartilage graft 25%, (5) costochondral graft 12%, and (6) sternoclavicular graft 21%. The success rate decreased in all autologous tissue groups, as the number of previous TMJ surgeries increased. Pain and ankylosis were the most common causes of failure. The results of TMJ reconstruction with a custom-made total joint prosthesis (Techmedica Inc., Camarillo, CA) were as follows: (1) 88% of patients had functional and occlusal stability; and (2) the level of pain reduction was rated as good in 46%, fair in 38%, and poor in 16%.

In one subgroup of the PT patients, a foreign body giant cell reaction was still present an average of 40 months (range 32 to 48 months) after implant removal, and after an average of 4.5 (2 to 9) additional debridement surgeries.

Studies by Bradrick and Indresano (1992), Henry and Wolford (1993), and Wolford et al. (1994) and indicate that after two operations, the success rate of TMJ reconstruction using autologous tissue approaches zero. In the complex multiply operated TMJ patient, and those with previously failed alloplasts, a total joint prosthesis using materials with proven safety and efficacy in orthopedic use may be the only option available to predictability improve the quality of life.

HUMAN LEUKOCYTE ANTIGEN (HLA) STUDIES

The association of certain arthropathies with an increased incidence of specific human leukocyte antigens (HLA) has been demonstrated in well-controlled human studies. We have performed HLA typing on 25 patients with TMJ dysfunction and failed PT implants to determine if an increased incidence of HLA types associated with a predisposition to connective tissue disease could be demonstrated. Most of the patients were experiencing chronic pain and dysfunction. Medical histories of the 24 female patients also included the following findings: 58% with fibrocystic breast disease; 50% with hypersensitivity to metals; 35% with endometriosis. Results showed that 10 of 25 patients (40%) had HLA-B locus antigens associated with psoriasis or psoriatic arthritis, versus 17.6% of 125 controls. Other patients demonstrated antigens associated with juvenile rheumatoid arthritis or sarcoidosis, ankylosing spondylitis, Reiter's syndrome, and/or systemic lupus erythematosus. If these findings are considered, then 20 of 25 patients (80%) have antigenic associations with various connective tissue diseases, which may have predisposed them to immune dysfunction and treatment failure.

IMMUNOLOGICAL STUDIES

We have performed a preliminary study evaluating the human immunological response to PT implants in 12 patients (Henry et al., submitted for publication). The total lymphocyte count was calculated and immune response assessed by immunophenotyping peripheral blood lymphocytes: IA, CD2, CD3, CD4, CD8, CD4:CD8 ratio, CD20, CD56, and surface Ig positive cells. The IA subset was below controls in 73% of patients, and CD4:CD8 ratio was decreased significantly below the normal range. By contrast, the CD56 subset was elevated in 60% of patients. An in vitro lymphocyte activation assay was used with six patients to determine the presence of activated T cells. Lymphocytic activation was present in four of six patients. The activated T cell response was greater in those patients experiencing more severe symptoms. The immunologic consequences of the activated T cell response remains to be investigated.

A small study followed four patients who had a significant decrease in their immunodeficiency panel prior to removal of the PT implant. Three of the patients who had reconstructions with the Techmedica custom-made total joint prosthesis demonstrated a significant improvement toward normal values at one year postsurgery.

SYSTEMIC DISEASES

Clinical observations suggest that some patients may have developed connective tissue diseases that may have been promoted or exacerbated by TMJ implant materials. Some conditions that have been recorded in TMJ patients with PT, Silastic, and PMMA implants include: chronic fatigue syndrome, chronic pain, impaired cognition, short-term memory loss, lupus, psoriasis, psoriatic arthritis, sarcoidosis, polyarthritis, fibromyalgia, human adjuvant disease, scleroderma, Sjögren's syndrome, rheumatoid arthritis, visual disturbances, localized and distant muscular disease, neurologic dysfunction, chronic low-grade fever, and significant hormonal imbalances. Undifferentiated or mixed connective tissue disease may be a common finding. Problems associated with these conditions, especially chronic pain, physical limitations, and diminished mentation often render these patients partially or totally disabled. Foreign body giant cell granulomas have been found in the TMJ, masticatory muscles, parotid and submandibular glands, regional lymph nodes, on the roof of the orbit, within the orbit, in the lung, and in breast biopsies. The extent of systemic involvement with alloplastic materials remains unclear and requires further investigation.

HISTOPATHOLOGIC DIFFERENCES OF ALLOPLASTIC TMJ IMPLANTS

Our series of patients suggests that foreign body giant cell reaction to PT implants is proliferative and worsens with time, as more PT particles are generated. Cartilage and bone degeneration and resorption occur. Heterotopic bone formation and/or reactive neo-ossification can develop. It is unknown what effect the aluminum oxide, used in some PT implants, has in the pathological process.

Silastic and PMMA particles appear to create a less proliferative foreign body giant cell reaction. Cartilage and bone resorption can occur. Particle size may be larger than the PT particles, resulting in fibrosis, sometimes with reactive cartilage, neo-ossification, and/or heterotopic bone formation. Local tissues may be affected by direct contact with the material, or leaching of monomer from the PMMA. Local reactions may in part be chemically mediated from the polymers, from cells releasing substances in an effort to degrade the polymers or upon cell death and lysis. An antibody to silicone has been identified (Goldblum et al. 1992), and unidentified antibodies may exist for other polymers.

CONCLUSIONS

The local and systemic effects of PT, Silastic, and other polymeric implants that undergo fragmentation and formation of particulate debris are not clearly understood. Further studies will be necessary to identify the effects of these materials, particularly in patients who may have a predisposition to connective tissue disease, and to develop treatment modalities that will pre-dictably help the unfortunate patients afflicted with these diseases.

REFERENCES

Bradrick, J.P. and Indresano, A.T., Failure rates of repetitive temporomandibular joint surgical procedures (abstract), J. Oral Maxillofac. Surg., 50, Suppl. 3, (1992) 145.

Goldblum, R.M., Pelley, R.P., O'Donnell, A.A., Pyron, D. and Heggers, J.P., Antibodies to silicone elastomers and reactions to ventriculoperitoneal shunts, Lancet, 340 (1992) 510–513.

Heffez, L., Mafee, M.F., Rosenberg, H., II and Langer, B., CT evaluation of TMJ disc replacement with a Proplast-Teflon laminate, J. Oral Maxillofac. Surg., 45 (1987) 657–665.

Henry, C.H. and Wolford, L.M., Treatment outcomes for temporomandibular joint reconstruction after Proplast-Teflon implant failure, J. Oral Maxillofac. Surg., 51 (1993) 352–358.

Ryan, D.E., Alloplastic implants in the temporomandibular joint, Oral Maxillofac. Surg. Clin. North Am., 1 (1989) 427–441.

Timmis, D.P., Aragon, S.B., Van Sickels, J.E. and Aufdemorte, T.B., Comparative study of alloplastic material for temporomandibular joint disc replacement in rabbits, J. Oral Maxillofac. Surg., 44 (1986) 541–554.

Wagner, J.D. and Mosby, E.L., Assessment of Proplast-Teflon disc replacements, J. Oral Maxillofac. Surg., 48 (1990) 1140–1144.

Wolford, L.M., Cottrell, D.A. and Henry, C.H., Temporomandibular joint reconstruction of the complex patient with the Techmedica custom-made total joint prosthesis, J. Oral Maxillofac. Surg., 52 (1994) 2–10.

Yih, W.Y. and Merrill, R.G., Pathology of alloplastic interpositional implants in the temporomandibular joint, Oral Maxillofac. Surg. Clin. North Am., 1 (1989) 415–426.

Correspondence to: Larry M. Wolford, DDS, 3409 Worth Street, Suite 400, Dallas, TX 75246, USA. Tel: 214-828-9115; Fax 214-828-1714.

Temporomandibular Disorders and Related Pain Conditions, Progress in Pain Research and Management, Vol. 4, edited by B.J. Sessle, P.S. Bryant, and R.A. Dionne, IASP Press, Seattle, © 1995.

Reaction Papers to Chapters 19–25

Jeffrey P. Okeson and Laurence A. Bradley

Jeffrey P. Okeson

Orofacial Pain Center, University of Kentucky College of Dentistry, Lexington, Kentucky, USA

The prevention of temporomandibular disorders (TMDs), as discussed by Fricton (this volume), is far more complicated than first appreciated. Numerous risk factors, such as anxiety, depression, somatization, and bruxism, have been identified, and I believe that we will learn of many more risk factors with time.

Fricton quotes an article that revealed that 34% of myofascial pain patients report an acute traumatic injury associated with the onset of their pain disorder. It would seem impossible to prevent such disorders, since the onset was unexpected. A case could be made, however, for early treatment, since it is likely that some of these patients would seek care following their trauma. Of greater concern may be the 66% who do not associate any trauma with the onset of their pain. Can these be prevented? What was the etiology? I suggest that Fricton not use the term *acute trauma* in his model, but instead refer to the etiology as "an event," which can imply both traumatic or other events such as stressful encounters or conditions.

Fricton reports that four items from the IMPATH questionnaire were found to be useful predictors of poor treatment outcome: "self esteem," "feel worried," "low energy," and "sleep activity." He reports that all of these predictors are associated with depression. These findings further emphasize the significant role of the clinical psychologist in the management of many painful TMDs.

Discussion of the prevention of TMDs at present can involve only insight, not data. The profession needs long-term general population studies that consider etiology and the natural course of these disorders before a report on prevention and early treatment can have true meaning.

Rudy and Turk (this volume) bring some very important methods and measurement instruments into the TMD field that are helpful in better evaluating our patients. They make an excellent case for why the mechanistic approach to treatment fails miserably with TMDs. Dentistry needs to embrace the biopsychosocial model of disease when approaching the management of complex orofacial pain problems.

Their chapter presents solid research methodology that assists the reader in understanding the relationship between dental and psychological therapies for managing TMDs and reveals that the combination of these therapies may in fact be the most effective management strategy. Their study also demonstrated the usefulness of categorizing patients as "dysfunctional," "interpersonally distressed," or "adaptive copers."

A question arises why Rudy and Turk selected only a portion of the Coping Strategies Questionnaire and Multidimensional Pain Inventory scales, instead of the entire scales. I would be most interested in seeing the rest of the results. I also wonder why the catastrophizing scale did not reveal any improvement in the study, when cognitive therapy is often directed toward this issue. It would also be useful to know if they used any training criteria to determine the effectiveness of the psychology therapy. I believe training criteria are needed to assure adequate learning by the patient. If not, the results of the study can be misleading. The same thing can happen if an occlusal appliance is studied but the subject fails to wear the appliance appropriately.

An issue that Dionne (this volume) did not discuss but that I feel needs to be presented is appropriate control of pain so as to avoid central sensitization. Work by Dubner and others has demonstrated the importance of controlling nociceptive input to the second-order neurons to avoid neuroplastic changes that lead to neuropathic pains. The issue of appropriate pain control is a difficult problem that presents questions between pain control, addictive considerations, and society's standards.

Clark et al. (this volume) present a thorough review of the scientific literature on the physical medicine therapies used for TMDs. Although the classification scheme used in that chapter is not necessarily widely endorsed by the profession, the categories can certainly be used to evaluate treatment modalities. Clark et al. review more than 30 different treatments in 15 categories to conclude that methodological flaws are common in nearly all of these studies; yet all boast significant success. This reflects the problems that propagate numerous treatment philosophies. These findings reinforce the need for controlled randomized clinical trials. Their review of the literature supports the viewpoint that TMDs are rarely disabling and therefore need to be approached conservatively and reversibly.

McNamara et al. (this volume) have done an outstanding job in assembling all the scientific evidence relating to occlusion, orthodontics, and TMDs. Their conclusion that occlusal factors are not a major contributor to TMDs is supported by the literature. Similarly, their assessment that routine orthodontic therapy does not pose any unusual risk factors to TMDs is in accord with the known body of scientific literature.

The reviewed studies do not completely rule out occlusal factors as etiology in TMDs. In fact, gross orthopedic instabilities between the occlusal condition and a stable joint relationship may be a contributor to TMDs. Certain conditions such as significant retruded contact position to intercuspal contact position slides and unilateral crossbites were significantly related to symptoms. Perhaps these studies have demonstrated that the static occlusal relationships and observed eccentric contact movements are not significantly related to TMDs. We have not, however, investigated dynamic jaw function, nor whether occlusal instabilities during these functions are significantly related to TMDs. The present data suggest that occlusal therapy not be considered for the routine management of TMDs.

Mercuri and Mercuri and Wolford et al. (this volume) emphasize how improper diagnosis is a major reason for treatment failure. He also discusses the importance of developing standard criteria for treatment outcomes so studies can be more standardized. The only area missing from his chapter is discussion of the natural adaptive capacity of the TMJ. Although we do not have great numbers of longitudinal studies, those by Boering, de Bont, and de Leeuw demonstrate the adaptability of the TMJ. These studies demonstrate that some patients adapt without the need for significant therapy.

Correspondence to: Jeffrey P. Okeson, DMD, Professor and Director, Orofacial Pain Center, University of Kentucky College of Dentistry, Lexington, KY 40536-0084, USA. Tel: 606-323-5500; Fax: 606-258-1042.

Laurence A. Bradley

Division of Clinical Immunology and Rheumatology, The University of Alabama at Birmingham, Birmingham, Alabama, USA

The development of treatment outcome studies for temporomandibular disorders (TMDs) has been hindered by a dearth of knowledge regarding the etiopathogenesis of these disorders. Indeed, Clark, Mercuri, Wolford, and McNamara and colleagues (this volume) have prepared excellent discussions of the long history of unsuccessful attempts to identify single factors (e.g., malocclusion, internal derangement) that might be related to the etiology of the TMDs. This history is not unique to the study of TMDs; research regarding rheumatologic and gastrointestinal disorders, for example, also has been characterized by failed attempts to find simple causes for complex pain perceptions and pain behaviors. But several innovative studies from these research areas have improved our understanding of the relationships among physiologic events, psychological and environmental factors, symptoms, and behavior. This chapter reviews these studies and provides suggestions for future research that may help us to develop better treatment interventions for TMDs and related pain conditions.

A great deal of effort has been devoted to examining pain associated with gastroesophageal reflux disease (GERD). This is the most common disorder of the esophagus (Henderson 1980) and is associated with a known and somewhat controllable physiologic event, reflux of gastric acid into the esophagus. The perception of pain among patients with GERD, however, is the product of complex relationships between acid production and several moderating factors. Thus, patients may report reflux symptoms when no acid is present in the esophagus, or may experience no symptoms despite prolonged acid exposure (Johnson et al. 1987).

Psychological stress often has been identified as a variable that increases painful symptoms among patients with GERD (Nielzen et al. 1986; Gallup Organization 1988). However, my colleagues and I recently performed the first controlled laboratory investigation of the influence of stress on symptoms of GERD (Bradley et al. 1993). We found that prolonged psychological stress, relative to neutral conditions, reliably increased several psychophysiologic stress measures (e.g., heart rate, blood pressure) but did not significantly increase esophageal acid exposure among patients with GERD. We also found that a subgroup of chronically anxious GERD patients reported significantly greater reflux symptom activity during the stressful periods relative to neutral conditions despite the fact that their total acid exposure did not vary across the stressful and neutral study phases. Patients with relatively low anxiety levels reported comparable amounts of reflux symptom activity during stressful and neutral conditions. These findings indicate that although a physiologic event (e.g., acid reflux) is known to cause tissue damage and pain among patients with GERD, psychological characteristics and environmental variables also may interact to produce symptoms that are not congruent with physiologic status. Therefore, it is likely that our understanding of TMD symptoms also will be enhanced by shifting the focus of our research efforts from single physiologic factors that may cause pain to interactions among physiologic, environmental, and psychological variables. An example of this shift in emphasis can be found in the "dual diagnostic" approach recommended by Rudy and Turk (this volume).

Patient selection bias also has hindered our understanding of TMDs. Many of the patient samples studied to date have consisted of persons who sought treatment from specialists at tertiary care medical centers or practices. These samples, members of which often have been characterized by high levels of psychological and physical distress, may not be representative of the population of persons with TMDs (Wolfe 1990).

An important example of selection bias is found in research on fibromyalgia (FM). Many investigations have shown that patients with FM, relative to healthy controls, have more psychiatric diagnoses and higher levels of psychological distress (Boissevain and McCain 1991). My colleagues and I recently examined psychiatric morbidity and symptom severity among three subject groups: (a) patients with FM recruited from a tertiary care medical practice, (b) individuals with FM recruited from the community who had not sought medical treatment for their pain within the past 10 years, and (c) healthy controls (Bradley et al. 1994). We found that patients with FM, relative to persons who had not sought medical care for their symptoms, reported significantly higher levels of pain, disability, and fatigue. Moreover, we found high levels of psychiatric morbidity only among the patients with FM; the other subject groups did not differ on this variable. These results suggest that high levels of psychological distress are not a primary feature of FM. Rather, psychological distress, in combination with high levels of pain and disability, may drive persons to obtain medical care at tertiary care practices.

These results also indicate that it may be necessary to modify treatment interventions for persons with FM as a function of the severity of their pain and psychological distress. For example, patients with high levels of psychological distress and pain may require behavioral interventions in addition to exercise and psychotropic medication, whereas those with relatively mild symptoms may benefit from medication or exercise alone. It seems likely that treatments for patients with TMDs also will require modification based on the severity of pain and psychological symptoms. Indeed, Turk and colleagues (1993) already have demonstrated that patients with TMDs differ in their response to a combined dental and psychological treatment package as a function of their psychosocial and behavioral characteristics.

The studies discussed above focused on the importance of tailoring treatment interventions to patient characteristics. However, it is imperative that we attempt to ensure the validity of our studies of the outcomes produced by these interventions with the use of appropriate control groups, adequate follow-up periods, and the determination of the clinical as well as statistical significance of patient change (see Clark et al., Dionne, Fricton, and Rudy and Turk, this volume). It is important to determine whether the treatment effects actually are mediated by the factors proposed to underlie the interventions. For example, relaxation training, relative to attention-placebo, produces a significant reduction in symptom reports among chronically anxious patients with GERD (Haile et al. 1994). It was assumed that this effect would be mediated by reductions in physiologic stress variables (e.g., heart rate) and subjective anxiety. Patients who received relaxation training did show lower heart rates and anxiety ratings; however, they also displayed a significant reduction in esophageal acid exposure. The effect of relaxation training on acid exposure may have been mediated by increased pressure in the lower esophageal sphincter produced by diaphragmatic breathing or by centrally induced reductions in gastric acid secretions. Regardless of the exact mechanisms underlying patient change, the results suggest that all intervention studies should include careful evaluation of mediating variables as well as outcomes.

In summary, the study of treatment outcomes for TMDs can advance only if investigators attend to interactions among physiologic, psychological, and environmental variables that influence symptoms and responses to interventions. Progress has been made in understanding these interactions within other areas of pain research. Research on gastrointestinal and rheumatologic disorders provides models that investigators could build upon to better understand the etiopathogenesis of TMDs and to develop effective treatments for these disorders.

ACKNOWLEDGMENT

Preparation of this paper was supported by National Institute of Arthritis, Musculoskeletal and Skin Diseases (2 P60 AR 20641-15), National Center for Research Resources (5 MO10032), and National Institute of Digestive Diseases and Kidney Disorders (R01 DK40490-01A1).

REFERENCES

Boissevain, M.D. and McCain, G.A., Toward an integrated understanding of fibromyalgia syndrome. II. Psychological and phenomenological aspects, Pain, 45 (1991) 239–248.

Bradley, L.A., Richter, J.E., Pulliam, T.J., McDonald Haile, J., Scarinci, I.C., Schan, C.A., Dalton, C.B. and Salley, A.N., The relationship between stress and symptoms of gastroesophageal reflux: the influence of psychological factors, Am. J. Gastroenterol., 88 (1993) 11–19.

Bradley, L.A., Alarcón, G.S., Triana, M., Aaron, L.A., Alexander, R.A., Stewart, K.E., Martin, M., and Alberts, K., Health care seeking behavior in fibromyalgia: association with pain thresholds, symptom severity, and psychiatric morbidity, J. Musculoskel. Pain, 2 (1994) 79–87.

Gallup Organization, A Gallup Survey on Heartburn across America, The Gallup Organization, Princeton, N.J., 1988.

Haile, J.M., Bradley, L.A., Bailey, M.A., Schan, C.A. and Richter, J.E., Relaxation training reduces symptom reports and acid exposure in patients with gastroesophageal reflux disease, Gastroenterology, 107 (1994) 61–69.

Henderson, R.D., Motor Disorders of the Esophagus, 2nd ed., Williams and Wilkins, Baltimore, 1980.

Johnson, D.A., Winters, C., Spurling, T.J., Chobanian, S.J. and Cattau, E.L., Esophageal acid sensitivity in Barrett's esophagus, J. Clin. Gastroenterol., 9 (1987) 23–27.

Nielzen, S., Petterson, K.I., Regnell, G. and Svensson, R., The role of psychiatric factors in symptoms of hiatus hernia or gastric reflux, Acta Psychiatr. Scand., 73 (1986) 214–220.

Turk, D.C., Zaki, D.S. and Rudy, T.E., Effects of intraoral appliance and biofeedback/stress management alone and in combination in treating pain and depression in patients with temporomandibular disorders, J. Prosthet. Dent., 70 (1993) 158–164.

Wolfe, F., Methodological and statistical problems in the epidemiology of fibromyalgia. In: J.R. Fricton and E. Awad (Eds.), Advances in Pain Research and Therapy, Vol. 17, Raven Press, New York, 1990, pp. 147–163.

Correspondence to: Laurence A. Bradley, PhD, 625 Medical Education Building, UAB Station, The University of Alabama at Birmingham, Birmingham, AL 35294, USA. Tel: 205-934-3883; Fax: 205-975-6859.

Part VIII

Biostatistical Commentary and
Research Recommendations

Temporomandibular Disorders and Related Pain Conditions, Progress in Pain Research and Management, Vol. 4, edited by B.J. Sessle, P.S. Bryant, and R.A. Dionne, IASP Press, Seattle, © 1995.

26

Statistical and Methodological Issues in Temporomandibular Disorder Research

Timothy A. DeRouen

Departments of Biostatistics and Dental Public Health Sciences, University of Washington, Seattle, Washington, USA

The nature of general clinical research methodology allows one to identify issues in that domain rather easily, whereas identifying statistical issues in basic science research usually requires considerable familiarity with specific research techniques. With that prologue, I now offer comments related to clinical research discussed during the conference.

FALLACIES OF UNCONTROLLED STUDIES, PUBLICATION BIAS, AND SMALL SAMPLE SIZES

It is remarkable to see multiple authors with differing backgrounds and interests reach the same conclusion when summarizing the clinical research into temporomandibular disorders (TMDs) done thus far in their area, especially with respect to treatment. They generally indicate that published reports suggest that there are treatments that may be efficacious, but because of the nature and quality of the studies published, the scientific evidence needed to reach a valid conclusion of treatment efficacy is lacking.

Most of the studies cited are case series, a design useful for providing preliminary evidence of possible treatment efficacy, but which is also fraught with potential biases. The most serious flaw in case series is the absence of a control group of similar patients who were untreated or who received a standard treatment. Without a control group, the only measure of efficacy is pre- versus posttreatment status in the treated patients. Other than providing preliminary evidence on which to base comparative studies, published case series are of dubious value. Although many investigators who publish case series try to be as scientifically honest as possible, they often allow bias to enter through methods they do not recognize as being problematic, such as by rationalizing that certain cases with untoward outcomes can be omitted because they don't meet a narrow definition of an appropriate case (even though they were treated).

In almost any area, published case series tend to show a positive outcome for a new treatment. That occurs because of the biases introduced at the investigator level, as described above, and because of the publication bias resulting from the lack of incentives for investigators to publish negative case series (after all, one interpretation of a negative case series is a set of documented treatment failures by a clinician). There is also likely to be publication bias against negative case series by editors, because publication of a clinical study of low credibility and that does not suggest treatment efficacy probably will be a low priority. Therefore, case series that are published tend to be positive with respect to treatment outcome.

An additional problem contributing to the lack of conclusive literature is the propensity for published comparative studies to involve small sample sizes. Unless the effect of a treatment is quite substantial, a small comparative study involving a treatment that truly is efficacious is likely to conclude that the trend is encouraging but the results not statistically significant. A small comparative study involving a treatment that is truly not efficacious is also likely to result in equivocal findings. Thus, although they do provide additional preliminary evidence of potential treatment efficacy, small studies are likely to be inconclusive regardless of the true efficacy of a treatment, and multiple small studies often merely add to the confusion rather than help find a definitive answer. Further discussion of issues associated with various kinds of study designs can be found in Feinstein (1985), Weiss (1986), and Fletcher et al. (1988).

LACK OF STANDARDIZED DISEASE DIAGNOSES, MEASURES, AND TREATMENT OUTCOMES

There seems to be fairly universal appreciation for the need to standardize the definitions of the diagnoses and measures of disease process used in studies of TMDs, as well as in the outcomes used to measure treatment efficacy. The myriad of diagnostic terminologies and outcome measures used up to this point make it difficult to make comparisons across studies. Presumably, the resulting confusion and frustration led to the development of the research diagnostic criteria (RDC) published in Dworkin and LeResche (1992), which can be viewed as the first stage in the standardization effort. To make the RDC more readily available and usable, a computer program that implements the algorithms used for the criteria has now been written in SAS and is available upon request. A description of the program and directions for its use are provided in Whitney and Zhu (1994). Although one of the recommendations from this conference is to study the validity of the RDC (which is not straightforward, as there is no "gold standard" with which to compare the RDC diagnoses), in my view the most important effect of the RDC is merely to standardize how patients are classified, regardless of whether some of the classifications are as useful prognostically as expected. The call for a conference to identify and define core standardized measures of disease process and treatment outcomes, prior to embarking on a series of recommended clinical trials, correctly identifies the next stage in the standardization process, which is crucial to maximize the amount of information to be learned from clinical trials.

THE CALL FOR RANDOMIZED CLINICAL TRIALS

There appears to be almost unanimity of opinion that it is time to subject the various treatment options for TMDs to the scrutiny of randomized clinical trials. A possible exception to this unanimity of opinion is the guidelines suggested by the oral surgeons for future studies, which lack any mention of randomized clinical trials. The reluctance of surgeons to subject their patients to randomized clinical trials when they feel that they know the best treatment is not a phenomenon unique to the oral/maxillofacial area. Studies in which I participated 15 to 20 years ago compared the efficacy of coronary artery bypass surgery with medical (nonsurgical) treatment of patients with coronary heart disease. Many of the opinions expressed at this conference regarding the need (or lack thereof) for surgical or nonsurgical treatment of TMDs sound similar to the arguments at that time surrounding coronary bypass surgery. However, as in other areas, the controversy surrounding the relative efficacy of surgical versus nonsurgical treatment is not likely to be resolved without conducting randomized clinical trials. Much can and should be learned about natural history and treatment sequelae from observational studies, including the identification of treatments that have obvious positive or negative effects. However, valid comparisons of treatment modalities for which differences in results are likely to be rather subtle, as is likely the case here, will require the scrutiny of randomized clinical trials.

ISSUES IN RANDOMIZED CLINICAL TRIALS

Randomized clinical trials to evaluate and compare the efficacy of various treatment modalities for TMDs clearly would be a new area for many clinicians. Those new to the area should be forewarned that many unfamiliar issues will be raised. For example, the rationale and importance of randomization in a clinical trial is not always understood. It is fairly widely understood that one purpose of the randomization is to provide balance among the patients in the treatment groups for characteristics that may affect the outcome, even when those characteristics have not been identified ahead of time. What is often not understood is that the randomization process allows the most valid inference to be made from the statistical tests. With randomization and the use of a test based on it, we can legitimately calculate the probability that any observed differences in outcomes between groups are merely due to chance assignment of patients to the groups when there are no real differences in effects of the treatments. Without randomization, a calculated P-value is an attempt to evaluate a similar probability, but it does not have the same underlying probabilistic basis, and therefore is not considered as valid scientifically.

An issue that will emerge in planning a randomized clinical trial is the necessity to define a priori a clinically significant treatment effect. Such a definition is needed to specify the sample size for the trial, because the investigator wants to have reasonable power to detect such a clinically significant treatment effect, if it exists. As opposed to merely indicating at the end of a study whether an observed effect that is deemed statistically significant can be interpreted to be clinically significant, proper planning of a randomized clinical trial will require specifying in advance the magnitude of effect that must be observed to consider the result clinically significant. That is often a very difficult task.

Another necessary methodological task before conducting a trial is the specification of a small number of primary endpoints or outcome variables. There is a natural tendency to include a large number of outcome measures, based on the rationale that the TMDs are multifactorial in nature. Nevertheless, the smaller the number of variables selected to describe primary outcomes, the easier it will be to minimize the overall Type I error rate (the probability of incorrectly claiming a treatment effect to be significant). The definition of a clinically significant treatment effect, mentioned earlier, should be based on these primary outcome variables. To specify the sample size using the definition of a clinically significant treatment effect in the primary outcome variables, we also need an estimate of the variability of the primary outcome variables in the population. All these points suggest that the design of valid clinical trials requires a consensus on which outcome variable or variables are most important. Prior experience with the outcome variables provides an estimate of the variability inherent in the outcome, and of the magnitude of change or difference in the outcome variable that would be deemed clinically relevant or significant.

With the information described above, we can calculate the sample size required to provide reasonable power for detecting what is deemed to be a clinically significant treatment effect. Such determinations are important, because studies with small sample sizes and low power for detecting clinically significant treatment effects that result in no statistically significant differences in treatments contribute little other than confusion and are probably a waste of resources.

Clinical trials that assess such subjective outcomes as pain must be conducted in such a manner that the outcome measures are as objective as possible. This usually means that any examiner who is assessing an outcome variable should be blinded, if at all possible, as to the treatment received by the patient being examined. Even when examiners are blinded, multiple examiners may not conduct the examinations and measure the exam items consistently. Therefore, it is usually necessary to conduct training and calibration sessions for examiners to ensure consistency.

One of the methodological issues that affects the design of a clinical trial is the question of whether the study is one of "efficacy" or "effectiveness." This terminology, while perhaps not universally used, can be employed to demonstrate the fundamental difference between two kinds of studies. A study of efficacy is one in which participants may be selected and even encouraged to be "high compliers," i.e., they are likely to follow through with all aspects of the treatment or intervention and they are likely to stay in the study until the end. Thus, in a study of efficacy the treatments are evaluated in the context of their effects on selected patients in an ideal setting. On the other hand, some aspects of the treatment may cause less-than-ideal patients to not comply with everything required by the treatment. If that is the case, the effect of the treatment on patients who are representative of the entire target population (i.e., not screened to be only high compliers) and to whom the treatments are applied as they ordinarily would be in practice, might be different than in the ideal setting of an efficacy study. This latter kind of study, which may more accurately reflect how well a treatment would work in the general population, can be termed a study of effectiveness. The study design (selection of patients, treatment protocol, and even the method of analysis) is affected by which concept, efficacy or effectiveness, is of primary interest.

A related analytical issue that is probably foreign to many investigators working in TMD research is the concept of conducting statistical analyses based on the "intent-to-treat" principle. As previously mentioned, in a randomized clinical trial the most valid type of statistical analysis used to compare group outcomes is the one that evaluates the probability of the group differences occurring by chance alone. In such an analysis, patients should always be included with the group to which they were originally assigned. In some studies, patients may not complete or comply with the treatments (e.g., they fail to attend all of the behavioral sessions required for an intervention, or they quit using a splint required for another intervention). More complex is the situation where a patient crosses over from one intervention to the other (e.g., after trying the nonsurgical treatment to which he or she was randomized, a patient decides to seek out and receive surgical treatment). Sometimes there are patients who, after being randomized to one treatment, decide not to undergo that treatment at all or even seek out the alternative treatment. If the intent-to-treat principle is employed, all patients and their outcomes will be included and analyzed as members of the group to which they were randomized, regardless of what subsequently occurred. This principle is often difficult to accept, especially if there are many deviations from the treatments to which patients are randomized. If the intent-to-treat principle is abandoned for the analysis, then the study must be evaluated as if it were an observational (i.e., nonrandomized) study, and the weight given to the results is greatly diminished. The key is to properly design and administer the study to minimize problems with respect to completion or crossover of treatment, so that employment of the intent-to-treat principle is not problematic.

Another analytical issue, related to the choice of outcome or endpoint variables, is the problem of multiple tests or comparisons. As previously indicated, investigators often want to use many variables to monitor the effect of treatment. If statistically significant observed differences in any one variable would be considered sufficient reason to declare a treatment successful or effective, then a penalty must be paid for doing tests on the multitudes of variables in order to avoid having a high overall probability of committing a Type I error. For example, suppose multiple studies were conducted in which the same 20 variables were declared to be primary outcome measures, and in each study two treatment groups were compared on each variable using a significance level of 0.05. Under that scenario, even when there are no true differences between treatments, one can expect to see an average of one variable per study for which group differences are declared to be statistically significant merely due to chance. Thus the probability of committing a Type I error is high.

To keep the overall probability of a Type I error under control (say 0.05), one type of adjustment called the Bonferroni method would require that each of the individual tests be conducted at the desired overall significance level divided by the number of tests. In the above example, to have an overall significance level of 0.05, each of the tests on the 20 individual variables would have to be conducted at a significance level of 0.05/20, or 0.0025, thus making it much more difficult for differences in any one variable to be declared statistically significant. The result is decreased power for detecting differences of fixed magnitude declared to be clinically significant, so that the sample size has to be increased to maintain reasonable power for detecting clinically significant differences. While the Bonferroni method is a conservative way of adjusting for multiple comparisons, it demonstrates the problems caused by trying to declare a large number of variables or outcomes to be of primary interest.

These and many other issues that arise in the planning and conduct of randomized clinical trials are discussed in texts such as Pocock (1983) and Meinert (1986). Fricton (1991) provides an incomplete but useful discussion of some of these issues as they specifically relate to studies of TMDs and orofacial pain. Future meetings and conferences should seek to standardize the diagnoses and outcomes used in future clinical trials and develop guidelines for conducting TMD clinical trials that consider methodological issues in the context of TMD research.

REFERENCES

Dworkin, S.F. and LeResche, L. (Eds.), Research diagnostic criteria for temporomandibular disorders: review, criteria, examinations and specifications, critique. J. Craniomandib. Disord. Facial Oral Pain, 6 (1992) 300–355.

Feinstein, A.R., Clinical Epidemiology: The Architecture of Clinical Research, W.B. Saunders, Philadelphia, 1985.

Fletcher, R.H., Fletcher, S.W. and Wagner, E.H., Clinical Epidemiology: The Essentials, 2nd ed., Williams and Wilkins, Baltimore, 1988.

Fricton, J.R., Chronic orofacial pain. In: M. Max, R. Portenoy and E. Laska (Eds.), Advances in Pain Research and Therapy, Vol. 18, Raven Press, New York, 1991, pp. 375–389.

Meinert, C.L., Clinical Trials: Design, Conduct and Analysis, Oxford University Press, New York, 1986.

Pocock, S.J., Clinical Trials: A Practical Approach, John Wiley and Sons, New York, 1983.

Weiss, N.S., Clinical Epidemiology: The Study of the Outcome of Illness, Oxford University Press, New York, 1986.

Whitney, C. and Zhu, X., A SAS computer program to evaluate the research diagnostic criteria for classification of temporomandibular disorders, Technical Report 9401, Biometry Core, Regional Clinical Dental Research Center, University of Washington, Seattle, 1994.

Correspondence to: Timothy A. DeRouen, PhD, Departments of Biostatistics and Dental Public Health Sciences, SM-35, University of Washington, Seattle, WA 98195, USA. Tel: 206-543-7304; Fax: 206-685-4258.

Temporomandibular Disorders and Related Pain Conditions, Progress in Pain Research and Management, Vol. 4, edited by B.J. Sessle, P.S. Bryant, and R.A. Dionne, IASP Press, Seattle, © 1995.

27

Workshop Recommendations on Research Needs and Directions

Edited by Patricia S. Bryant[a] and Barry J. Sessle[b]

[a]National Institute of Dental Research, National Institutes of Health, Bethesda, Maryland, USA, and [b]Faculty of Dentistry, University of Toronto, Ontario, Canada

Despite a proliferation of papers over the past twenty years discussing presumed causes or treatments for jaw dysfunctions, and dramatic expansions in the scope and intensity of health care services delivered for these conditions, solid scientific knowledge on conditions associated with pain or dysfunction in the jaw region has developed slowly. Recognizing this, the National Institute of Dental Research and several other components of the National Institutes of Health in the United States convened two meetings in 1994 to stimulate the critical synthesis of available information and to accelerate research progress.

More than 100 scientists, clinicians, and government officials participated in the International Workshop on the Temporomandibular Disorders and Related Pain Conditions and a later workshop, TMJ Alloplastic Implants: Local/Systemic Effects. At each meeting a substantial amount of time was reserved for the development and discussion of research directions and recommendations. This chapter presents the specific recommendations that resulted.

Because distinct content areas were covered by each of the working groups, each group's recommendations are presented here separately. Seen as a whole, however, the recommendations strongly emphasize the need to expand knowledge of basic etiologic mechanisms underlying conditions producing temporomandibular pain and dysfunction. These recommendations also highlight the need to elucidate factors accounting for the higher prevalence of temporomandibular disorders (TMDs) among women, to assess relationships between the TMDs and other disorders (e.g., fibromyalgia, other disorders of connective tissues, osteoarthritis), and to appropriately integrate information on normal and pathological muscle and joint function.

Recommendations from each of the six working groups convened at the International Workshop on the Temporomandibular Disorders and Related Pain Conditions (IWOT) and from the two working groups convened at the workshop on TMJ Alloplastic Implants (TMJI) are presented below. Only those recommendations voted as having high or excellent priority are included; their order of presentation does not reflect relative priority. While some recommendations from different groups are similar, only limited editing has been done so as to preserve the intent, emphasis, and priority given to each recommendation by each group.

I. EPIDEMIOLOGY AND HEALTH SERVICES WORKING GROUP (IWOT)

Co-chairs: Drs. Gunnar Carlsson and Linda LeResche
Members: Drs. Alexia Antczak-Bouckoms, Katherine Atchinson, Ernest Glass, Mr. Milton Glass, Dr. Isabel Garcia, Mrs. Rene Glass, Drs. James Lipton, Joseph Marbach, Michael Von Korff, Alexander White, Frederick Wolfe

RECOMMENDATIONS

A. Examine and test standardized diagnostic criteria such as the temporomandibular disorder research diagnostic criteria (TMD/RDC) and other criteria in various settings, including primary care (e.g., family practice of general dentistry), specialty care, and tertiary care (e.g., pain clinic), and evaluate the stability of the diagnostic categories over time.

B. Develop and validate measures of process and outcome for the TMDs in categories that include physical examination; pain; psychological status; functional, social, and vocational disability; direct and indirect costs; and adverse effects of treatment. Develop a schema for collecting and reporting demographic, psychosocial, and current and past physical and mental comorbid conditions.

C. Assess the economic impact of various TMDs from the perspective of the patient, insurers, employers, and society, including both direct and indirect measures of costs.

D. Assess the cost-effectiveness of various interventions targeted toward the prevention, diagnosis, management, and treatment of the TMDs. Such interventions include preventive services, diagnostic tests, surgical and nonsurgical procedures, and self-help interventions.

E. Drawing on automated claims and data bases from health care and insurance systems representing diverse regions and delivery systems, develop a national reporting system that monitors the frequency of patients being treated for the TMDs per unit population, the diagnoses assigned to patients, tests and treatments administered, utilization of services, and costs of care. Within the national reporting system, settings should be identified where it is possible to use automated data to track treatment histories of patients over time, in order to assess outcomes of care for TMDs of varying types and severity.

F. Develop a registry of treated TMD patients from various health care settings (both primary and specialty care) in order to carry out long-term studies of treatment trajectories and clinical course. Samples of patients exposed to specific surgical, nonsurgical, and behavioral therapies should be identified, assessed prior to treatment, and followed up for short-term and long-term outcomes.

G. Create a registry of completed and ongoing clinical trials. Drawing on this data base, apply decision-analytic methods to the diagnosis and treatment of the TMDs in order to aid clinical decision making and identify critical areas for future research. Communicate results to patients and clinicians so they have better information regarding potential treatment effects before treatments are rendered.

H. Conduct randomized controlled clinical trials to assess the effectiveness of various treatments for the TMDs through:

1. Use of a standardized core data set including an assessment of clinical signs and symptoms, quality of life, and costs.

2. Assessment of treatments rendered by various providers and measures evaluating self-care.

3. Establishment of priorities for such studies that take into account current evidence of effectiveness and the frequencies with which the treatments are used.

I. Use longitudinal and prospective designs to assess onset rates, age of onset, risk factors for, and the natural history of specific TMDs. Age and gender differences in rates of TMDs should be investigated epidemiologically by examining possible age- and gender-related biological, psychologic, and social risk factors.

J. Conduct epidemiological studies of co-occurrence of TMDs and other pain conditions to measure the extent of comorbidity and to evaluate and refine diagnostic criteria. These studies could be followed by studies of the effectiveness of treatments for patients with comorbid conditions.

II. BASIC SCIENCES WORKING GROUP (IWOT)

Co-chairs: Drs. Kenneth Hargreaves and Steven Milam
Members: Drs. Lynda Bonewald, Brian Cooper, Ronald Dubner, Susan Herring, Douglas Jackson, Sunil Kapila, Sigvard Kopp, Siegfried Mense, Sukhbir Mokha, Afsael Nikaen, Anthony Ratcliffe, Barry Sessle, Arthur Storey

RECOMMENDATIONS

Preface. This working group noted that all research recommendations were intended to include the temporomandibular joint (TMJ), muscle, ligaments, and other orofacial tissues, even when not specifically stated. They also emphasized that studies comparing the TMJ with other joints and tissues could contribute to understanding of the TMDs and noted that their recommendations were intended to include analyses of developing, normal, and pathological tissues, with issues of gender and age to be examined at each level. Additionally, they noted that implementation of these recommendations could help define relationships between peripheral tissue pathology and the TMDs and would be expected to include markers that differentiate between pathological states and adaptive processes.

A. Define the molecular mechanisms that cells use to synthesize, maintain, and degrade the extracellular matrix and tissues. This is to include genetic regulation and the effects of hormones, mediators, pharmacological agents, mechanical loads, aging, and developmental changes.

B. Determine the molecular and cellular composition of each tissue (e.g., expression of genes, level of proteins) in normal and dysfunctional tissues.

C. Determine the mediators and inhibitors of inflammation, including mechanisms regulating their release, and mechanisms of action. This is to include mechanisms of immunological modulation of normal tissue function as well as injury, degeneration, and repair.

D. Clarify the mechanisms used by the nervous system to detect and regulate the functional and dysfunctional state of the orofacial tissues. This is to include nociceptors, other afferents, the autonomic nervous system, and the effects of the peripheral nervous system on tissue repair. It would also include the role of the nervous system in regulating jaw function in both health and disease, since both joint loading and stabilization depend on neural feedback.

E. Define central nociceptive pathways and modulatory mechanisms that are activated in response to injury of joint, muscle, and other orofacial tissues. This is to include various neurotransmitters, neuromodulators, and transcellular and intracellular messengers involved in nociception and plasticity.

F. Define neural plasticity at physiological, cellular, molecular, and pharmacological levels in response to injury or placement of devices in the orofacial region. Such studies should characterize plasticity at peripheral and segmental levels in ascending pathways and descending pathways, and in processes involved in sensorimotor integration. They should include consideration of various neurotransmitters, neuromodulators, and transcellular and intracellular messengers involved in nociception and plasticity.

G. Delineate mechanisms underlying sensorimotor integration of the TMJ with associated muscles and other orofacial tissues. Included would be studies on the relation between reflex activity and pain, as well as studies evaluating responses to various TMJ replacements.

H. Define the molecular and cellular responses of local and systemic tissues to different types and forms of biomaterials and the impact of those responses on acute and chronic tissue interactions and pain.

I. Define the structural (e.g., dimensions, anatomy), biomechanical (e.g., displacement. force, stress, strain, plasticity, cycles), and physical (e.g., density, modulus, conductivity) parameters for normal and dysfunctional temporomandibular conditions.

J. Determine the effect of systemic, genetic, and hereditary diseases on structure and function of joint and muscle, and the mechanisms underlying associated developmental aberrations.

K. Define those factors of gender that predispose women to develop TMDs and related orofacial pain conditions.

L. Develop and validate animal, in vitro, and biomechanical models to study disease processes in the TMJ.

M. Develop indicators (markers) for disease processes affecting the TMJ. These indicators should differentiate between pathological states and adaptive processes and should include markers of early pathology (both molecular markers and other diagnostic markers, such as imaging).

III. MUSCLE DISORDERS WORKING GROUP (IWOT)

Co-chairs: Drs. Charles Greene and James Lund
Members: Drs. Norman Capra, Dean Dessem, Roger Eng, Arthur English, Ms. Tamara Hemingway, Drs. Rigmor Jensen, Alan Hannam, Richard Ohrbach, Octavia Plesch, Kevin Reid, Charles Widmer

RECOMMENDATIONS

Preface. The following proposals include a mixture of possible animal and human studies. In all experiments involving human subjects with pain, this group recommends that both TMD/RDC Axis I and Axis II variables, as well as American College of Rheumatology (ACR) criteria for fibromyalgia, be evaluated.

A. Compare metabolic changes in jaw-closing muscles of patients with TMD and control subjects. Recent advances, such as magnetic resonance imaging and magnetic resonance spectroscopy, have made it possible to study these phenomena noninvasively.

B. Investigate the effects of altered muscle use on muscle and TMJ performance.

C. Define the intrinsic properties of small-diameter masticatory muscle afferents and their representation and effects in the CNS.

D. Quantify muscle tenderness in TMDs. Conduct cross-sectional and longitudinal assessments using palpation of masticatory muscle, tendon, and control sites in TMD patients and control subjects to determine whether muscle tenderness reflects the local hypersensitivity of the underlying muscle or connective tissue or a generalized hyperalgesic state. Determine whether painful human masticatory muscles are associated with increased sensitivity to pain in distant muscular and cutaneous sites.

E. Test the hypothesis that fibromyalgia and TMDs associated with myofascial pain are diseases of connective tissue.

F. Determine the comorbidity and relationships between TMDs and fibromyalgia, and TMDs and tension-type headache.

G. Investigate oral parafunctional behaviors, their relation to nociception and pain, and their relation to diurnal and nocturnal states of consciousness.

IV. JOINT DISORDERS WORKING GROUP (IWOT)

Co-chairs: Drs. Franklin Dolwick and Jeffrey Okeson

Members: Dr. Ronald Attanasio, Ms. Terrie Cowley, Drs. Lambert de Bont, Richard Heinegard, Howard Israel, Sigvard Kopp, Regina Landesberg, Jack Lemons, Van Mow, Eric Schiffman

RECOMMENDATIONS

A. Develop suitable animal models for the study of normal TMJ function and TMJ pathobiology.

B. Characterize normal development and aging processes within the TMJ.

C. Investigate the biological and biomechanical factors affecting loading forces in the TMJ.

D. Determine the role of motion and function in the maintenance of the molecular, cellular, and morphological features of the TMJ.

E. Determine how biochemical events in the synovial fluid and synovial membrane reflect the morphological appearance of tissues in the TMJ. Identify metabolic events in the TMJ, as well as in other joints, in early osteoarthritis and develop specific markers for these events.

F. Study the relations among disk position, osteoarthritis, and masticatory muscle pain. This should include studies to clarify whether disk displacement is a *sign* of osteoarthritis or the *cause* of osteoarthritis and to determine the relation between disk position and/or osteoarthritis and growth disorders.

G. Conduct a long-term prospective study to determine the natural course of disk displacement and osteoarthritis.

H. Evaluate the relative role of biological, behavioral, and psychosocial factors in the initiation and/or perpetuation of disk displacement and osteoarthritis.

I. Evaluate the prevalence, etiology, natural history, and correlation of diagnostic tests for avascular necrosis.

V. ASSESSMENT AND DIAGNOSIS WORKING GROUP (IWOT)

Co-chairs: Drs. Christian Stohler and Sharon Brooks
Members: Drs. Donald DeNucci, Timothy DeRouen, Robert Gatchel, Marc Heft, David Keith, Charles Widmer

RECOMMENDATIONS

A. Develop a comprehensive sensory assessment paradigm for systematic evaluation of sensory functioning. This should include evaluation of dysesthesia, allodynia, hyperpathia, and/or hypopathia. Sensory assessments could contribute to evaluation of underlying pain mechanisms (e.g., nociceptive vs. neuropathic pain) and have direct implications for treatment.

B. Evaluate the potential overlap between myofascial pain associated with TMDs and similar muscle pain conditions, such as regional and widespread muscle pain, fibromyalgia, and headaches.

C. Determine whether there are physical or psychosocial risk factors at the acute stage of TMDs that predict the development of chronicity.

D. Develop selection criteria for various imaging modalities, including tomography, MRI, and other techniques, for the evaluation of TMDs.

E. Define indicators (markers) that can be used to determine progression or regression of various TMDs, and develop markers for disease processes affecting the TMJ, masticatory muscles, and related structures.

F. Develop techniques to assess the role of the sympathetic nervous system in the TMDs.

G. Develop a comprehensive orofacial motor assessment paradigm.

H. Evaluate the diagnostic validity of the TMD/RDC.

I. Determine what major forms of psychopathology or other psychosocial variables (i.e., coping ability, life stressors) are associated with chronic TMDs, and how these factors relate to TMD/RDC subtypes.

J. Evaluate the relations among physical characteristics, psychological status, pain, and disability measures as assessed by the TMD/RDC, and determine whether there are different subgroupings for acute and chronic conditions (i.e., longitudinal changes in characteristics over time).

K. Develop discriminating diagnostic criteria for non-TMD orofacial pain conditions.

VI. TREATMENT WORKING GROUP (IWOT)

Co-chairs: Drs. James Fricton and Thomas Rudy
Members: Drs. Laurence Bradley, Charles Carlson, Donald Chase, Glenn Clark, Barry Cooper, Timothy DeRouen, Raymond Dionne, Samuel Dworkin, Mark Fontenot, James Kelly, James McNamara, Charles McNeil, Louis Mercuri, John Rugh, Larry Wolford

RECOMMENDATIONS

A. Convene an interdisciplinary conference to define a minimum multidimensional set of measures for documenting treatment outcomes, which could be widely accepted for use in evaluating treatment interventions. In addition, the conference should develop guidelines for the planning and implementation of randomized controlled trials in TMDs, and highlight methodological issues to increase study validity.

B. Conduct randomized controlled clinical trials, or other study designs as appropriate, to determine the immediate and long-term multidimensional outcomes (e.g., pain, muscle and joint function, psychosocial/behavioral status) of interventions for patients fitting criteria for the diagnosis of muscle disorders (TMD/RDC Axis I, Group 1), independent of or in combination with other Axis I diagnoses. Potential interventions include self-care strategies with minimal therapist contact, intraoral orthotic appliances (splints), physical medicine, pharmacotherapy, psychological/behavioral therapies, intramuscular injections, and combined modalities.

C. Conduct randomized controlled clinical trials or other study designs as appropriate to determine the immediate and long-term multidimensional treatment outcomes of interventions for patients fitting criteria for the diagnosis of joint disorders (RDC Axis I, Groups 2 and 3), independent of or in combination with muscle disorders. Potential interventions to be studied include self-care strategies with minimal therapist contact, intraoral orthotic appliances (splints), physical medicine, pharmacotherapy, psychological/ behavioral therapies, intraarticular injections, and combined modalities.

D. Carry out randomized clinical trials and other clinical studies to determine the relative effectiveness of surgical therapies for the various stages of TMJ disk displacement, arthralgia, osteoarthrosis, and osteoarthritis, as compared with each other and with nonsurgical therapies. Potential surgical therapies include arthrotomy, arthroscopy, arthrocentesis, therapeutic joint infusion, joint reconstruction (e.g., autogenous tissue grafts), and the use of adjunctive nonsurgical therapy.

E. Conduct clinical and basic science studies to determine the pathophysiology associated with alloplastic implants, the status of patients who have had an implant relative to those who have had other treatments, and the most effective management of patients with failed alloplastic implants. Such studies are urgently needed.

F. Complete randomized clinical trials and other clinical studies as needed to determine outcomes and other issues related to rehabilitation of patients with chronic orofacial pain who are dysfunctional and have high levels of use of health care. Integrated interdisciplinary pain management strategies should be studied, including multiple modalities in single or multiple settings.

G. Conduct clinical trials and other studies as appropriate to determine the prognostic factors that influence treatment outcomes. Prognostic factors to be studied may include gender, physical diagnoses (RDC Axis I and other orofacial pain disorders), behavioral and psychosocial factors (RDC Axis II, depression, secondary gain, significant life events, sleep disorders, careseeking behavior, bruxism, and others), physiological factors (hormonal, systemic disease such as connective tissue abnormalities), local factors (occlusion, biomechanical factors, degree of pathology), provider practices and behavior, and iatrogenic effects of treatment.

H. Conduct multisite clinical studies on TMDs. Such studies are needed to determine the influence of factors such as ethnicity, gender, and age on TMDs; to assess the diagnostic and clinical utility of the RDC/TMD; to characterize less prevalent disorders, treatments, and etiologic factors; to evaluate the impacts of health care delivery and costs; and to demonstrate differential effects of geographic regions and practitioner behavior.

I. Conduct longitudinal randomized controlled clinical trials and other clinical studies that consider the relation of orthodontic treatment, orthognathic surgery, and TMDs. Studies could address the influence of orthodontics or orthognathic surgery on the etiology of TMDs, the role of orthodontics in the treatment and prevention of TMDs, and the long-term contribution of occlusion to maintaining normal masticatory function.

VII. CLINICAL RESEARCH GROUP (TMJI)

Co-chairs: Drs. Larry Wolford and Claudia Miller
Members: Drs. Thomas Aufdemorte, Iris Bell, Patricia Bryant, Andrew Campbell, Donald DeNucci, James Fricton, Sharon Gabriel, Ms. Jennifer Hutchinson, Dr. James Kelly

RECOMMENDATIONS

A. Define the magnitude of the problem of TMJ implant failure compared with failure of other orthopedic devices through:

1. Collection of descriptive epidemiologic data on the use of these devices.

2. Completion of outcome studies regarding:

a. short- and long-term outcomes (both favorable and unfavorable) associated with alloplastic implants,

b. the incidence and prevalence of various types of implant failure according to the type and site of the implant,

c. prospective controlled analyses of both local and systemic implant complications, and

d. analyses of the risk factors for implant complications and/or failure.

3. Gathering of estimates of the economic impact, both direct (e.g., medical costs of removal/revision) and indirect (e.g., work loss), of implant failure.

4. Gathering of estimates of the functional status and quality of life of implant patients, including both those with successful and those with failed devices, to provide a balanced evaluation of implant-related gains and losses in the population.

B. Develop interventions to improve the treatment of persons with failed implants. Specific interventions include pain medications, including opioid analgesics; physical medicine treatments; multidisciplinary pain rehabilitation; and surgical therapies. Studies should evaluate short- and long-term outcomes, cost-effectiveness of specific interventions, and compliance or relapse rates with various treatments.

C. Conduct a workshop on the management of patients with failed alloplastic implants, with the objective of fostering accelerated progress toward innovative or improved approaches for the treatment of persons with failed implants.

D. Develop improved mechanisms for the evaluation of new alloplastic devices, including their safety, effectiveness, and cost-effectiveness.

VIII. BASIC SCIENCE GROUP (TMJI)

Co-chairs: Drs. Steven Milam and Mir Kossovsky
Members: Drs. Norman Braveman, Elaine Collier, Ms. Terrie Cowley, Drs. Raymond Dionne, Regina Landesberg, Cato Laurencin, Kathryn Merritt, Thomas Namey

RECOMMENDATIONS

A. Establish contract sites to procure and categorize research materials (i.e., tissues, retrieved implant materials, blood samples, and patient data records) obtained from TMJ surgery patients, particularly those who have had alloplastic implants.

B. Identify the nature of the cellular response(s) associated with alloplastic materials used to reconstruct the TMJ. Such analyses may include, but are not limited to, phenotypic, functional, and biochemical assays.

C. Identify suitable methods, materials, and designs for partial and total TMJ reconstruction, taking into consideration the biomechanics and tissue properties intrinsic to the TMJ.

D. Identify methods to modulate the biological response(s) to alloplastic materials in the TMJ. These may include both systemic and local methodologies such as pharmacological regimens and novel delivery systems.

E. Define the role(s) of cellular, humoral, genetic, and neuroendocrine/hormonal factors that are associated with the biological response to alloplastic materials used in TMJ repair.

F. Investigate the role of genetic, neuroendocrine, and hormonal interactions in the cellular response(s) to alloplastic materials. (The female preponderance to diseases of the TMJ suggests that hormonal regulation may play an important role in the generation of TMJ disease and in the cellular response to alloplastic implant materials).

G. Evaluate the interactions among the immune, genetic, and peripheral and central neural systems and behavioral factors as they affect the cellular response to alloplastic materials and as they affect TMJ-associated pain.

H. Identify the nature of the systemic response(s) associated with alloplastic materials used to reconstruct the TMJ. Such analyses may include, but are not limited to, studies of both the cellular and the humoral arms of the immune system.

I. Identify or develop appropriate imaging methods to localize alloplastic particulate debris within the tissues.

CONCLUSION

The above recommendations have already provided the National Institute of Dental Research with the foundation for two research initiatives. Both a request for small grants relevant to women's health disorders, including the TMDs, and a request for research grant applications focusing on the etiology of the TMDs are being issued in 1995. The breadth of the recommendations provides a conceptually strong framework for involving oral health researchers and other scientists in efforts to understand conditions leading to persisting pain in the masticatory muscles and TMJ. These recommendations also provide a foundation for developing more sound, scientifically based approaches to the prevention, diagnosis, and treatment of TMDs.

Correspondence to: Patricia S. Bryant, PhD, National Institute of Dental Research, National Institutes of Health, Westwood Bldg., Rm. 506, 5333 Westbard Ave., Bethesda, MD 20896. Tel: 301-594-5500; Fax: 301-480-8318.

Index

Temporomandibular disorders *(cont.)*
classification of, 8–10, 138, 190,
193–194, 197–198, 353–354
degenerative joint disease
articular tissues, changes in,
96–97, 141
chondroblasts, role of, 97–98
cytokines, role in, 99–100
enzymology, 97
etiology, 92, 113–114
fibronectin, role in, 98
macrotrauma in, 113
models for, 92–93
depression in, 187, 352–353, 356
diagnosis, 4, 20–21
differential, 199–200, 250–252
research diagnostic criteria, 21, 185,
194–195, 201, 203–208, 220
research recommendations, 474
disability evaluation, 186–188,
221–222
disk displacement
absence of joint sound in, 165
animal models, lack of, 91–92
clicking in, 79–80, 83–84, 218
with crepitus, 81
definition of, 436
and degenerative joint disease,
91–92
etiology, 85
imaging of, 81–82
incidence of, 89
locking jaw in, 79–80
and mandibular growth disturbances,
84–85, 114
neuropeptides release in, 100
occlusal appliances for, 384–385
and osteoarthritis, 83, 84, 91
overview, 79–80
with perforated disk, 81
prevalence of, 434
primary versus secondary, 114
progression of, 84, 114, 218
relationship to pain, 83–84,
431–434
repositioning in, 384
research recommendations, 473
stages of, 80–81
surgery, 83, 344, 431–434
drug therapy, 363–374
economics, 468
in elderly adults, 219–220
epidemiology, 211–226, 247,
252–253
etiology, 337–339, 413–415, 450–451

evidence-based medicine in, 237–245
extra-articular disorders, 429–430
and fibromyalgia, 31–32, 41–42, 472
geographic distribution of, 222–223
and headache, 472
health seeking behavior in, 188, 249
HLA typing in implant failure,
444–445
inflammatory diseases. *See also*
Osteoarthritis; Rheumatoid
arthritis
clinical aspects, 119–131
metabolism, 134
pain in, 120
physiopathology, 133–140,
155–156
therapeutic goals, 119–120
types of, 119, 133
injuries causing, 339, 449
intra-articular biomechanical disorders,
430–431
lack of disability in, 387
literature reviews, 237–245
misdiagnosis of, 249, 451
occlusal factors in
etiology, 406–409
functional relationships, 404–405
literature reviews, 403
morphological relationships,
403–404
multifactorial analysis of, 405–409
normal, 406
study design, evaluation of,
401–402
occlusal therapy, history of, 399–400
occurrence, 320
and orthodontics
gnathologic principles in, 419
literature reviews, types of,
409–412
long-term effects of, 413–415
posterior condylar displacement by,
417–418
preventive use, 419–420
procedure type affecting, 415–417
pain. *See* Pain, temporomandibular
pathogenesis, 141
patient selection bias in, 453
physical assessment (Axis I),
161–172, 200–202
diagnostic reliability and validity,
167–172, 200–201
gold standard for, 200
imaging studies, 165–166, 172
joint sounds, 165, 171–172, 201